HOW THE BODY WORKS

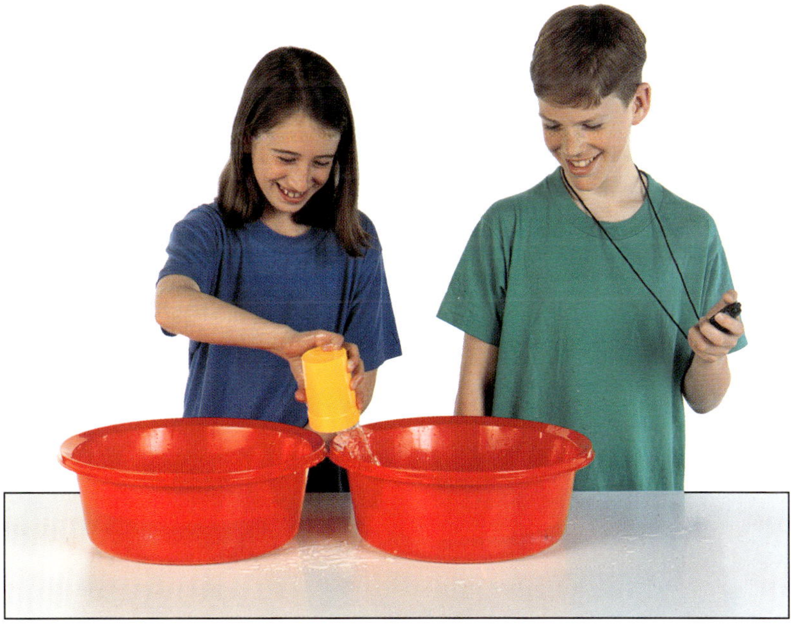

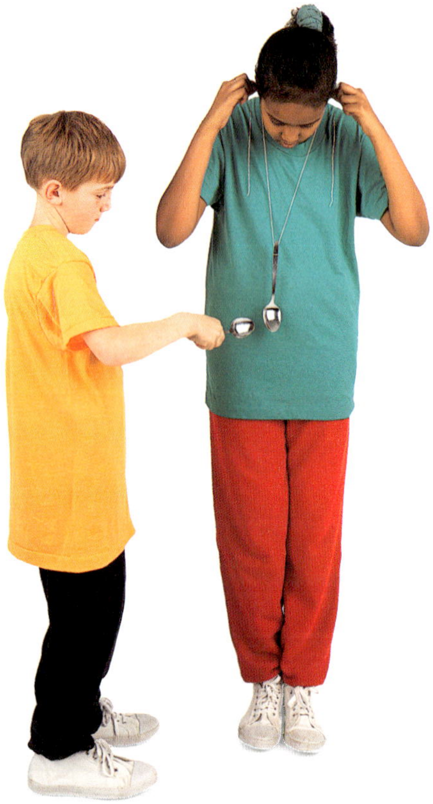

Hearing through a piece of string

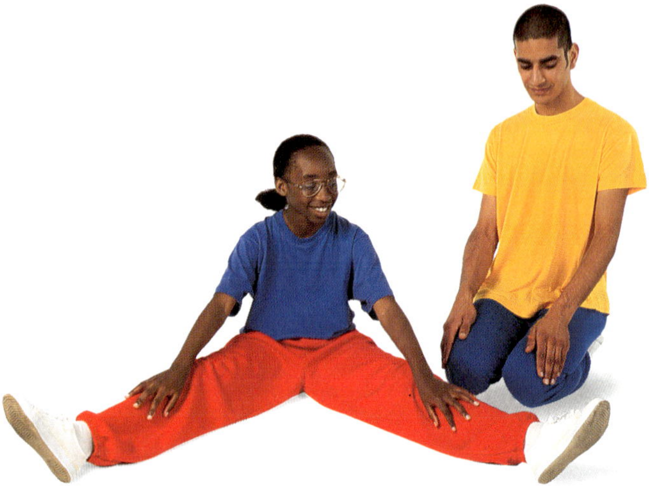

Learning how flexible your joints are

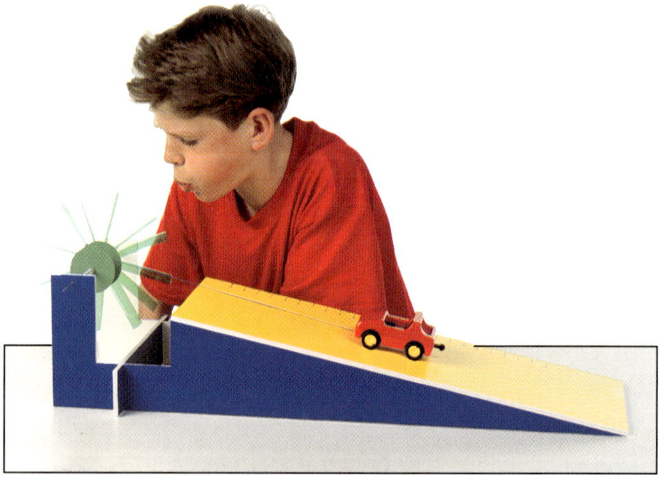

Building a turbine to test your lung power

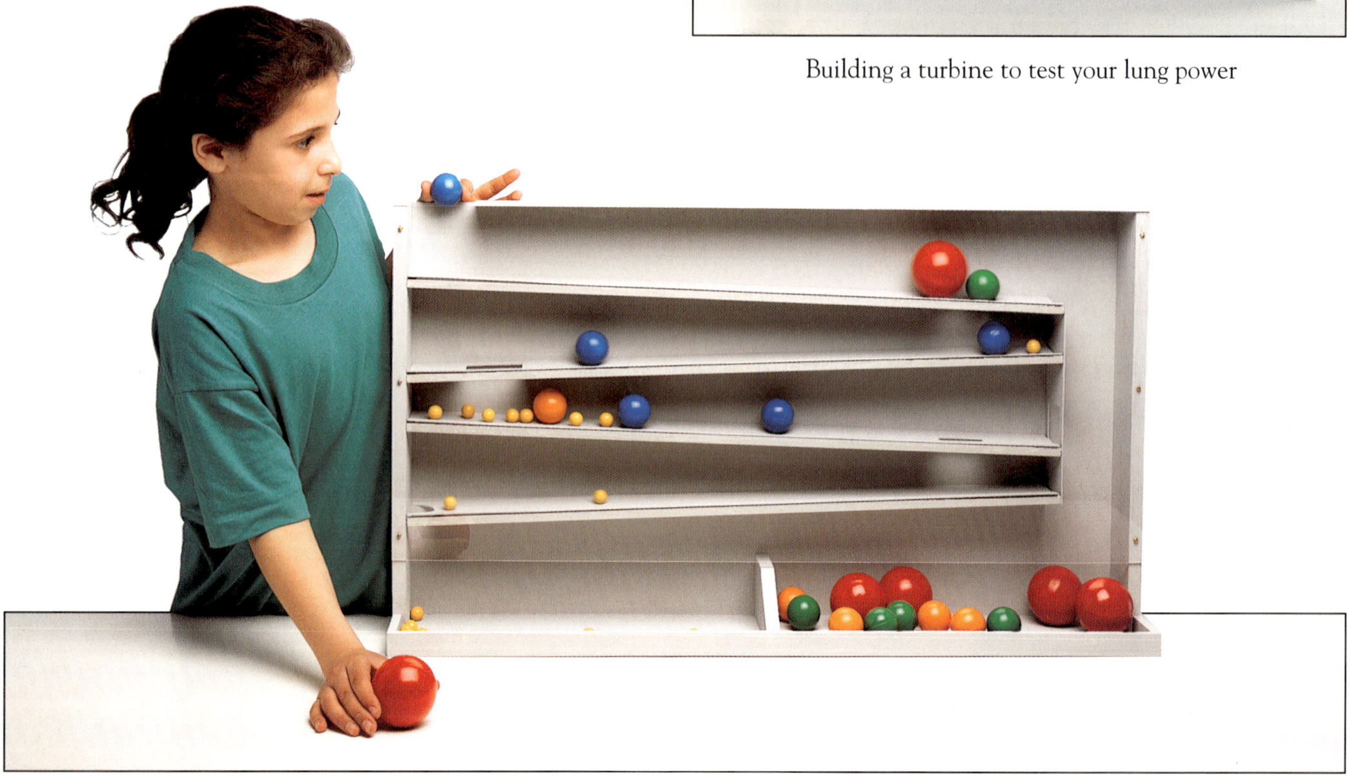

Seeing how your kidneys filter wastes from your blood

HOW THE BODY WORKS

Steve Parker

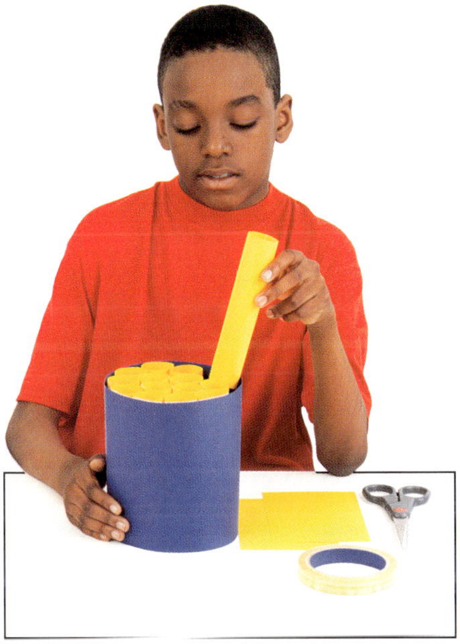

Finding out about your lung's inner surface

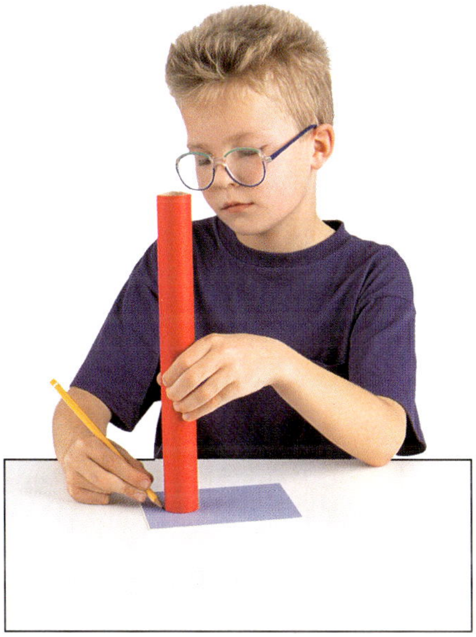

Observing your pupil's reflex action

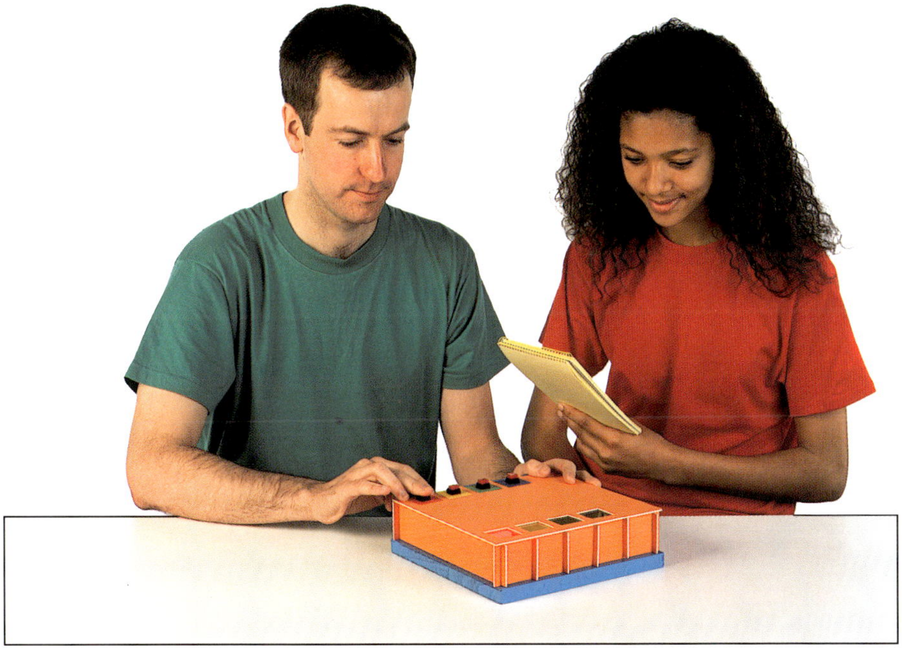

Following sequences of lights to test your short-term memory

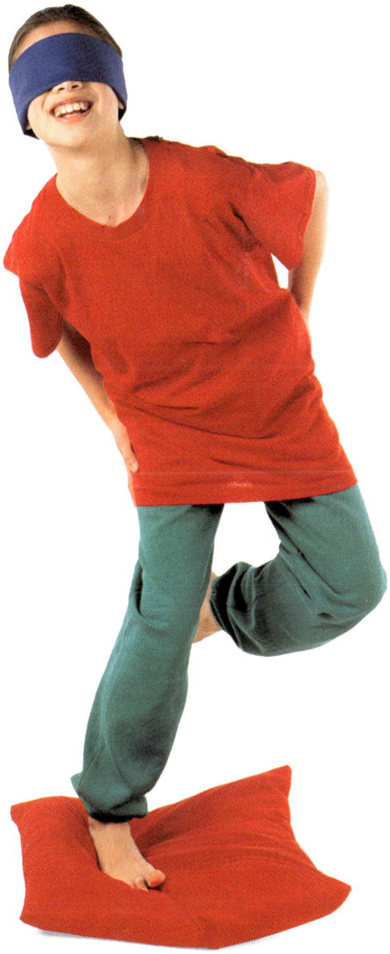

Discovering how you balance

Reader's Digest
YOUNG FAMILIES

Reader's Digest
YOUNG FAMILIES

Designed and edited by Dorling Kindersley Limited, London

Project Art Editor: Bryn Walls
Project Editor: Roger Tritton

Designer: Christina Berts
Editorial Assistants: Emily Hill and Mukul Patel
Production: Sarah Fuller
Managing Art Editor: Phillip Gilderdale
Managing Editor: Ruth Midgley

This edition published by
Reader's Digest Young Families, Inc.
Pleasantville, NY 10570
www.readersdigest.com

The credits and acknowledgments that appear on page 192 are hereby made a part of this copyright page.

Printed in Hong Kong.

Contents

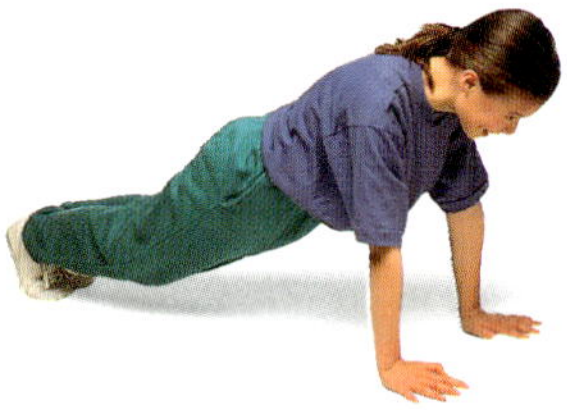

The body

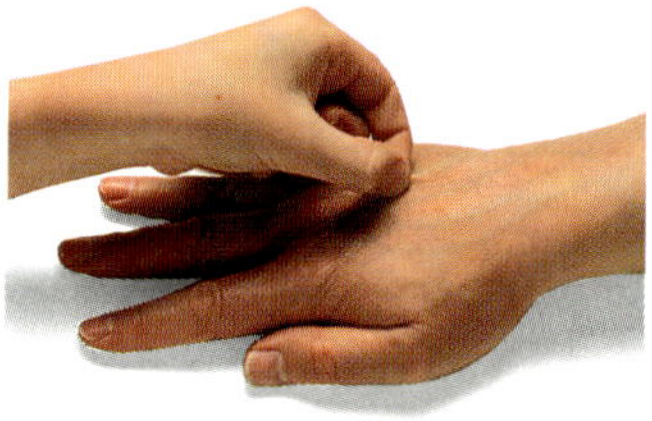

The body's surface

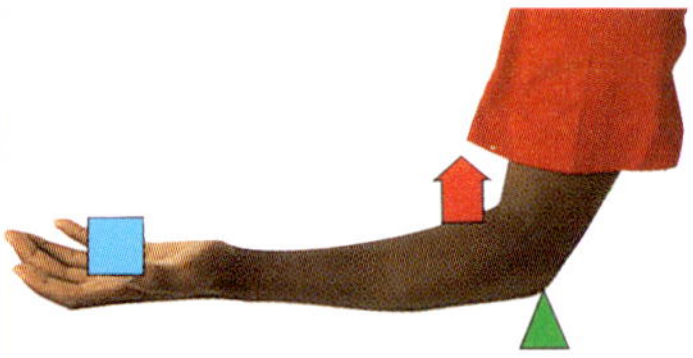

The body's framework

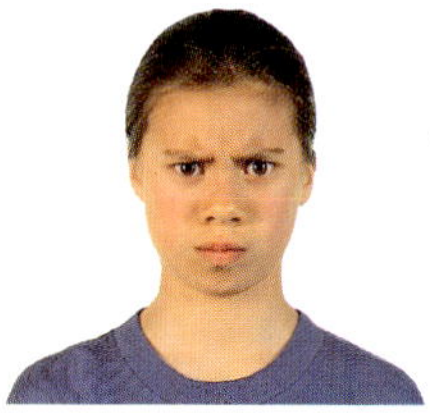

The moving body

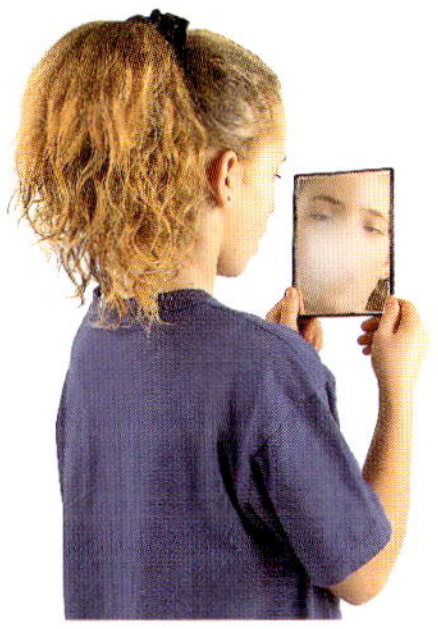

The oxygen supply

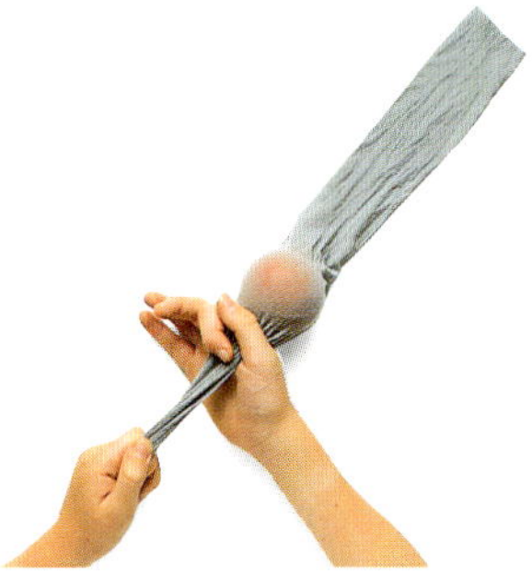

Fueling the body

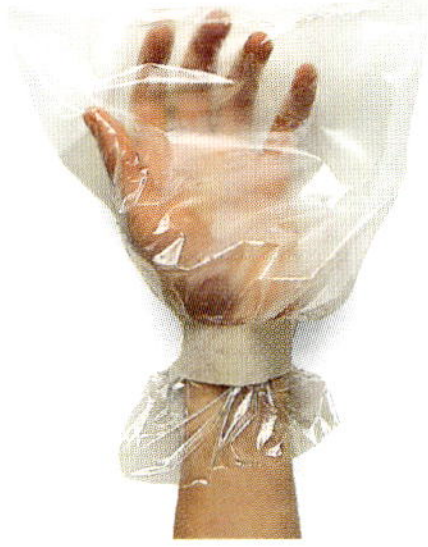

Transport and maintenance

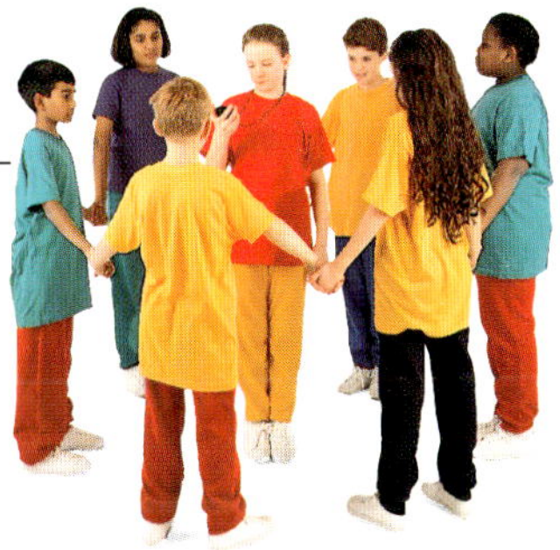

The control network

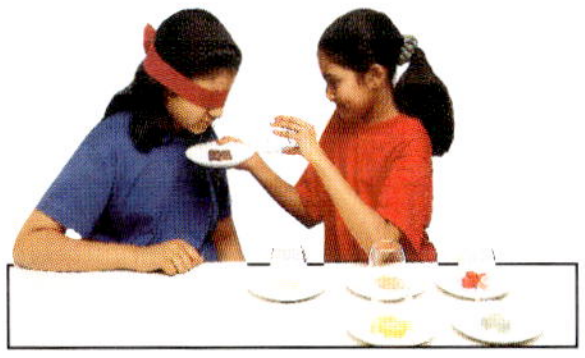

Sensing the surroundings

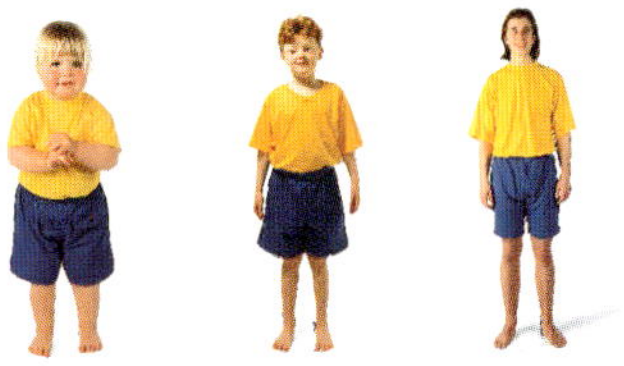

The body's life cycle

INTRODUCTION

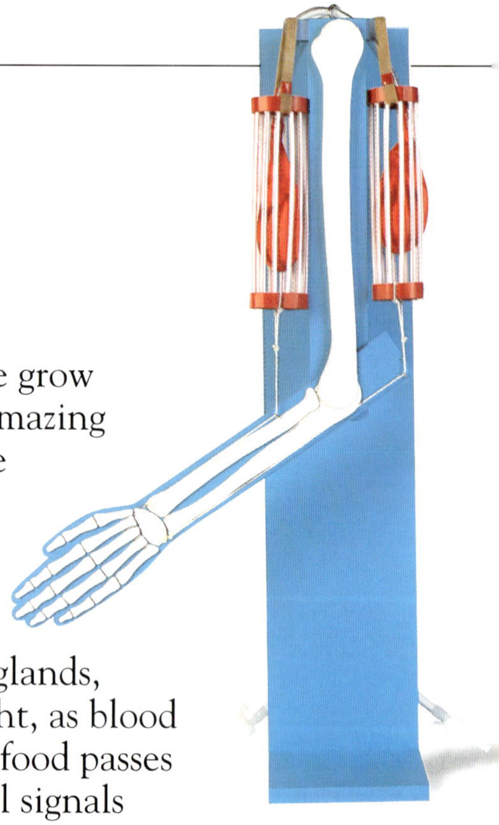

WE OFTEN TAKE THINGS FOR GRANTED as we grow more familiar with them. No matter how amazing something may be, we stop noticing it if we encounter it every day. The human body is a perfect example.

Your body is an incredible masterpiece of bioengineering. Under its skin lie hundreds of muscles, bones, blood vessels, glands, and other parts. These work day and night, as blood pulses through the arteries and veins, food passes through the intestines, and electrical signals flash along the nerves.

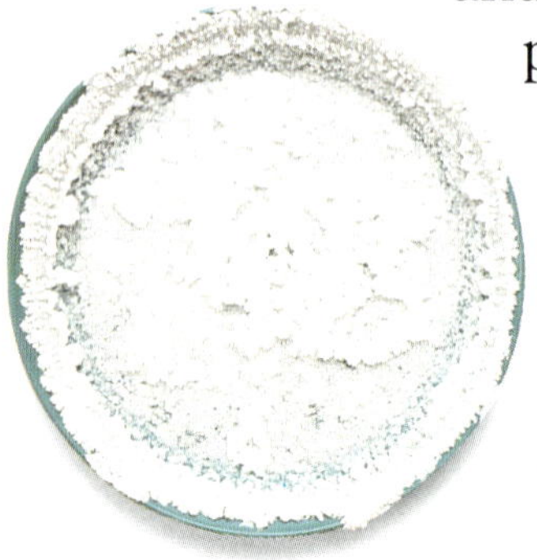

But do you think very much about the amazing and complex hive of activity that is your body when you look in the mirror each morning and see that familiar face? Probably not.

As you begin to learn about the structure and workings of the body, endless questions occur. How do your muscles move your body? Why do you breathe? What happens to food when you swallow? Why is your blood red? When is the body fully grown? Why do you resemble your parents? This book answers these questions and many, many more in an exciting visual and practical way.

The first chapter in this book describes the whole body and its main structures and features. Each of the following chapters is devoted to a major body system. A body system is a set of organs and other body parts that work together

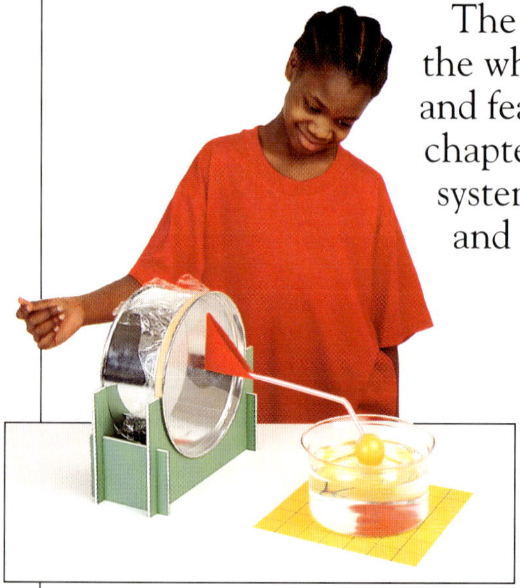

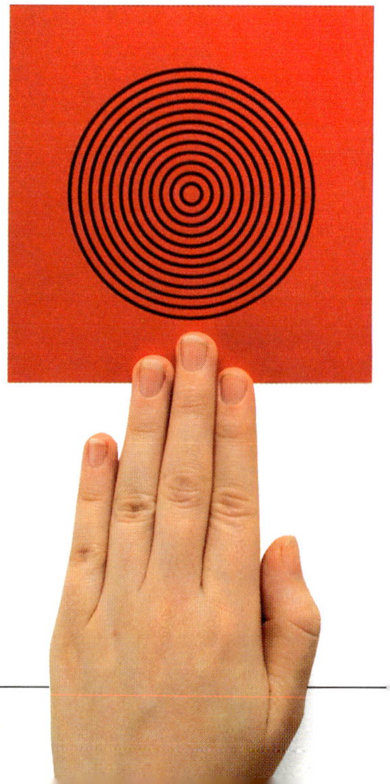

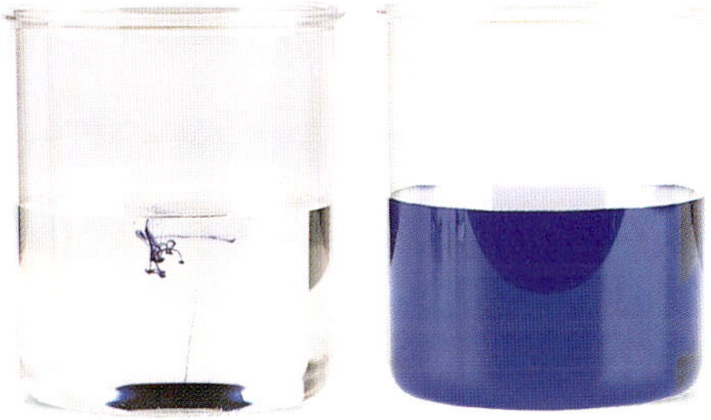

to carry out a major function within the whole body—such as making the body move, swallowing and digesting food, delivering and collecting blood, or seeing, hearing, and smelling what is happening in the world around us.

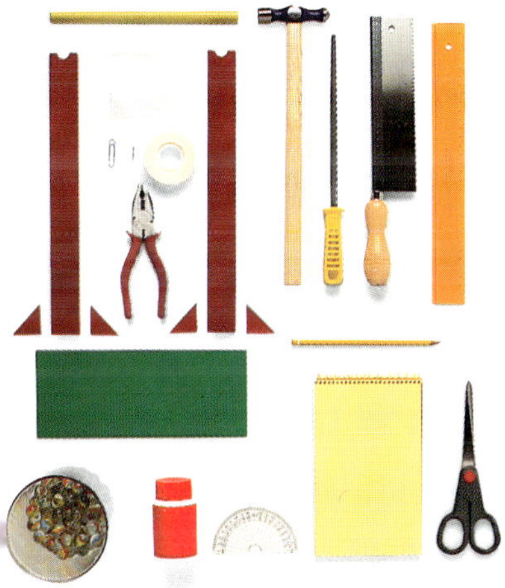

Organs themselves are made of body tissues, which are in turn made of microscopic cells. Every second, even as we sleep, millions of cells are being born and dying as the body maintains and repairs itself. This book includes detailed microscope photographs showing what the cells look like and how they work.

The book is packed with experiments and projects for the whole family. Some of them are safe for young people to carry out. When an adult's help is advised, this is clearly stated at the beginning of the experiment.

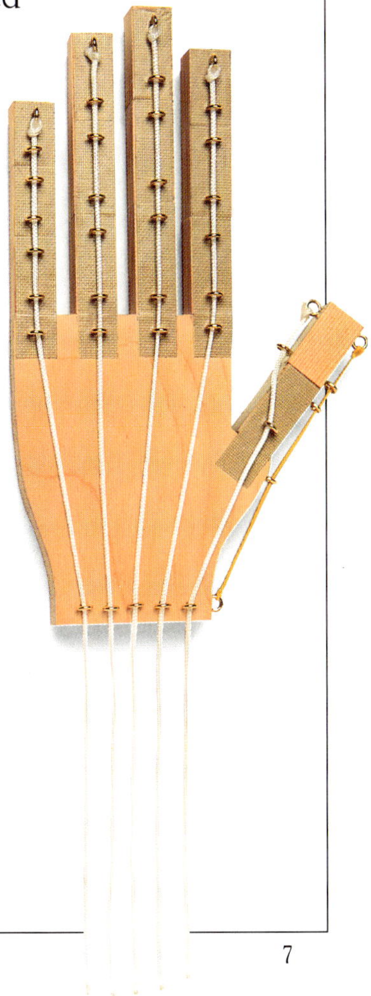

Many experiments in the book need only a few everyday items that can be found around the home. Others are more elaborate and call for greater time and effort. But all of the experiments require one vital piece of equipment—*you*. Find out directly about the way you grow and develop, and how your body works inside.

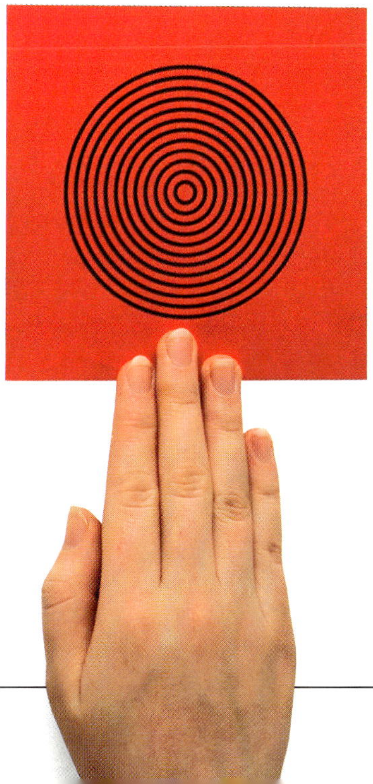

The more that you learn about the body and the way it works, the more fascinating it becomes. Also, the more you know, the better you can look after yourself, stay healthy, and live a long and active life.

The home laboratory

THE EXPERIMENTS in this book do not require specialized equipment. Most of the items can be found in the kitchen and around the house, or obtained easily and inexpensively. Alternatives that work just as well are often given in the list of materials for an experiment. The most important piece of equipment is your own body! You will also need some friends to help you. Shown on these two pages are some items you may find useful to help you to explore the human body.

Safety precautions

For some experiments you will need containers that are heat-proof. Always use protective goggles and oven mitts where indicated. NEVER put chemicals in any containers where they might be mistaken for food or drink items.

Glass bowl

Heat-proof jar

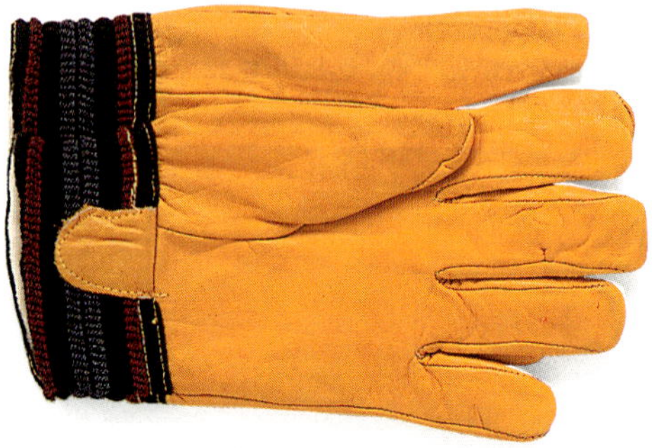

Oven mitts

Heat-proof tile

Cutting mat

Plastic-edged mirror

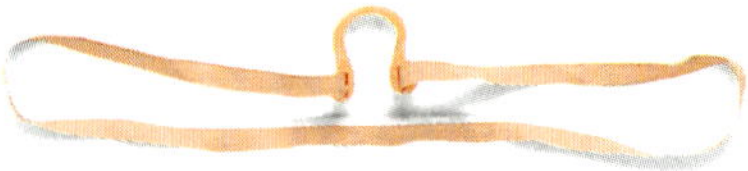

Nose clip

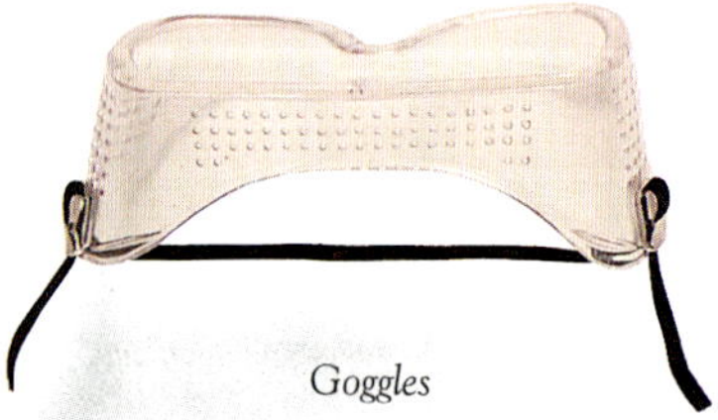

Goggles

Plastic bag

Saucer

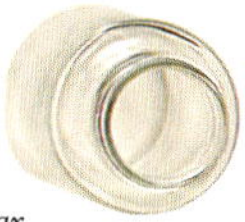

Glass jar

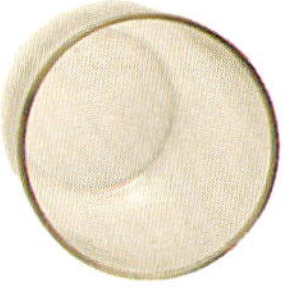

Glass

Measures

You will need measuring instruments in some of the experiments. All of the measurements in this book are given using two measurement systems. Use one system or the other—do not mix them. Make sure that you use a metal ruler as a cutting edge when you are cutting paper or poster board.

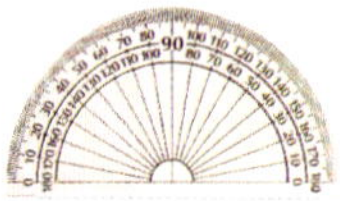

Protractor

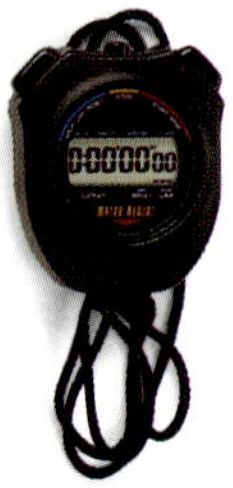

Stopwatch

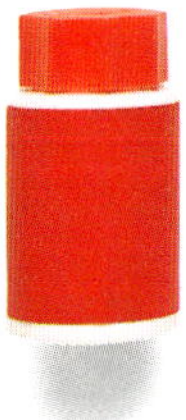

Glue

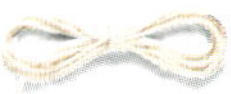

String

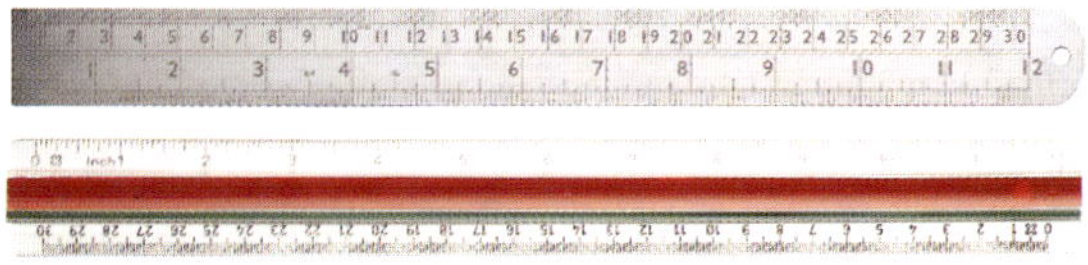

Metal and plastic rulers

Thermometer

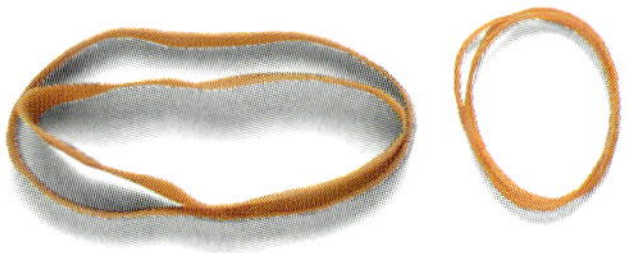

Assorted rubber bands

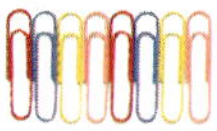

Paper clips

Materials

Most of the materials you need for the experiments and models are everyday items. You may already have some in your home, such as drinking straws. An assortment of differently colored sheets of paper and poster board is very useful. Other materials, such as wood, dowels, and screws, can be bought from a hardware or lumber store.

Tools and instruments

You will need colored pens, scissors, pencils, paints, and a good craft knife. Different types of tape are also very useful. You may need to borrow some ordinary household tools, such as saws, pliers, and screwdrivers. Ask an adult for help if these tools or other sharp instruments are required.

A simple light microscope allows you to examine exterior parts of the body in amazing detail, although it is not essential to have one for most of the experiments in this book. Advice on setting up and using a light microscope is given on page 178.

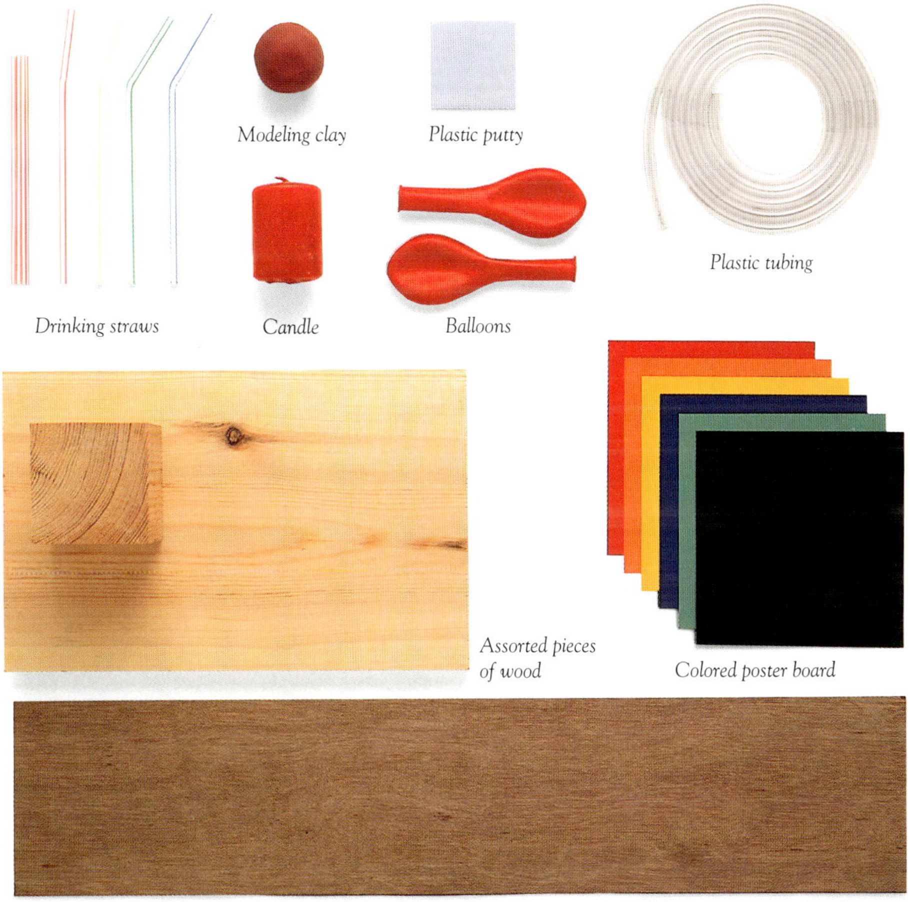

Drinking straws · *Modeling clay* · *Candle* · *Plastic putty* · *Balloons* · *Plastic tubing* · *Assorted pieces of wood* · *Colored poster board*

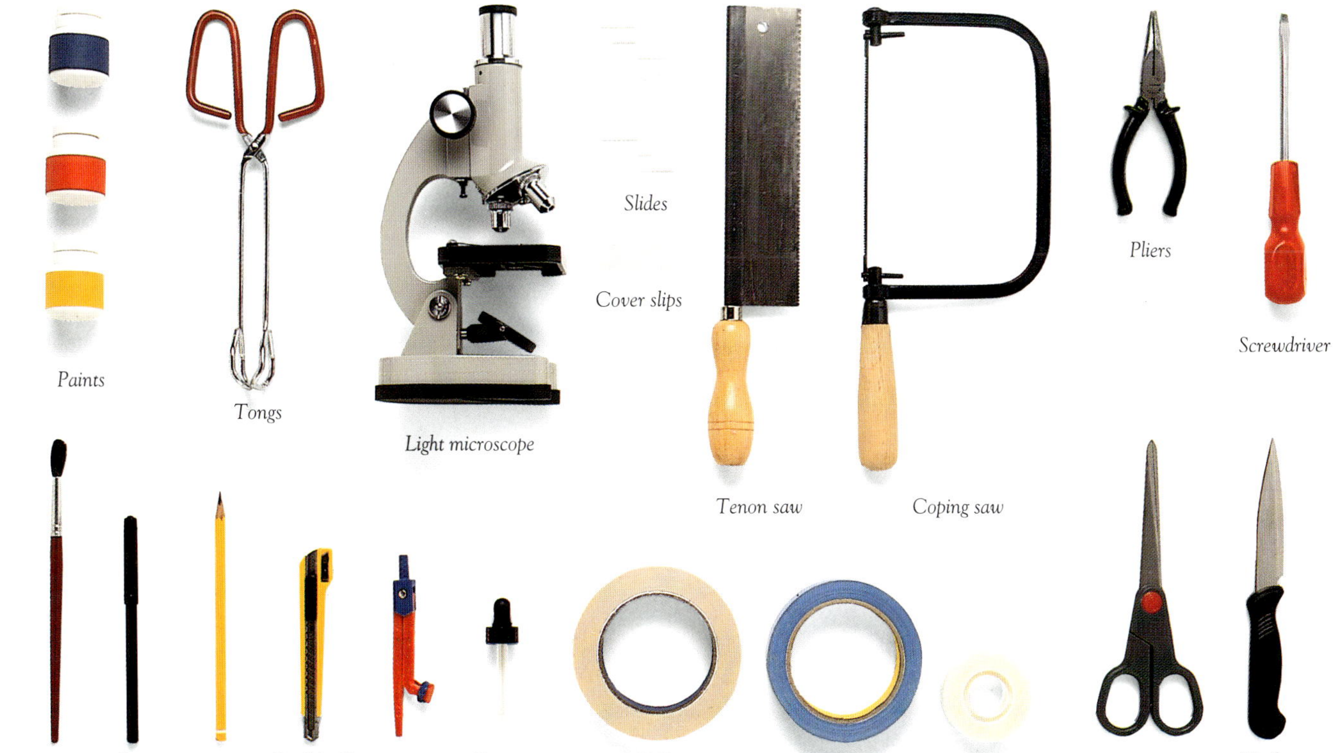

Paints · *Tongs* · *Light microscope* · *Slides* · *Cover slips* · *Tenon saw* · *Coping saw* · *Pliers* · *Screwdriver* · *Paintbrush* · *Pen* · *Pencil* · *Craft knife* · *Compass* · *Dropper* · *Masking tape* · *Duct tape* · *Cellophane tape* · *Scissors* · *Kitchen knife*

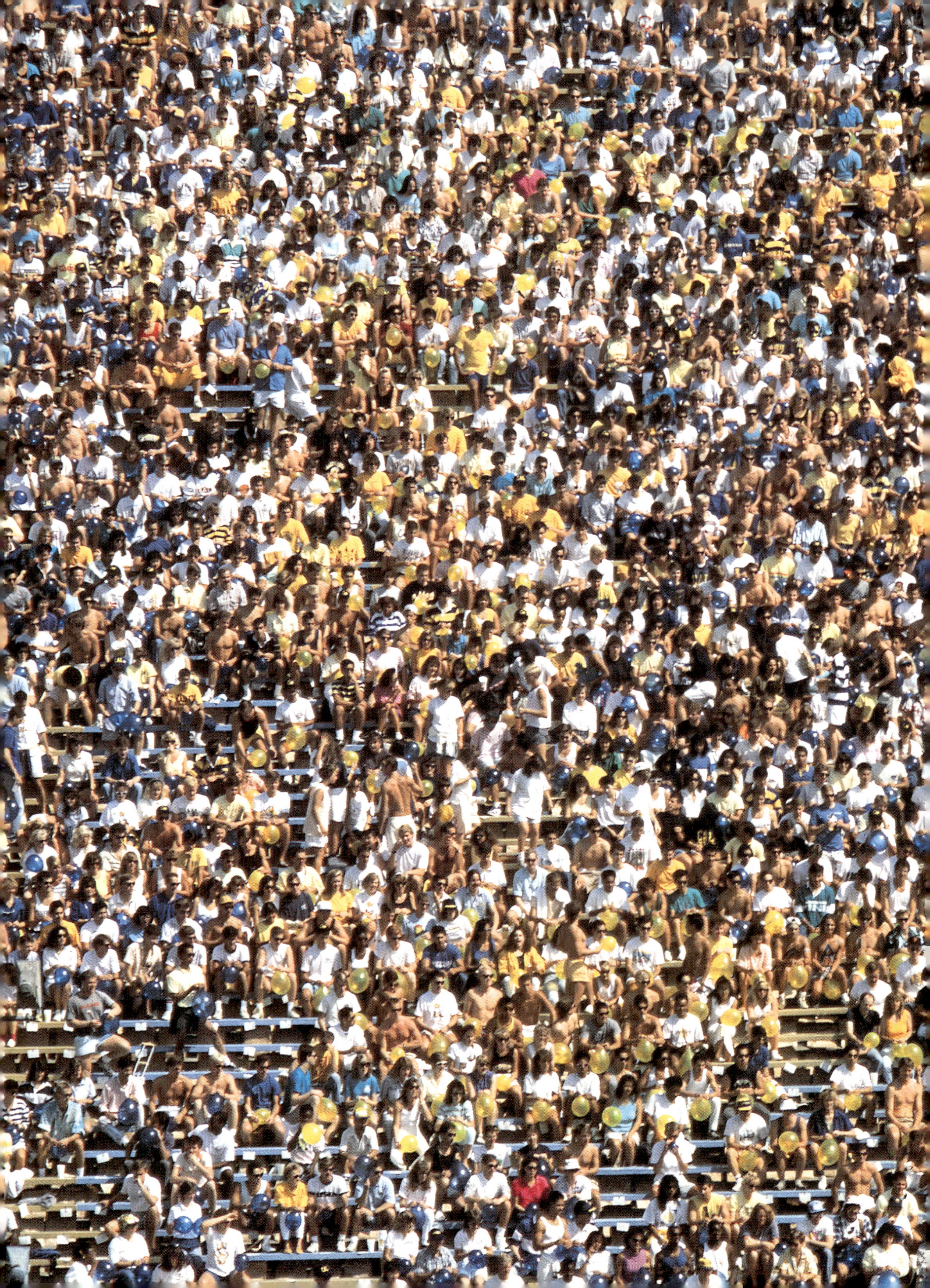

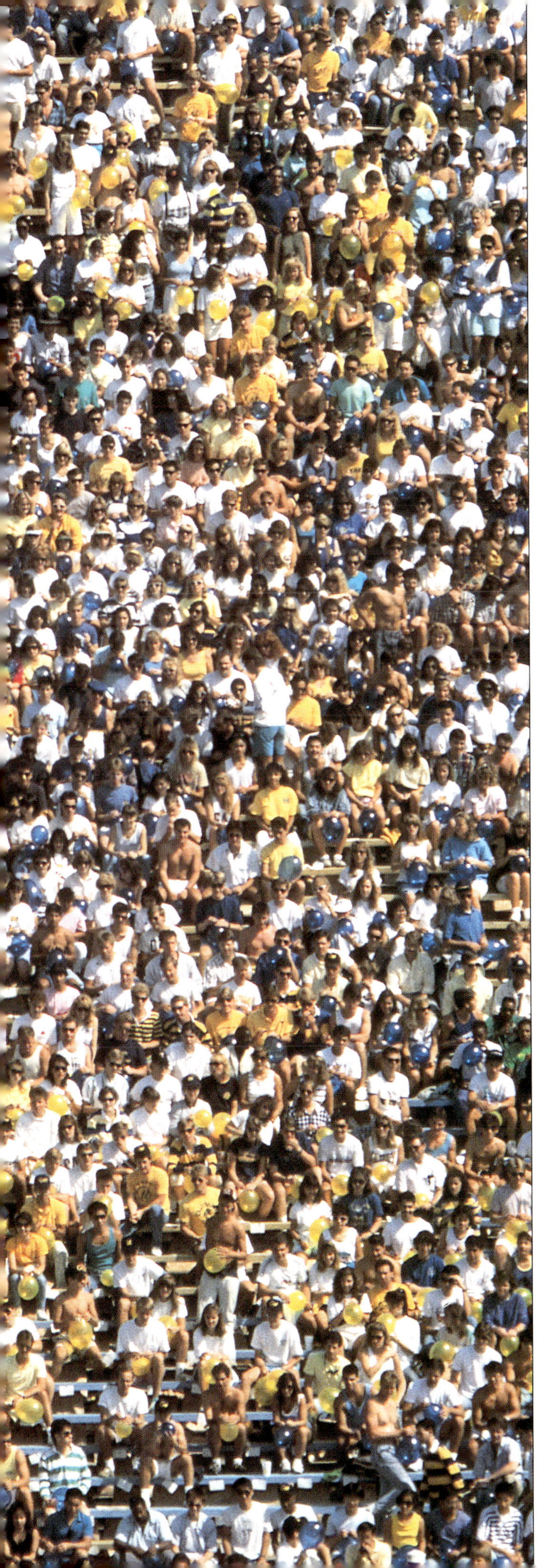

The BODY

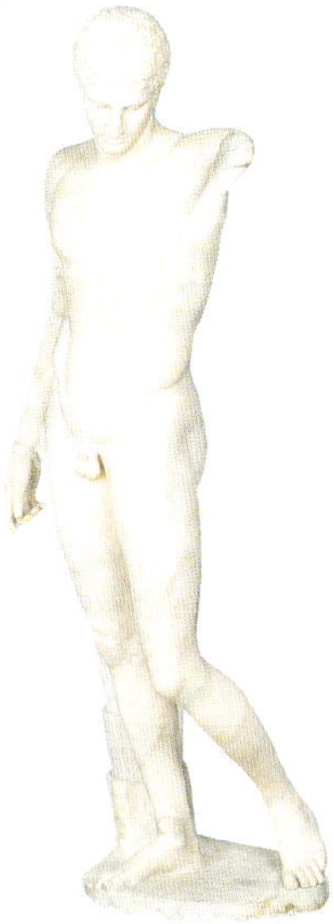

Variations on a theme
From ancient times, people have celebrated the beauty of the human form in painting and sculpture. The ancient Greeks carved an ideal body shape in stone (above). But every person is different. The unique shapes and curves of each body allow us to pick out individuals in a crowd of thousands (left).

EACH HUMAN BODY HAS the same basic design: two eyes, two ears, a nose, a mouth, a chest, an abdomen, two arms, and two legs. Even so, there is incredible variation in body shapes and sizes. All of our bodies are miracles of engineering, far more sophisticated than the most up-to-date computers. The body grows and develops, feeds and maintains itself, senses the world around it, and deals with the countless challenges of life.

WHAT MAKES A BODY?

THERE ARE MANY POSSIBLE WAYS to approach the question "What makes a body?" The science of biology suggests that humans are relatives of other mammals and that the human body we know today was made by millions of years of evolution. The science of anatomy shows that the body is made of main parts, called organs, composed of millions of cells. And the science of genetics reveals how, in a sense, the body makes itself—from instructions hidden in its genetic blueprint (pp.176–177).

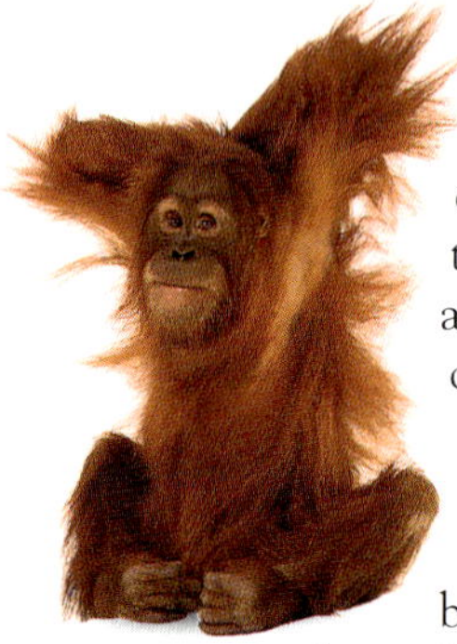

The orangutan *(above), chimpanzee, and gorilla—the great apes—are our closest animal relatives.*

To understand what makes a human body, we can compare it with other, similar bodies in the world around us. There are many parallels between our bodies and those of other mammals. Just like the 4,000 other mammal species, we have warm blood, hairy skin, and a bony skeleton. Also like other mammals, we feed our babies on mother's milk. We belong to the group of mammals called primates, which also includes lemurs, monkeys, and apes. Indeed, the great apes—the orangutan, gorilla, and chimpanzee—resemble us in incredible detail. Our genetic material, made up of DNA (p.180), is over 98 percent identical to a chimpanzee's. Therefore it makes scientific sense to view humans as close relatives of the great apes.

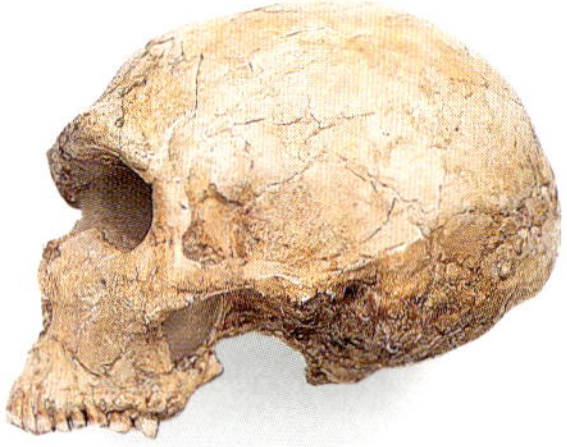

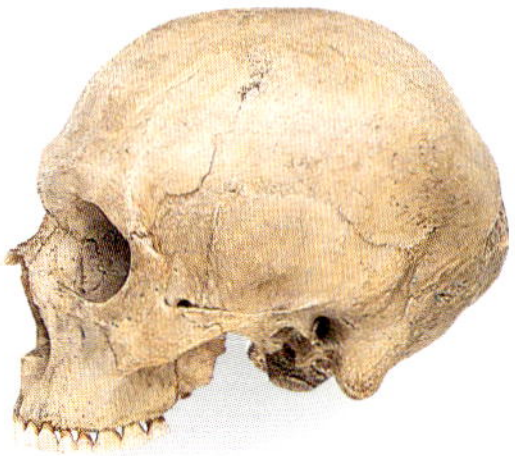

The fossil skull of a Neanderthal *human (top) is longer from front to back and is made of thicker bone than the skull of a modern person (above).*

Human origins

The ancient Greek philosopher Aristotle (384–322 B.C.) taught that in order to understand something thoroughly, we should know its origins (where it comes from). So to understand what makes a body, we must look at the body's origins.

Some people believe that human beings are specially created by a Deity or Supreme Being. Modern biological science sees the human body, like all natural living things, as the result of evolution. It holds that the human body has developed over millions of years, through a long sequence of changes that have made it better adapted to its environment. Since we have the most similarities with the apes, it is likely that both we and the apes evolved from a common apelike ancestor.

In 1859, the English naturalist Charles Darwin (1809–82) announced his theory of evolution in great detail in his book *On the Origin of Species by Means of Natural Selection*. This book caused a great deal of controversy at the time.

Fossils of human bones and teeth show how the human species may have evolved over several million years. An early human predecessor was the small-brained, chimplike creature known as *Australopithecus* ("Southern Ape"), which walked upright 3 million years ago in Africa. Almost 2 million years ago came the bigger-brained, tool-using *Homo habilis* ("Handy Human"). Then, about 1 million years ago, came the larger, more skilled tool maker *Homo erectus* ("Upright Human"). People who look like us, modern *Homo sapiens* ("Wise Human"), probably first appeared about 200,000 years ago.

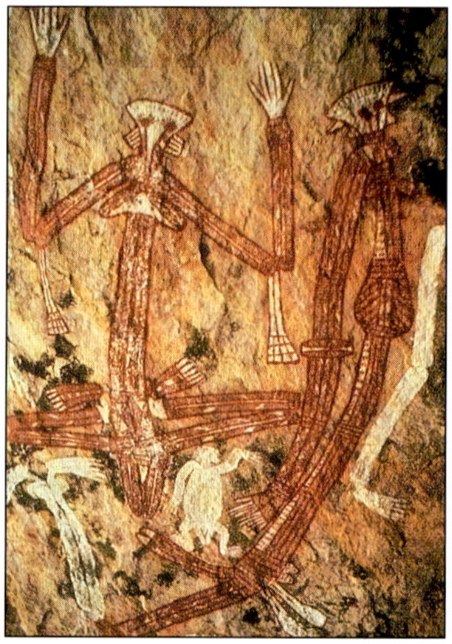

In their own image, the Aboriginal *people of Australia drew "X-ray" pictures of humans, with rods representing limb bones. Australian rock art is thousands of years old.*

However, some evolutionary branches were a dead end. One such branch was probably the Neanderthals of what is now Europe and the Middle East. Although the Neanderthals were well adapted to the intense cold of the ice ages, they died out by about 30,000 years ago.

Early anatomy

People have been fascinated by the body's inner structure for thousands of years. Cave art from prehistoric times shows that the artists knew about the inside of the body. In ancient civilizations in Egypt, Greece, China, India, and elsewhere, people studied and wrote about the twin sciences of anatomy (the body's structure) and physiology (how the body works). They did this partly from curiosity, but also to understand how the body became ill, so that they could treat and cure people. These scientists—including the Father of Medicine, Hippocrates (c.460–c.377 B.C.) of ancient Greece—were the first doctors.

The first person to write in great depth about anatomy was Galen (A.D. 129–c.201) of ancient Rome. Although he was a doctor, tradition prevented him from dissecting (cutting open) dead people, so many of his descriptions are adapted from animal studies. So great was Galen's authority that people blindly accepted all of his teachings, including the mistaken ones, for over 1,000 years.

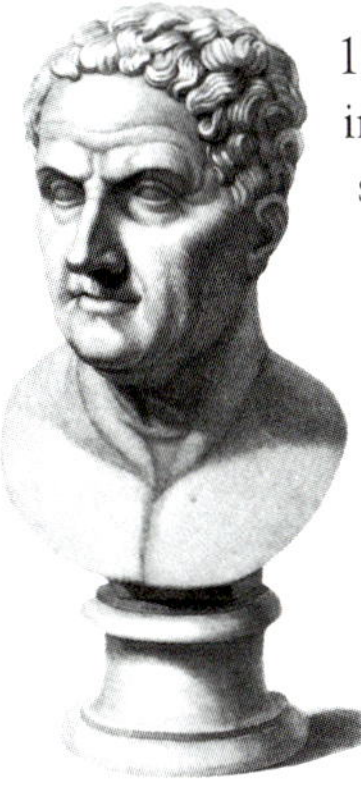

Galen was physician to *the gladiators in the Colosseum in Rome.*

In Europe, from about 1300, there was a new interest in the arts and sciences. During this Renaissance (French for "rebirth") period, people began to study the body more thoroughly. They dissected human corpses to see exactly what the body was made of. The major anatomical book of this period was *De Humani Corporis Fabrica* ("The Fabric of the Human Body") by Andreas Vesalius (p.22), professor of anatomy at Padua, Italy. Vesalius drew and described what he actually saw, rather than what tradition taught should be present. His work brought the science of anatomy into the modern world.

Microanatomy

By about 1600 the body's basic anatomy was understood in detail. But the invention of the microscope opened up a new microscopic world to see and study. Microscope pioneers such as the Dutchman Antony van Leeuwenhoek (p.172) and the Italian Marcello Malpighi (p.104) studied human organs under the microscope and saw that, like other living things, the body is constructed of cells—the "building blocks" of life (pp.24–25).

Each individual cell is a living entity: it uses nutrients and energy, carries out chemical processes, controls its own cellular contents, and reproduces itself. Each cell also has a special role to play in keeping the body running smoothly.

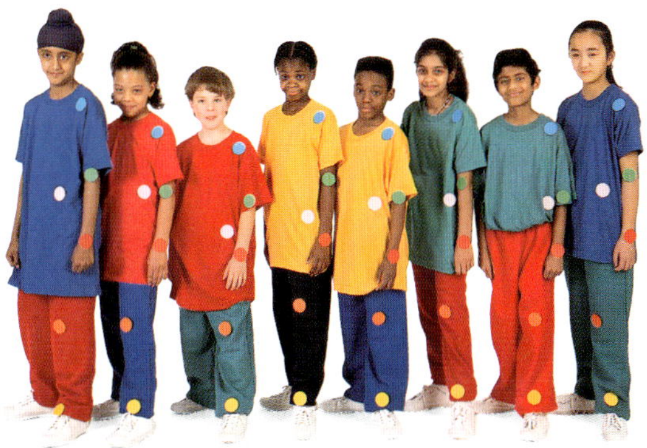

All bodies have the same basic plan, but the *variety in physical proportions and features, and in our personality, emotions, and experiences, makes each of us an individual.*

Genes

Over the last century, we have gained a far more detailed knowledge of what makes a body. A new type of microscope (p.24)—called an electron microscope—can magnify an object a million times or more. It has revealed the structures from which cells are made and even their molecules (p.182).

One of these molecules is deoxyribonucleic acid (DNA), the "blueprint for life." In 1953 the English scientist Francis Crick and the American biologist James Watson unraveled the structure of DNA (p.176). Inside each cell, long strings of DNA carry instructions, in a chemical code, for growth from an embryo (p.173) to an adult human and for running and repairing the body. Each instruction is in the form of a gene. In a single cell there are perhaps more than 100,000 genes, on DNA totaling almost 10 ft (3 m) in length.

When an egg cell is fertilized by a sperm cell (p.172), a new baby is conceived. The egg cell and sperm cell pass on, in the form of genes, the instructions that determine the general shape and size of the new person, and what features he or she will have.

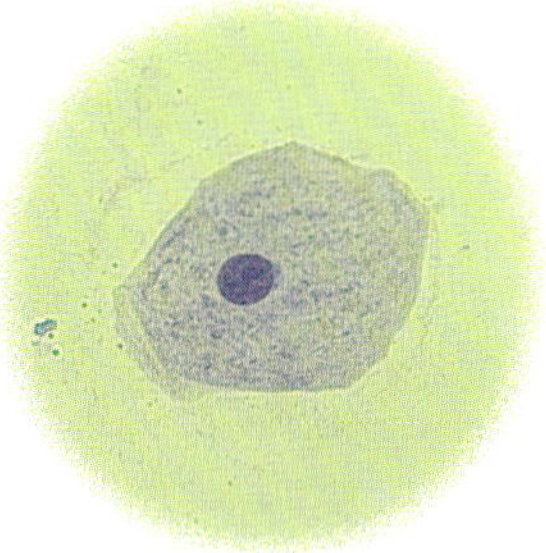

A single body cell *(pp.24–25) from the lining of the cheek has a life of only a few hours before it is rubbed away as you chew.*

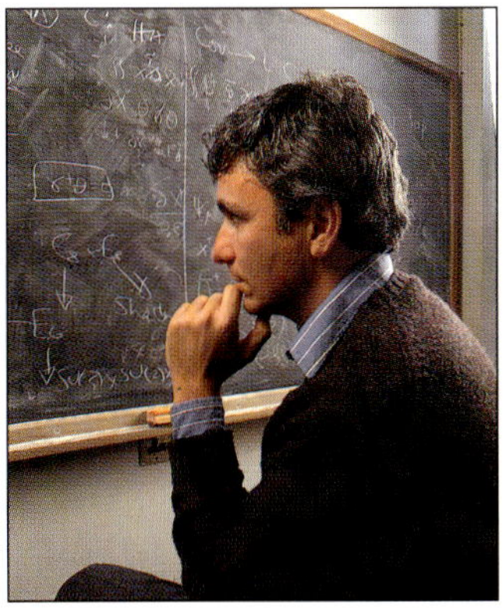

What sets humans apart from other *animals is the capacity of our brains (pp.126–127) for abstract thinking, planning, problem solving, and other aspects of what we term "intelligence."*

The body's ingredients

HOW YOU VIEW the ingredients of the body depends on which science (type of knowledge) you are interested in. To the biologist, the body is built up from millions and millions of cells that help the body to grow and to maintain itself. To the chemist, the body is an amazingly complicated combination of atoms and molecules—undergoing millions of chemical reactions every second. To the dietary expert, the body is a collection of substances such as proteins, minerals, and carbohydrates, and it needs to take in correctly balanced types of food to keep itself healthy and in good working order. And to a mechanical engineer, the body is an incredibly sophisticated, self-controlling, self-repairing machine.

An artificial body?

Many science-fiction stories feature robots, androids, or other humanlike machines. But the technology needed to build such sophisticated machines is still far in the future, if it will ever exist. Robots have never successfully copied the body's ability to walk in a well-balanced way on two legs, let alone its huge variety of fast-action, precise movements and its range of sight, hearing, touch, and other senses. Even the most advanced computers do not come close to the human brain's capacity for intelligent thought, learning, and creativity.

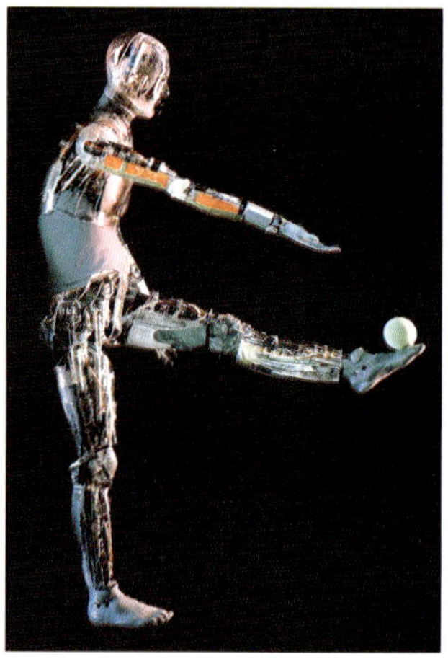

In the human image
Human-shaped robots are built for research purposes. But the balanced, upright, two-legged posture of the human body is very difficult for a robot to mimic.

From body to atom

Like all of the matter in the universe, the body is made of tiny particles called atoms. Collections of atoms make up molecules, molecules make up organelles, organelles make up cells, and so on, in a level-by-level hierarchy (organization) in the body. When early anatomists (p.13) studied the whole body, they were interested mainly in its large structural parts, the organs. Later, microscopists studied the body at a different level of its hierarchy—its microstructural parts, the cells. Other scientists developed a greater understanding of the body's functions (what it does). These scientists were particularly interested in the nature of body systems and tissues. Only in this century, with the development of the electron microscope, have we been able to view the smallest, most basic units in the body hierarchy—organelles and molecules.

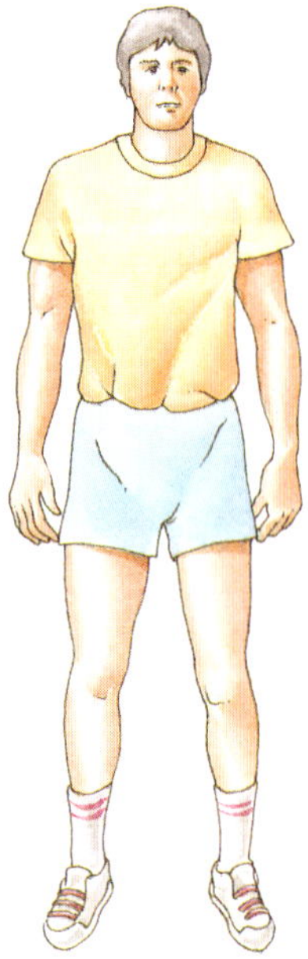

Body
There are more than 5 billion human bodies on the earth. Each is a unique individual. But all bodies have the same basic outer design, and inside they all have the same main parts in the same places.

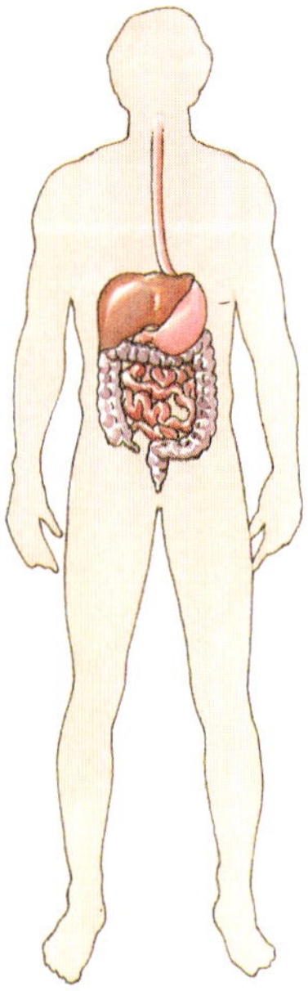

System
The body can be thought of as a collection of systems (pp.22–23). Each system has one major role. For the digestive system above, this is to digest food so that it can be absorbed by the body.

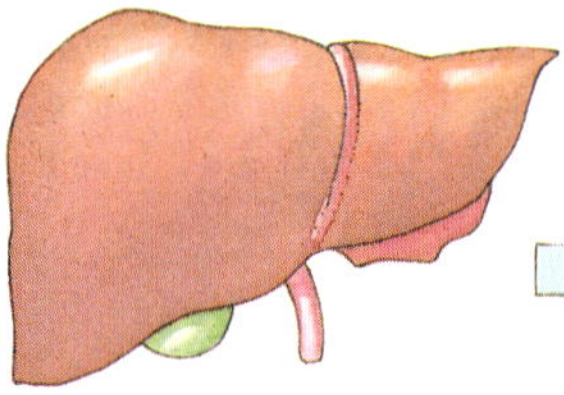

Organ
An organ is a distinct body part that carries out one or more main functions. Several organs working together make up a body system. For example, the liver is an organ that is part of the digestive system.

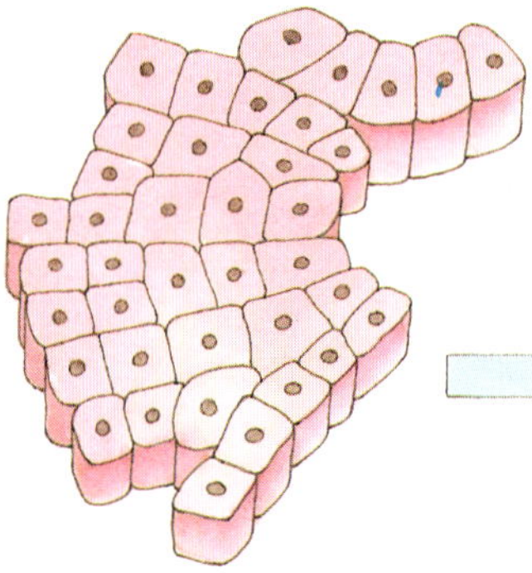

Tissue
Each organ is composed of one or more kinds of tissue. A tissue is a group of similar cells that carry out a specialized job. The liver is mostly made of sheets of hepatocytes—cells that process nutrients.

The body's chemical contents

The chemical substances that make up the human body can be divided into different groups, which are similar to the groups of substances—called nutrients—in the food we eat (p.83). The main nutrients in the body are carbohydrates, proteins, lipids (fats and oils), and minerals. If these main nutrients and other substances could be taken from the body and transformed into more familiar forms, they might look something like the collections of ingredients shown here:

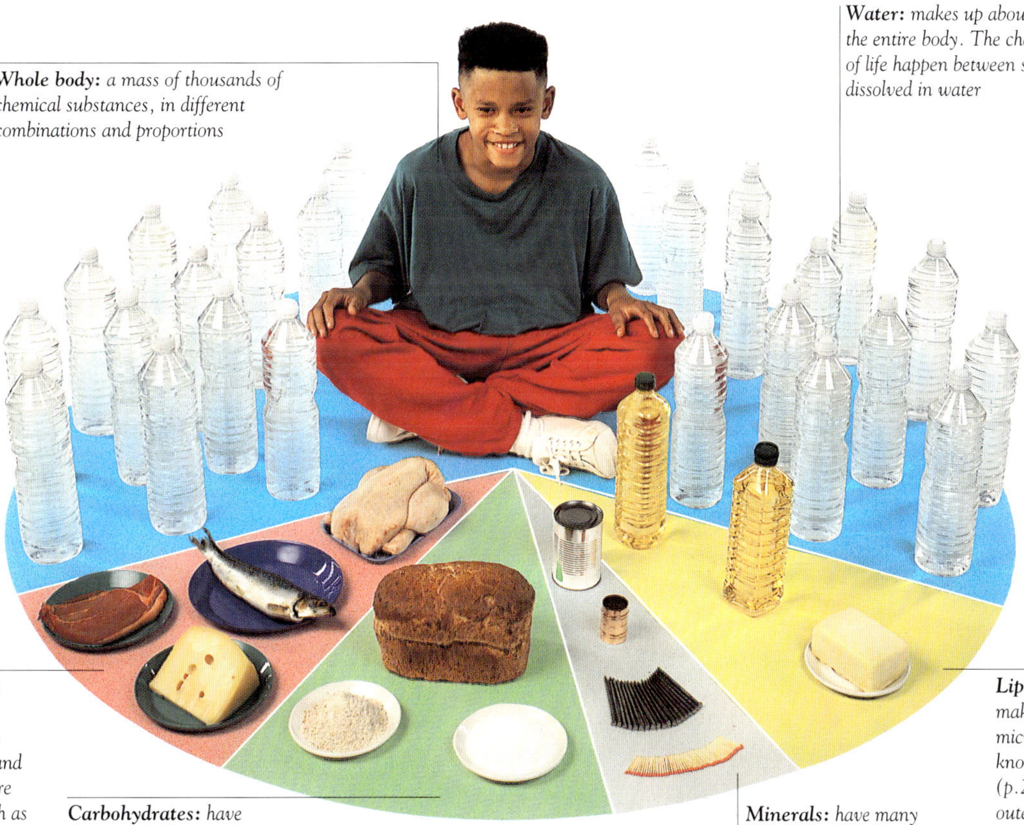

Whole body: *a mass of thousands of chemical substances, in different combinations and proportions*

Water: *makes up about two-thirds of the entire body. The chemical reactions of life happen between substances dissolved in water*

Proteins: *the body's main structural molecules, forming a living framework in and around cells. They are plentiful in foods such as meat, fish, and cheese*

Carbohydrates: *have mainly energy-providing functions in the body. They are abundant in sweet or starchy foods such as flour, bread, rice, and sugar*

Minerals: *have many specialized roles in body chemistry. Body minerals include copper (as in hot-water pipes), iron (as in nails), sulfur (as in match heads), and trace elements such as zinc (as in tin cans)*

Lipids (fats and oils): *make up the thin microscopic sheets, known as membranes (p.28), that form the outer "skin" of each cell and most organelles. They are similar to the fats and oils used for cooking and those in butter*

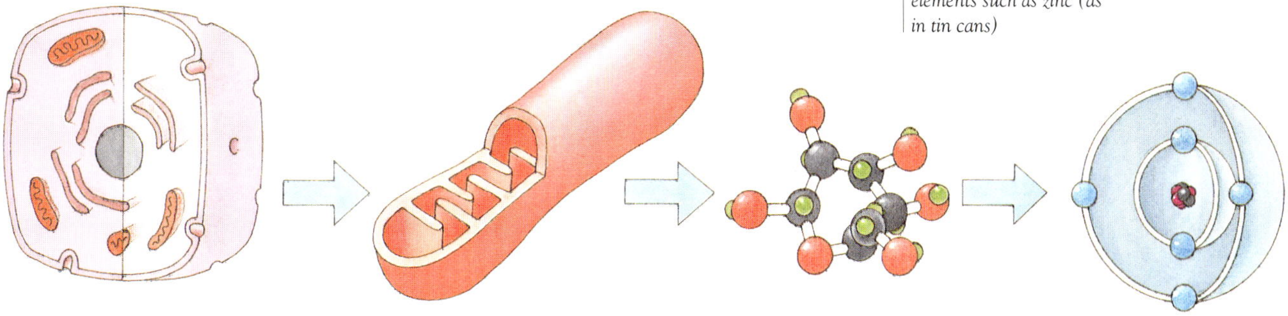

Cell
The cell (pp.24–25) is the basic unit, or building block, of all living things, plant or animal. A hepatocyte is 1/900 in (0.03 mm) wide and is shaped like a box with rounded corners.

Organelle
The cell contains structures called organelles (p.26). An important example is the sausage-shaped mitochondrion. Inside it, energy is released from nutrients and made available for the cell's use.

Molecule
Each organelle contains thousands or millions of molecules. This molecule is glucose, the body's main energy-rich ingredient. The gray balls in this model of a glucose molecule are carbon atoms (right).

Atom
A molecule is a combination of particles known as atoms. A glucose molecule has 24 atoms (including 6 carbon atoms like the one above). All life is based on organic (carbon-containing) molecules.

Body shapes and sizes

HUMAN BODIES COME IN ALL SHAPES, sizes, and proportions. The kind of figure you have depends in part on whether you are a child or an adult, a female or a male. Your figure is mostly the result of the size and shape of the bones of your skeleton. This is especially true for height. Total body height is only about 1 in (2.5 cm) more than the skeleton's height. In an adult, a quarter of this height is taken up by one bone in each thigh, the femur. Body proportions also depend mainly on bone size. For example, some people have broad shoulders; others have narrow ones. Some people have a short torso (trunk) and long limbs; others have a long torso and short limbs. Diet, exercise, and living conditions also affect your shape and size. Excess food is stored as fat that pads out the body, while regular exercise can lead to large, bulging muscles.

Food and conditions

The body's genes play a large part in controlling how it grows and develops. But the amount and quality of food that a person eats are also important. Babies and children who do not get proper nourishment grow more slowly than they would if they had a healthy diet. As adults, they may not be as tall or as well developed as they would have been if they had been well nourished. Cramped, unhealthy living conditions, with a lack of light and fresh air, can also have an effect on growth.

Body measurements

Far back in history, people did not have rulers or tape measures. But they did have body parts, such as hands and arms, which they could use for measuring. The size of the body parts varied from one person to another. But they were an accurate-enough guide for the building methods of the day. The ancient civilizations of Egypt (c.3300–c.1000 B.C.), Greece (c.900–c.350 B.C.), and India (c.2300–c.1700 B.C.) all had measuring systems that were based on parts of the body, although they often used different names for the same measurement. The names they used are shown in this table.

Geometric shapes

Great artists and sculptors noted that the head, torso, arms, and legs of the human body are in proportions that please our eyes. "Vitruvius man," by the Italian artist Leonardo da Vinci (1452–1519), showed how the arms and legs of a human body mark points on both a circle and a square.

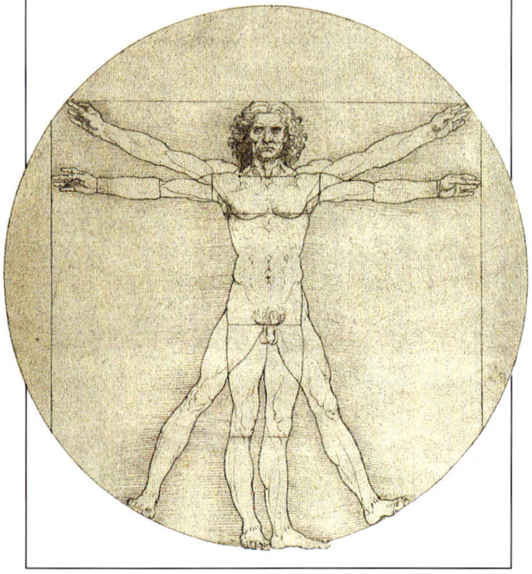

		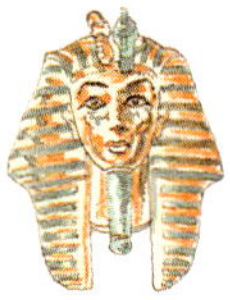 EGYPTIAN	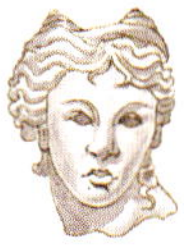 GREEK	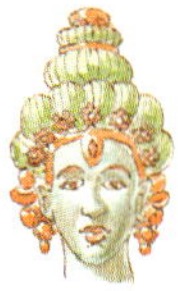 INDIAN
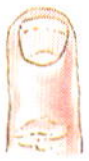	*Width of finger*	*Zebo*	*Daktyloi*	*Angula*
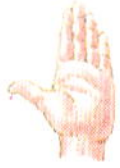	*Width of palm*	*Shep*	*Palaste*	*No equivalent measurement*
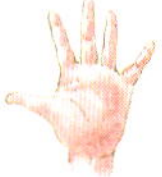	*Width of spread-out fingers*	*Span*	*Spithame*	*Pradesa*
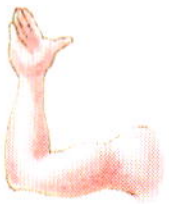	*Fingertip to elbow point*	*Royal cubit*	*Olympic cubit*	*Vitasti*
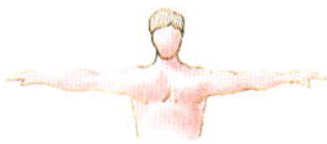	*Tip to tip of outstretched arms*	*No equivalent measurement*	*Orguia*	*Vyayama*

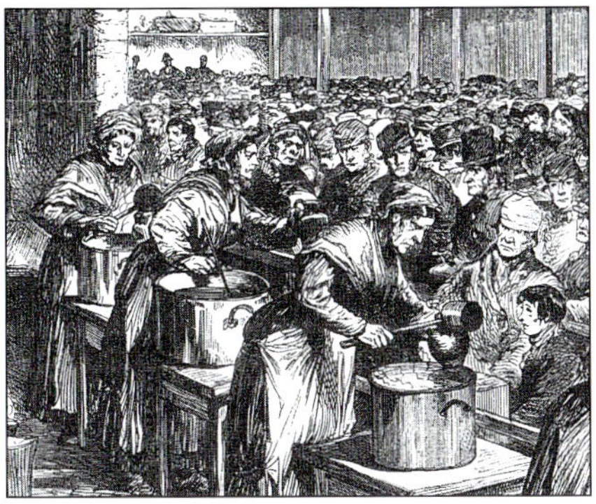

Poor living conditions

If food is in short supply and conditions poor, as in this 19th-century soup kitchen, people's heights tend to be lower than normal.

EXPERIMENT

Body proportions

Even if you are the same height as a friend, you may have longer legs or shorter arms. Variations like these depend mainly on the sizes of the bones in your skeleton. Using poster-board disks, make a "human graph" to show how body proportions vary. Photograph the lineup to study it. Measure distances between different disks with a ruler.

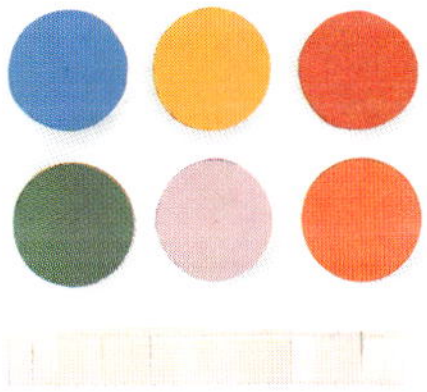

You Will Need

- *sets of 6 colored poster-board disks*
- *adhesive pads or double-sided tape*

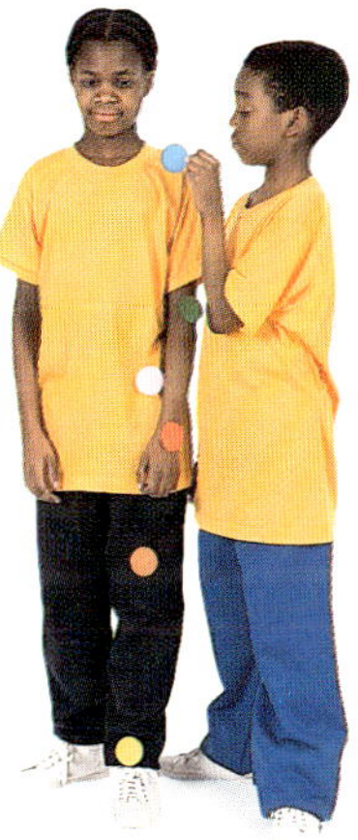

1 Ask a friend to stand up straight, with his or her shoulders square. Press to find the hard, bony points on the shoulder, elbow, wrist, hip, knee, and ankle. Stick a different colored disk on each of these parts.

2 Stick disks on a whole line of friends. Measure distances between disks on each person. How much of the body height is made up of legs? Is the upper arm longer than the lower arm? Do tall people always have longer arms than shorter people?

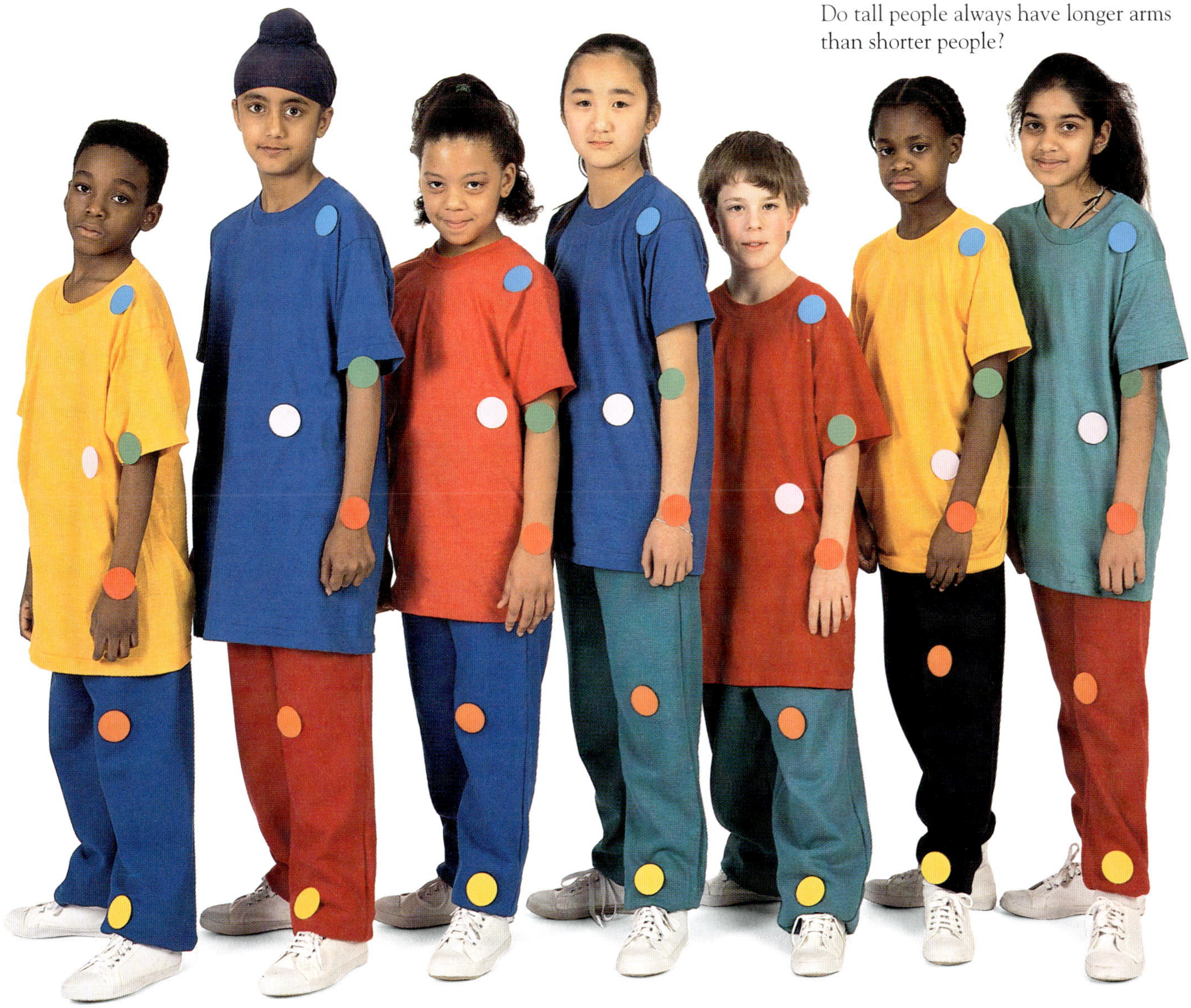

Faces and features

HOW EASY IS IT TO RECOGNIZE people you know? You can often identify family and friends from far away by their body sizes and proportions, and the ways they stand and walk. If they are closer, you probably look at their faces. You do this not only to identify people, but also to assess their emotions and what they are thinking. In particular, you concentrate on the eyes and mouth, since these reveal a lot about a person's moods and intentions. It is amazing how easily people can change their appearance—and even become unrecognizable—just by altering the face with glasses, make-up, or mustache.

EXPERIMENT

Revealing faces

Which of the face's features helps you to recognize someone most easily? Is it the eyes, the nose, or the mouth? Take photographs of familiar people, or cut out famous faces from magazines. Test your friends by revealing different face features one at a time.

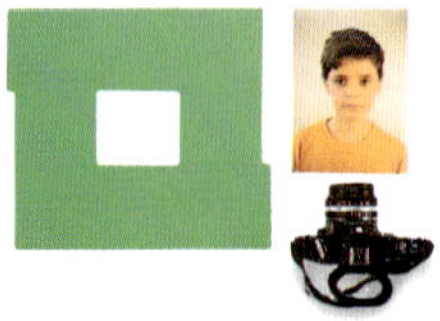

YOU WILL NEED

- *L-shaped cards*
- *camera and film or photographs of faces*

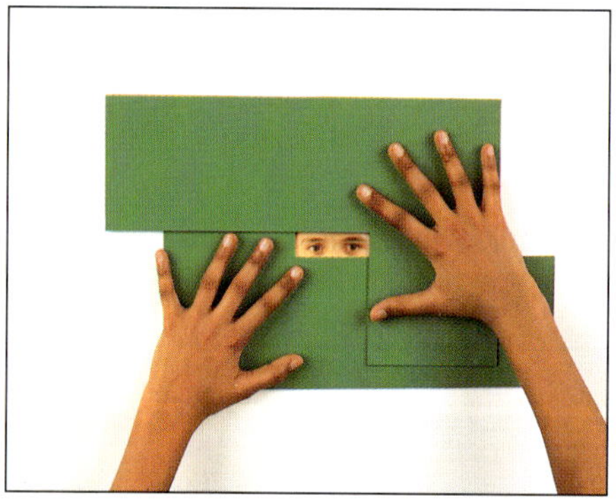

Reveal the parts
Lay the cards over a photograph to reveal only the eyes. Can your friend identify the person pictured? Try again with a new face or a different facial feature. Which feature helps you to recognize people most easily?

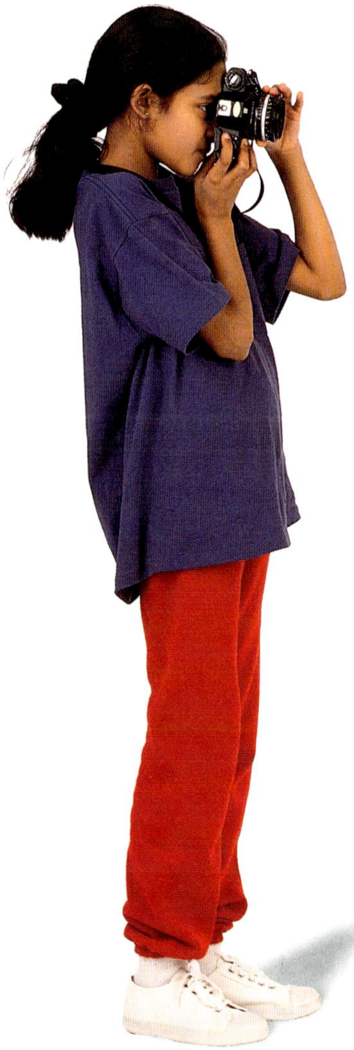

Photographing a friend's face
To take a photograph of a face for these experiments, hold the camera directly in front of your friend and level with his or her eyes. Turn the camera so that it is vertical. Make sure your friend's face fills the frame and that she or he is looking into the lens. Then click. You may want to ask an adult to take the picture.

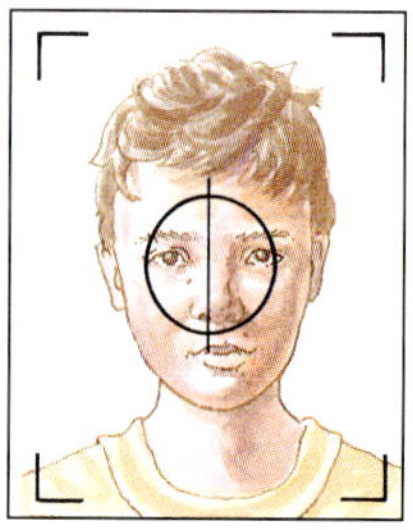

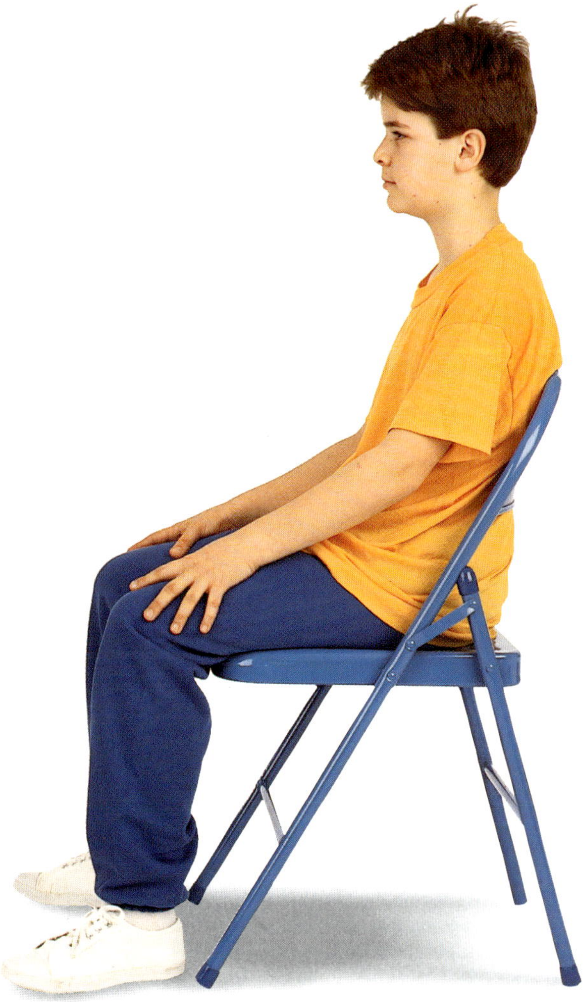

EXPERIMENT

Mirror-image faces

Adult help is advised for this experiment

Is a face exactly symmetrical? In other words, is one side an exact mirror image of the other? Are your eyes or your ears level with each other? Is your mouth the same shape at both corners? Find out with this experiment, which uses photographs of faces. When you get your film developed, ask for a normal set of prints and a set printed with the image reversed. (Make sure the photographs are taken head-on, as on the opposite page.)

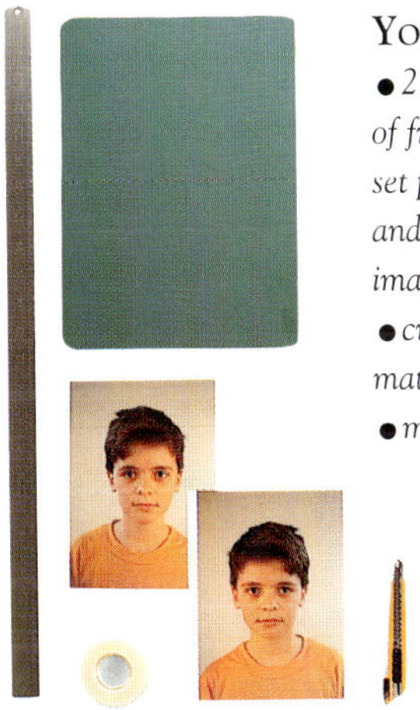

YOU WILL NEED

- *2 sets of photographs of friends' faces, one set printed normally and the other with the image reversed*
- *craft knife*
- *cutting mat*
- *cellophane tape*
- *metal ruler*

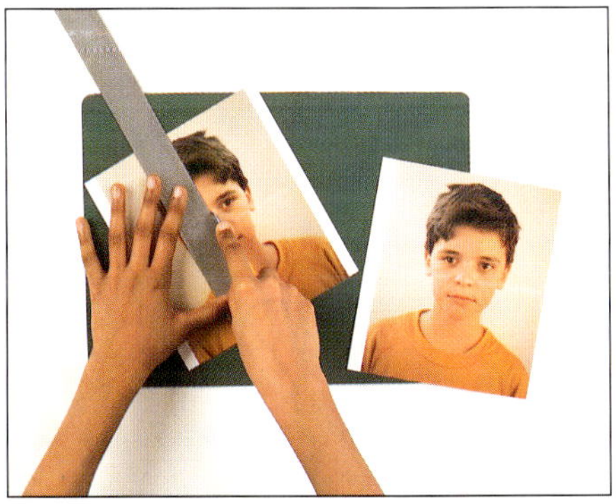

1 PLACE THE RULER down the center of each photograph, exactly through the middle of the eyes, nose, and mouth. Carefully cut along this line.

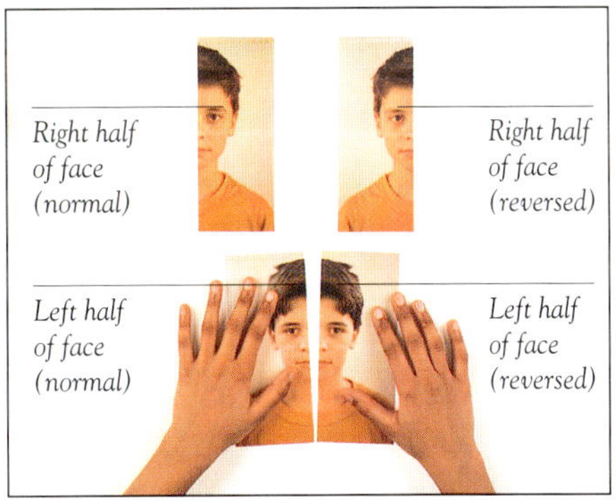

2 PLACE HALF of one photo next to the reversed version of the same half. Tape together the backs of these two halves. Repeat for the other halves.

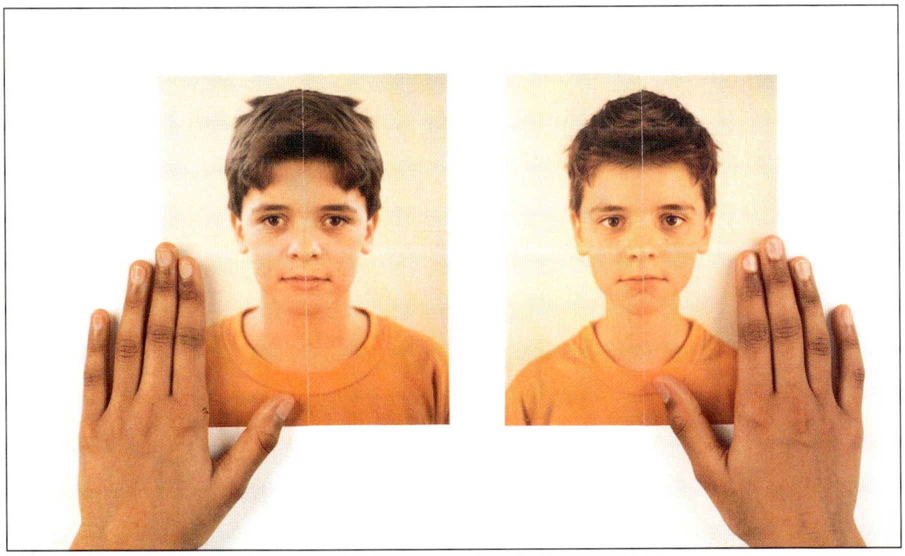

3 YOU HAVE MADE each picture exactly symmetrical. Each picture has one side of the face and its mirror image. See how the two faces look different from each other—often dramatically so! This experiment shows that people's faces are never exactly symmetrical. One eye or eyebrow is always higher than the other, or one side of the mouth or the nose is shaped differently from the other.

Recalling a face

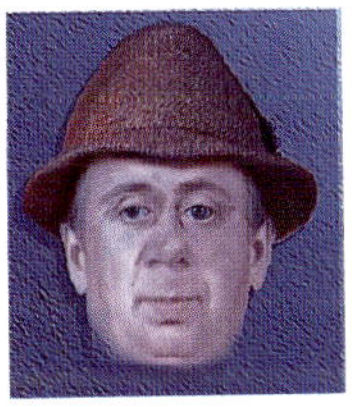

Computer face
Human faces like this one can be built up feature by feature using a special computer program.

Although it may be easy to recognize faces, it can be difficult to describe or draw them. So to re-create the faces of missing people, or to help people to identify suspects in a crime, the police use special pictures of faces. These are built up from face parts—such as hair, forehead, and eyes—of varying shapes and sizes. The viewer concentrates on recalling each of the suspect's facial features in turn. Then he or she selects the best likeness for each feature from a collection of photographs or a choice of images on a computer screen. These parts are gradually put together to build up a whole face, like the one above.

How identical?

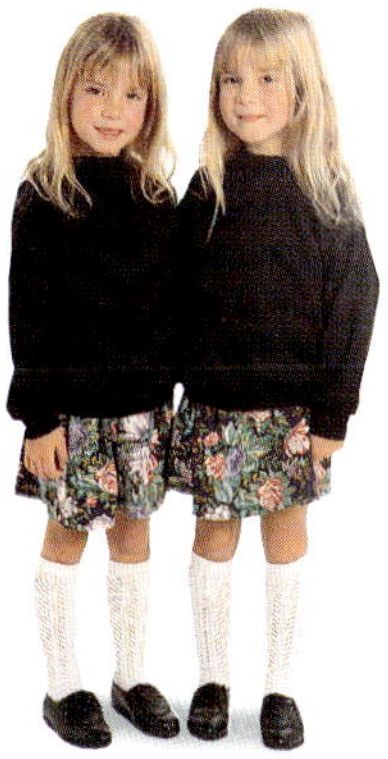

Identical twins have exactly the same genes (the "blueprints" of the body, p.181). When they are babies, and even when they are at school, the twins may be very hard to tell apart. But, like two identical cars rolling off a production line, they can never have exactly the same experience. During their lives, they eat different foods and they are exposed to different types of wear and tear. These different living conditions affect the appearance of their bodies in different ways. Usually, the older the twins become, the more different from each other they look.

The body's limits

DO YOU THINK you would win a running race against a cheetah? Or a diving competition against a dolphin? Probably not. But what about a running race against the dolphin? Compared to other animals, humans may not excel at any single event. But we are good at a variety of physical feats and skills. Imagine a well-trained human athlete taking part with various animals in a decathlon competition, comprising 10 different events such as running, jumping, throwing, and swimming. The human would almost certainly receive the overall prize—and would definitely win the throwing event, since very few animals are able to throw an object any distance.

EXPERIMENT

Finding your limits

Adult help is advised for this experiment

It is true that "practice makes perfect," especially with such muscle-developing actions as push-ups (opposite, below). But sometimes we are not aware of what our bodies can do. For example, this experiment shows that your joints may be more flexible than you realize. *Caution: If you feel dizzy, sick, or in any discomfort or pain, stop at once and rest.*

Animal champions

Here are some of the best performers from the mammal group—but only at their own events. An elephant hardly excels at high jumping! The human is the most capable all-around athlete.

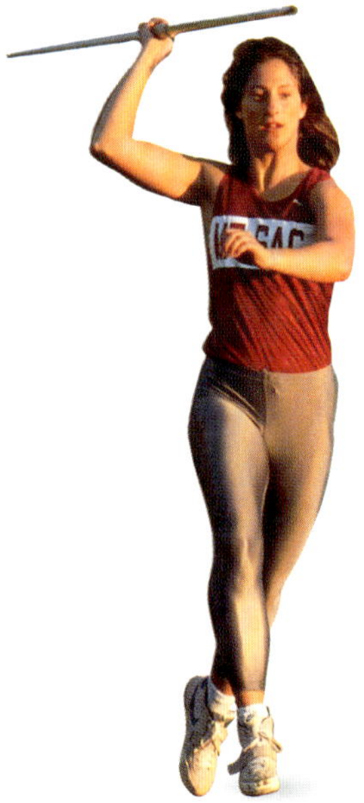

Throwing
A human athlete throws a javelin over 295 ft (90 m). Few animals could even hold it.

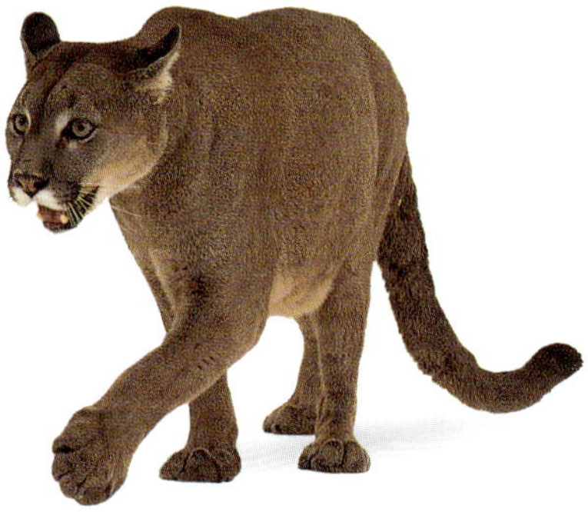

High jump
Big cats such as the puma can clear 15 ft (4.5 m), nearly twice our record.

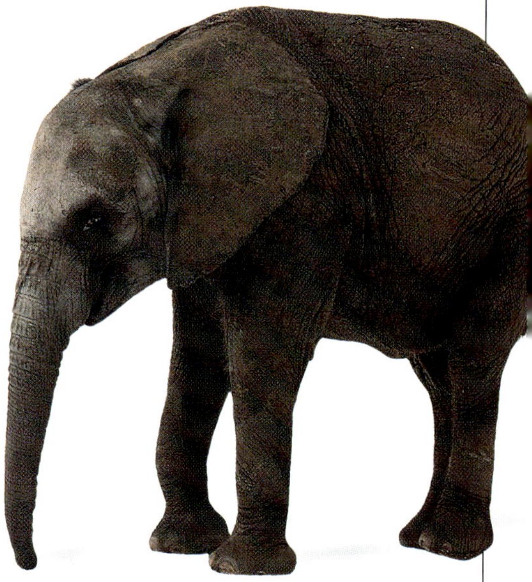

Weight lifting
An elephant uses its trunk to lift over 1,100 lb (500 kg), about twice the human record.

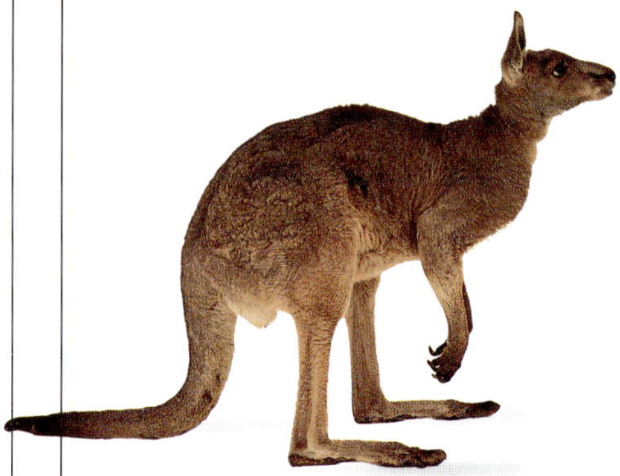

Long jump
A kangaroo can leap more than 39 ft (12 m), 10 ft (3 m) more than the human record.

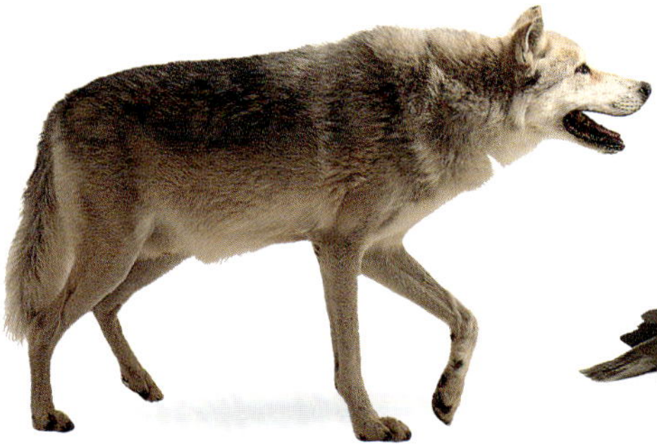

Long-distance running
Wolves can trot on and off at about 5 mph (8 kph) for several days. No human can do this.

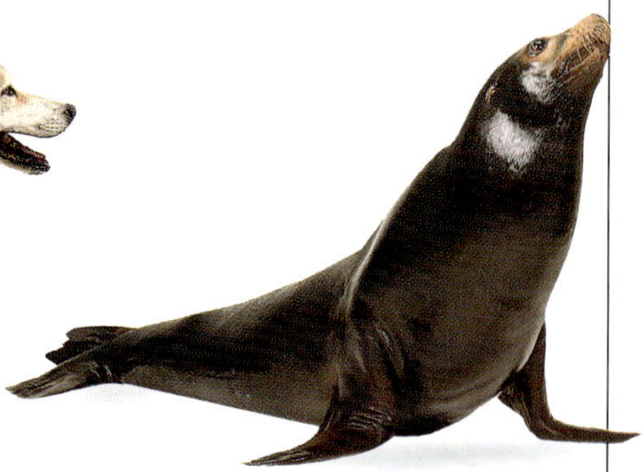

Swimming
A sea lion swims at about 15 mph (24 kph), three times faster than the fastest human.

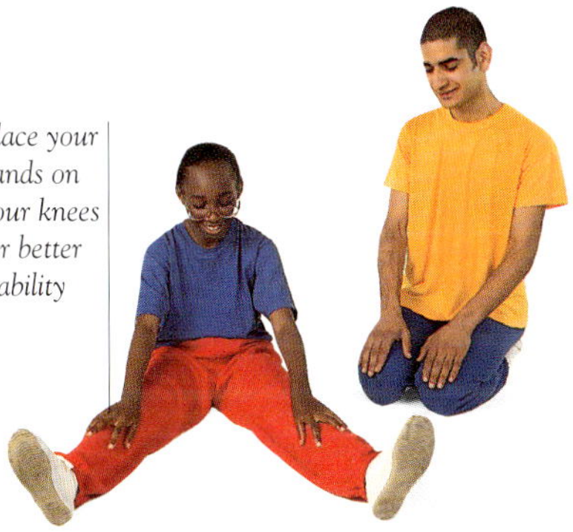

Place your hands on your knees for better stability

1 SIT ON THE FLOOR, your back upright and legs straight out in front. Slowly move each leg out to the side. Keep moving your legs slowly sideways until you feel you cannot go any farther. Stop moving. Rest and relax in this position.

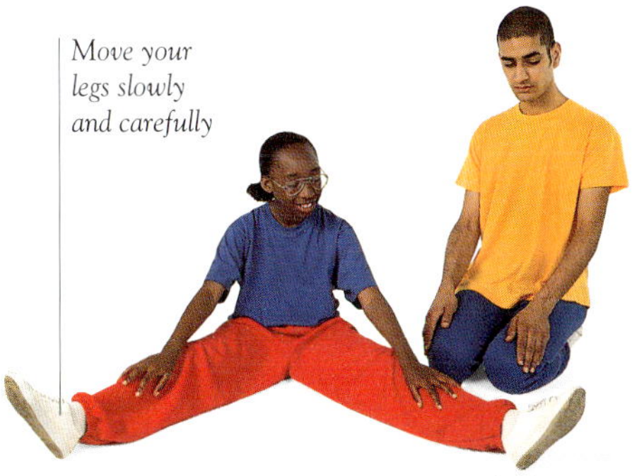

Move your legs slowly and carefully

2 THIRTY SECONDS LATER, carefully try to move your legs slightly more. You may be surprised at how much farther they go. You can do this because the muscles, tendons, and ligaments in your hip joints have stretched and relaxed into the extended position.

Artificial aids

Through the ages, by ingenuity and inventiveness, humans have created aids to improve and extend the body's physical capabilities. In the Stone Age rock axes and spears allowed people to hunt bigger, more powerful animals. Today, wearing the latest running shoes saves split-seconds in races.

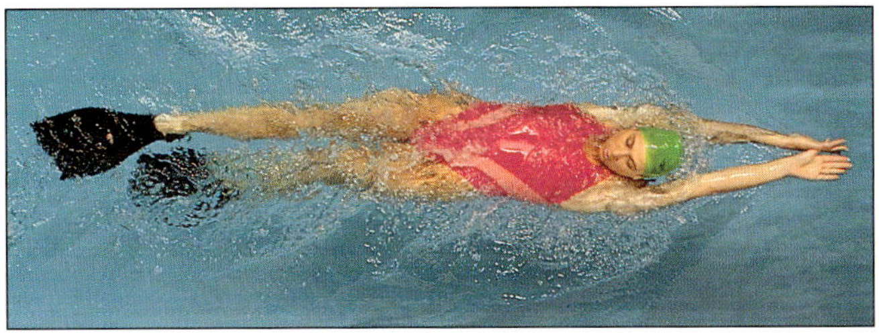

Webbed feet
Flippers copy the webbed feet of seals and otters. They give swimmers greater speed and power in the water.

A better way

Occasionally, humans develop a completely new way of doing something familiar. For example, U.S. high jumper Dick Fosbury developed a new leaping technique in the 1960's, which was more effective than the old methods. Other high jumpers took up his technique, and records rose rapidly.

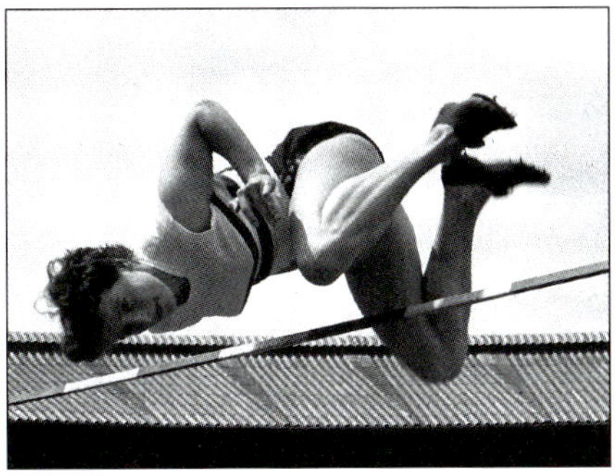

Pre-Fosbury
Most high jumpers "straddled" the bar, sideways and face down.

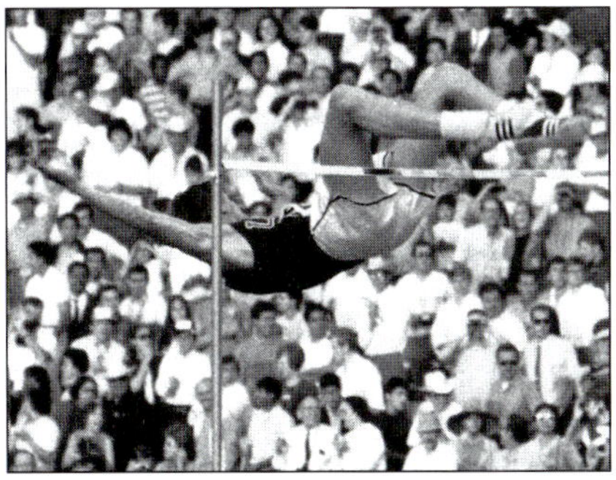

The "Fosbury flop"
With his innovative headfirst, face-up style, Dick Fosbury won gold at the 1968 Olympics.

EXPERIMENT

Improving your ability

Adult help is advised for this experiment

Many parts of the body respond to the demands put on them. For example, regular physical activity increases the strength and stamina of muscles. It also improves the efficiency of the lungs and heart. If you do an activity such as push-ups (press-ups) regularly, you should soon find that you have improved. In a safe place, count how many push-ups you can do without too much strain. For one push-up, bend your arms to lower your chin so that it touches the floor, then straighten your arms and lock your elbows. Repeat the test each day. Does the exercise become any easier? Caution: *If you feel dizzy, sick, or in any discomfort or pain, stop at once and rest.*

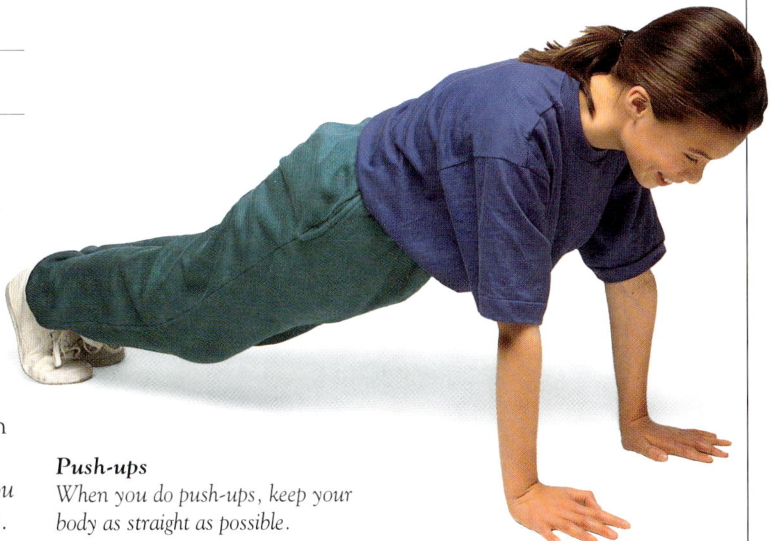

Push-ups
When you do push-ups, keep your body as straight as possible.

Body systems

IF YOU LOOK AT THE OWNER'S manual for a car, you will probably find that it is arranged in chapters, each dealing with one particular system—a set of closely connected parts inside the machine. One chapter is about the electrical system, another about the fuel system, another about the brakes, and so on. You could arrange the "owner's manual" of the human body in the same way. Each of the body's main systems has a major job to do, such as getting oxygen, digesting food, or disposing of waste. The systems work together to make sure that the whole body runs smoothly.

■ DISCOVERY ■

Andreas Vesalius

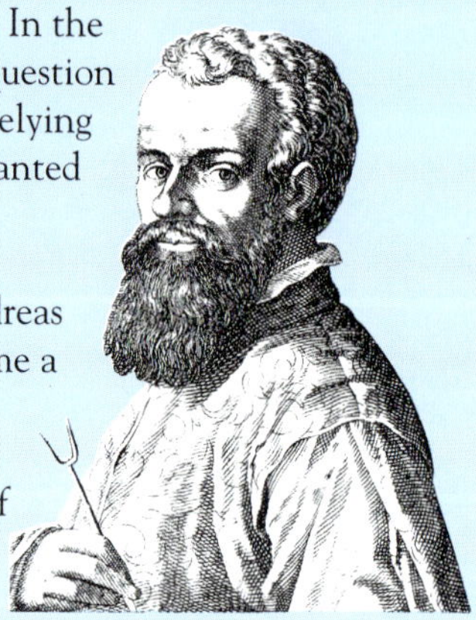

Until the Renaissance period of the late 14th to mid 17th centuries, people's ideas about the body had changed very little for over a thousand years. In the Renaissance, people began to question the old knowledge. Instead of relying on pictures from books, they wanted to open up bodies and look for themselves. The greatest early anatomist was the Belgian Andreas Vesalius (1514–64), who became a professor at Padua in Italy. His book of 1543, *De Humani Corporis Fabrica* ("The Fabric of the Human Body"), portrayed the body in amazing detail.

Skin, hair, and nails (integumentary system)
Skin protects the body from wear and harmful rays, keeps in body fluids, and senses touch. Skin and hair also help in the control of body temperature.

Muscles (muscular system)
All body movement is caused by the contraction of muscles. Most of these muscles move bones, for actions such as walking or lifting, but some move other body features, such as the eyebrows.

Bones (skeletal system)
The bones of the skeleton are the supporting framework of the body. Bones also protect some inner parts. The skull shields the brain, and the ribs form a cage around the heart and lungs.

Heart, blood vessels, and blood (circulatory system)
These parts make up the body's transport network. The heart pumps blood, which distributes hundreds of substances, such as life-giving oxygen and body-building nutrients.

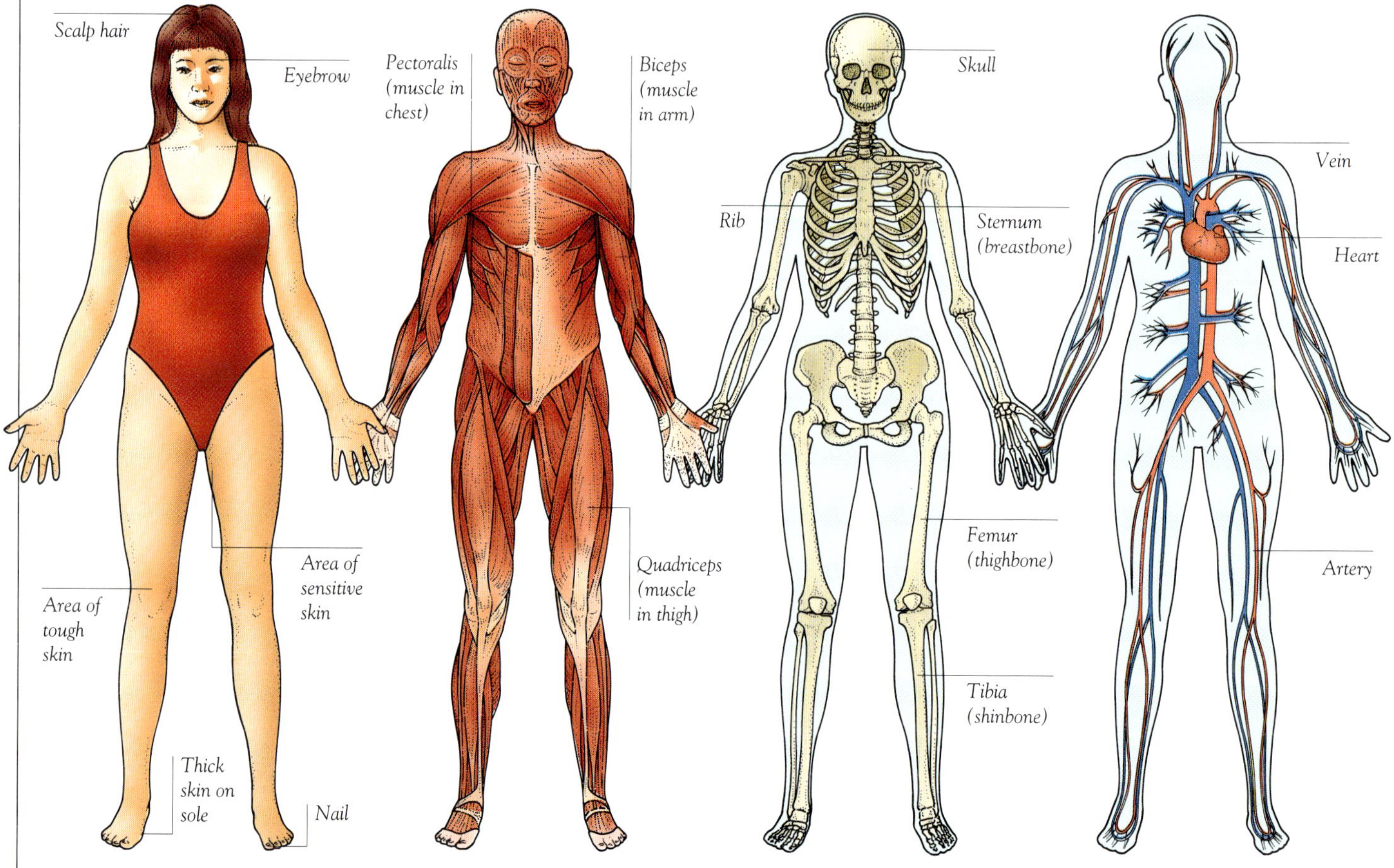

Nose, windpipe, and lungs (respiratory system)
Oxygen is vital for life. This system breathes fresh air into the lungs and transfers the oxygen from that air into the blood for distribution.

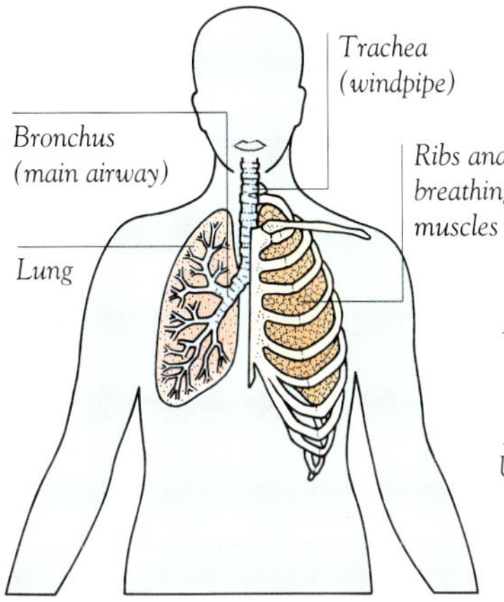

Kidneys and bladder (urinary or excretory system)
These organs excrete (get rid of) waste substances. The kidneys filter them from the blood as a liquid, urine, that is stored in the bladder.

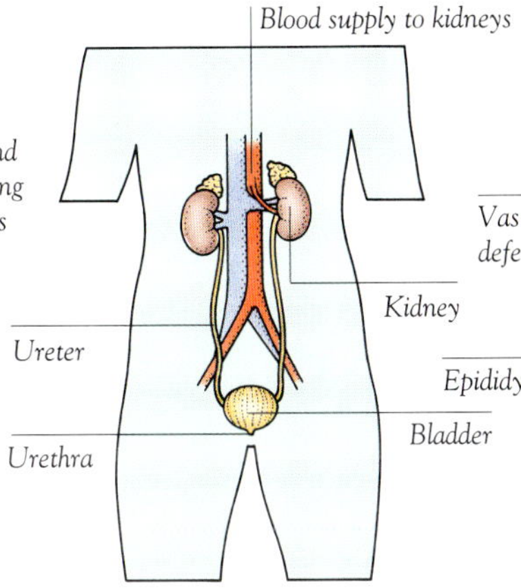

Male sex organs (reproductive system)
The male organs make microscopic tadpole-shaped sperm. If one of these joins with an egg cell in a female (right), a baby may develop.

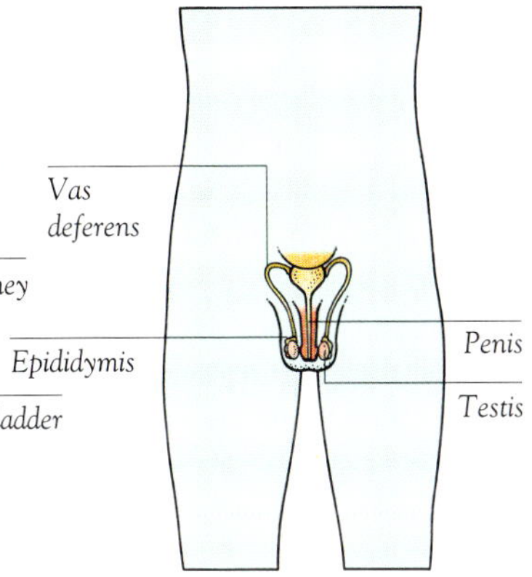

Female sex organs (reproductive system)
The female organs are designed to produce egg cells and nourish a baby as it develops from an egg cell and grows in the womb (uterus).

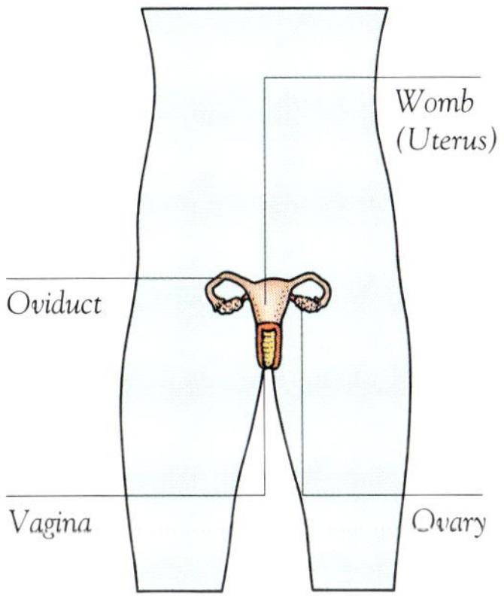

Brain, nerves, and senses (nervous and sensory systems)
The brain is the body's control center, "wired in" by the nerves. It receives information from sense organs, such as the eyes and ears, and decides what to do.

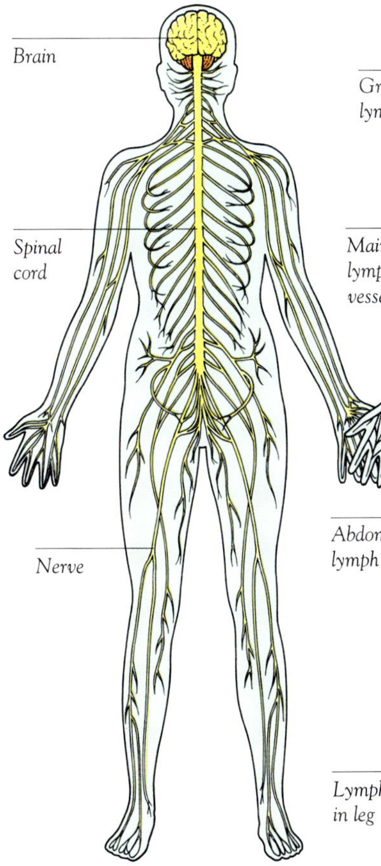

Lymph nodes and vessels (lymphatic system)
Lymph is a pale fluid collected from body tissues by a network of tiny vessels. It carries germ-fighting cells and is cleaned in "glands" called lymph nodes.

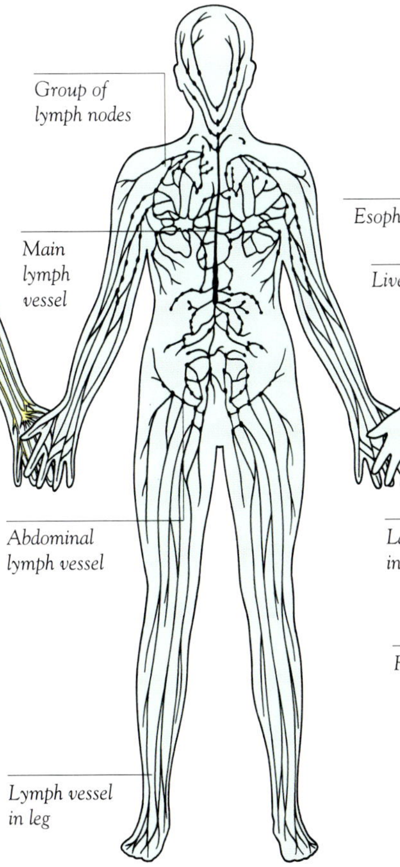

Mouth, stomach, and intestines (digestive system)
After the teeth cut and chew, this system digests food until the pieces are small enough to be absorbed by the body. Leftover bits of food leave the system as feces (solid wastes).

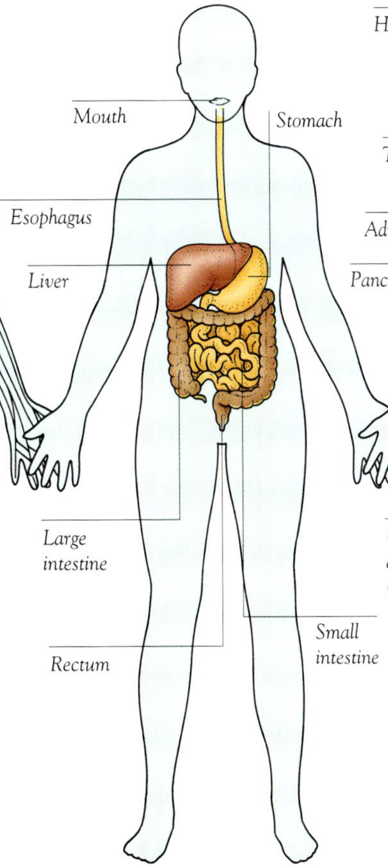

Hormonal glands (endocrine or hormonal system)
Hormonal glands, including the male and female sex organs, make hormones—chemicals that control body processes such as growth and blood cell production.

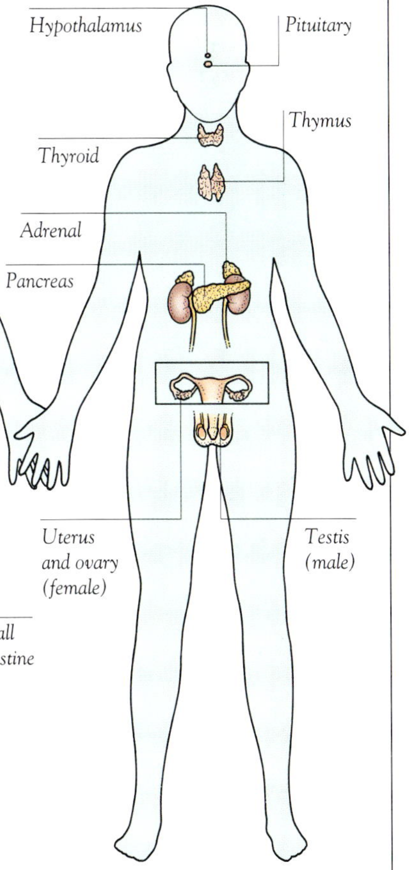

THE BODY'S BUILDING BLOCKS

THE BODY IS MADE OF UNITS CALLED CELLS. Most of them are tiny—you can see them only through a microscope. Several hundred cells could fit on the period at the end of this sentence. They are also incredibly numerous. There are about 100 million million cells in a human body, around 20,000 times the number of people in the world today. Cells are enormously varied too. There are dozens of cell types in the body, each with a particular shape and size, and each designed for a special job.

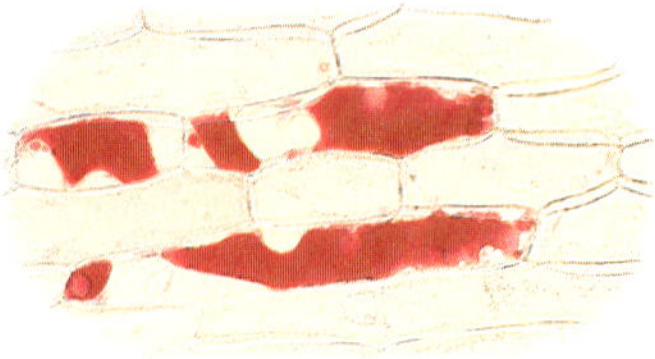

Cells from an onion can easily be *studied under a microscope (p.178). They carry out the same basic processes as human body cells.*

The cell is often called the "basic unit of life." This is because all living things are made of cells. Indeed, some living things, such as amoebas, consist of only a single cell. Amoebas look like minuscule bags of jelly as they ooze along the bottom of ponds. The amoeba's single cell contains all the amazingly complex chemical machinery that it needs to carry out the basic tasks of life, such as sensing its surroundings, moving about, feeding, disposing of its waste products, and reproducing.

A small worm that is as thin as a hair and as long as a rice grain is built out of many hundreds of cells. Insects such as mosquitoes have tens of thousands of cells. Large living things, from human bodies to oak trees, are built out of many billions (thousands of millions) of tiny cells.

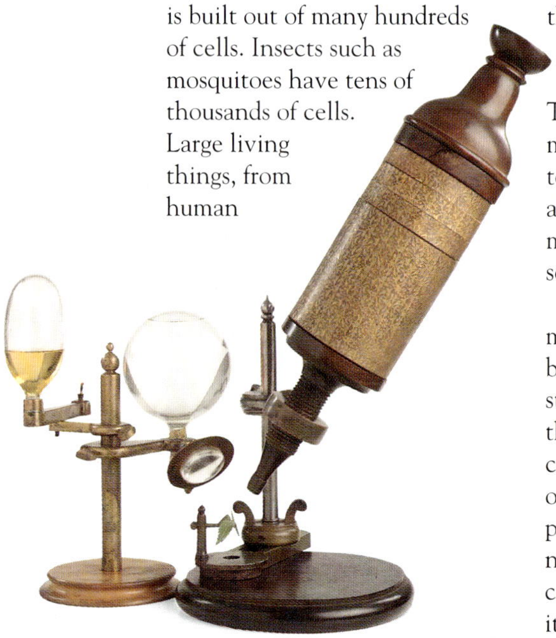

Robert Hooke's light microscope used an oil-fueled flame as *a light source. A water-filled globe acted as a lens to focus the light onto the specimen—in this case a small leaf.*

Seeing cells

The technology needed to see what typical cells look like did not exist until the early 1600's, when the light microscope was invented. During the 17th century, pioneering microscopists such as the Dutch cloth dealer Antony van Leeuwenhoek (p.172) observed the huge number and variety of cells in nature. The Italian microscopist Marcello Malpighi (p.104) was one of the first scientists to concentrate on studying the cells in the human body. He described their basic structure and suggested theories about how they might function.

Looking closer

The light microscope is still the most common microscope in use today. It can magnify an object about 1,000 times. A simple light microscope (p.178) is used for several experiments in this book.

If you look through a light microscope at body cells, you may be able to see a few vague structures inside them. Each of these structures within a cell is called an organelle ("little organ"). One of the most prominent is a dark blob—the nucleus. This is the control center of the cell and the site of its genetic instructions (p.176).

For around three centuries, microscopists studied the hazy outlines of organelles, but they could only guess at what cells look like in detail.

The development of the electron microscope in the 1930's meant that far greater magnifications became possible. Some electron microscopes can magnify objects by more than a million times. Instead of rays of light, the electron microscope uses beams of atomic particles called electrons, which are fired at the specimen. (These are the same particles that are fired at the inside of a television screen to make it glow.) The specimen is not studied through an eyepiece. Instead, an image of it appears on a visual display screen.

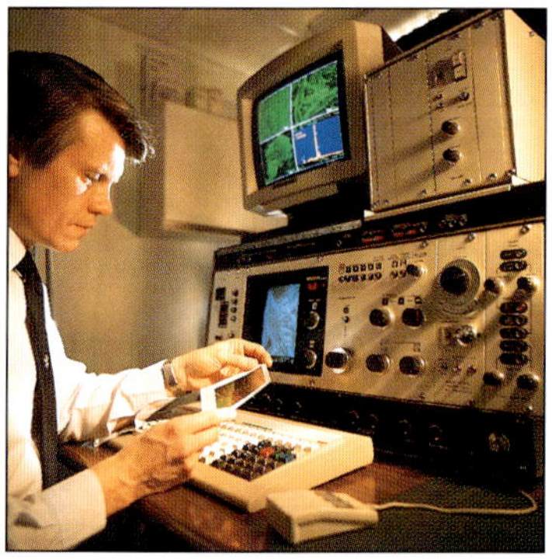

Scientists do not look through *glass lenses in an electron microscope, as they do with a light microscope. Instead, an image of the specimen can be focused on a monitor screen.*

Using an electron microscope, the modern microscopist can see cells and the organelles inside them in amazing detail. Although many mysteries concerning cells remain, we now understand more than ever before about the way they work.

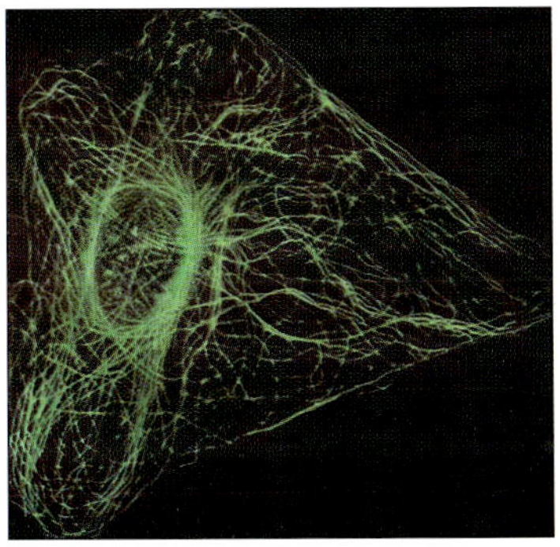

***The microtubular network that** forms the skeletal framework of a cell shows up in this microscope photograph taken in ultraviolet light.*

Watery environment

Like amoebas, human cells live in a watery environment. There is water both inside and outside the membrane (the cell's outer barrier). Individual water molecules (p.15) are small enough to pass between the molecules in the cell membrane by osmosis (p.28), a process that the cell cannot control.

Although water can pass in and out of the cell in this uncontrolled way, nutrients, minerals, and other essential items cannot, because their molecules are too large to pass through the membrane. If, as a result, the concentrations of these substances became too low or too high inside or outside the cell, water would flood into or out of the cell by osmosis. Such a flood would destroy the cell and damage the body.

The reason that this does not normally happen is that each cell membrane can regulate the passage of larger molecules through a kind of "door" (p.28) in the membrane. Molecules of nutrients and minerals are continually being passed through these "doors" as the cell works to keep a healthy balance of body substances.

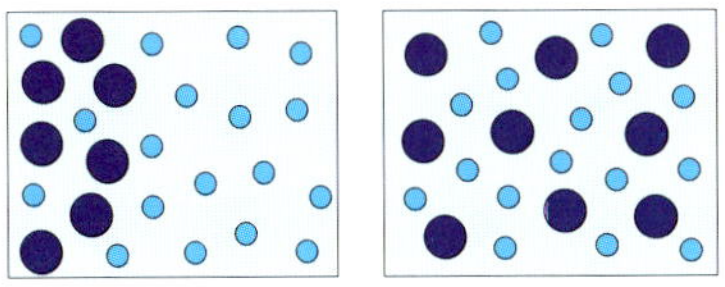

***The process of diffusion (p.27)** allows cell chemicals to spread through the watery cellular environment.*

Chemical factory

Living things are like vast, complex chemical factories. Hundreds of chemical changes and reactions occur every second in each living cell. These changes can take place only if the chemical substances are in the form of a watery solution (dissolved in water). So water is vital for life of any kind. In solution, chemical substances are free to drift around the cell, spreading by processes such as diffusion (p.27).

A cell is not a random collection of chemicals floating about as if they were in a bowl of soup. Instead, just as the interior space of an office building is organized into useful sections by walls, floors, doors, elevator shafts, windows, and stairways, the cell's interior is highly structured too. Membranes are found not only surrounding the cell as a barrier, but also inside the cell. These membranes curve, bend, and fold back on themselves, to create tubes, channels, compartments, organelles, and other structures in which chemicals are organized.

And in the same way that the whole body has a framework of bones to give it shape and strength, a cell also has a framework. This is made of scaffolding-like microtubules of protein found in the clear fluid of the cytoplasm (p.27).

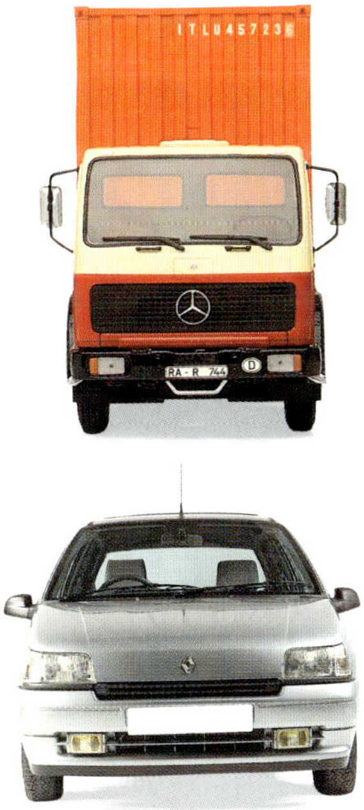

***Like motor vehicles, from** trucks to family cars, cells have different designs for the different jobs that they do.*

Cell types

If you want to carry a heavy load from one place to another, you might use a truck. If, however, you need to make a quick trip alone, you might use a small car instead. In the same way there are many different types of body cells for different tasks. For example, nerve cells carry tiny electrical signals around the body, while blood cells carry oxygen from part to part, and epithelial cells form protective coverings or linings. Each different type of cell has a unique design, with a different number of organelles.

The lifespans of the different types of cell vary too. The epithelial cells that line the intestine are rubbed away by digested food squeezing through the intestine tube. These cells die within a few hours of being formed and pass out of the body in feces.

In contrast, cells called osteocytes make a hard substance around themselves. This substance is bone (pp.44–45). As the bone builds up, it traps the cells that manufactured it. Unable to move, the osteocytes live in their self-built prisons for many years.

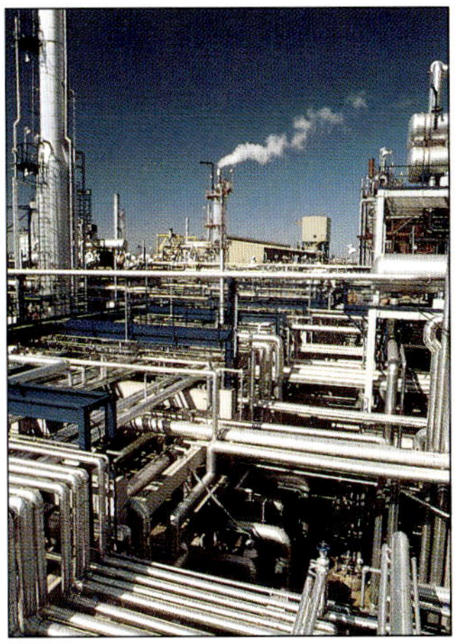

***A giant chemical factory** breaks down substances and builds them up, just like a tiny cell.*

Body cells

A CELL IS A HIGHLY ORGANIZED unit. Just as your body as a whole has important organs that carry out specific tasks, each cell also has individual parts—called organelles—for different functions. The most important organelle is the nucleus. This is the control center for all that goes on in the cell. Another type of organelle, a sausage-shaped structure called a mitochondrion, is like a power station. It transforms nutrients from food into energy that the cell can use. The cell's outer boundary, called the membrane, regulates the flow of substances into and out of the cell by processes such as osmosis (p.28). Inside the cell, many substances move around by a spreading-out process called diffusion (opposite).

■ DISCOVERY ■

Robert Hooke

In the 1600's the invention of the microscope opened up a new world for scientists. With a microscope, researchers could see things that were too small to see with the naked eye. One of the earliest explorers of the microscopic world was the English scientist Robert Hooke (1635–1703). His 1665 book *Micrographia* ("Small Drawings") included many engravings of tiny things, from the insides of insects to plant parts. Hooke noticed that cork wood was made of tiny boxes, which he called cells—because they looked like the rows of monks' rooms in a monastery. It was the first time that the word "cell" was used in this way.

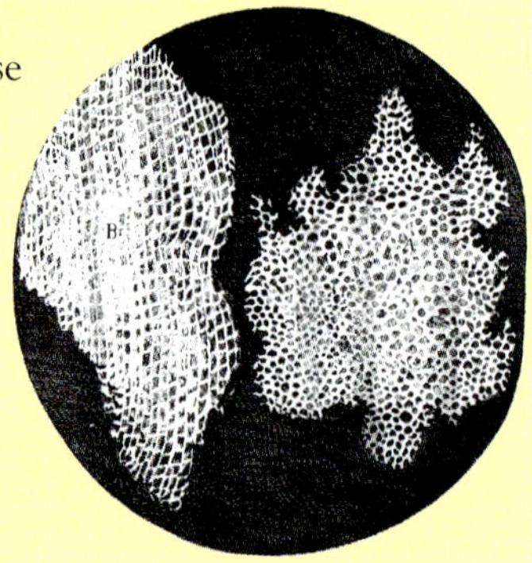

Cells in cork
Drawings of cells in thinly sliced cork, from Hooke's book Micrographia.

Types of cell

This chart shows some of the types of cell in the body. Each type of cell has a specific function. Nerve cells, for instance, have thin wirelike extensions, called axons (p.119), that carry nerve signals through the body. In some nerve cells in the arms and legs, the axons are over 3 ft (1 m) long. Epithelial cells are wide and flat, like paving stones. They form the coverings or linings of many body parts, including the insides of the nose, mouth, lungs, and intestines. In the chart, the sides of each small grid square are just 1/25,000 in (0.001 mm) long. On the same scale, one page in this book is as thick as the pinkish-gray strip that runs down the center of the chart.

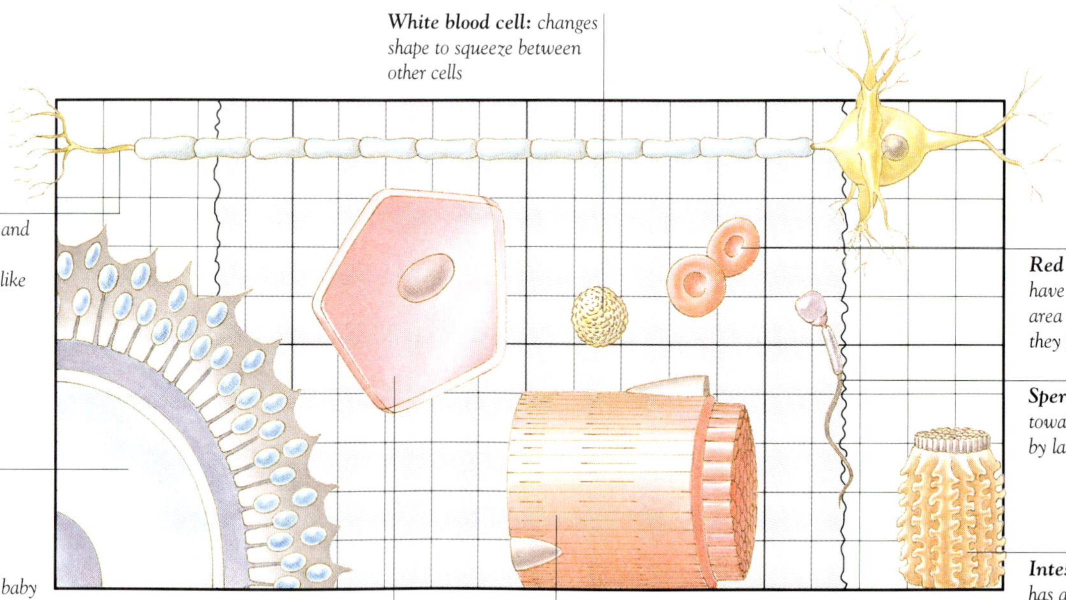

Inside a cell

It is hard to see the organelles of a cell through even the most powerful light microscope. But you can see them through an electron microscope (p.24), which magnifies objects a million times or more. Many of the organelles have their own membranes (p.182), which work in similar ways to the main cell membrane. Some organelle membranes are folded many times, like the endoplasmic reticulum here. The organelles form numerous compartments within the cell. Substances can spread from one compartment to another through pores (holes) and "doors" in the membranes.

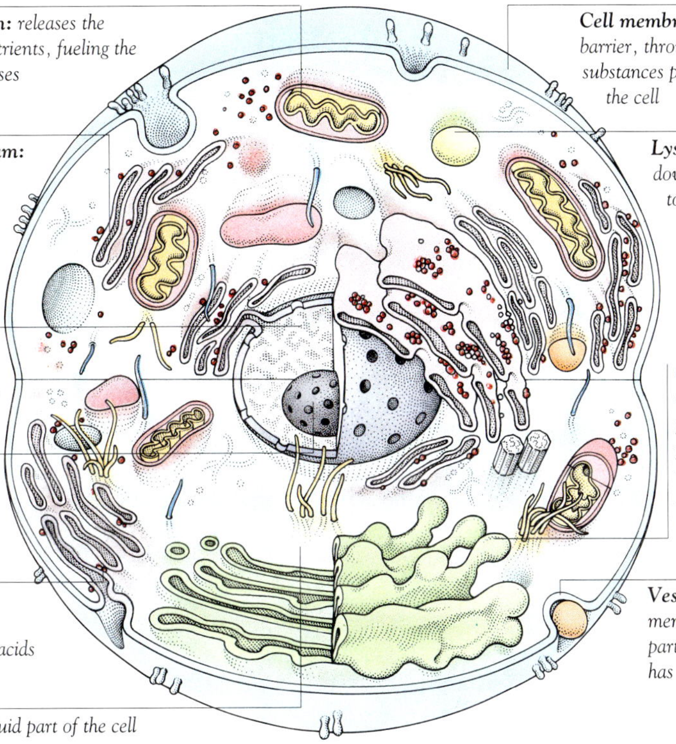

EXPERIMENT

Diffusion in action

Many chemicals move through the fluid inside a cell by "spreading out" in a process known as diffusion. They move from places where they are highly concentrated to places where they are less concentrated. For example, as oxygen is used up in one part of a cell, it becomes less concentrated there. So more oxygen diffuses to that place from the rest of the cell. Carbon dioxide, glucose, and minerals such as calcium move around a cell in the same way. In this experiment you can see diffusion in action—by adding a small amount of water-soluble ink (ink that mixes with water) from a dropper into a jar of water.

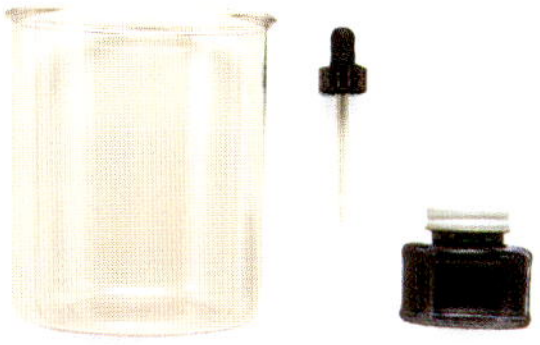

YOU WILL NEED

- jar of water • dropper • water-soluble ink

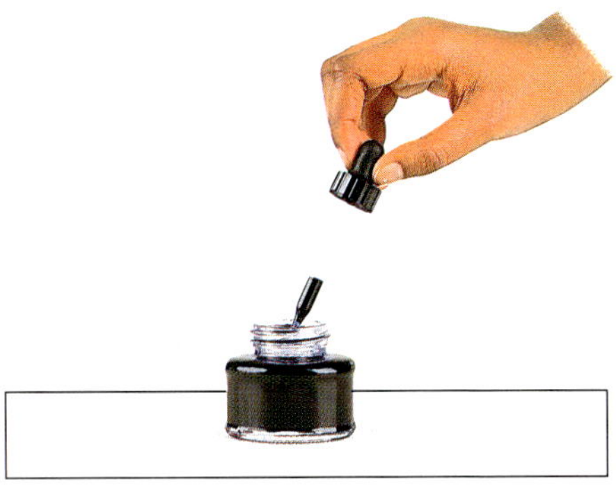

1 PLACE THE TIP of the dropper into the surface of the ink, and squeeze to fill it. Tap the dropper gently to remove air bubbles from near the tip.

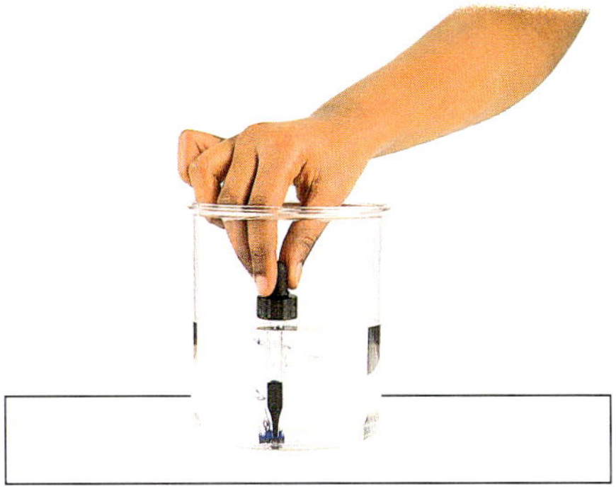

2 CAREFULLY LOWER the dropper to the bottom of the jar. Slowly squeeze out a large blob of ink. Then lift out the dropper without disturbing the ink.

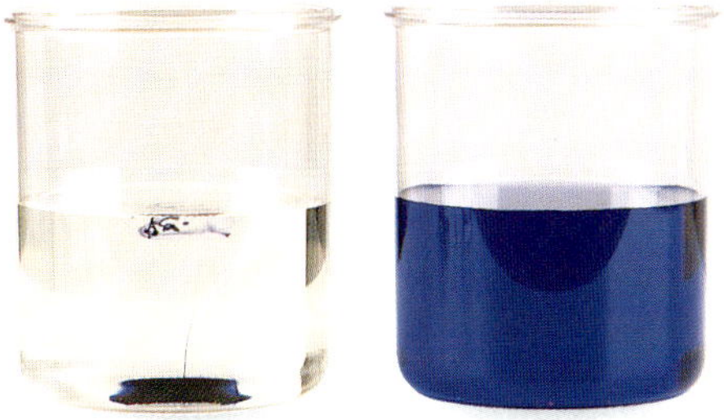

3 LEAVE THE JAR in a safe place, where it will not be knocked or shaken. Examine it the next day. Is the blob of concentrated ink still there?

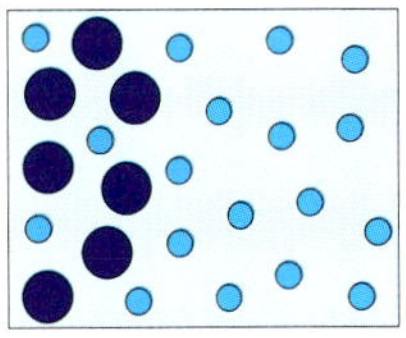

At first
Molecules (tiny particles) of ink (shown as dots of dark blue) stay in a concentrated blob among the water molecules (light blue).

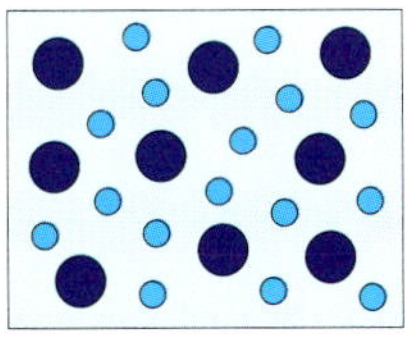

Later
As diffusion occurs, the ink molecules spread throughout the water. Eventually the ink molecules and the water molecules are evenly spaced.

The cell membrane

LEFT ALONE, THE SPREADING-OUT process of diffusion (p.27) would distribute water, and the substances dissolved in it, evenly throughout the body. But this does not happen, due to the cell membrane, the barrier around each cell. The cell membrane is semipermeable, which means that it lets molecules of water permeate (pass through) freely because they are very small, but it does not allow larger molecules to pass freely. The free passage of water molecules through a semipermeable membrane is called osmosis. Larger molecules, such as proteins and lipids, can pass through the membrane only at certain sites, which are like entrance and exit "doors." By opening and closing these "doors," the cell regulates some of its contents.

■ DISCOVERY ■

Camillo Golgi

The Italian microscope expert Camillo Golgi (1844–1926) was a professor of histology (the study of tissues and cells) at Italy's University of Pavia. Golgi devised new methods of staining cells with chemicals to reveal what their membranes and inner structures look like. In 1898 he showed how certain membranes are folded over many times to form a stack, like a pile of pillows all joined to each other. These stacks are now called Golgi bodies (p.27) in his honor. Golgi also devised a silver-containing stain that revealed nerve cells and the fibers from which they are made very clearly. This allowed him to classify nerve cells into types (p.119) and to show the tiny gaps called synapses between these cells. In 1906 Golgi received the Nobel Prize for Physiology or Medicine.

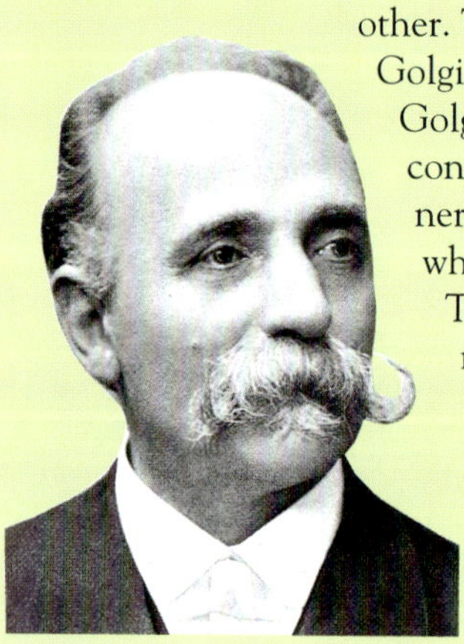

EXPERIMENT

A selective barrier

Adult help is advised for this experiment

Some freezer bags are semipermeable—like a cell membrane. Gaps between the molecules of the bag let small molecules pass through the bag by osmosis, but not larger ones. Show this using tincture of iodine, obtainable from a drugstore.

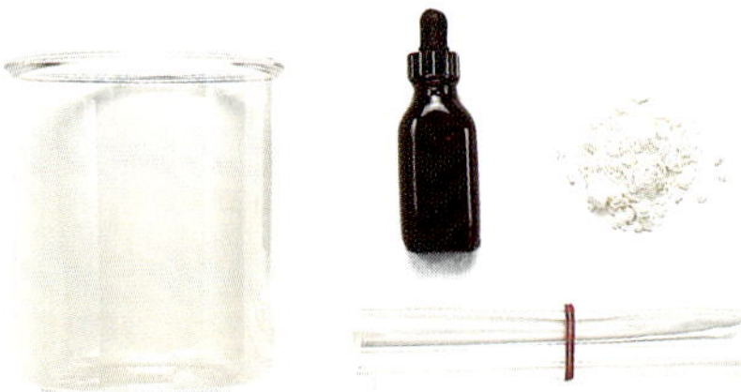

YOU WILL NEED
- *large clear jar of water*
- *tincture of iodine*
- *freezer bag*
- *freezer bag tie*
- *cornstarch*

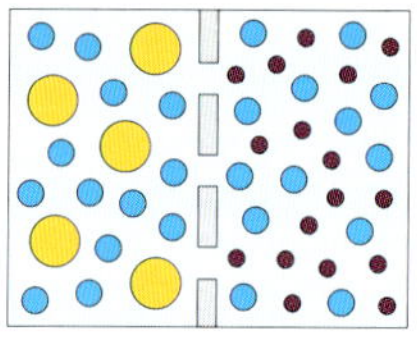

At first
The bag is shown as a dashed line. Water molecules are blue, starch molecules yellow, and iodine molecules purple.

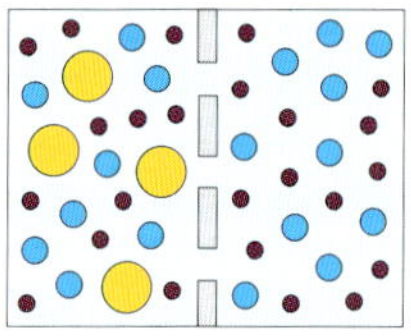

Later
Starch molecules are too big to exit the bag, but iodine ones are small enough to enter.

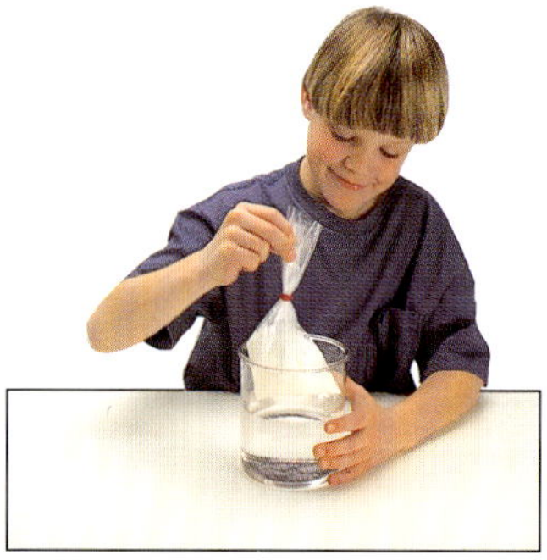

1 PUT 2 tablespoons of cornstarch into the bag. Mix enough water with the starch to make the bag sink when it is put in the jar. Tie the bag very securely, and lower it into the jar of water.

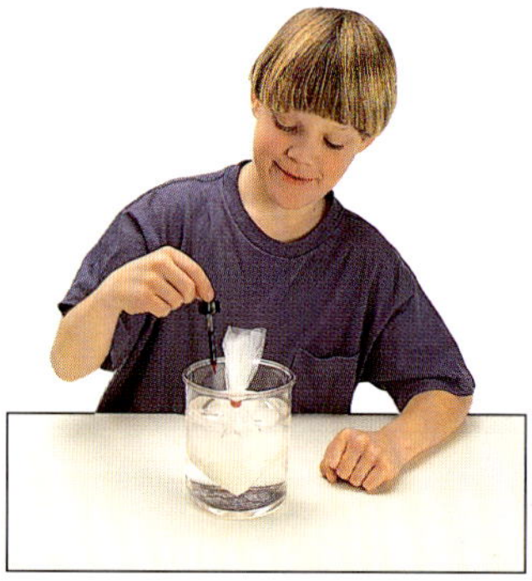

2 MAKE SURE that the tied part of the bag remains above water, to prevent water from leaking in. Add a few drops of iodine to the water, turning the water pale brown-orange. Leave overnight.

Starch in the freezer bag

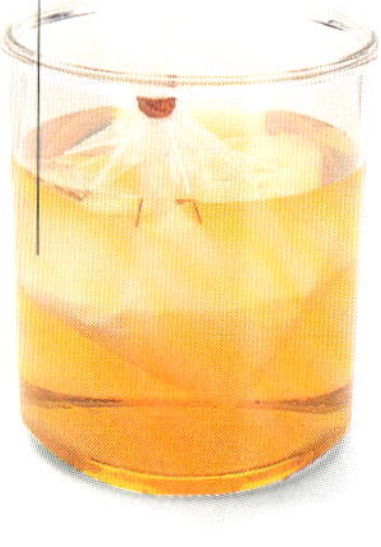

Iodine begins to color the starch blue-black

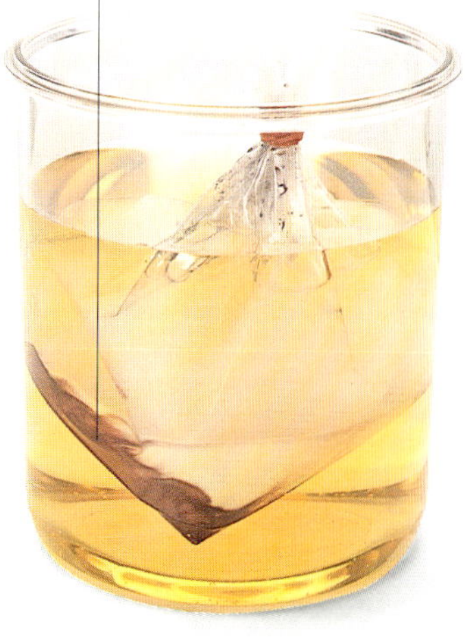

3 IODINE MOLECULES are small enough to pass into the bag. They react with the starch, making it blue-black. But starch molecules cannot leave the bag, so the color outside does not change.

EXPERIMENT

Osmosis in action

Adult help is advised for this experiment

If the solution of chemicals outside a cell is stronger than the chemical solution inside it, water passes out of the cell by osmosis. The cell contents shrink as water is lost. If the shrinkage is too great, it can endanger the life of the cell. In this experiment onion cells are exposed to a very strong salt solution. Onion cells have a different structure from human cells but behave in a similar way.

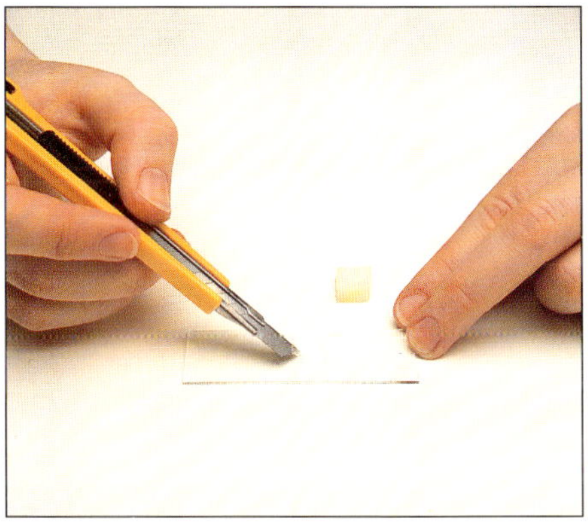

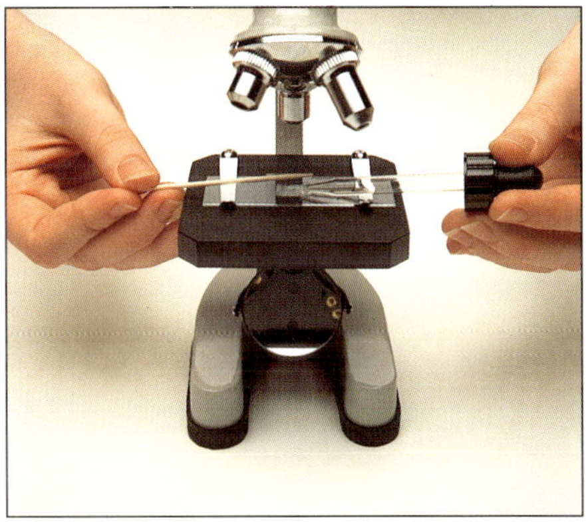

1 ASK AN ADULT to cut a wedge from the onion using the knife. Peel off the dry outer skin. Underneath the dry skin is a very thin see-through layer, which is only one cell thick. Carefully tease off a portion of this layer with the knife, and spread it flat on the slide.

2 PUT A DROP of water on the onion cells on the slide, then gently lay the cover slip on top. Adjust the microscope (p.178) so that you can see rows of onion cells. Next, make a strong salt solution by stirring 2 teaspoons of salt into 1 cup of water.

3 LIFT THE COVER slip with the toothpick, and add a drop of the salt solution to the cells. At once, gently replace the cover slip and look through the microscope, adjusting as necessary. Watch the area in the middle of each onion cell, where the cell fluids lie. Does it shrink? Read the captions (right) to find out why. If nothing happens, add stronger salt solution.

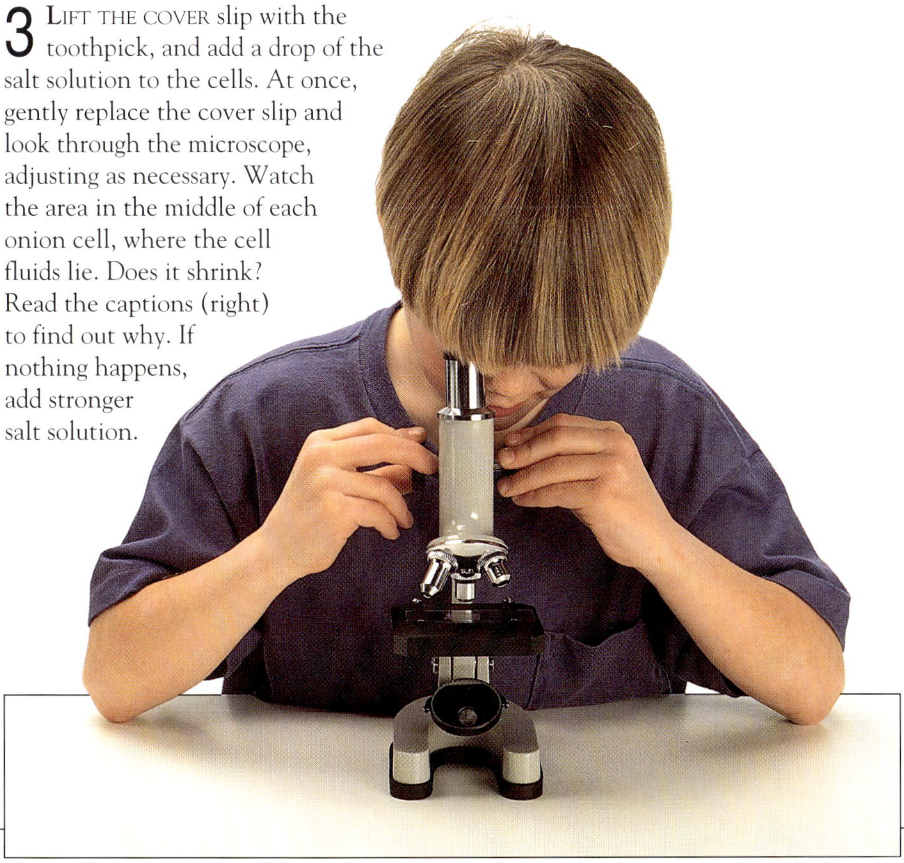

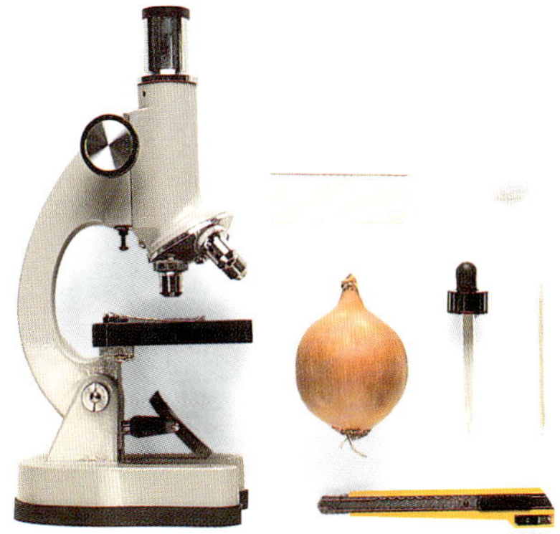

YOU WILL NEED

- microscope • slide • cover slip • salt • onion • dropper • toothpick • craft knife • water

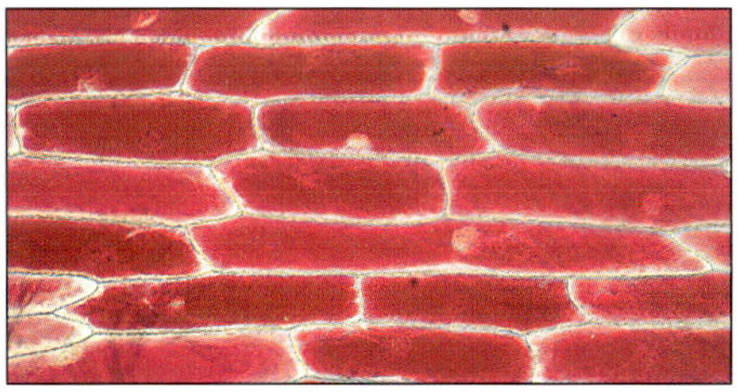

Normal red onion cells
Cells from a red onion are especially clear when you look at them through a light microscope. Like all plant cells, they have a stiff outer cell wall and a cell membrane within this. The red cell fluids lie inside the cell membrane.

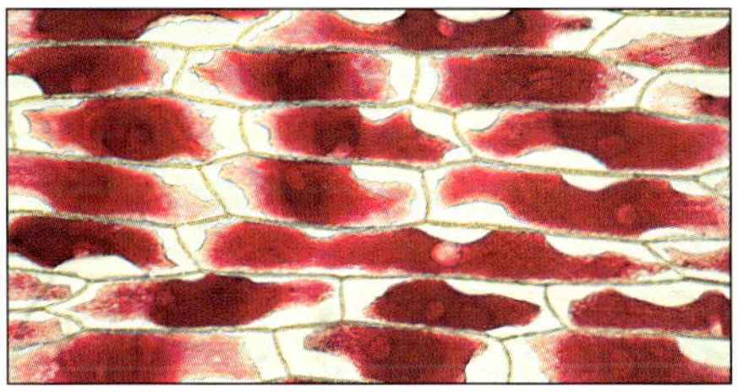

Shrunken red onion cells
When you add the strong salt solution, this solution is much more concentrated than the solution of chemicals inside the cells. So water passes out through the membrane by osmosis, and the cell fluids shrink.

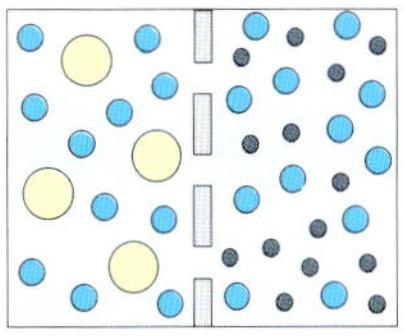

At first
Water molecules are blue, cell chemicals yellow, and salt gray. Outside the cell, to the right of the membrane (dashed line), the solution is stronger.

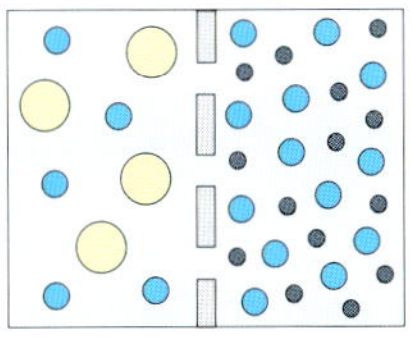

Later
Water osmoses out of the cell to try to make the two solutions equal. The cell fluids become more concentrated and the salt solution less so.

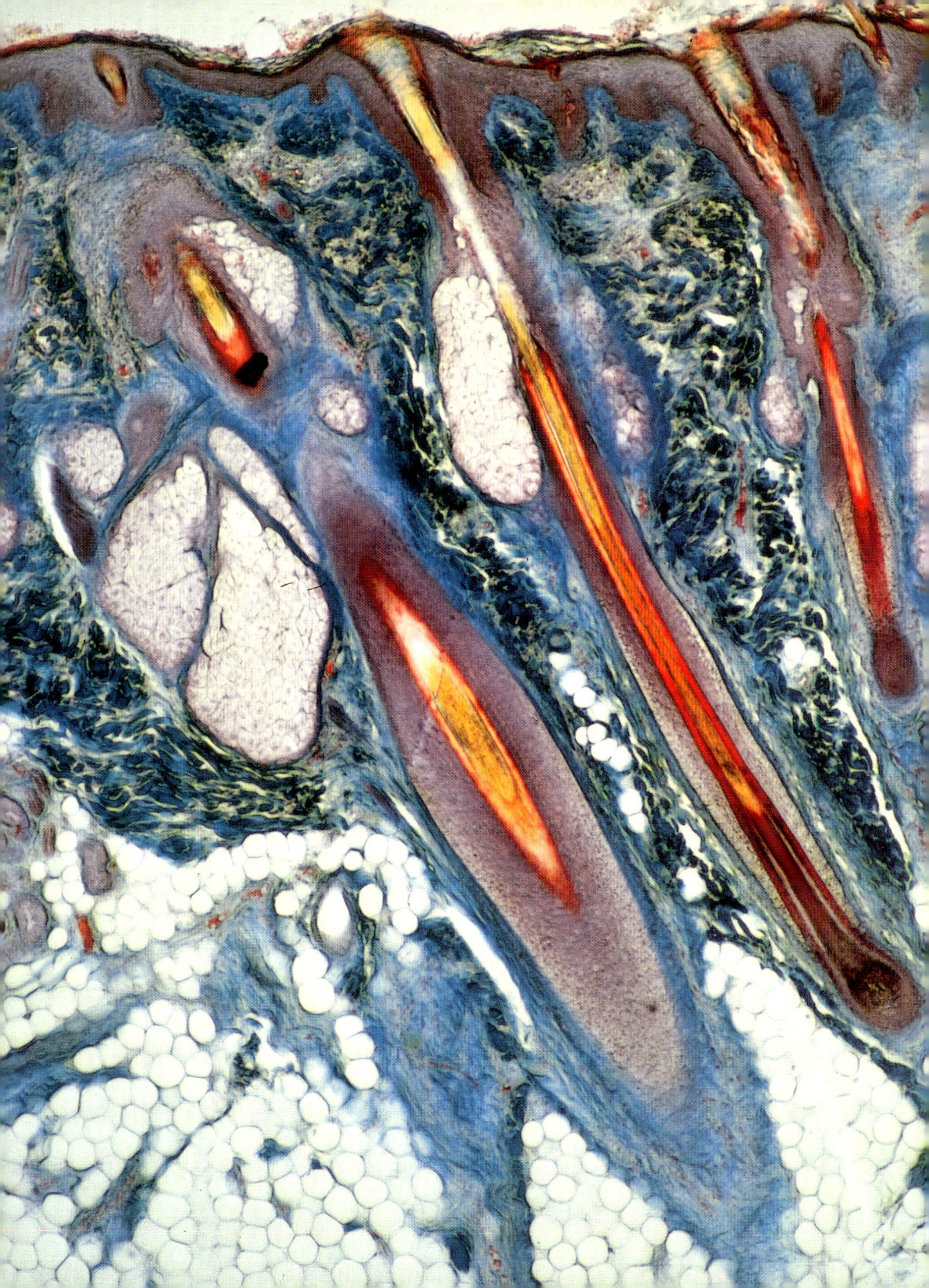

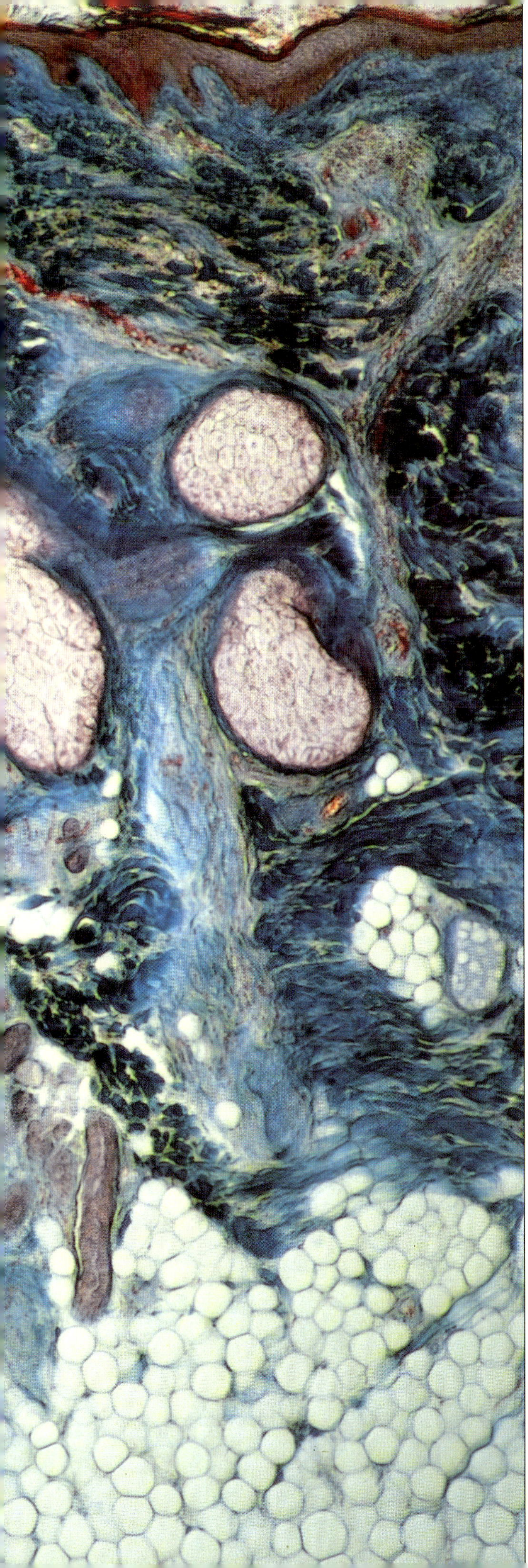

The BODY'S SURFACE

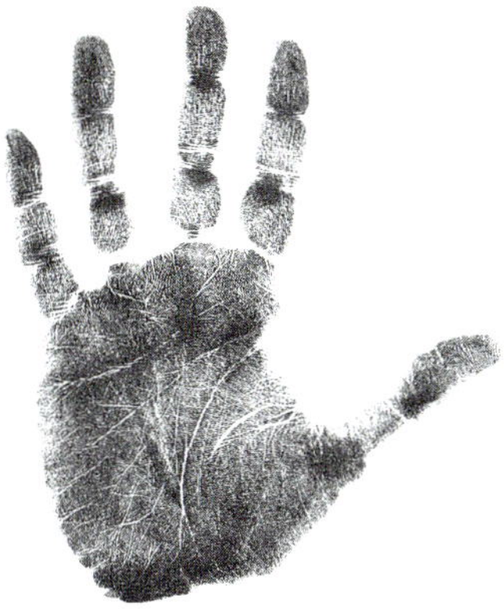

Getting a grip
The ridged skin of the fingers and palm (above), slightly moistened by sweat, gives the hand its nonslip grip. Under a microscope the hairs that sprout from skin over most of the body look like thin yellow pipes (shown sliced through, left).

WHEN YOU LOOK AT A human body, nearly everything you see on the surface is dead. The outer skin, hair, and nails are all composed of cells that died weeks ago. Yet just beneath this outer layer, millions of cells are multiplying, making skin one of the body's busiest parts. Throughout your life, your skin continues to renew and repair itself. It protects the delicate inner parts of your body from wear and tear, from excess heat and cold, and from water and germs—and it gives you your sense of touch (p.164).

THE LIVING BARRIER

A LAYER OF SKIN, usually less than one-fourth of an inch (5 mm) thick, is the only barrier between the body's interior, with its delicate cells and finely balanced fluids, and the harsh, changing conditions of the outside world. Yet we rarely give our skin a second thought—unless it becomes bruised, cut, or otherwise damaged.

Few of the great scientists of the Renaissance period, such as Leonardo da Vinci (1452–1519) and Andreas Vesalius (p.22), took any interest in the workings of the skin. They thought of it as an uninteresting covering that had to be removed in order to study the much more fascinating parts that lay underneath. Perhaps this is not surprising, since there were no microscopes at that time. To the naked eye, the skin and the parts that grow from it, hairs and nails, do not look particularly complex or interesting.

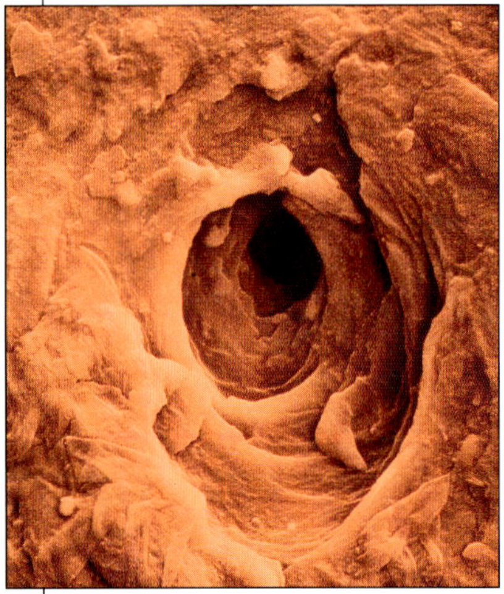

***Sweat oozes up this hole from** the sweat gland (p.34) beneath it. This aerial view of a sweat pore in the skin's surface is seen through an electron microscope.*

The invention of the microscope in the early 17th century meant that for the first time scientists could see the cells (pp.24–25) that make up the skin. From this point on, people could see how intricate the skin is and what a vital role it plays. They could see how the epidermis (outer layer) of the skin continually renews itself with new cells, and how tiny sensors in the dermis (inner layer) give the body its sense of touch.

Skin coat

The skin is the body's heaviest organ. The skin of an average adult weighs around 9 to 15 lb (4 to 7 kg)—about one-twelfth of the body's total weight. If you wore an overcoat that heavy, you would soon appreciate how heavy your skin is.

Your wrap-around coat of skin protects your body from water and from general wear and tear. Like a showerproof raincoat skin keeps out most of the water and other fluids to which it is exposed, although it is not fully waterproof. Water is repelled by the natural oils and waxes made in the tiny sebaceous glands (p.34) just under the surface of the skin. These sebaceous products also keep the skin flexible and supple.

Skin insulates the body too. When pioneer anatomists cut open the skin, they found a soft, yellowish layer beneath. This layer is called subcutaneous ("under-skin") fat. It works like the padding in a quilted coat to keep the body warm and also absorbs knocks and bumps.

Keratin

One reason that skin is so tough is that skin cells contain a robust body protein called keratin. Sometimes keratin is flexible—for example, in epidermal skin cells. But elsewhere it can be much thicker, stiffer, and harder—for example, in fingernails and toenails. Keratin is also the material which makes up the human "fur" that we call hair.

Like the cells at the skin's surface, those in hair and nails are dead. The only living parts of hair and nails are the growing points in their roots. Any sensations you feel through your hair and nails come from sensors wrapped around the hair roots or in the skin under the nails.

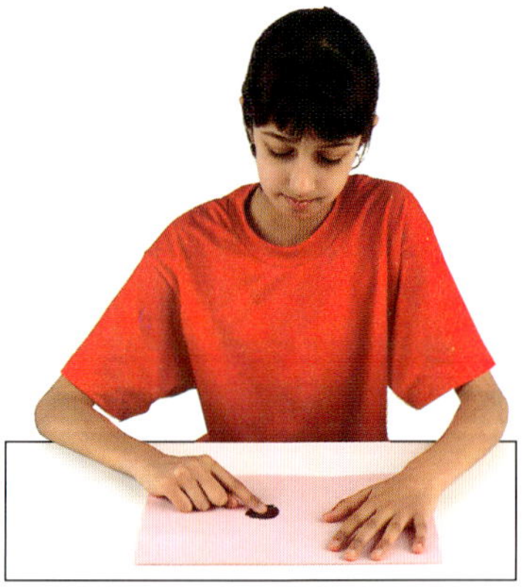

***Fingers are slightly tacky from** natural skin oils and sweat. Use your fingertips to pick up powdered graphite to make fingerprints (p.38).*

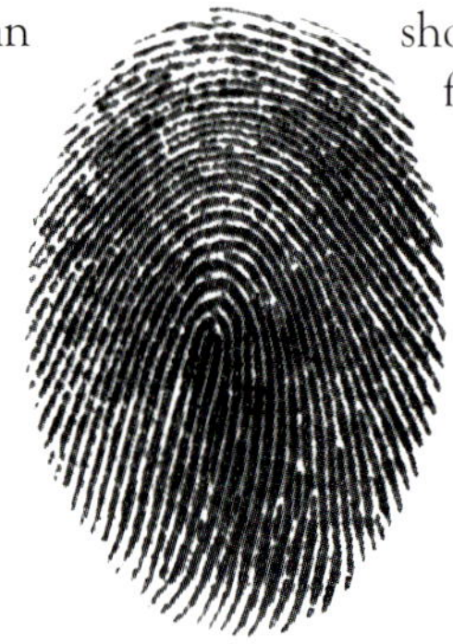

***Each and every** fingerprint has a special pattern that is unique.*

Germ barrier

The world is full of microscopic germs. They float in the air and lie on the things we touch. Even objects that are apparently clean have germs on them or in them.

Skin prevents germs from entering the body. Under a microscope, the skin's surface shows many dead, flattened cells that interlock and overlap tightly, like tiles on a roof. Few germs can penetrate this barrier, which completely covers healthy skin. However, they can enter the body through cuts or breaks in the skin.

The natural waxes and oils on the skin's

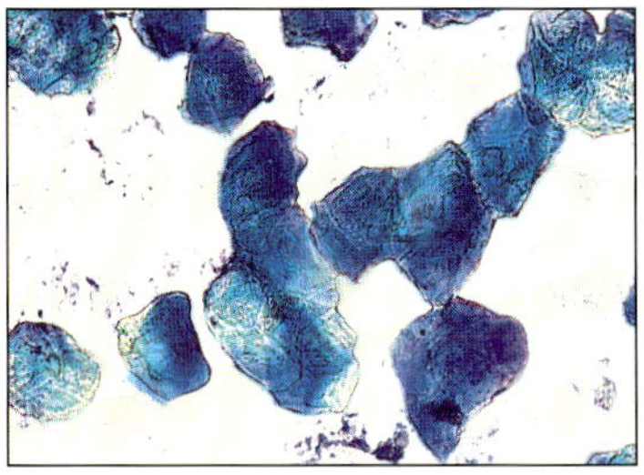

Like tiles blown from a roof in a *gale, hard, dead epidermal cells fall off the skin surface. You can dye cells with blue ink so that they can be seen under a light microscope (p.35).*

surface contain germ-killing chemicals. These are the body's own disinfectants, giving added protection against bacteria, yeasts, and other potentially harmful microscopic organisms.

Sensitive skin

Before the invention of the microscope, one of the great puzzles for scientists was what role the skin plays in the sense of touch. The microscope showed that in the dermis there are millions of tiny sensors of several different types. These sensors are attached to nerves. The sensors respond to being pressed, squeezed, heated, or cooled, and they send tiny electrical signals along nerves to the brain, where the signals are processed. This gives you the sense of touch (p.164).

Most of the types of microscopic sensor in the skin are named in honor of the person who first described or studied them. These were mainly the Italian and German microscopists of the 19th century. Pacini's endings are an example. Shaped like tiny onions, these sensors—at most about $\frac{1}{24}$ in (1 mm) wide—are named after Filippo Pacini (1812–83), a professor of anatomy at Pisa in Italy. They respond to heavy pressure when the skin is squeezed. Meissner's endings are named after German anatomist Georg Meissner (1829–1903).

Today, scientists know that the skin is a multisensitive organ: that is, it can detect light touch, heavy pressure, vibrations, heat, cold, and pain. But they are still not sure exactly how the skin does this.

Early in this century, researchers tried to show that each element of this multiple sense was detected by one kind of microscopic sensor. However, they were not able to prove this. More recently, scientists have suggested that some sensors in the skin respond to more than one type of stimulation, but also that each sensor is particularly sensitive to one or more types of touch. From the billions of nerve signals coming to it every second from the millions of sensors in the skin, the brain assembles an overall picture of the type of touch being experienced.

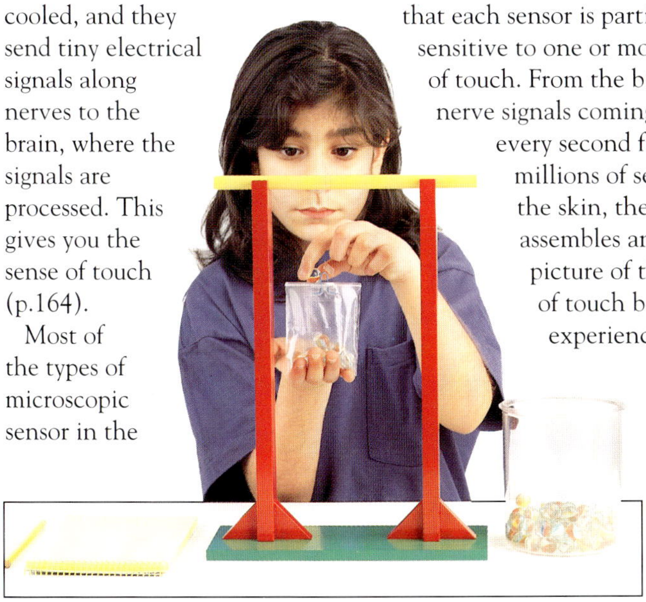

Human hair is surprisingly strong, considering that it is so thin. *People once used hair for making rope and twine. You can test the strength of hair using marbles (p.41).*

Cooling skin

Skin has other functions too. For example, when the sun shines on it, it produces vitamin D. This vitamin is used by the whole body, particularly the bones. Lots of sunlight stimulates the skin to make more of its dark pigment, called melanin, so that when it is exposed to sun its color gradually becomes darker (p.36).

Skin also has a vital role in keeping the temperature of your body stable. If the body becomes too hot, a watery fluid called sweat oozes from tiny coiled tubes (sweat glands) onto the surface of the body, where it evaporates. This evaporation draws heat from the body and so you feel cooler.

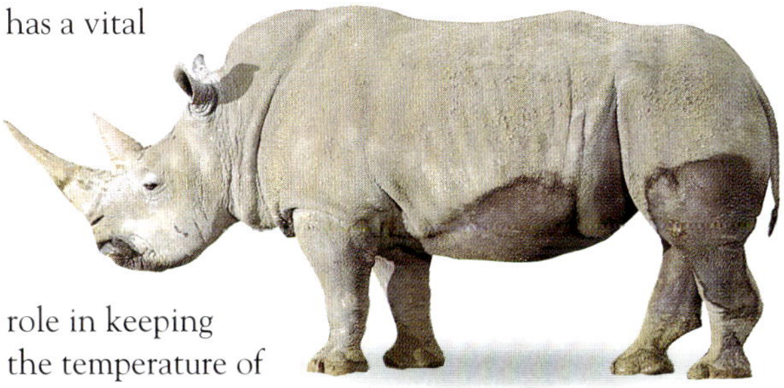

We are not as thick-skinned as *creatures such as rhinoceroses. Their skin may be more than 1 in (2.5 cm) thick. Rhino horn is made of matted, compacted hair.*

Lost skin

Did you know that much of the dust in almost any room, from a bedroom to a classroom, is made of tiny fragments of human skin? In a minute, 30,000 to 40,000 microscopic skin cells fall unseen from your body. This shedding is a natural part of the skin's renewal system. Cells are lost continually as skin rubs against clothes, soap and water, sheets, and other objects.

But your skin is not worn away, because while dead cells are being rubbed away, the cells just below the surface of the epidermis are busy reproducing themselves. As soon as they are produced, the new cells begin rising to the surface to replace those that have been lost, like people moving to the front of a line.

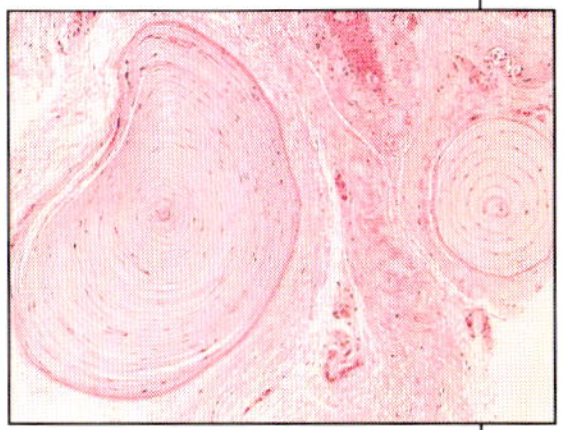

Pacini's endings *are the biggest of all the touch sensors in the skin (p.164). Some are just visible to the naked eye.*

The skin

EACH YEAR UP TO 9 lb (4 kg) of your skin wears away and flakes off your body's surface. The skin that falls from your body collects as dust, which you can find around the house. You do not lose this amount of weight, because your skin is constantly renewing itself. This renewal takes place in the skin's outer layer, the epidermis. Cells in the lower part of the epidermis are always multiplying. Their "offspring" pass upward, gradually becoming filled with a tough fibrous substance called keratin. By the time they reach the surface, the cells are hard, flat, and dead—ready to be worn away. This continual cell sacrifice in the epidermis protects the lower layer, the dermis, which contains delicate blood vessels, nerves, and touch sensors.

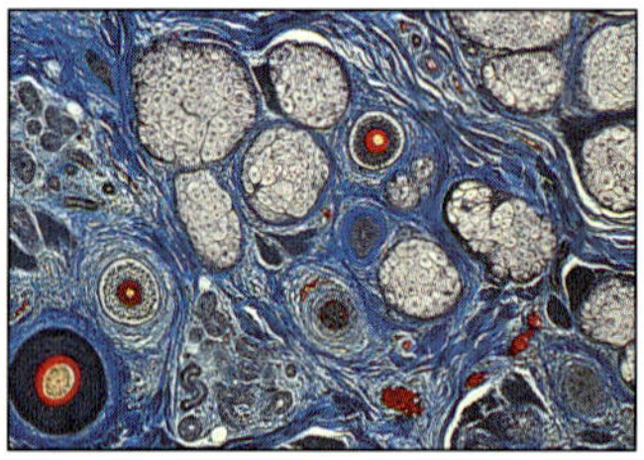

Hairy skin
This microscope photograph of skin, sliced horizontally and seen from above, shows the hair shafts and smaller sweat pores.

At the skin's surface

The hard, tough cells in the upper part of the epidermis become wide and flat as they fill with keratin. When they reach the surface, they flake off like tiles blown from a roof in a strong wind. This is due to wear and rubbing, and also to being pushed up by more cells from below.

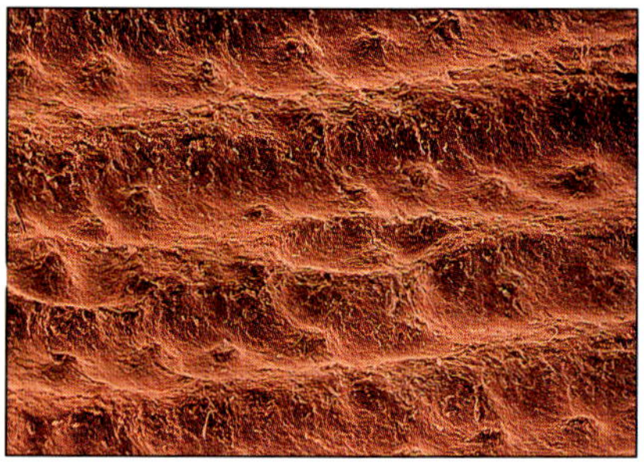

Microscopic mountain ridges
When seen through an electron microscope, the ridged skin on the palm looks like a range of mountains. The tiny pits are sweat pores.

Under the skin

This diagram shows the numerous touch sensors, blood vessels, and other parts in a piece of skin less than 1/24 in (1 mm) deep. This type of skin is from the back or thigh, where the outer layer, the epidermis, is considerably thinner than the inner layer, the dermis. These layers are fixed firmly together at a line of small bumps, called papillae. Next to each hair is a sebaceous gland, which makes the natural skin oil, sebum. The busily multiplying cells in the lower epidermis have no direct blood supply. They receive nutrients and oxygen by diffusion (p.27) from blood vessels in the dermis.

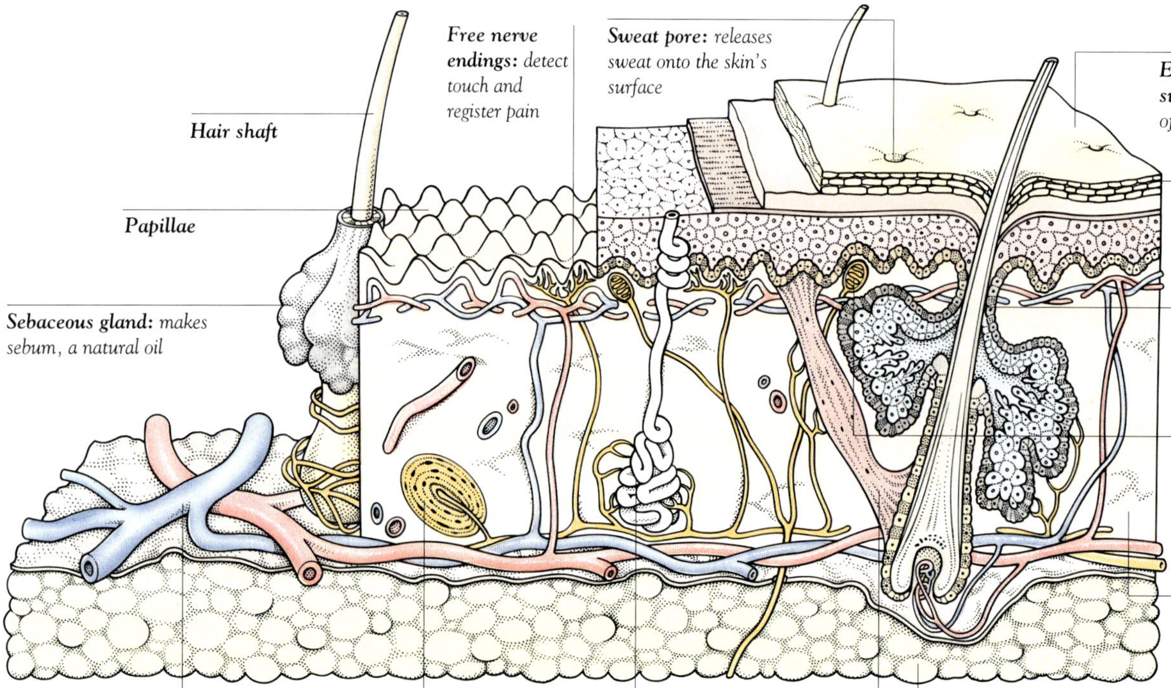

EXPERIMENT

Is all skin the same?

Do you know the back of your hand as well as the old saying suggests? What skin looks like varies from one part of the body to another and from person to person. Look at the skin on the back of your hand through a magnifying lens. Then look at the skin on your palm, fingers, wrist, arm, leg, and sole. Where is the skin smoothest? Which part has the most hairs? Are there any truly hairless areas?

YOU WILL NEED

- *magnifying lens*

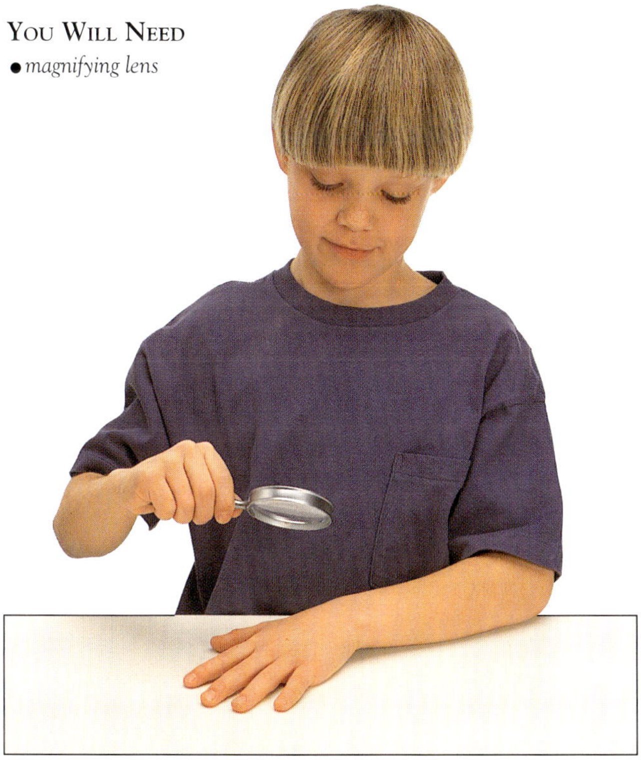

EXPERIMENT

See skin cells

Adult help is advised for this experiment

Use a microscope (p.178) to see some of the dead cells that fall off your skin by the million daily. Lift the cells safely from your hand with tape. Individual skin cells are almost transparent, so use ink to make them visible. *Caution: Make sure that the ink you use is nontoxic.*

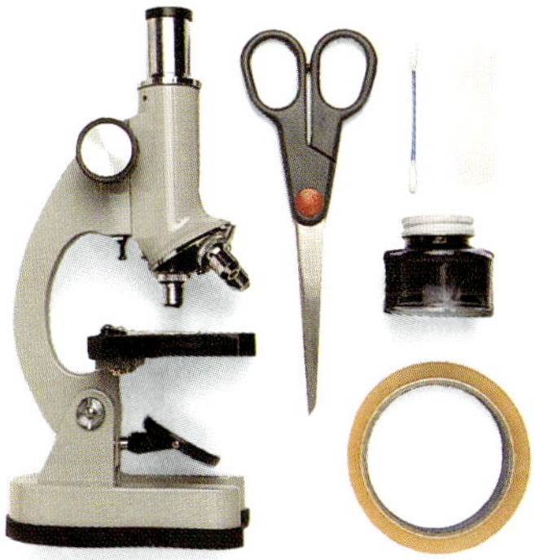

YOU WILL NEED

- *microscope*
- *slide*
- *scissors*
- *cotton swab*
- *nontoxic blue ink*
- *clear cellophane tape*

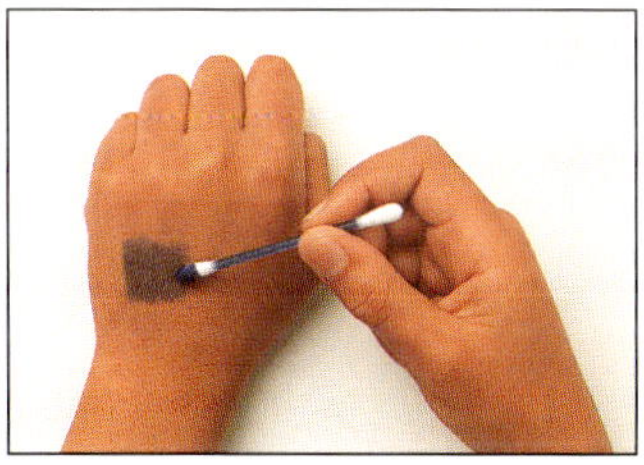

1 SPREAD A FEW drops of ink on the back of your hand with the cotton swab. Let it dry for a few minutes.

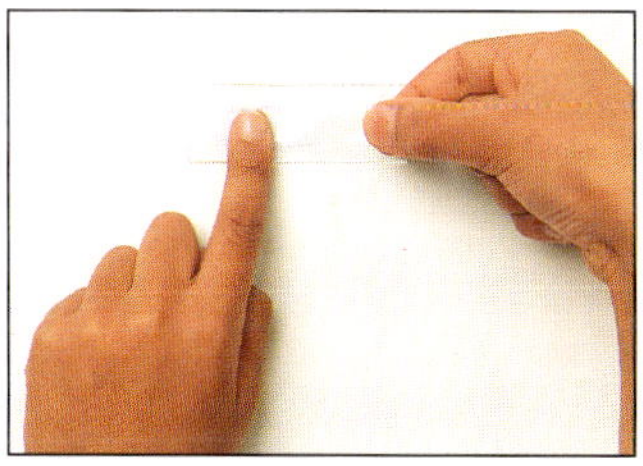

2 PRESS A LENGTH of tape onto the inked area. Peel it off, and place it sticky side down on the slide.

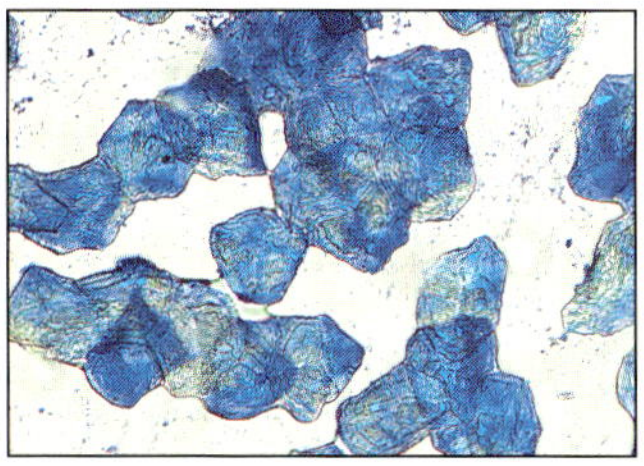

3 TAKE CARE not to put any fingerprints on the tape. Look at the tape with the cells stuck to it through the microscope. Can you see any blue flakes, like those in the photograph on the left?

How hairy are humans?

Our closest cousins in the animal world are the great apes—gorillas and chimpanzees. Their bodies are similar to our own in many ways. One of the most obvious differences, however, is in the skin. Humans seem almost hairless compared with apes (we have been called "naked apes"), except for on the scalp. However, if you examine the skin on your body closely with a magnifying lens, you will find that you have many hairs too. The difference is that human body hairs are small and fine, while the body hairs of apes are long and thick. In fact, a human has just as many hairs as an average great ape—about 3 to 5 million.

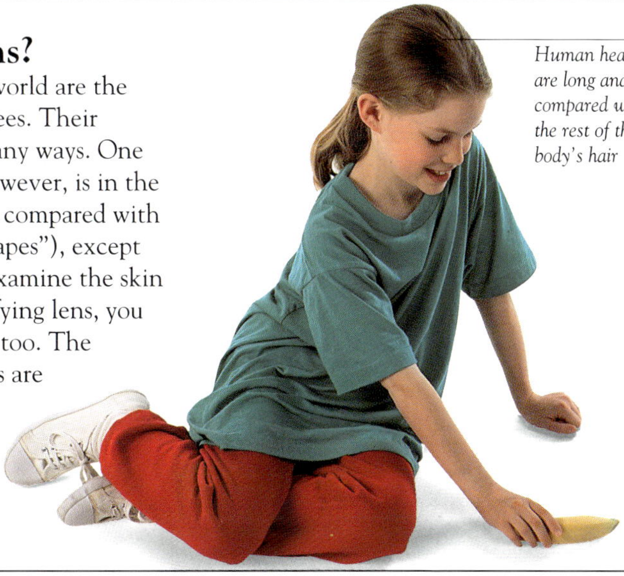

Human head hairs are long and thick, compared with the rest of the body's hair

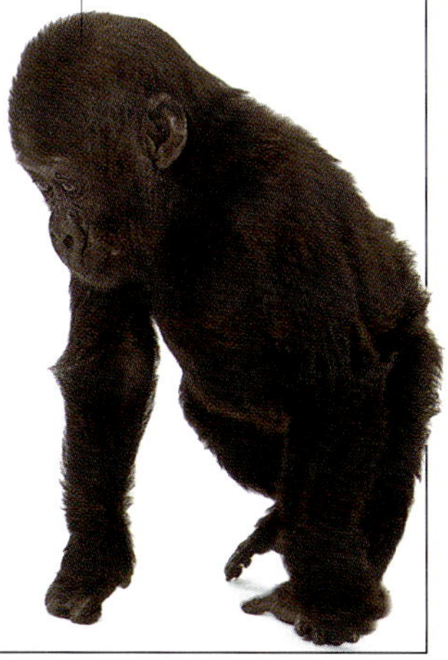

A gorilla's hairs are long and thick, and cover most of its head and body

Skin changes

MANY PARTS OF THE BODY can change and adapt, depending on how much they are used. For example, if you exercise your muscles often, they get bigger and stronger. Skin also adapts to the demands made on it. Patches of skin that receive great wear and tear respond by becoming thicker and tougher. This happens on the fingertips of a guitarist and on the soles of the feet of someone who often walks barefoot. Hard patches called calluses may develop as natural shields to protect the parts beneath. Skin color also adapts to changing conditions. Skin that is exposed to more sunlight than usual tends to darken in color. The darker color helps to filter out the sun's ultraviolet rays. Too much exposure to these rays can be harmful, causing sunburn and increasing the risk of skin cancer.

Changing texture

The texture of skin (how it feels to the touch) varies from one person to another. Some people have skin that is smoother or more supple than that of other people. Skin texture also changes through the years. Our skin tends to become less supple and more lined with increasing age. These changes are due mainly to the way that elastin fibers in the dermis (p.34) shrink and become less flexible over the years. The changes are also due to the way that, as you get older, the subcutaneous fat layer under the dermis becomes thinner, making the skin's underlayer less supple and less resilient.

EXPERIMENT

Skin color

You may have noticed that someone who has been indoors for a long time, away from natural sunlight, looks paler than normal. Just as skin may darken when exposed to more sunlight, it may also lighten when exposed to less light. You can investigate this process by using an adhesive bandage to prevent light reaching a small patch of skin. For this experiment you need to leave a bandage on your finger for several days. If the bandage becomes dirty, replace it with a new one on the same part of the finger.

YOU WILL NEED

- *adhesive bandages (use hypoallergenic ones)*

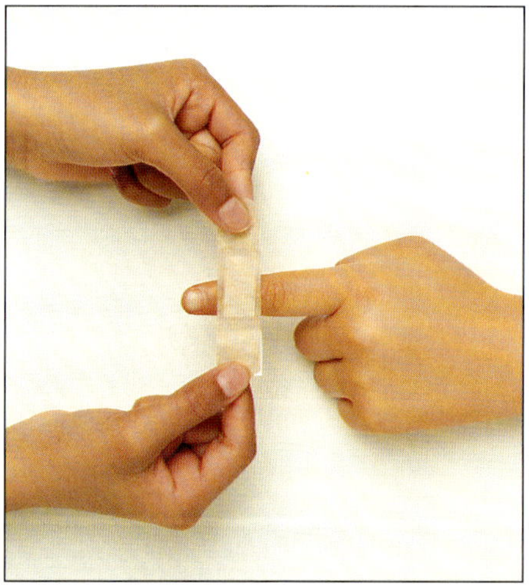

1 WRAP THE bandage around one of your fingers in the usual way. Put it between the knuckle joints, so that it is less likely to fall off.

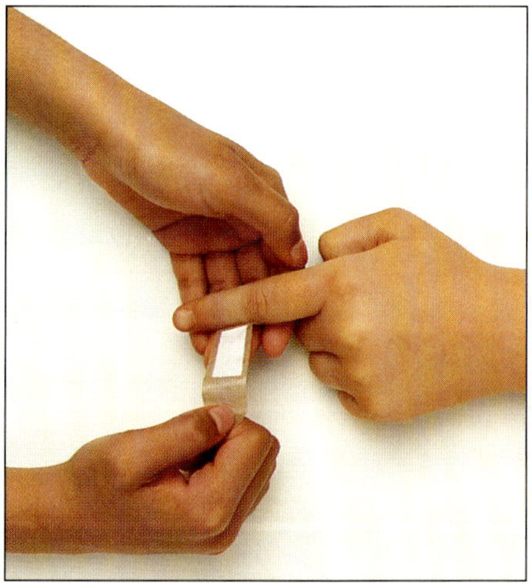

2 AFTER SEVERAL DAYS, remove the bandage. Has the skin under it changed color? How long is it before this area returns to its normal color?

Melanin

The skin's color comes from melanin, a very dark brown natural pigment (coloring substance). Melanin is made in melanocytes, special cells scattered in the lower epidermis (p.34). The amount of melanin that melanocytes make is controlled chiefly by the body's inherited genes (p.176). Melanocytes are stimulated to make extra melanin by ultraviolet light—particularly from the sun—falling on the skin.

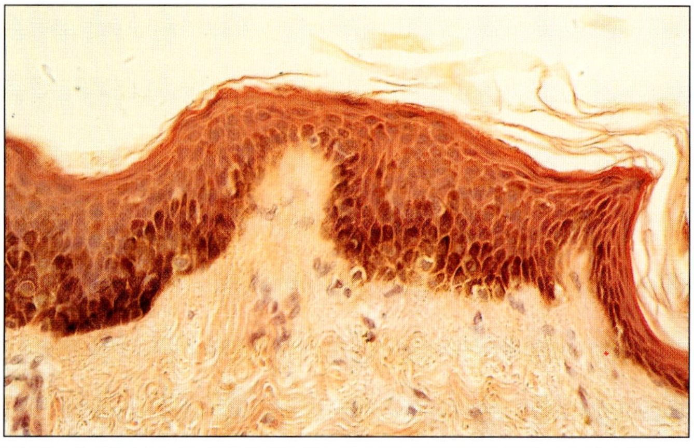

Melanin grains
This microscope photograph shows a piece of cut-through skin viewed from the side. The melanin shows up clearly as dark grains. The melanocytes make the melanin grains and then pass them out into the cells of the epidermis surrounding them.

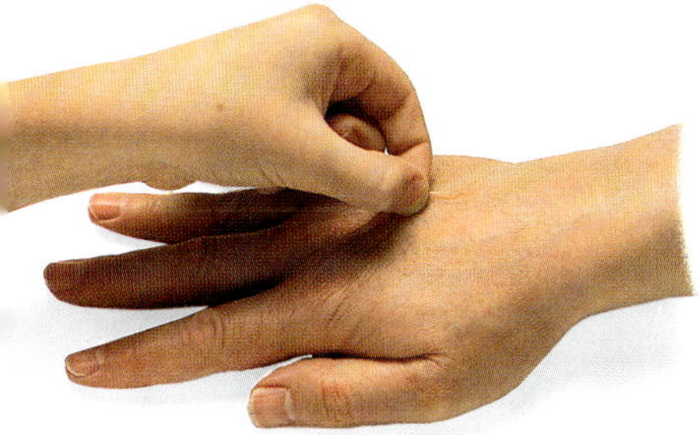

Testing texture
The "pinch test" gives an idea of the general texture of someone's skin. Grasp a small fold of skin from the back of the hand. Grip firmly enough to hold the skin away from the hand, but do not pull too hard! Hold for 30 seconds and release. Note how quickly the skin becomes flat again. Test people of widely differing ages. Do you notice any differences?

Ancient skin

The skin's proteins—keratin, collagen, and elastin—are tough and durable. Treated with special chemicals, skin becomes even longer-lasting. Ancient Egyptian "mummies"—bodies prepared for burial—were treated with certain chemicals, which have preserved them for thousands of years. The ancient Egyptians believed that souls could then revisit their bodies after death.

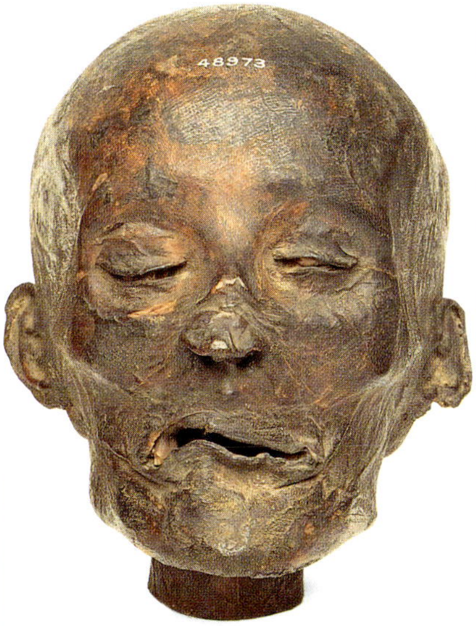

Long-lasting face
The preserved skin of this Egyptian mummy is still intact after more than 4,000 years.

EXPERIMENT

The sebum layer

Adult help is advised for this experiment

Sebaceous glands (p.34) make an oily substance called sebum, which mingles with sweat and spreads over the skin, helping it to stay supple and water-repellent. Find out what happens when you remove the sebum layer.

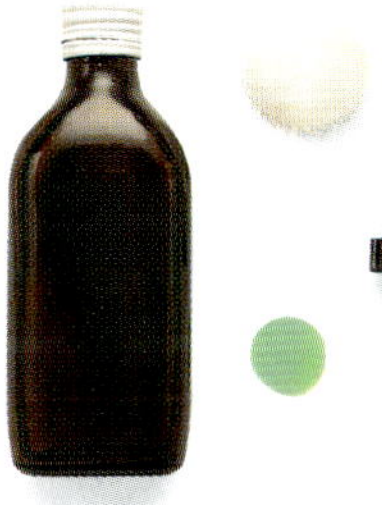

YOU WILL NEED
- *rubbing alcohol (from a drugstore)*
- *cotton balls*
- *weak solution of dishwashing liquid in water (a single drop in a beaker of water)*
- *dropper*

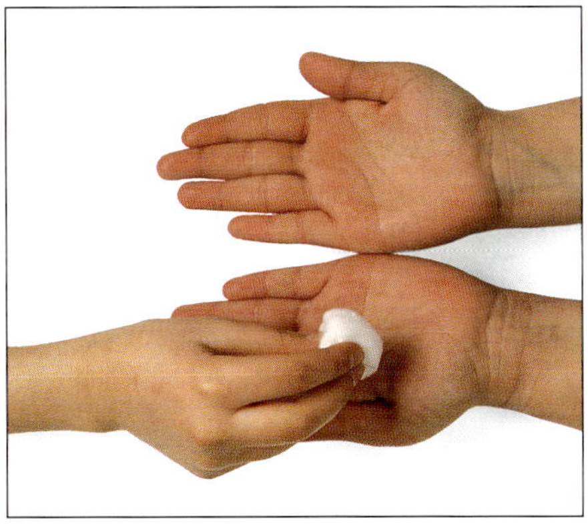

1 ASK A FRIEND to place his or her hands on a table. Rub one hand thoroughly with a cotton ball soaked in rubbing alcohol. This dissolves and cleans away the sebum and sweat layer.

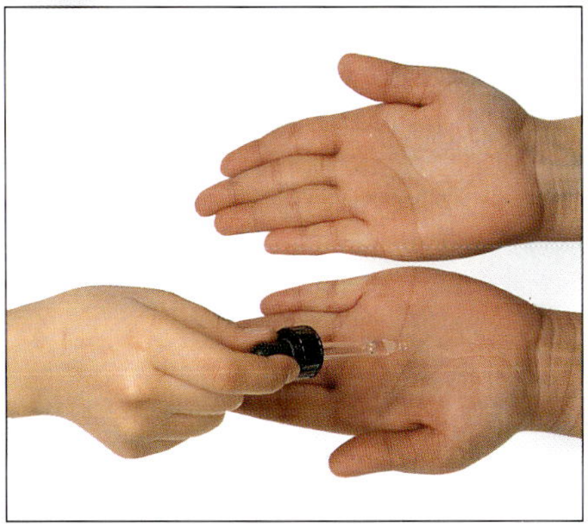

2 ON EACH HAND, place two or three drops of the weak dishwashing liquid solution. (This solution will give you a clearer result than water alone.)

3 WATCH WHAT HAPPENS to the drops on each hand. Do they stay as rounded blobs, repelled by the waterproofed skin? Or do they spread out and soak into the skin, because the skin has lost its natural water-repelling properties? In fact, human skin is "showerproof" rather than fully waterproof. After a long soak in the bathtub, the sebum is washed away. Water can then get into the skin and make it soggy and wrinkled.

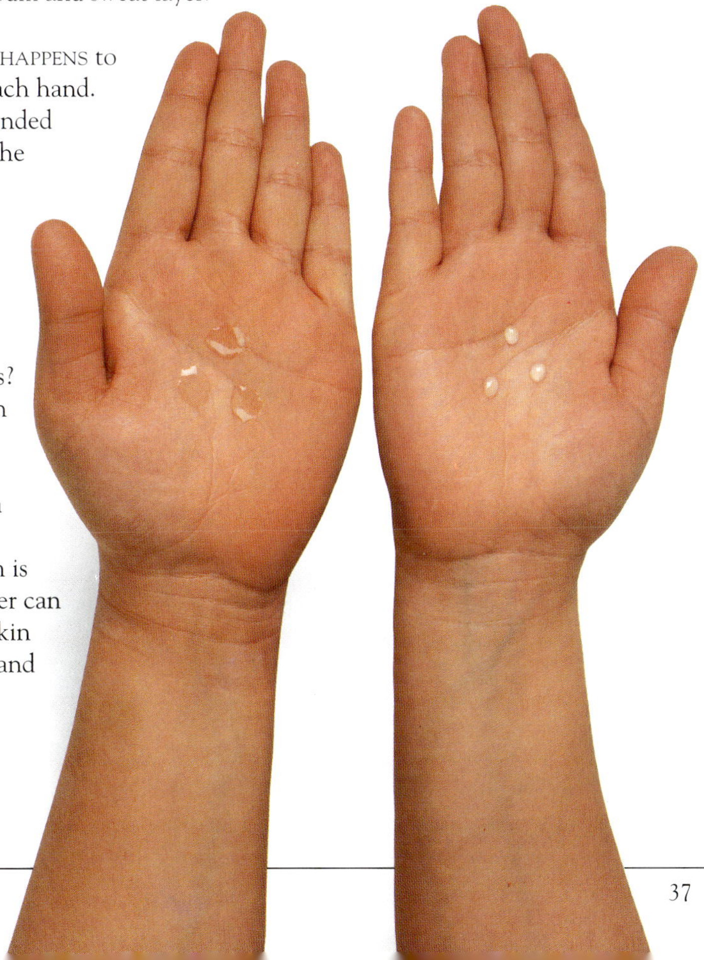

Fingerprints

WASH AND DRY YOUR HANDS. Now try to pick up a pin. It is difficult because you have washed away the film of sweat and natural skin oils that covers your fingertips. This sticky film coats the swirling ridges on your fingers and palms, helping you to grip objects. The word "fingerprint" means both the pattern on the skin of the finger and the impression left when you touch an object, especially one that is smooth. Each person in the world has a unique pattern of fingerprints. Scientists can help police catch criminals by studying the fingerprints of suspects.

EXPERIMENT

Making fingerprints

Adult help is advised for this experiment

Collect friends' fingerprints on paper, and use them for some simple detective work —to find out which one of your friends secretly picked up an empty glass. Keep the prints on file, and make new ones as you and your friends grow older. Although the newer fingerprints will be bigger, the patterns will hardly change.

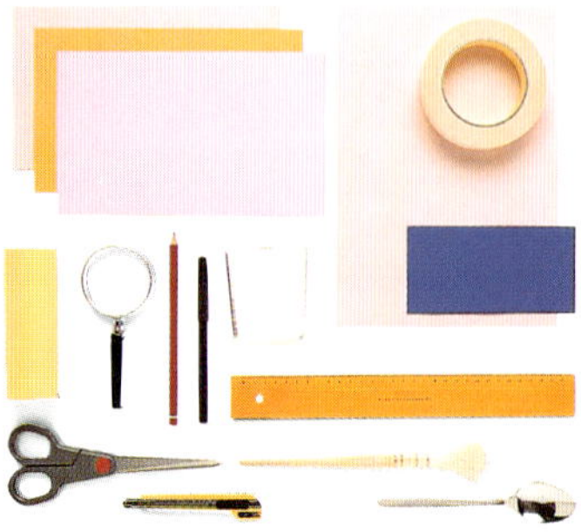

YOU WILL NEED

- *sheets of colored paper*
- *wide double-sided tape*
- *talcum powder*
- *magnifying lens*
- *soft (3B) graphite pencil*
- *spoon*
- *felt-tip pen*
- *glass*
- *ruler*
- *scissors*
- *soft brush*
- *craft knife*

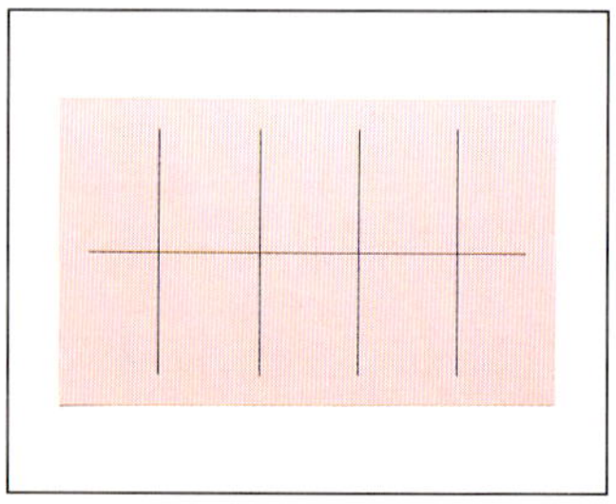

1 DRAW A GRID of four vertical lines and one horizontal line, so that you have two rows of five spaces.

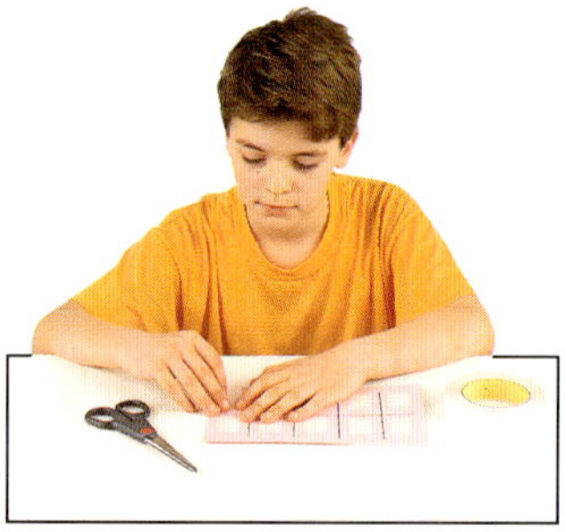

2 CUT 10 PIECES of tape, each about 1 in (2.5 cm) long. Peel off one side of each and stick it into a space.

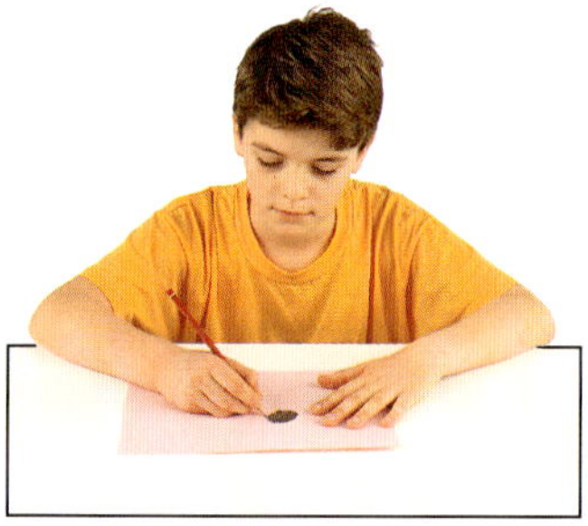

3 RUB THE TIP of the pencil on another piece of paper until it leaves a patch of loose, powdery graphite.

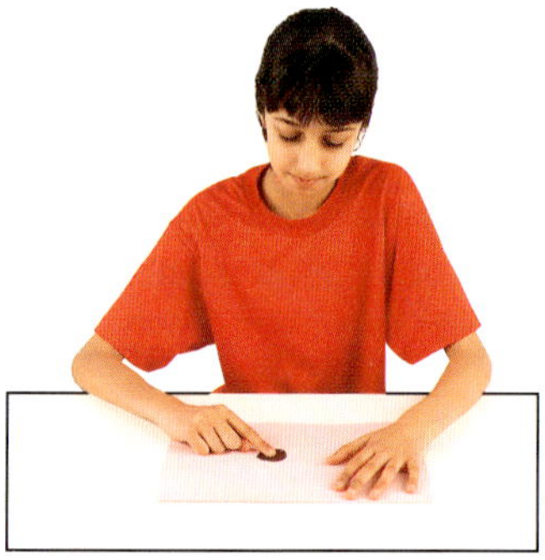

4 GET A FRIEND to dab one fingertip into the patch of pencil graphite until it has a light-black coating.

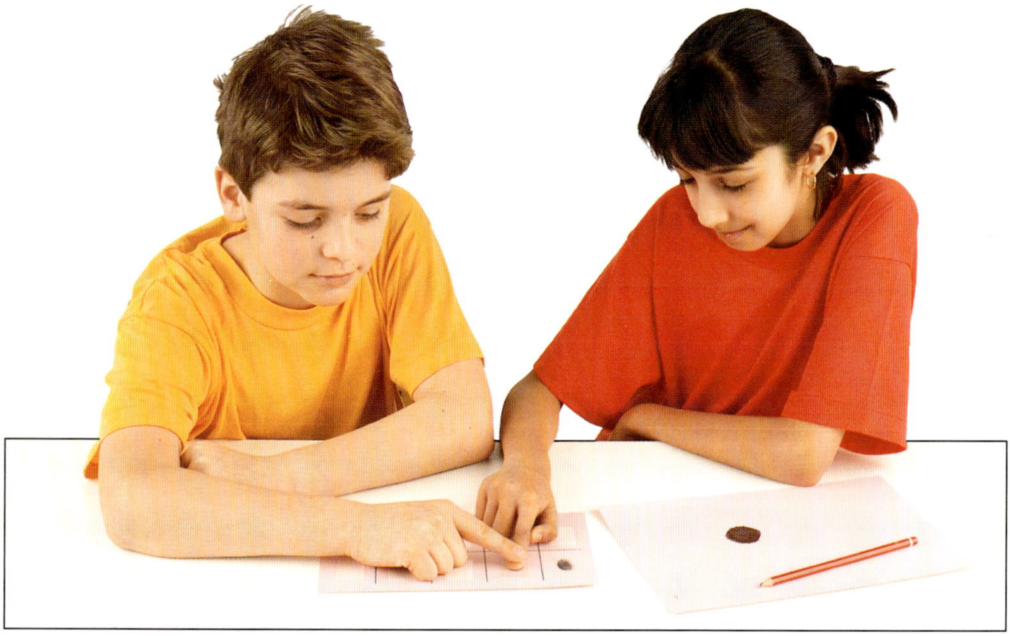

5 PEEL OFF the other side of a piece of tape, and press the finger firmly on the sticky surface to make a fingerprint. Repeat with all fingers and thumbs to make a full set of fingerprints for each hand. Write your friend's name on the back of the piece of paper. Note which fingerprints were taken from the left hand and which from the right hand. Ask your friend to wash his or her hands. Make "fingerprint galleries" like this for other friends. Wait for a few hours, to give time for a new sticky film of sweat and oil to form on your friends' hands.

Fingerprint features

The scientific study of fingerprints began in about 1900. Edward Henry of the police headquarters at Scotland Yard, London, devised a system based on three main print patterns called whorls (spirals), arches, and loops. A fourth pattern, called a composite, has combined features of the others. Detectives look for similarities in the fingerprint patterns and the number of ridges. If they find a certain number of similarities between a suspect's prints and prints left at the scene of a crime, they can be sure the suspect was there.

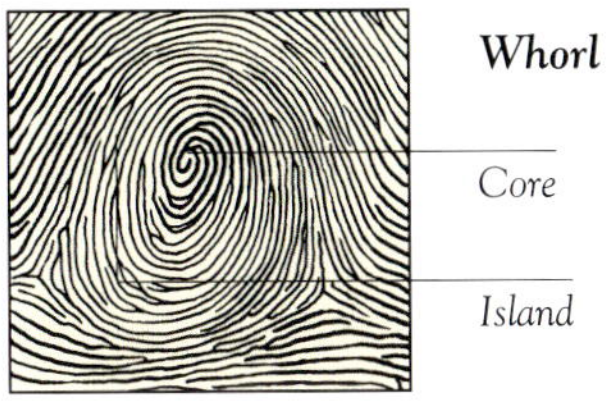

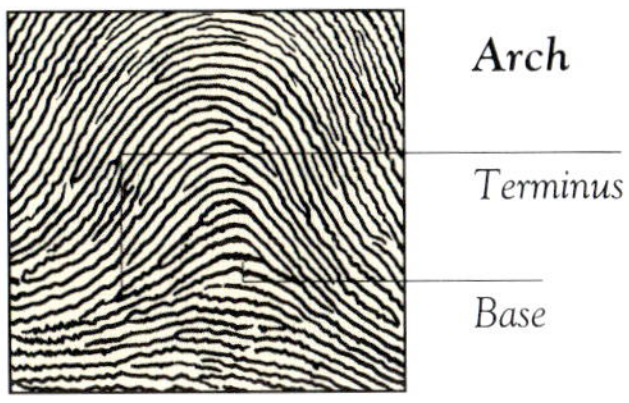

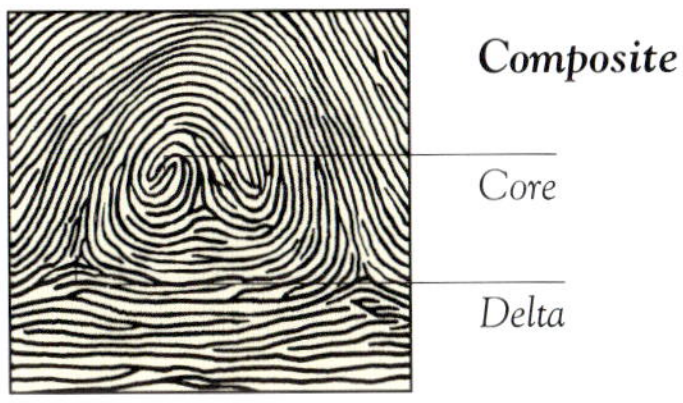

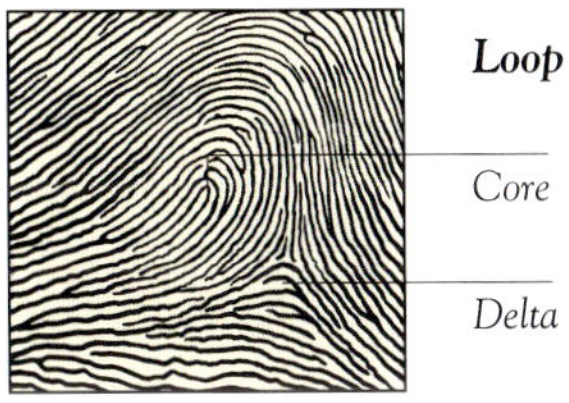

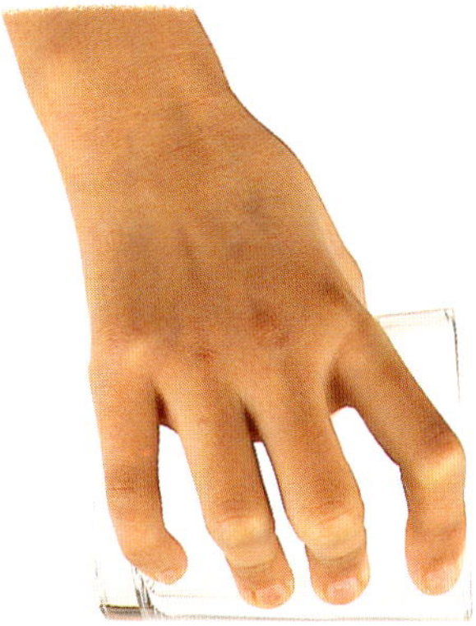

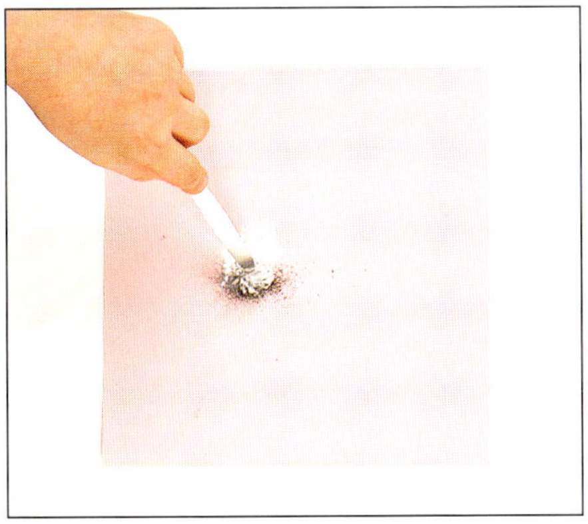

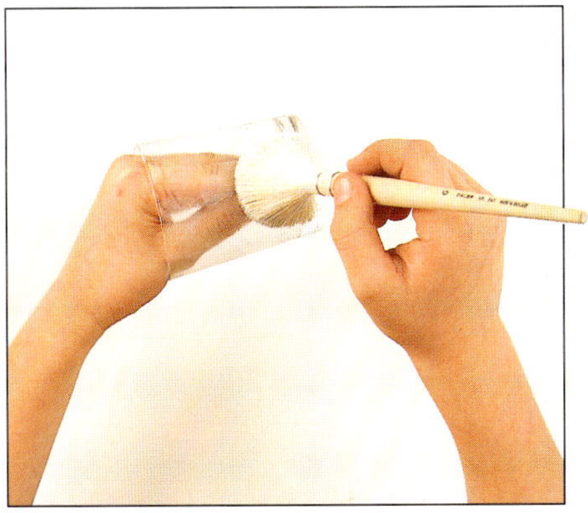

6 NOW YOU ARE READY for the mystery! While you look away, one of your friends picks up the glass, touching the outside.

7 USING THE KNIFE, carefully scrape some more graphite from the tip of a pencil. Using the end of a spoon, mix this with a teaspoon of talcum powder.

8 HOLD THE GLASS from the inside, so as not to disturb the invisible fingerprints. Lightly brush the mixture of graphite and talcum powder onto the outside. This will reveal the prints.

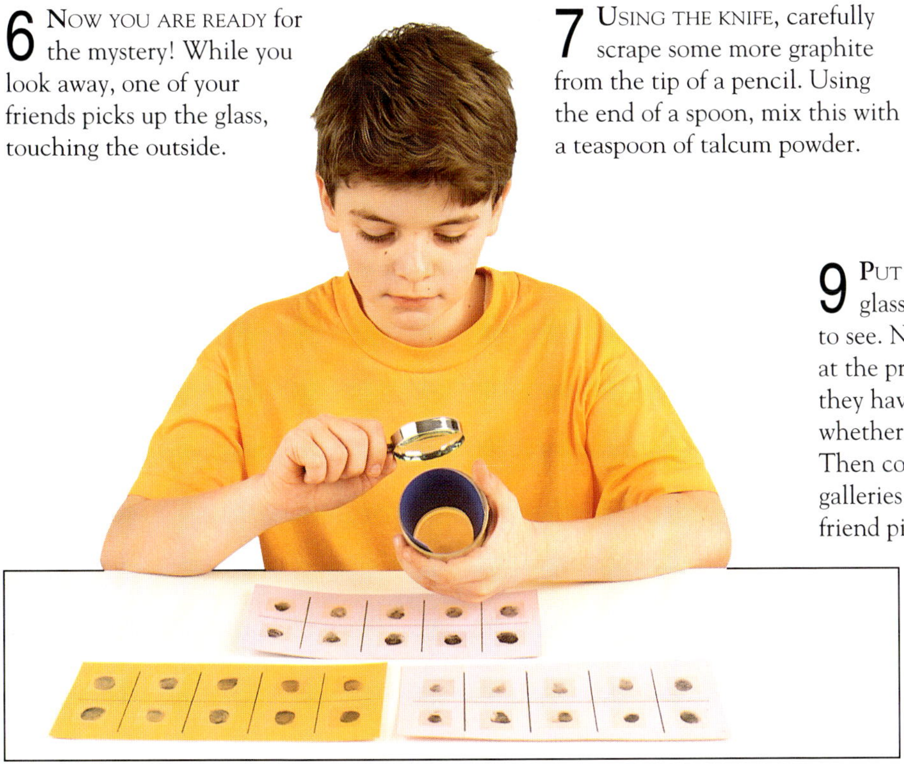

9 PUT A PIECE of dark paper inside the glass, to make the fingerprints easier to see. Now for the detective work! Look at the prints on the glass to see whether they have whorls, arches, or loops, or whether they are composites (above). Then compare them to the fingerprint galleries that you have made. Which friend picked up the glass?

Hair and nails

NEXT TIME YOU PET a friendly dog or cat, remember that you too have "fur" and "claws." The hairs on your head are your most obvious "fur," but most of your skin is also covered with hairs—over 3 million of them, spread over your whole body. The hairs grow out of the skin (pp.32–33) in exactly the same way that animal fur grows. Your fingernails and toenails also grow from the skin, just like dogs' and cats' claws. The main difference is that your nails are broad and blunt while claws are thin and pointed—to help animals run, climb, and hunt. Hair and nails are both made mainly of a tough, hard body protein called keratin. This strong yet light substance is also found in the skin, and it has many uses in the animal world. Horses' hooves and birds' feathers are made of keratin.

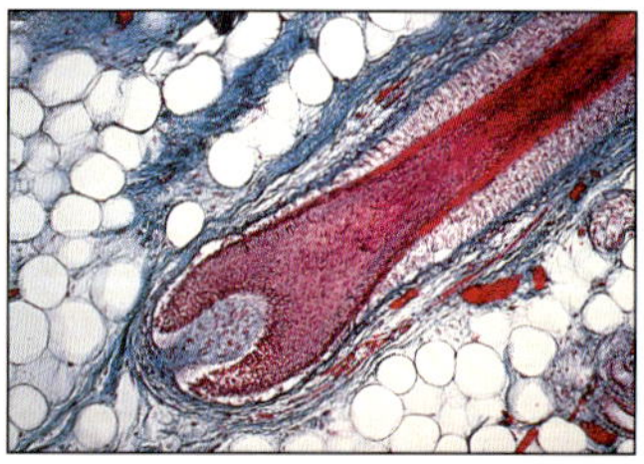

Root of the hair
Hairs grow from pits in the skin called hair follicles. A hair grows by adding new cells at its root. Under a microscope these cells appear as a gray bulge in the hair base. The hair shaft (the pink area) is dead.

EXPERIMENT

How thick is hair?

You can measure how wide a hair is using a microscope (p.178). Ask an adult to cut a strand of hair. Put the hair on the slide, and place a cover slip over the hair to hold it still. Now lay a transparent plastic ruler over the cover slip. Look at the hair and the markings on the ruler through the microscope, and judge how wide the hair is. How much do the hair widths vary on one head, and how much do they vary from person to person?

YOU WILL NEED
• *hair* • *microscope* • *slide* • *cover slip* • *ruler*

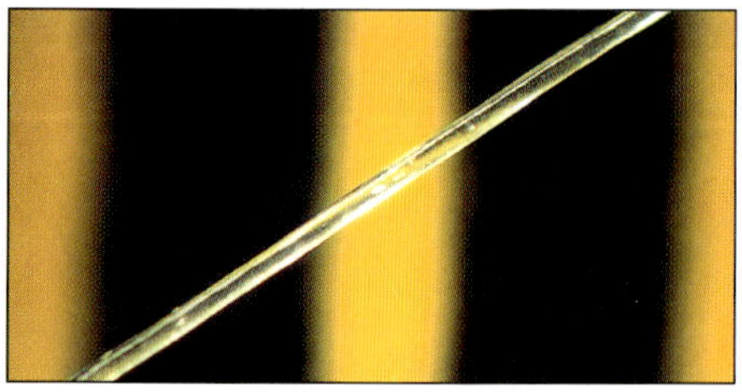

Hair raising

In furry animals, a tiny muscle in the skin—the erector pili muscle—is attached to the base of each hair. It can pull the hair base to make the hair stand on end. This happens when the animal wants to look big and fierce. It also happens when it is cold. Air becomes trapped between the erect hairs, creating an air blanket to keep in body heat. Our hairs are smaller than animal hairs, but they stand on end in exactly the same way when we are scared or cold.

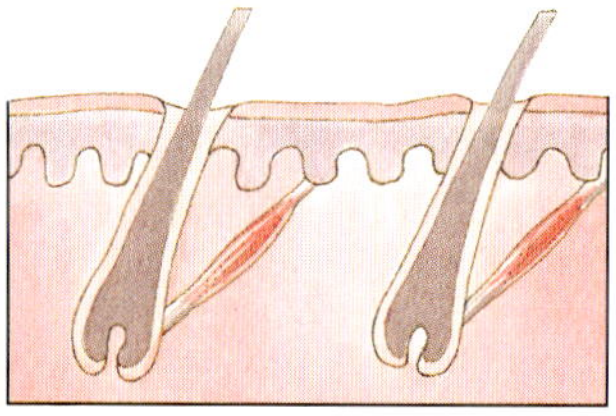

Normal skin
The erector pili muscles attached to your hair roots are relaxed, so your body hairs lie fairly flat.

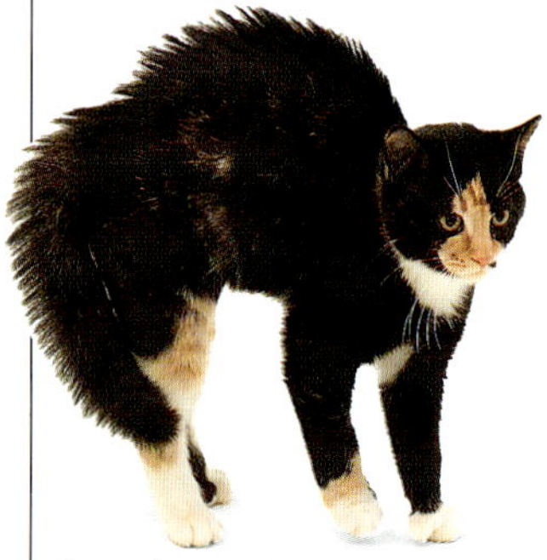

Scared cat
A cat's fur stands on end when it is scared to make it look bigger.

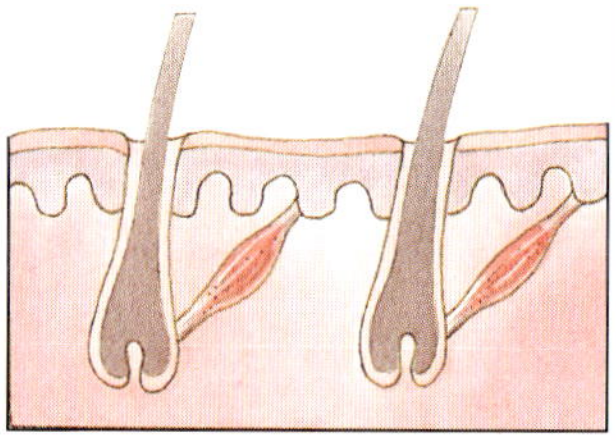

Hairs on end
If you are cold or frightened, your erector pili muscles contract and pull your skin hairs upright.

EXPERIMENT

How fast do your nails grow?

Nails grow faster on some people than others. They may also grow faster when warm—in summer rather than winter. Nails on the hand you use most may grow faster than those on your other hand, because the greater activity of that hand keeps them warmer. How fast do your own fingernails grow?

YOU WILL NEED
• *ruler with 1/16 in or 1 mm divisions* • *graph paper* • *pen*

1 MEASURE the nail length of each finger. Include all of the nail, from base to tip.

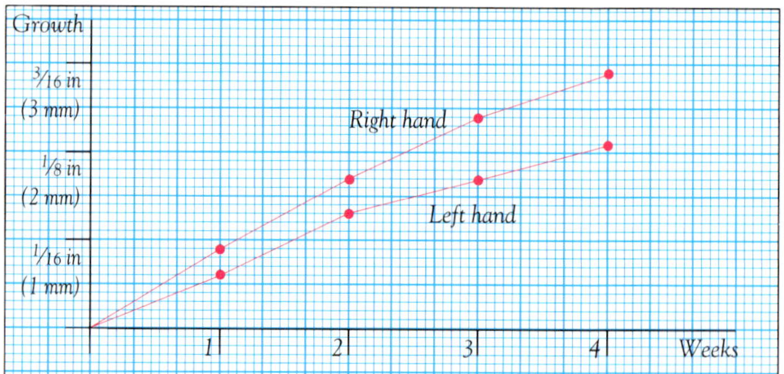

Nail growth chart: middle fingers

2 A WEEK LATER, measure the nail lengths again. Make 5 charts (one for each finger and the thumb, on both hands) to see how much your nails grow each week. Do not bite your nails! Is there a difference between the growth rates in different seasons or between your left and right hands?

EXPERIMENT

How strong is hair?

Adult help is advised for this experiment

Is hair as strong as other materials, such as cotton? Use marbles to test hair strength. Find out also whether some colors of hair are stronger than others.

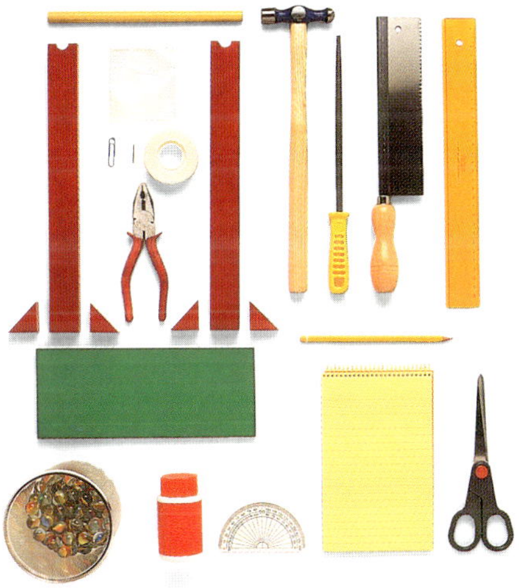

You Will Need

- *tools (file, saw) to make a wooden stand* • *for the stand supports: 2 wooden strips 1 ft (30 cm) long* • *for the base: wood 10 in x 4 in (25 cm x 10 cm)* • *4 small triangular blocks* • *dowel rod* • *pin* • *small plastic bag* • *paper clip* • *pliers* • *cellophane tape* • *ruler* • *pencil* • *marbles* • *wood glue* • *protractor* • *notepad* • *scissors* • *hammer* • *hair*

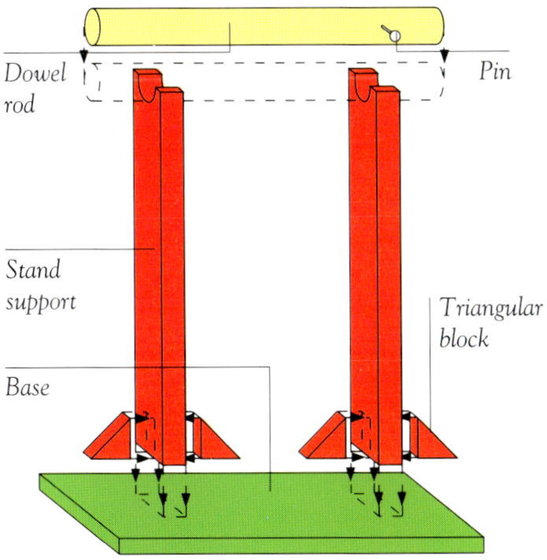

Assembling the stand

File a large groove in the top of each stand support. Glue the supports to the base and strengthen the joints by gluing on the triangular blocks. Lay the dowel rod in the grooves in the supports, with the pin resting against one groove.

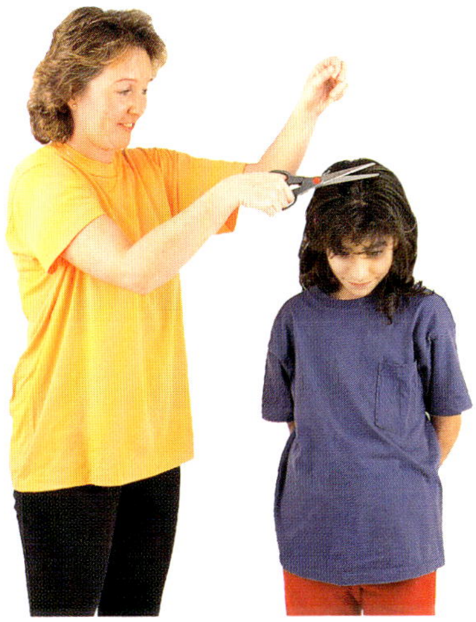

1 ASK AN ADULT to cut some strands of hair using the scissors. You need long strands for this experiment.

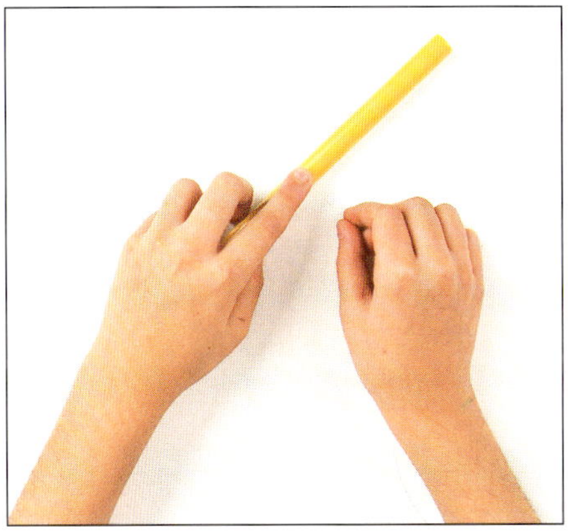

2 ATTACH ONE END of the hair to the rod with tape. Wrap the hair around the rod twice.

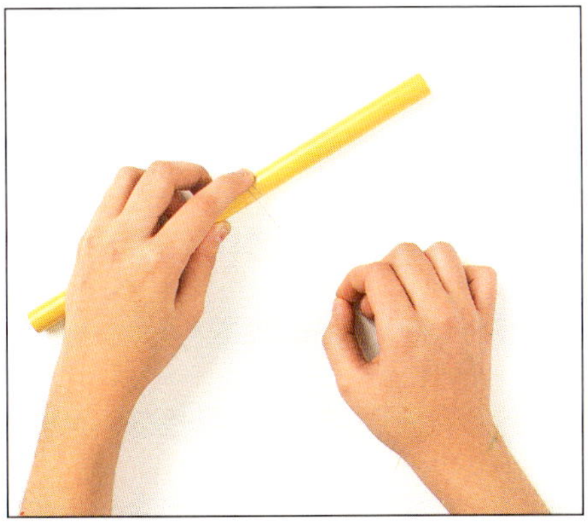

3 TAPE THE HAIR to the rod again. Carefully tap a pin into one end of the rod with the hammer, so that the rod will not spin in the stand (left).

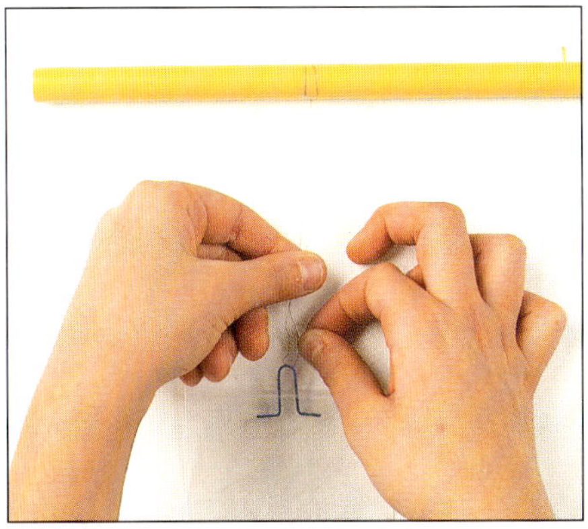

4 USE THE PLIERS to bend the paper clip into a U-shape, and tape it to the plastic bag. Loop the hair around the clip, and tape it together securely.

5 LAY THE ROD in the grooves in the stand. Support the bag with your hand, and add one marble. Then slowly take your hand away. Repeat by adding another marble, then another. How many marbles can you add before the hair breaks? Now test hair of different colors and from different parts of the head. Try cotton and other fibers too. Measure the thickness of the strands of hair and the other fibers (opposite). Is hair stronger than other materials of similar width?

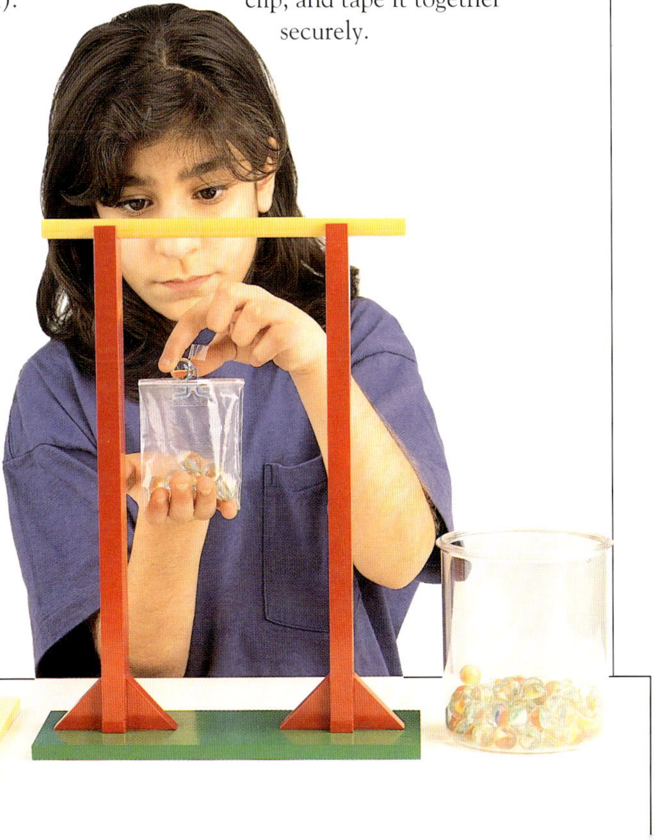

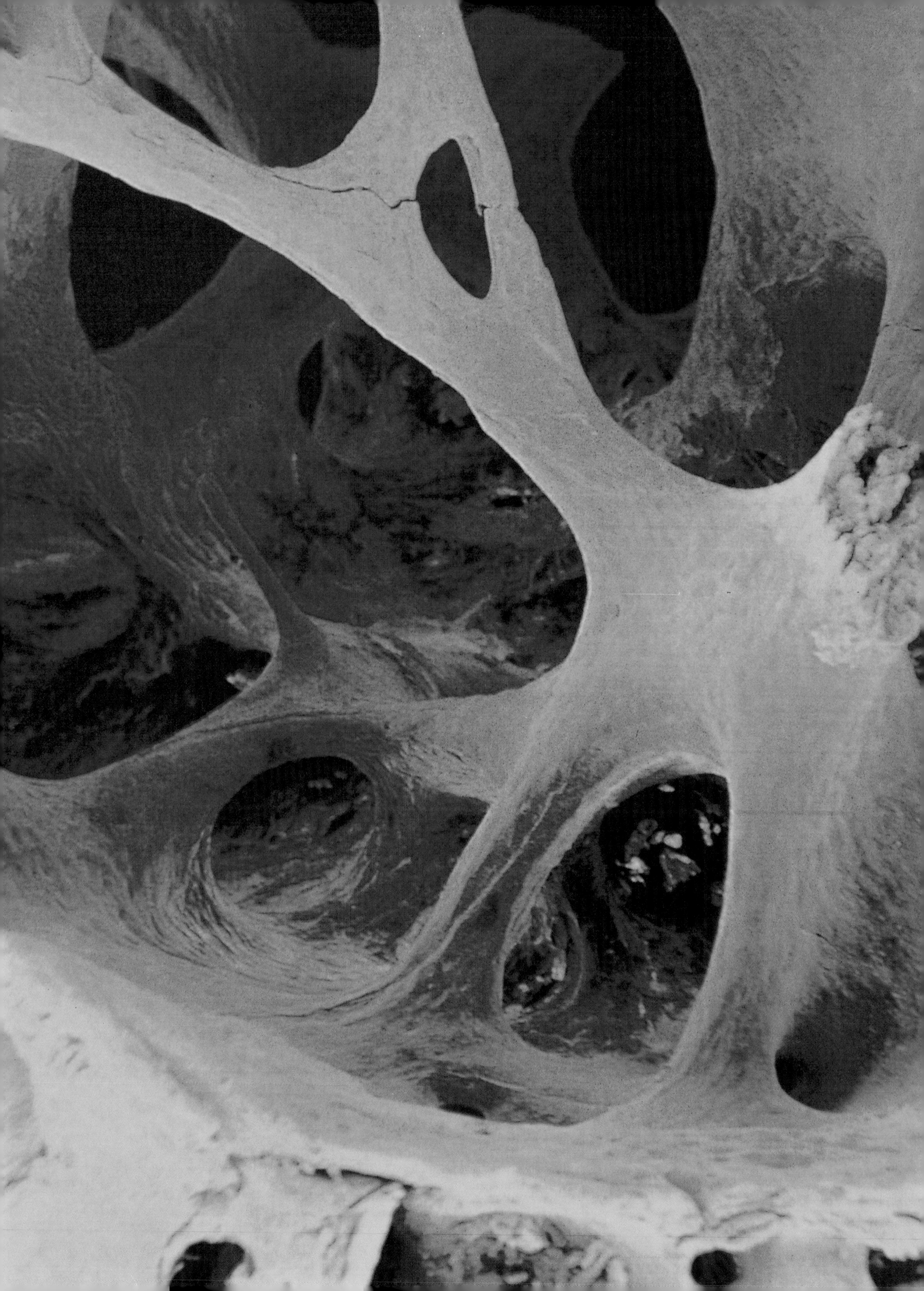

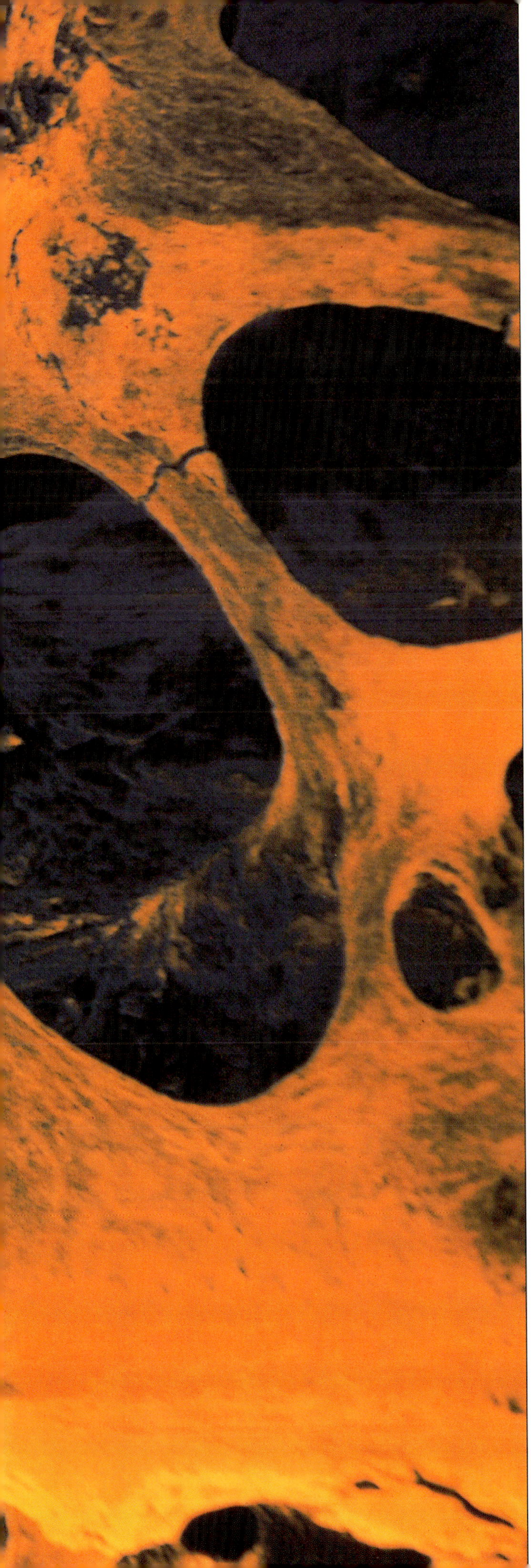

The BODY'S FRAMEWORK

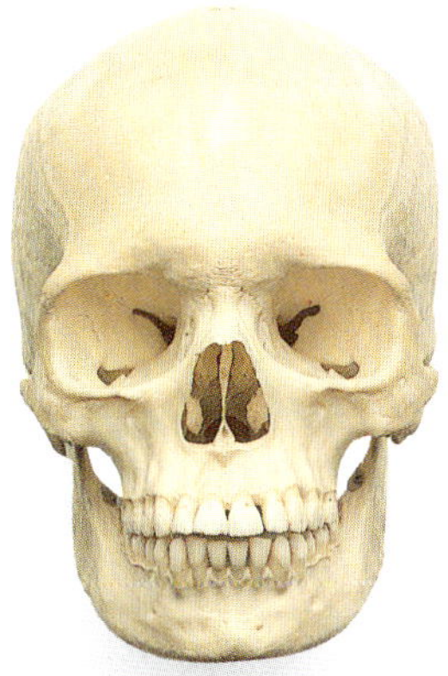

A head case
Bones support and protect. The large dome of the skull (above) is actually made from eight separate bones. They grow and fuse together during early childhood to form a rigid case, the cranium, which shields the brain. The interior of a rib (left) is shown magnified many times. The jellylike bone marrow has been removed, leaving the hard honeycomblike scaffolding of proteins and minerals.

YOUR MUSCLES, GUTS, BLOOD vessels, and other body parts would collapse into a soggy heap if it were not for the body's supporting framework—the skeleton. In an adult, this consists of 206 bones, linked at flexible joints, which allow movement. Bones also contain the marrow that makes millions of new blood cells each second, and they act as reservoirs of minerals, which other parts of the body can call upon when deprived of nourishment.

THE FLEXIBLE FRAME

THE BONES AND JOINTS TOGETHER form the inner framework of the body. This highly flexible, constantly moving, internal scaffolding is designed to work nonstop for your whole lifetime. Unlike most structures built by humans, the body's framework can adapt to the demands placed on it. For example, reasonable amounts of activity and exercise help to make the bones stronger and more resilient, and encourage the joints to stay supple and healthy for longer.

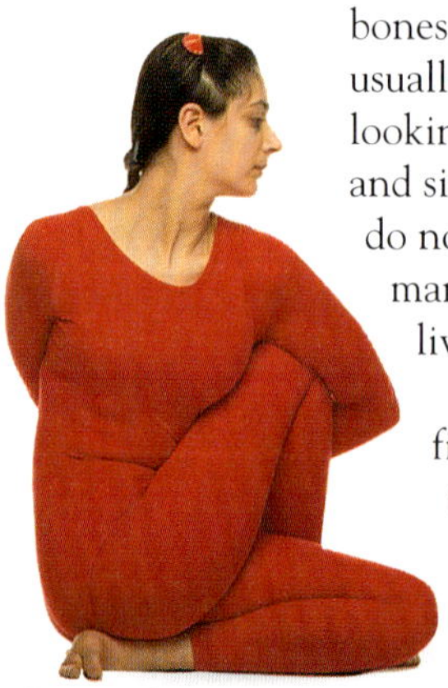

With enough practice, most *people could increase the flexibility of their joints and become as supple as this yoga expert.*

Have you seen animal or human bones in a museum? They are usually pale, dry, and brittle-looking. They show the shapes and sizes of the bones, but they do not give a true picture of the many active roles fulfilled by living bones.

Bones were probably the first parts of the human body to be studied in detail by anatomists. Although the flesh and other soft parts of the body soon rot away after death, bones are hard and tough, and can last for hundreds of years without decaying. So early anatomists had no problem in finding a supply of skeletons to study. Bones were among the earliest parts of the body to be given formal scientific names, many of which are still used nearly 2,000 years later (p.46).

Living parts

In studies by early anatomists, bones were likened to the stone columns and wooden beams in a building. They were thought of as lifeless internal supports that held up the nerves, muscles, vessels, and other soft, floppy parts of the body.

However, as the science of anatomy advanced during the Renaissance period, this view of bones gradually changed. Anatomists realized that bones in the body are not dry and brittle. They discovered instead that up to one-third of a bone is water, that bones are slightly soft and flexible, and that they have their own blood vessels and nerves, like any other organ. In other words, a bone is alive, it uses energy and nutrients, and it can detect sensations.

Physiologists realized that bones also store extra mineral reserves for the body. If the body runs short of food, essential minerals can be transported from the bones to places where they are needed more urgently, such as the blood or the nerves.

Strength by design

Anatomists discovered that the construction of bones can take different forms. A typical bone consists of a hard, dense outer shell containing a "filler," which resembles a honeycomb. The outer shell is called compact bone, and the inner type is known as spongy, trabecular, or cancellous bone.

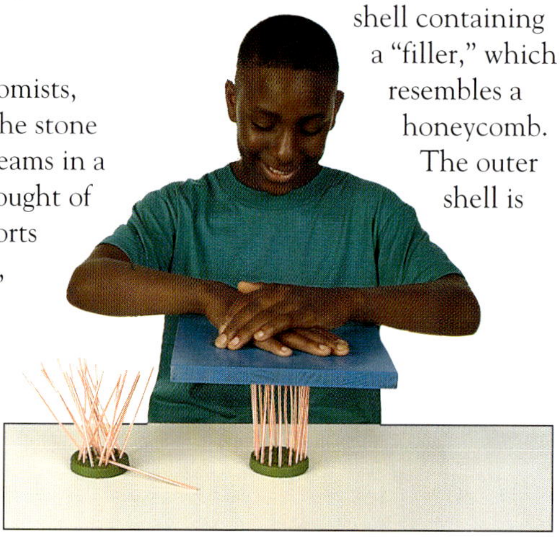

Bone is formed of bundles of microscopic tubes, *which are themselves arranged in tubes. A simple model shows how the design of bone makes it very strong (p.48).*

The strength of bone comes from its design. The Italian astronomer and physicist Galileo Galilei (1564–1642) knew that if hollow tubes and solid rods are both made from the same weight of material, the hollow tube is stronger. Following the same principle, the long, slim bones in the body's limbs, such as the femur (thighbone), are not solid rods but tubes, with hollow chambers along their shafts. This makes them both light and strong.

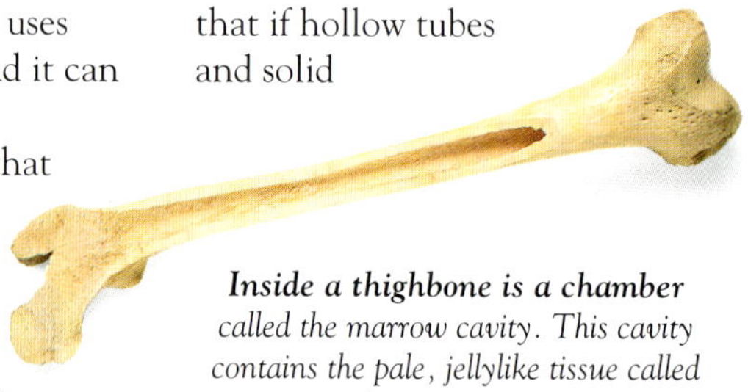

Inside a thighbone is a chamber *called the marrow cavity. This cavity contains the pale, jellylike tissue called bone marrow.*

The spongy centers of other bones, such as the breastbone and ribs, do not have to be as strong as the femur, but it is important that they too are light.

Bone-making cells

The invention of the microscope in the 1600's had a great impact on osteology (the study of the bones). Microscopists discovered that bone is built from hundreds of tiny cylindrical units called Haversian systems (p.48), which are also known as osteons. Haversian systems are constructed from cells, like all other body parts.

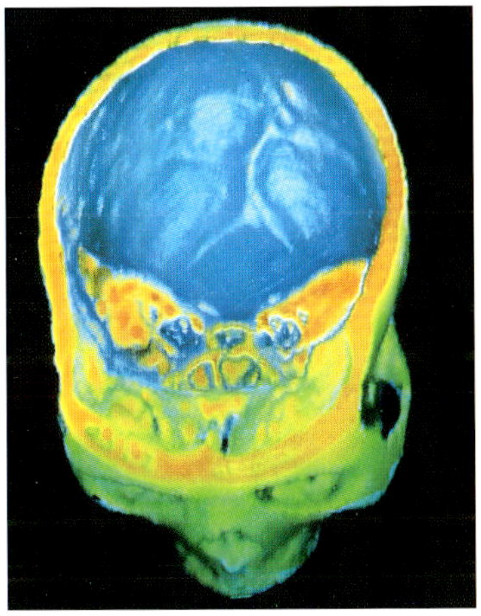

A modern medical scanning *machine can produce a computerized three-dimensional image from X-rays of the skull of a living person.*

Bone-making cells are called osteocytes. These cells, which look like tiny spiders, produce a complex substance known as bone matrix. This has two main components. One component is a mixture of microscopic crystals containing minerals such as calcium, phosphorus, magnesium, and sodium. The other component is bundles of fibers, made from the body protein collagen, which is also found in the skin and muscle tendons. The minerals make the bone hard and fairly rigid, but the collagen gives it some elasticity and resilience. As a result, bones are slightly flexible, and under a small amount of stress they tend to bend rather than snap.

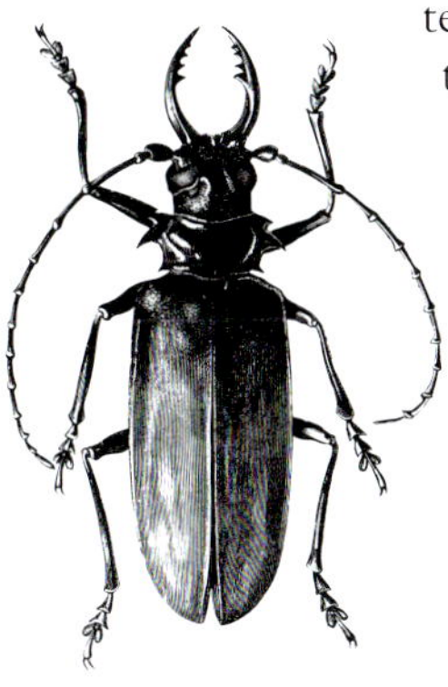

Unlike humans, insects *such as beetles wear their skeletons on the outside of their bodies, as hard protective cases.*

Bone marrow

In the body the centers of bones are filled with a soft, jellylike substance called bone marrow, of which there are two main types.

The first is red marrow, which makes nearly all of the body's new blood cells (p.103). When you are young, red marrow occurs in all the bones of your skeleton. Red marrow is found in the spaces in the spongy interiors of bones and in the large marrow cavity of long limb bones.

From the time you are about 5 years old, the red marrow in your limb bones is gradually replaced by the second type, called yellow marrow. This consists mainly of fibrous connective tissue and fat, and it produces far fewer blood cells than red marrow.

By the time you are about 25 years old, the production of blood cells takes place in only a few bones—mainly the spine, sternum, collarbones, hipbones, and skull.

Mechanical devices

Giorgio Baglivi (1668–1707), an Italian physician, held the opinion that the human body was a collection of mechanical devices. He thought that the lungs were bellows, the teeth were scissors, and the bones were a variety of beams, girders, rods, and plates. Baglivi's "mechanical body" ideas brought him into conflict with those colleagues who argued correctly that the body could not possibly be made from nonliving machines.

However, then and now, both anatomists and engineers could see many parallels between the body's bones and the structural frameworks and mechanical joints of various machines.

One principle of engineering is that a system of levers gives an object a mechanical advantage (p.50). Mechanics recognize that there are three orders (types) of lever, which can be used for various purposes. The human body has examples of each of these orders (p.51) for lifting objects and moving itself around.

Where bones meet

You can nod your head, walk, run, and reach out and grasp objects, because your bones are linked together by movable joints (p.182). Human joints are very similar to mechanical joints, from door hinges to computer joysticks. In a well-designed joint there are special smooth, hard-wearing substances where the two parts come into contact. In the body this is cartilage. This shiny, hard substance is made by cells called chondrocytes. Also, in the same way that a machine bearing needs grease or oil to keep its parts moving smoothly, the human joint has its own "oil," which is called synovial fluid (p.51).

Together the body's joints work as a smooth unit, constantly maintaining—and occasionally repairing—themselves, to give the body a lifetime of service.

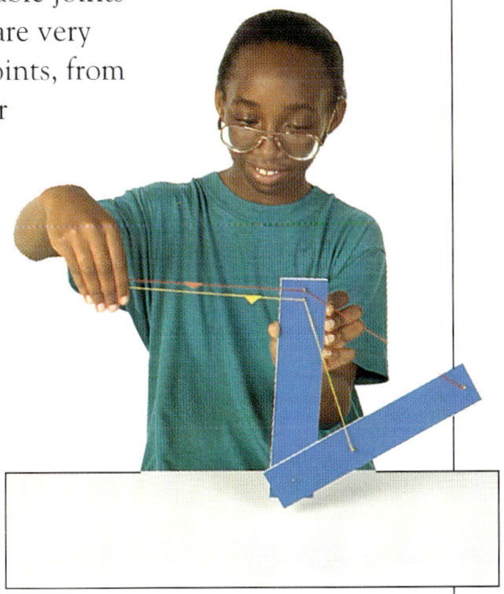

Bones and muscles work *together using the lever-based principle of mechanical advantage. Make a model joint to see mechanical advantage in action (p.50).*

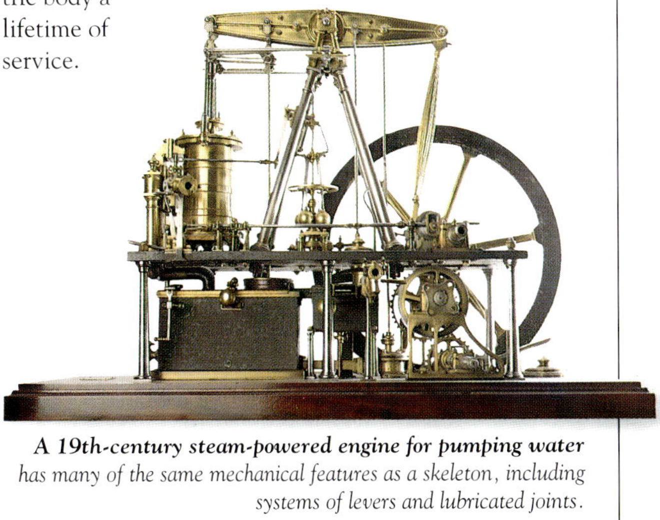

A 19th-century steam-powered engine for pumping water *has many of the same mechanical features as a skeleton, including systems of levers and lubricated joints.*

The skeleton

IF A BABY HAS A FALL, the baby is much less likely to break the bones of his or her skeleton than an adult. This is partly because a baby is lighter than an adult, but more important, it is because a baby's skeleton is very different from the skeleton of an adult. The newborn baby has more than 300 parts that we call bones, yet some of these contain very little true bone at all. They are made mainly of the slightly softer, more flexible cartilage. In a fall, cartilage bends rather than breaking. During childhood, true bone gradually replaces nearly all of the cartilage. Some of the separate bones fuse together, as in the skull, reducing the total number of parts. The skeleton continues to get larger and harder in the teenage years. By the age of 20 to 25 years it has the final number of 206 fully mature, hardened bones.

Rebuilding from the bones

Bones hold many clues to the size, age, and features of a person. For example, the shape of the mandible (lower jawbone) gives a face its characteristic jawline. Using clay, experts are able to rebuild the muscles and the exterior features of a person from clues given by a skull and other bones. This work helps scientists to reconstruct the faces and bodies of people long dead, like the owner of the skull below.

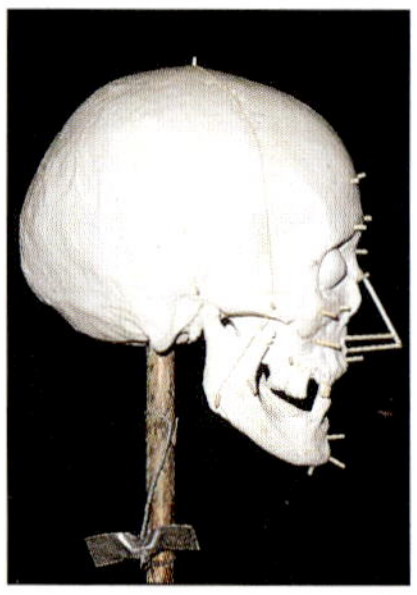

The bones
First, plaster casts are made of the bones to avoid damaging the originals, which may be fragile. Cracks, chips, and missing fragments can be filled in at this stage.

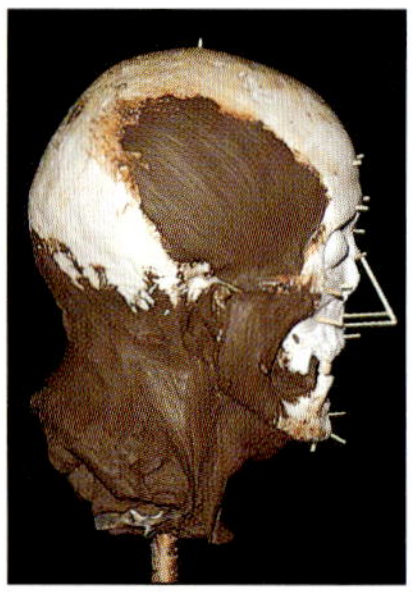

The muscles
Using their knowledge of anatomy, the experts reconstruct the muscles of the neck and jaw. Roughened patches on the bones indicate where the muscles joined them.

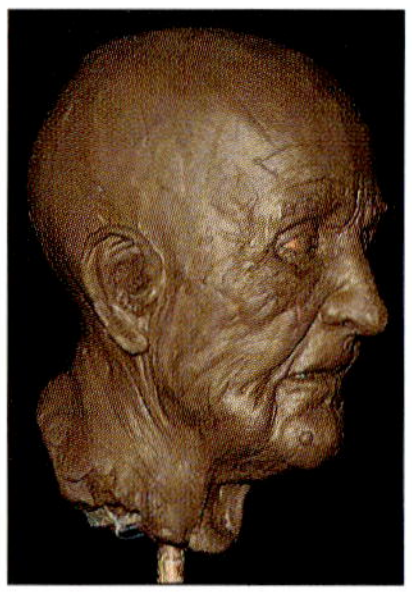

The skin
The shape and size of the skeleton and the changes in bone due to aging show how old the subject is. Skin of a suitable texture is added to complete the reconstruction.

Naming the bones

Every bone has its own anatomical name, usually in Latin. Some names are given here. Most of these names were introduced by anatomists of ancient times, especially the Roman physician Rufus of Ephesus, in his book *The Names of Different Parts of the Human Body* (about A.D. 100), and Galen (p.13). Many bones also have everyday names.

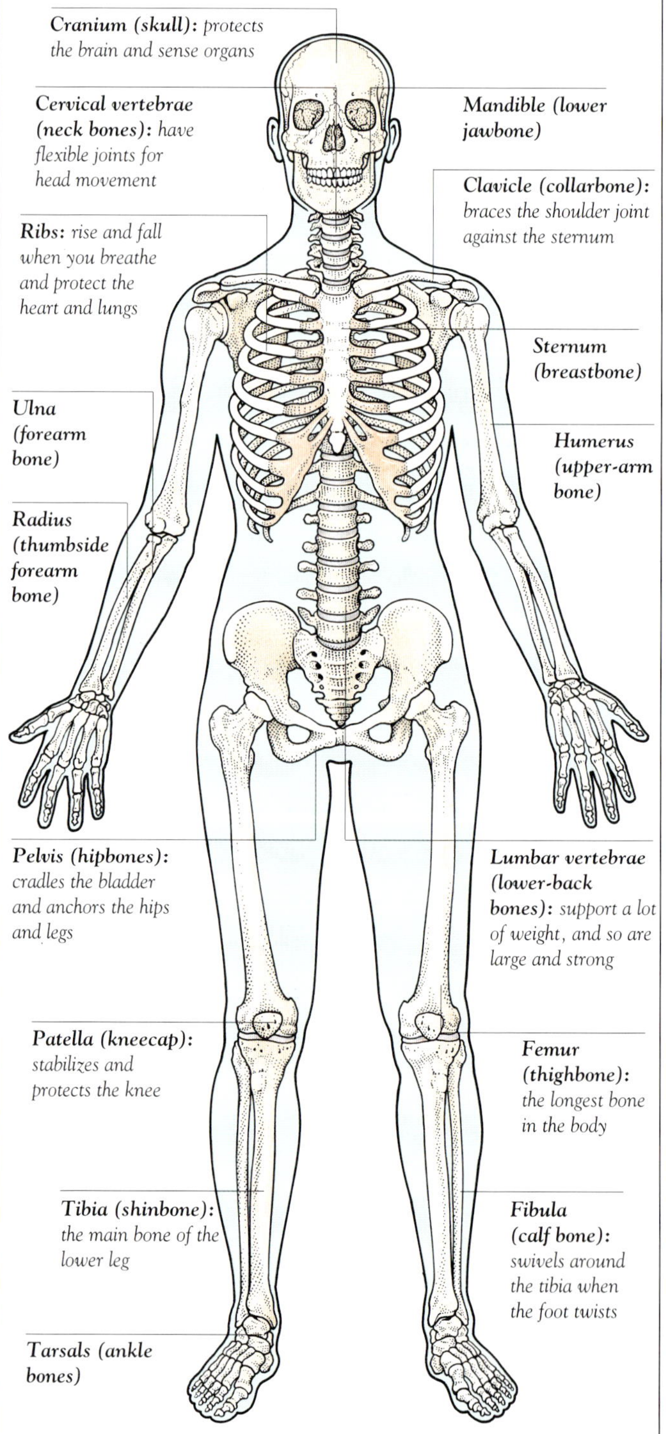

■ DISCOVERY ■

Wilhelm Röntgen

X-rays were discovered in 1895 by the German physicist Wilhelm Röntgen. He detected mysterious electromagnetic rays created by streams of high-speed electrons. He found that the rays, although invisible, could "shine" through living flesh and form an image on a photographic plate on the other side. X-rays pass easily through soft body parts, such as muscles and nerves. But they cannot pass through hard, dense bones. So an X-ray photograph, called a radiograph, shows bones as distinct shapes against a contrasting background. However, X-rays can damage living tissues, so their use is carefully controlled.

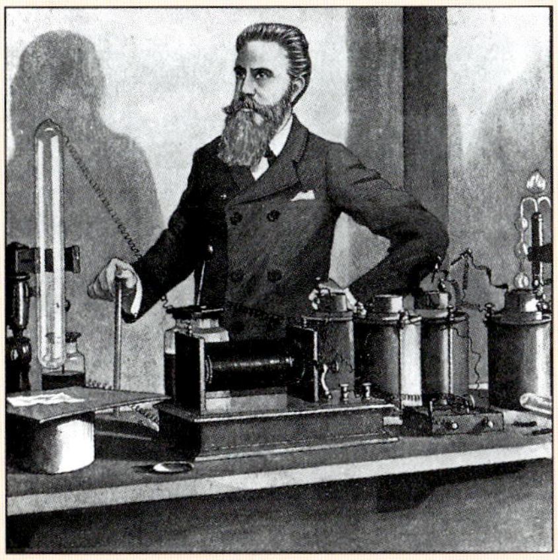

X for unknown
Röntgen, a 1901 Nobel Prize recipient, called the rays "X" due to their mysterious nature.

Bone growth

This sequence of X-rays shows how bones grow and develop during childhood.

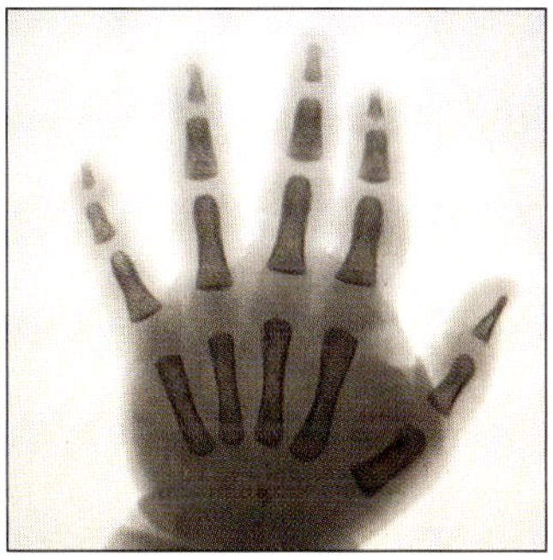

Hand of a 2-year-old
The skeleton is formed, but much of it is made of cartilage, which does not show on the X-ray.

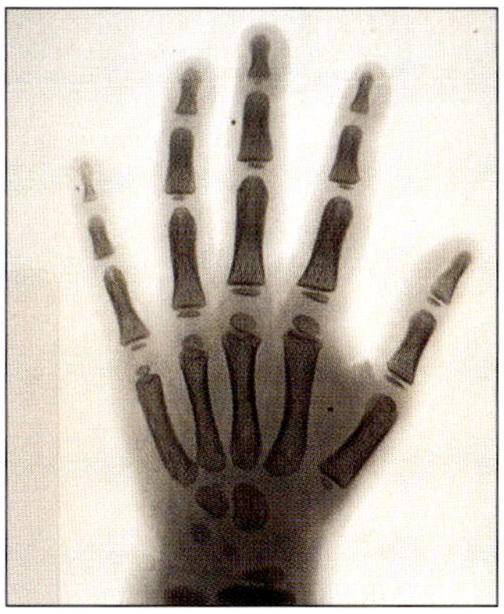

Hand of a 3-year-old
The cartilage is gradually being replaced by bone. Note that the wrist is still mostly cartilage.

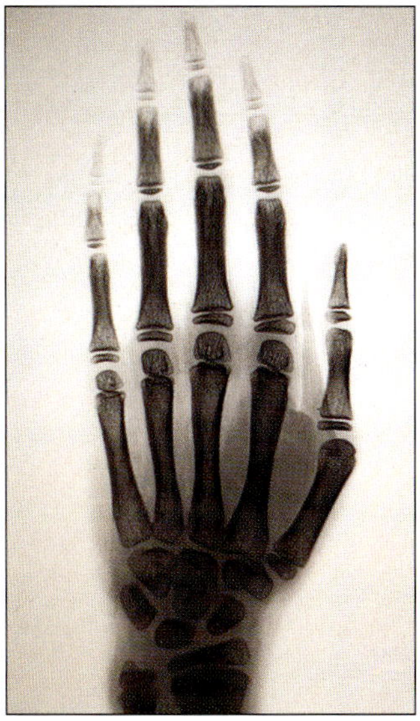

Hand of a 14-year-old
The skeleton of the wrist and hand is now made of mature, hard bone (see also the bones on the left).

Hands and feet

According to the theory of evolution (p.12), our distant ancestors of millions of years ago walked on four legs, like other mammals. Early humans started to walk on two legs 5 to 10 million years ago, leaving their arms free for carrying and manipulating objects. But the bones of our arms and hands are still similar to those of our legs and feet. The upper arm and thigh each have one long bone. The forearm has two bones, like the shin. On the hand and foot there are five fingers and five toes respectively, each with the same pattern of bones inside. The main difference is that the wrist has eight bones, but the ankle has only seven.

Bones of the foot

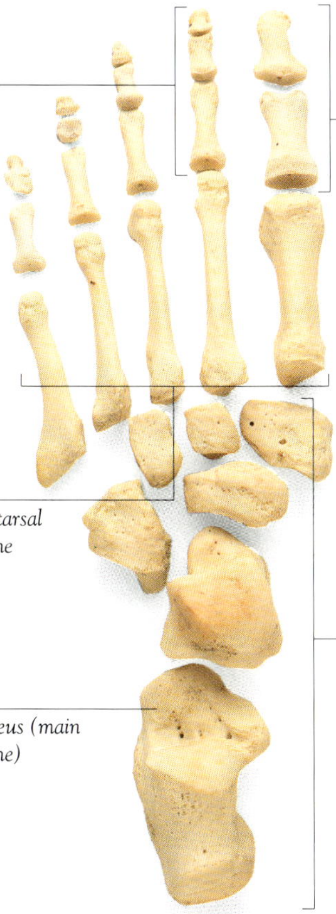

Bones of the hand and forearm

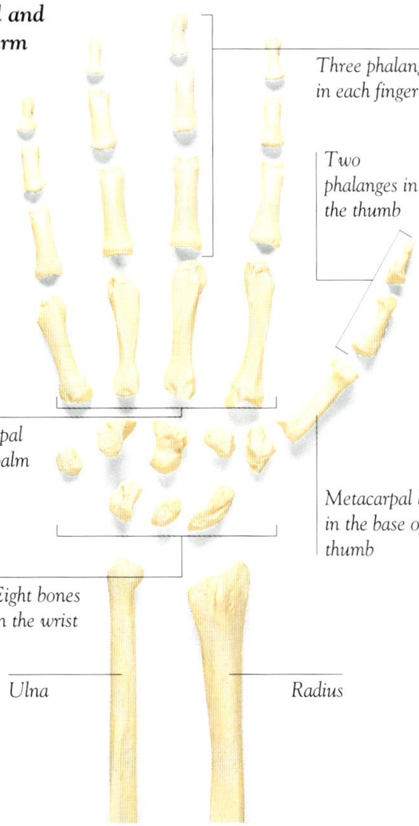

Inside bones

STRUCTURAL ENGINEERS have long acknowledged the combination of strength and lightness given by bone. Pound for pound, bone is stronger than wood, concrete, or steel. If the human skeleton were made of enough steel to equal the strength of bone, it would weigh five times as much. The strength of bone comes mainly from its inner structure. It is built up from thousands of compactly arranged tube-shaped units, each called a Haversian system. The units are named after the English physician Clopton Havers (1650–1701), who published his bone studies in 1691. The bone tissue in the walls of these tubes is made of fibers of the protein collagen, which give it elasticity, and mineral crystals, which make it hard. Haversian systems lie in the direction of the greatest stresses on the bone. In a long bone, such as the femur (thighbone), the tubes lie lengthwise in the bone shaft, so the bone resists buckling.

EXPERIMENT

Tower of strength

Adult help is advised for this experiment

When engineers work on the design for a large structure, such as a skyscraper or big crane, they know that the strength of the building material to be used is only one consideration. Other factors are the size, shape, and arrangement of the main supporting parts, such as steel girders or concrete pillars. This experiment shows how you can arrange structural parts in different ways: some arrangements may be weak, but others can have surprising strength. A structure may have a good supporting capacity even if its individual structural parts—in this case drinking straws—are quite weak. The ring-of-straws design that you build here is similar to the way that Haversian systems (left) are arranged in bone.

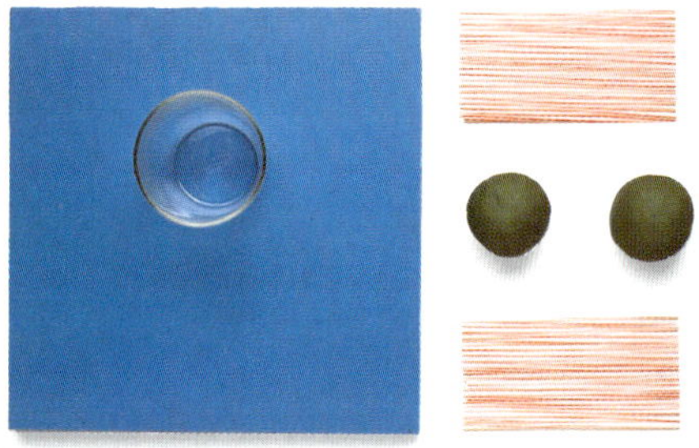

YOU WILL NEED

- *wooden board or book*
- *plastic beaker*
- *2 egg-size lumps of modeling clay*
- *about 50 plastic drinking straws*

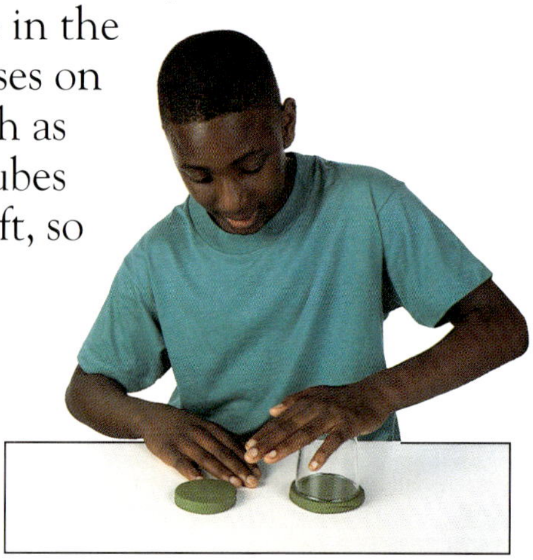

1 FLATTEN EACH LUMP of modeling clay into a disk just larger than the beaker mouth. Press the beaker rim into one disk to make a slight indentation.

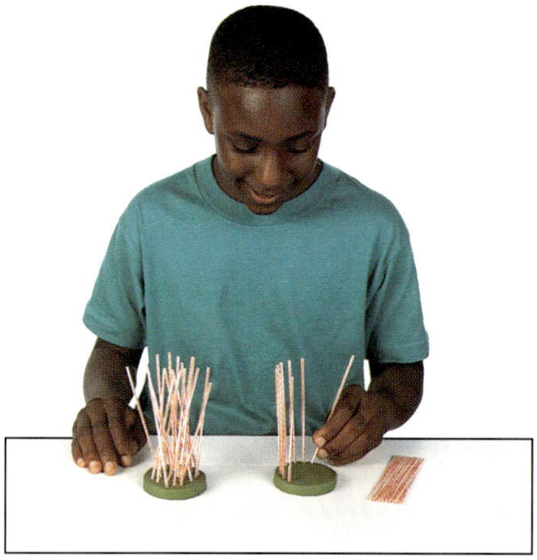

2 MAKE A TOWER of straws pointing in all directions. Then make a second tower with the same number of straws, placed upright around the indentation.

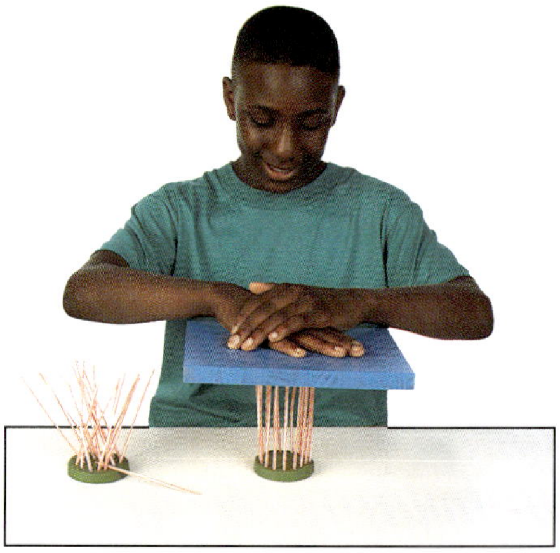

3 TEST THE STRENGTH of each tower by pressing the board or book on it. The random arrangement soon collapses. The ring-of-straws design is much stronger.

Haversian systems

A Haversian system is only $\frac{1}{100}$ in (0.25 mm) in diameter. It is made from thousands of fibers of collagen, embedded in mineral salts of calcium and phosphorus. The fibers are laid in circular layers known as lamellae, like the growth rings you see in a sliced-through tree trunk.

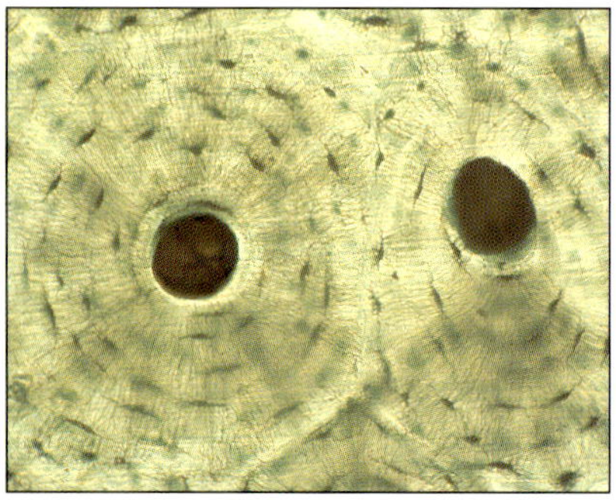

Lamellae, blood vessels, and nerves
This microscope photograph shows a cross section through two Haversian systems with their lamellae. The central dark areas are canals for blood vessels and nerves. The spots that ring the canals are bone cells (p.44).

EXPERIMENT

A tube of tubes

Adult help is advised for this experiment

The arrangement of Haversian systems is only part of bone's structural strength. These tube-shaped units are also stuck firmly to each other by the bone matrix, which acts as a "living glue." Extend the experiment opposite by sticking the straws together—in this case using a paper tube as a container. See how a very strong structure can be built from lightweight materials. Real bones are covered by a kind of flexible "skin"—like the paper tube. This is called the periosteum.

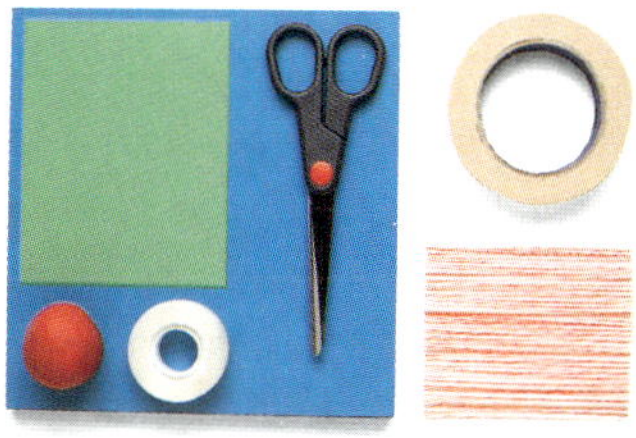

YOU WILL NEED

- *wooden board or book*
- *stiff paper*
- *modeling clay*
- *scissors*
- *single- and double-sided tape*
- *drinking straws*

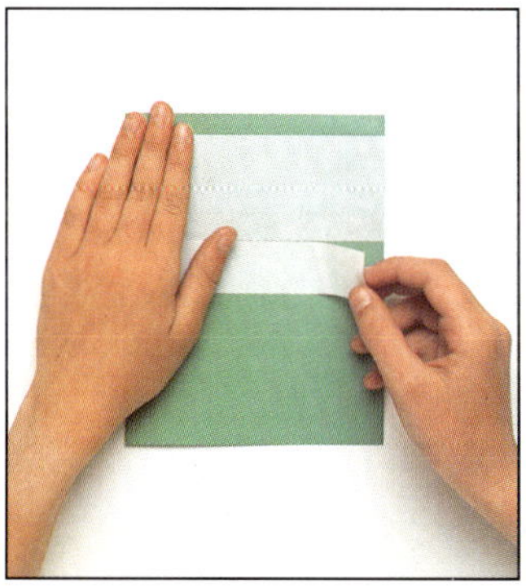

1 TRIM THE PAPER so that its width equals the straws' length. Cover one side of the paper completely with double-sided tape.

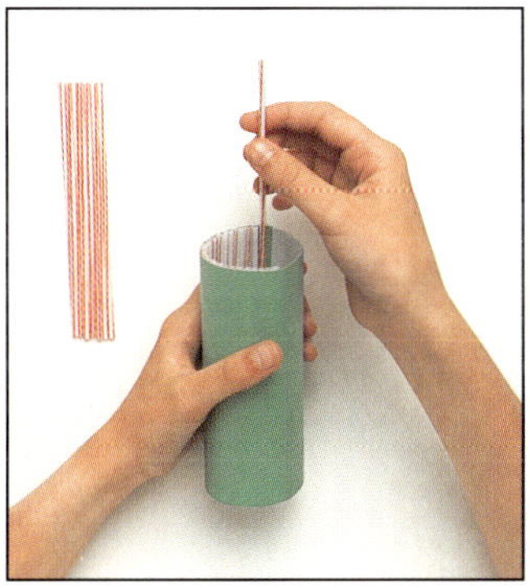

2 ROLL THE PAPER into a tube with the tape inside. Tape its edges together. Stick a closely packed layer of straws around the inside.

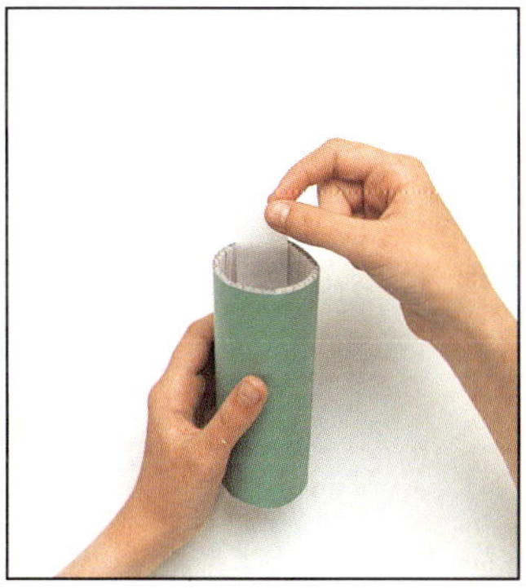

3 STICK MORE double-sided tape to the inward-facing parts of the straws. Now stick more straws to this tape to make a second layer.

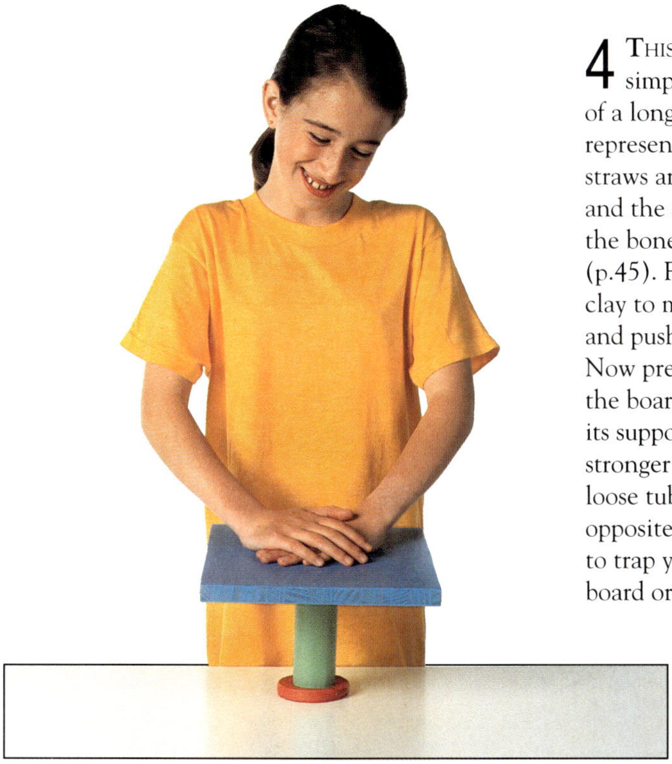

4 THIS TUBE of tubes is a simple model of the shaft of a long bone. The paper represents the periosteum; the straws are Haversian systems; and the space in the middle is the bone marrow cavity (p.45). Flatten the modeling clay to make a nonslip base, and push the tube into it. Now press on the tube with the board or the book to test its supporting strength. Is it stronger than the circle of loose tubes in the experiment opposite? (Be very careful not to trap your hands under the board or book.)

How bones heal

Bone has a great advantage over structural materials such as steel and concrete. If it breaks, it can mend itself. The self-healing process is more effective if the bone's broken ends are brought back into their natural alignment, a process doctors call "reducing a fracture."

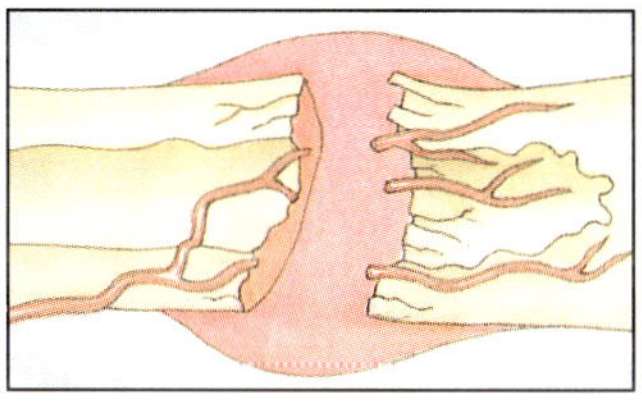

Within an hour
Healing of a fracture (break) begins almost at once. Leaking blood from the broken bone ends forms a clot.

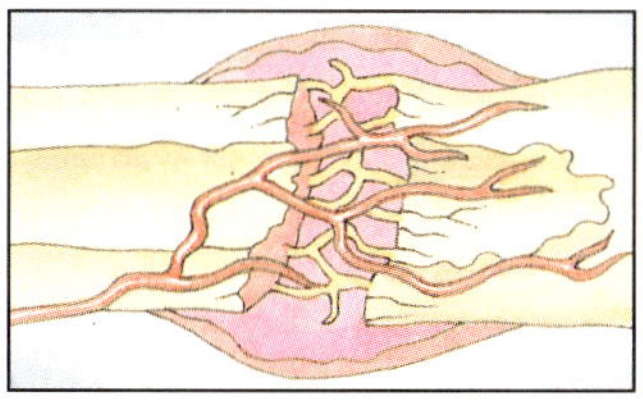

After a few days
Cells called fibroblasts and osteoblasts make an open network of spongy bone (p.44) in the gap.

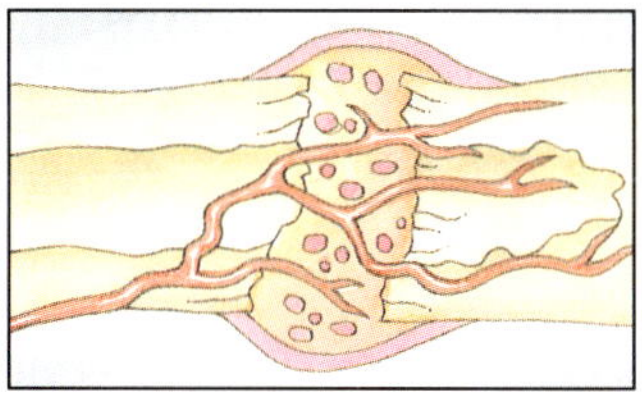

A week or two later
The spongy bone gradually fills in and becomes harder. Blood vessels have regrown and healed.

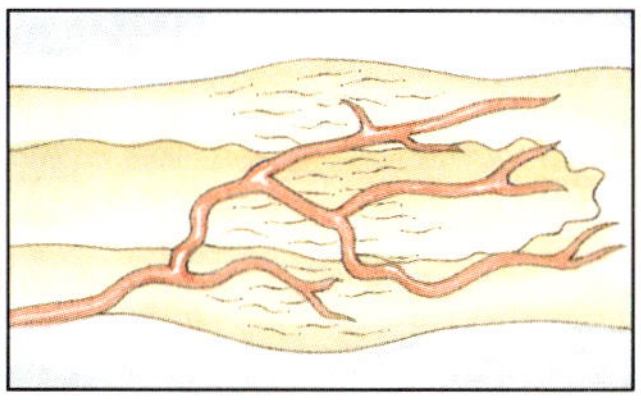

After 2 or 3 months
The bone is almost mended. The bulge at the break shrinks away, a process called bone remodeling.

Joints and levers

MANY OF YOUR BONES work as levers. They tilt to lift and move various parts of the body. The bones are connected by flexible joints, which allow them to move freely. To make body movements, your muscles pull on certain parts of the bones. The muscles, bones, and joints in the body work according to the same principles as those used by engineers who design lifting and moving machines, such as cranes and mechanical diggers.

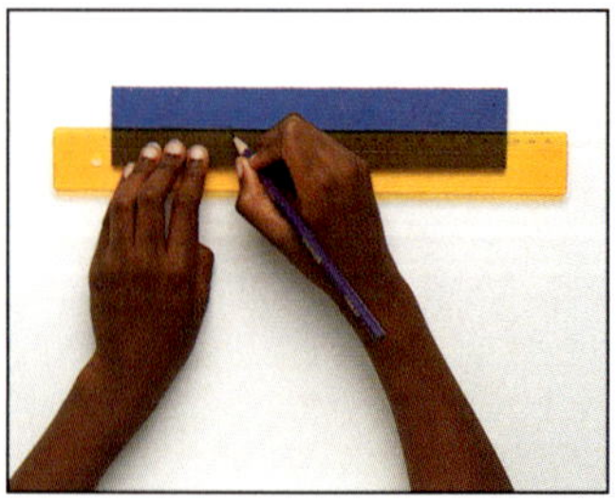

1 WITH THE PENCIL, draw a line along the middle of each poster-board strip. On one strip, make marks on this center line at $\frac{1}{2}$ in (1 cm) and 6 in (15 cm) from one end. Put marks on the other strip at $\frac{1}{2}$ in (1 cm) and 1 in (2.5 cm) from one end.

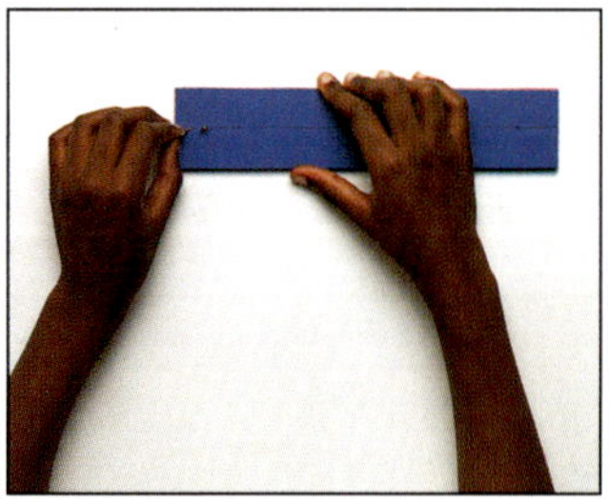

2 SCREW ONE EYE into each of the four marks that you have made. At the other end of each strip, make a new pencil mark 1 in (2.5 cm) from the end. This will be the site of the joint that is the "elbow" between two poster-board "arm bones."

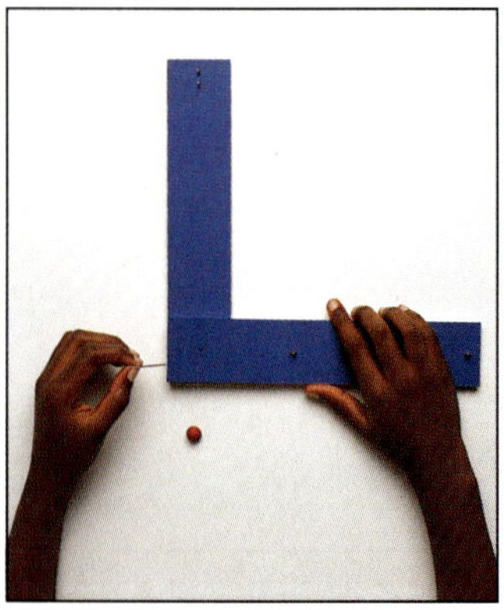

3 WITH THE NEW pencil marks on top of each other, form an L-shape with the strips. Carefully push the pin through the marks. Place a blob of clay on the sharp pin end, to cover the point and make it safe. Check that the "arm bones" move easily.

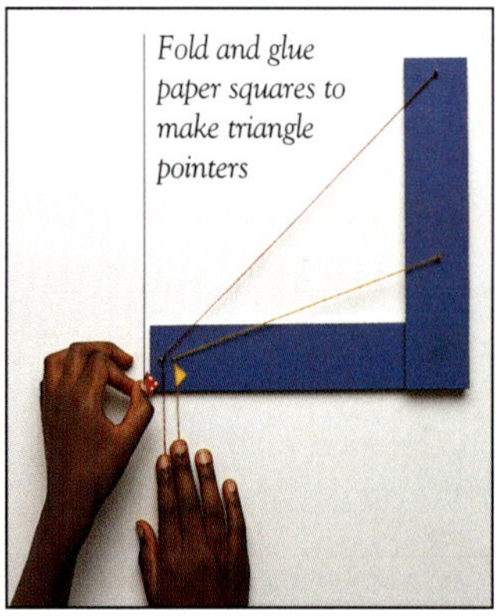

4 TIE A PIECE of string to each of the widely spaced eyes. Feed the strings through the corresponding eyes on the other strip. With the strips at right angles, glue a paper triangle pointer to the string of the same color, at a point just past the closely set eyes.

EXPERIMENT
Living levers

Adult help is advised for this experiment

Like all levers, many bones work by mechanical advantage; that is, when your muscles pull part of a long bone near a joint a small distance, the other end of the bone moves a much greater distance. A small movement is turned into a large one, so an advantage is gained. In this experiment you see the mechanical advantage of the biceps muscle, which moves the elbow.

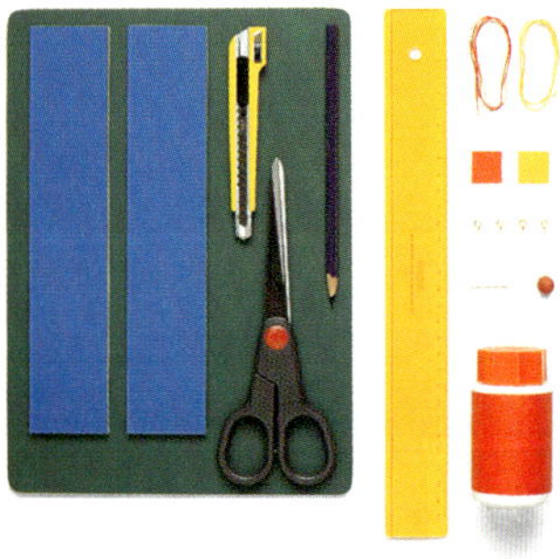

YOU WILL NEED

- *2 strips of stiff poster board 10 in x 2 in (25 cm x 5 cm)*
- *cutting mat*
- *craft knife*
- *ruler*
- *pencil*
- *scissors*
- *2 lengths of string in 2 colors*
- *small squares of paper colored to match the strings*
- *4 small metal screw eyes*
- *pin*
- *modeling clay*
- *glue*

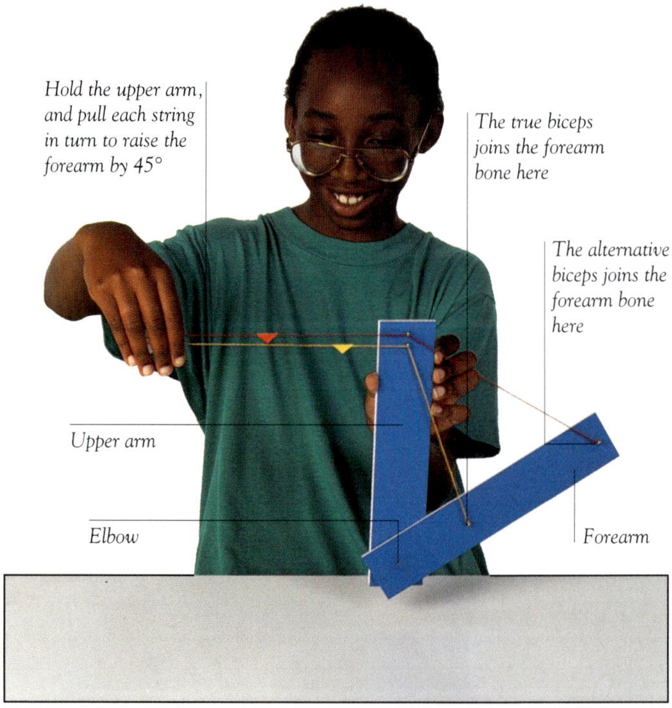

5 ONE STRING (yellow in the photograph above) represents the biceps (p.59), which pulls on the forearm when you lift things. The other string (red) represents an alternative muscle, which does not exist in the body. This muscle would also pull on the forearm, but at a point nearer the hand. Lift the forearm halfway, using each string in turn. Which pointer travels the shortest distance? This shows which string "muscle" raises the arm with the least amount of contraction, and so has the greatest mechanical advantage.

EXPERIMENT

Smooth-moving joints

Adult help is advised for this experiment

If the ends of bone pressed directly on each other in a joint, their rough surfaces would grate together and wear away. So inside a typical joint, the bone ends are covered with a smooth, glossy substance called cartilage. There is also a slippery "oil" called synovial fluid. These features greatly reduce friction (resistance or rubbing) in your joints, as this experiment shows.

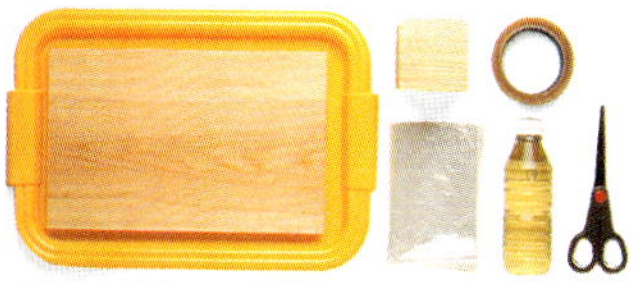

YOU WILL NEED

- *tray*
- *wooden board*
- *wooden block with natural sanded finish (not varnished or polished)*
- *cellophane tape*
- *plastic bag or plastic sheet*
- *cooking oil*
- *scissors*

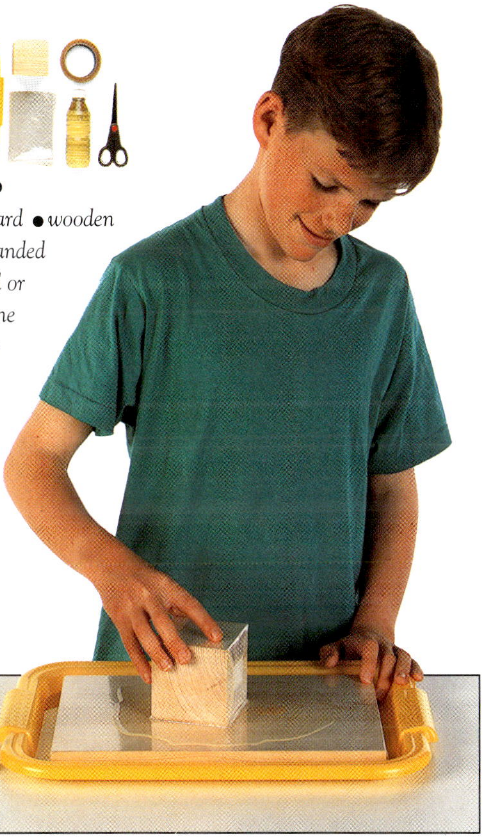

1 THE BOARD and block represent two bone ends in a joint. Press them together hard, and slide one against the other. Feel the friction.

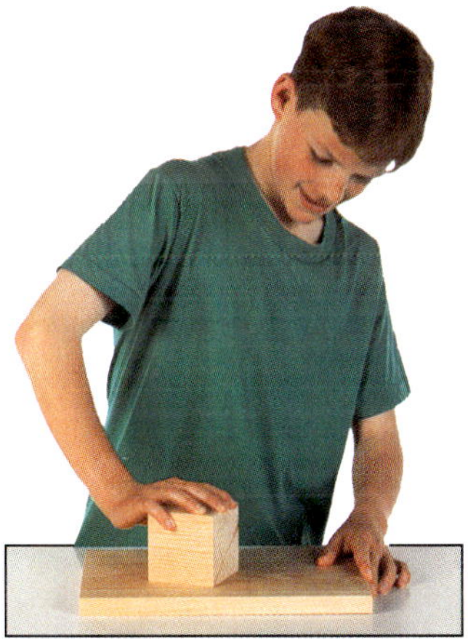

2 WRAP THE BOARD and block in plastic, taped in place. The plastic is smooth like cartilage. Feel how the "bone ends" slide more easily.

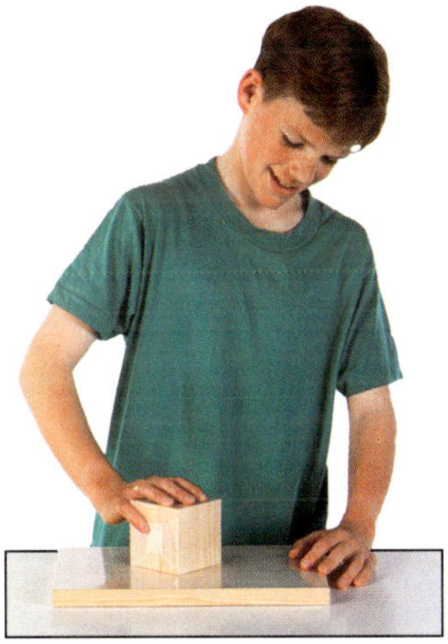

3 SMEAR SOME COOKING OIL on the plastic. Now feel how easy it is to slide the block over the board. The cooking oil works like the synovial fluid in the body's joints. It lubricates the cartilage surfaces to help them slide past each other, with little effort or wear.

Orders of lever

A lever is a rigid bar or rod that turns on a certain point, called the fulcrum. The lever moves a weight called the load, using a moving force known as the effort. There are three main orders (types) of lever—and the body has examples of all of them. In the body, the lever is a bone, the effort is supplied by a muscle, and the load is the weight of the body parts supported by the bone. Gently move your various body parts around, and see if you can identify which types of lever are involved in the movements you make.

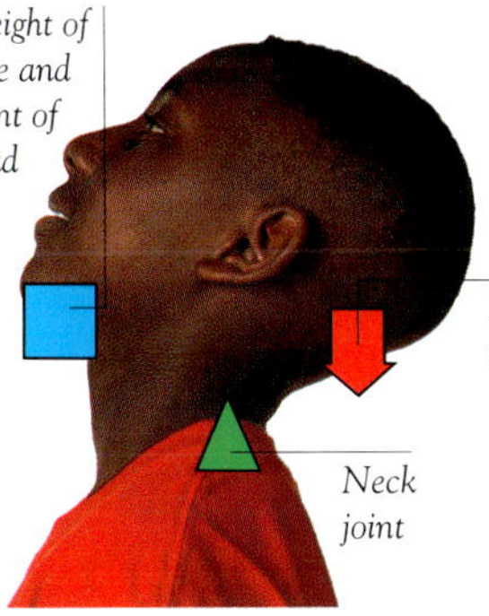

First-order lever

The fulcrum is between the load and the effort. The neck joint is an example of this, as the skull nods up and down, pulled by neck muscles.

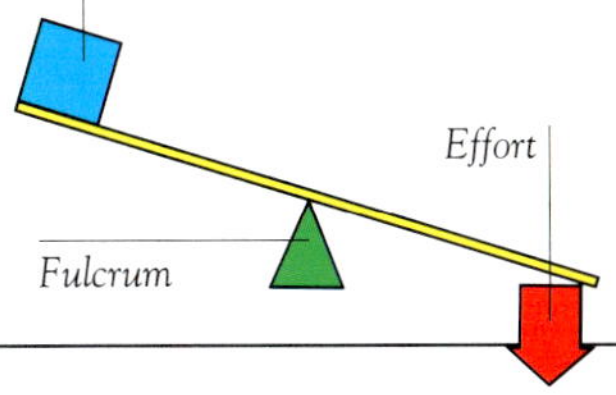

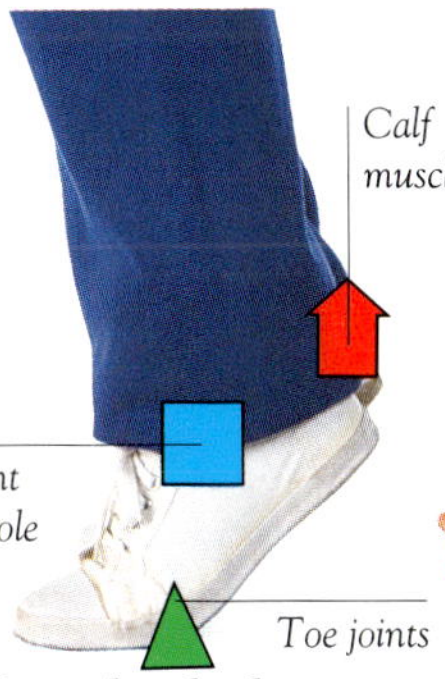

Second-order lever

Another possibility is for the load to be placed between the fulcrum and the effort. This happens when you stand on tiptoe.

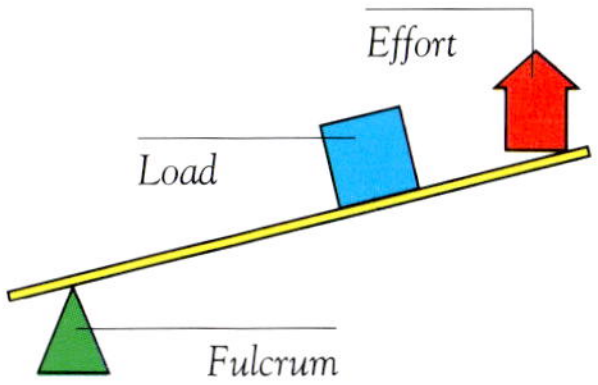

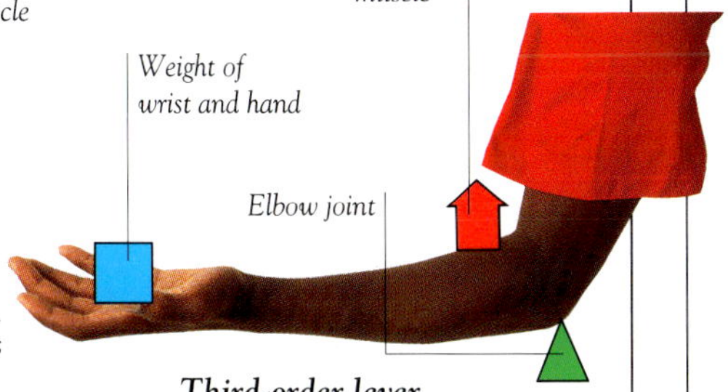

Third-order lever

In this type of lever the effort is in the middle, between the fulcrum and the load. This happens at the elbow joint in the arm.

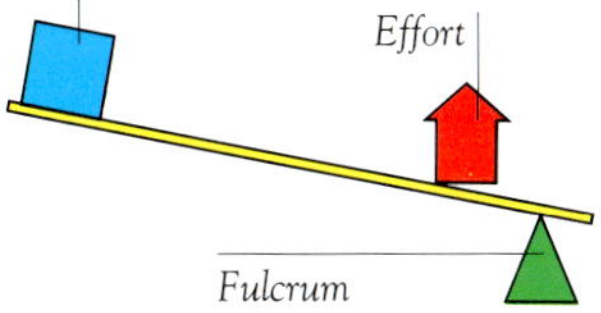

Types of joint

PEOPLE DESIGN different mechanical joints for different types of job. The hinge joint on a door, for example, could not replace the ball joint on a computer joystick. The body has many joints, and each is designed for a special job too. Your shoulder can move in almost any direction, like a joystick. Your elbow is less flexible, moving only to and fro, like a hinge. A joint that has high mobility usually has low stability. For example, a shoulder is more likely to be dislocated (put "out of joint") than an elbow.

EXPERIMENT

Knee joints

Adult help is advised for this experiment

The knee joint is the body's largest single joint. It is a hinge, which allows the leg to swing backward. The bottom of the femur (the main bone in your upper leg) and the top of the tibia (the main bone in your lower leg) are shaped so that, as the knee straightens, the femur slips into and sits in the tibia, "locking" the joint (below). Make a knee joint out of poster board that shows how the leg locks.

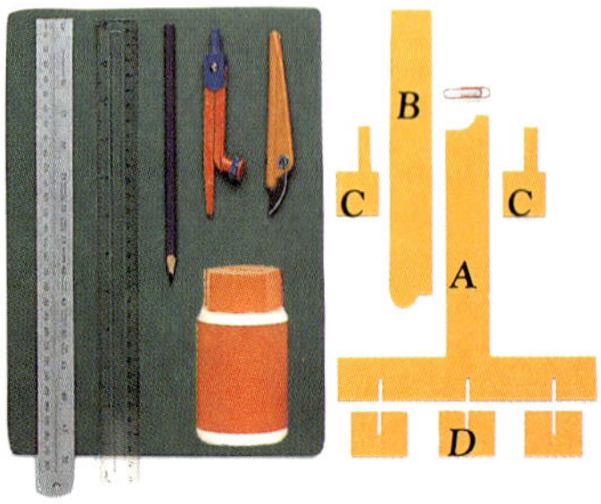

YOU WILL NEED

*● cutting mat ● metal ruler ● glue ● plastic ruler ● pencil ● compass ● craft knife ● paper clip ● thick poster board about 16 in x 8 in (40 cm x 20 cm) for cutting into 7 pieces; lower leg and foot (**A**), upper leg (**B**), 2 knee sides (**C**), and 3 foot supports (**D**)*

Shoulder and arm joints

There are many types of joint in your shoulder and arm. A bone often has more than one joint type. For example, the humerus has a ball and socket at the shoulder and a hinge at the elbow. The main joints have been color-coded below, with simplified representations showing their range of movement.

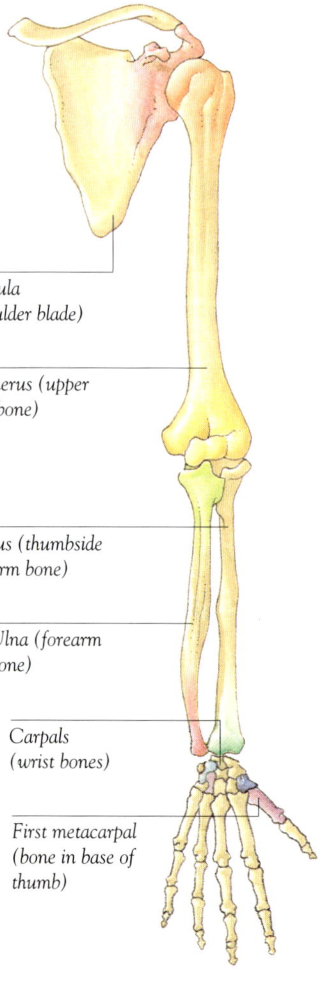

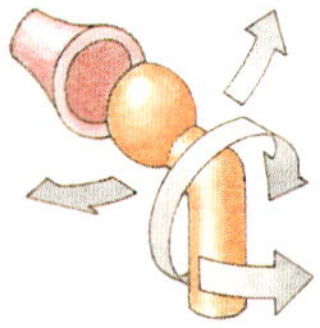

Ball and socket
The top of the humerus (orange) has a ball-shaped head that fits into a shallow, cup-shaped socket formed by the scapula (red). This gives good all-around mobility.

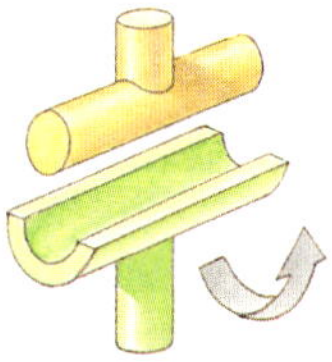

Hinge
The humerus (yellow) and the ulna (green) move to and fro in one plane only, like a door hinge. Other elbow movements are made by twisting the shoulder or forearm.

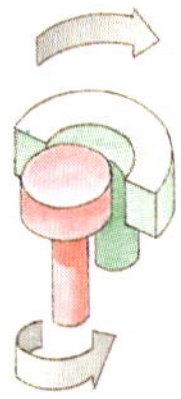

Pivot
As the wrist twists, a C-shaped notch in the end of the radius (green) pivots around the rounded end of the ulna (red). This joint is also called a swivel joint.

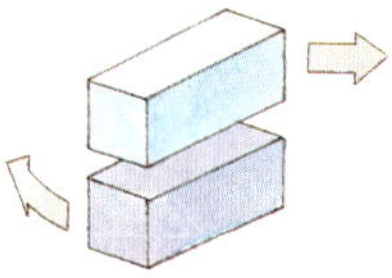

Plane
There are about 20 joints between the eight carpal bones. The plane joint between the bones colored light blue and violet allows small amounts of sideways movement.

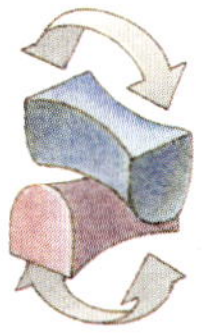

Saddle
Wiggle your thumb at its joint with the wrist. It can tilt in all directions. The bone ends (dark blue and maroon) are shaped like saddles and slide smoothly over each other.

Stable positions

Each joint has a position in which its bones fit together most securely. For example, when you stand upright, your knee joints are "locked" and your muscles do not have to use up valuable energy to prevent your body from collapsing to the floor.

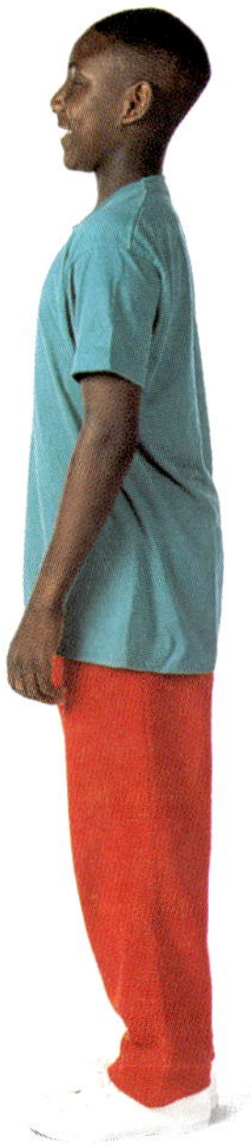

Knees straight
In their locked position, little muscle power is required.

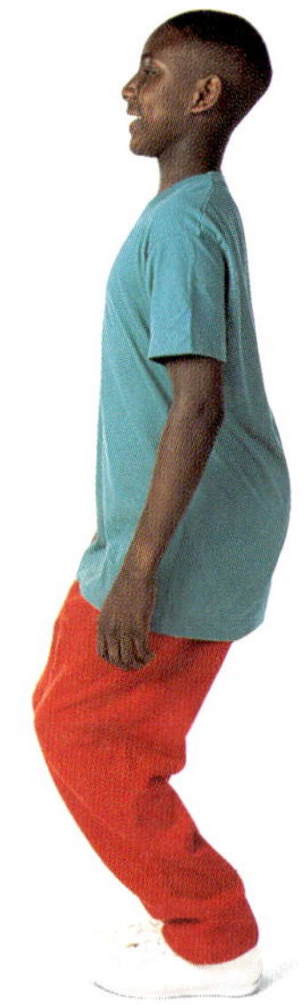

Knees bent
Muscles take the strain. How long can you stand like this?

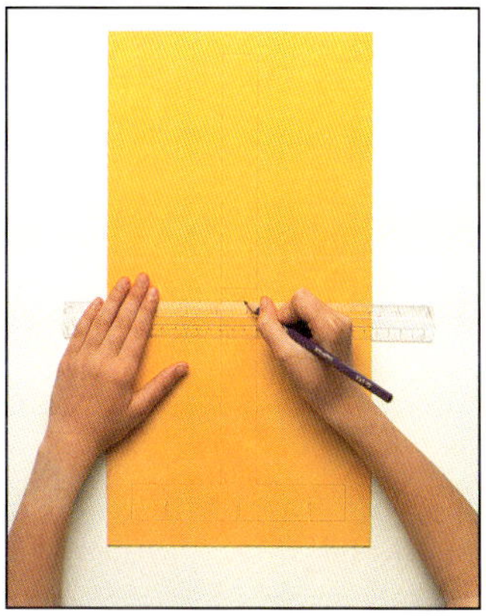

1 DRAW AN upside-down "T," 1½ in (3 cm) wide, 14 in (35 cm) tall, with a base of 7 in (18 cm). Draw three slots in the base and a line halfway up the upright. Below this line, against the left edge, draw a half circle of radius ½ in (1 cm). Draw a short line from the lowest point on the half circle to the left edge.

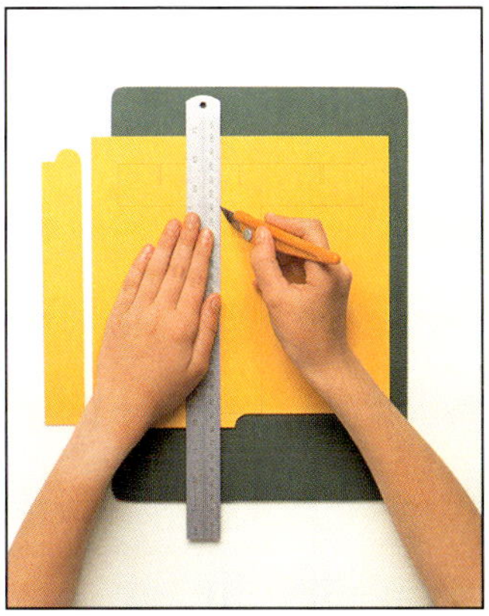

2 CUT ACROSS the short line, around half of the half circle, and along the long horizontal line to the other side of the "T." This divides the "T" into a lower leg (**A**) and an upper leg (**B**). For **B**, trim the rest of the half circle to leave a knob as above. Cut off excess poster board and cut out the slots in the base.

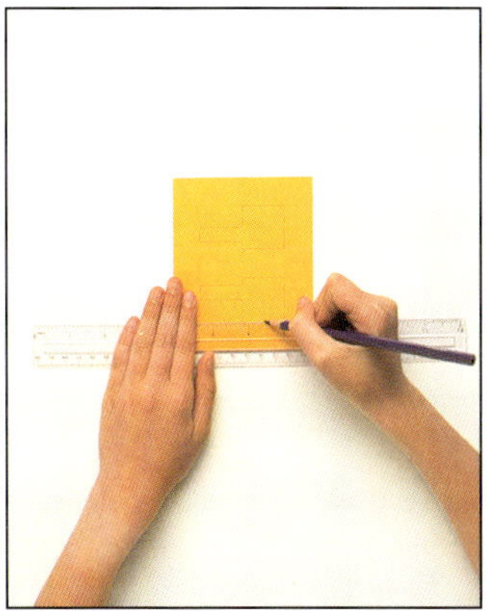

3 DRAW TWO shapes for the knee sides (**C**). Each is a square with 1½-in (3-cm) sides, and a 1½ in x ½ in (3 cm x 1 cm) rectangle set ¼ in (0.5 cm) from a corner of the square. These shapes must be mirror images of each other.

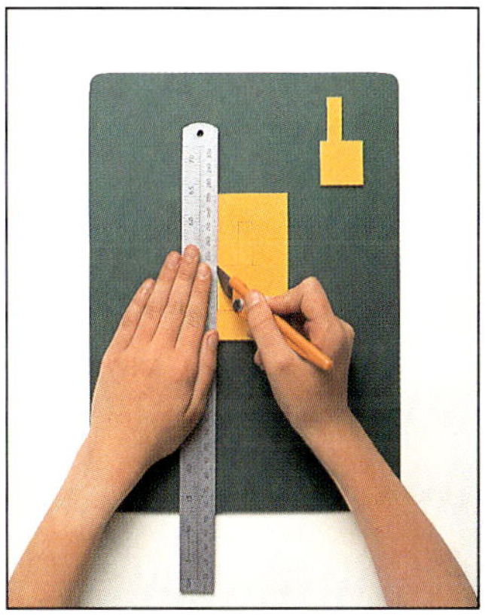

4 CAREFULLY CUT out each knee side. In the model they keep the upper leg from collapsing sideways. In the real knee this job is done by ligaments—bundles of taut fibers attached to bone or cartilage (p.179).

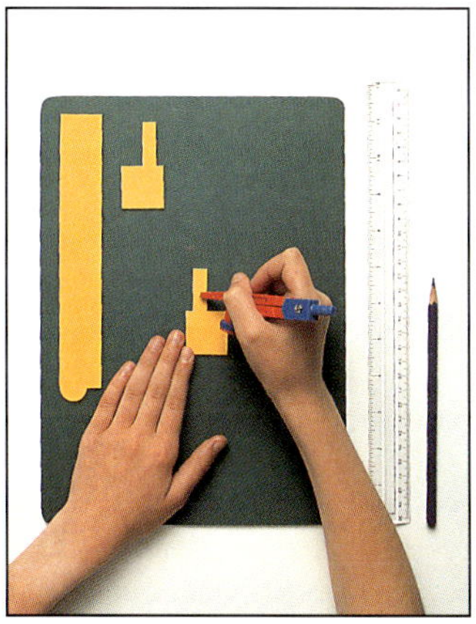

5 CAREFULLY make a hole in each knee side, using the compass. Make it in the midline of the projecting rectangle, ½ in (1 cm) from the square. Now make a hole in the center of the knob on the upper leg (**B**).

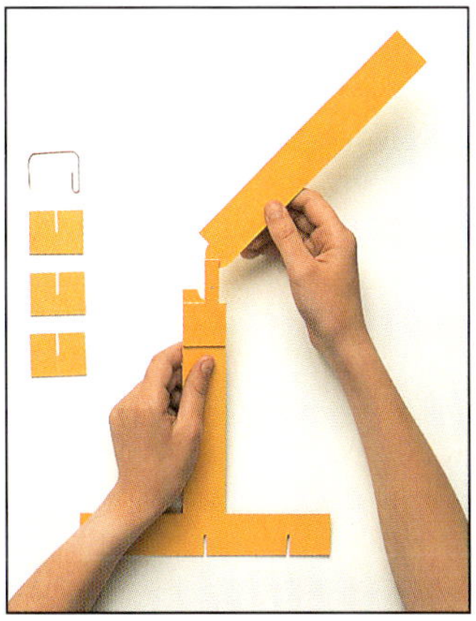

6 GLUE THE KNEE sides to **A**, with the holes in line with the top of **A**, at the center of the cutaway half circle. Cut out supports (**D**), each 2 in x 1½ in (5 cm x 3 cm), with a small slot. Unbend the paper clip.

7 SLOT THE UPPER LEG between the knee sides, so that the three holes line up. Push the paper clip through the holes, and bend it to secure the joint. Slot in the supports (**D**). Now stand your model knee upright. See how the upper leg balances on the lower leg. The flat part of the top of the upper leg (on a real femur this is a knuckle-like part called a condyle) prevents the body from falling forward. Now push the upper leg backward. The upper leg collapses. There is no "lock" there.

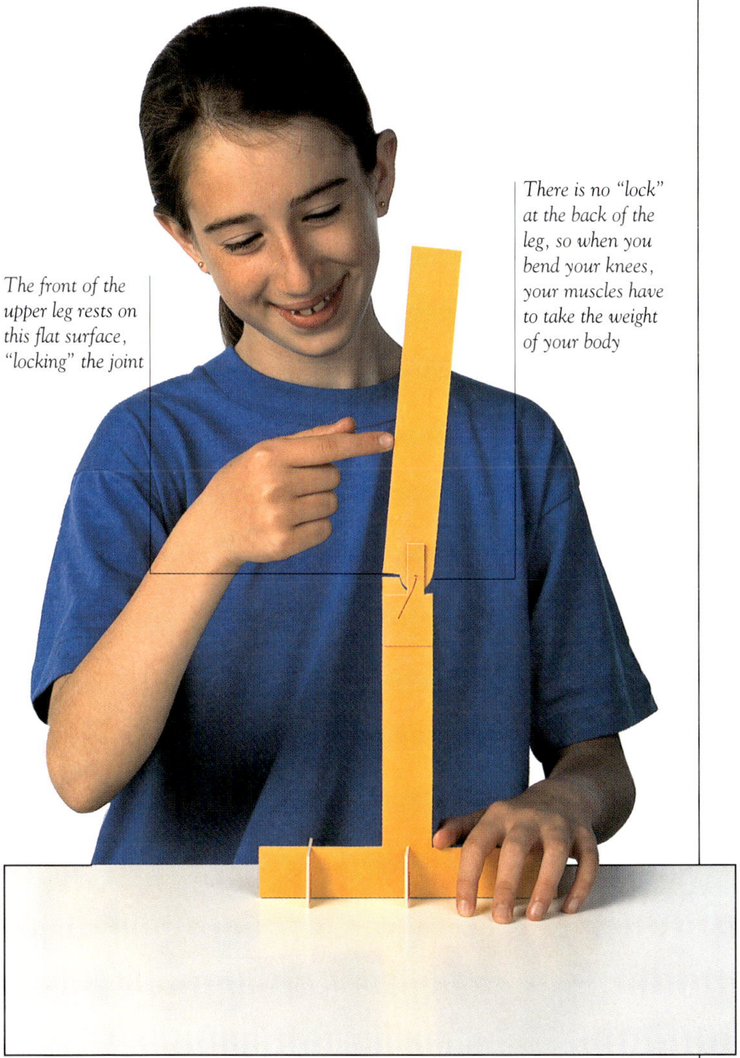

The front of the upper leg rests on this flat surface, "locking" the joint

There is no "lock" at the back of the leg, so when you bend your knees, your muscles have to take the weight of your body

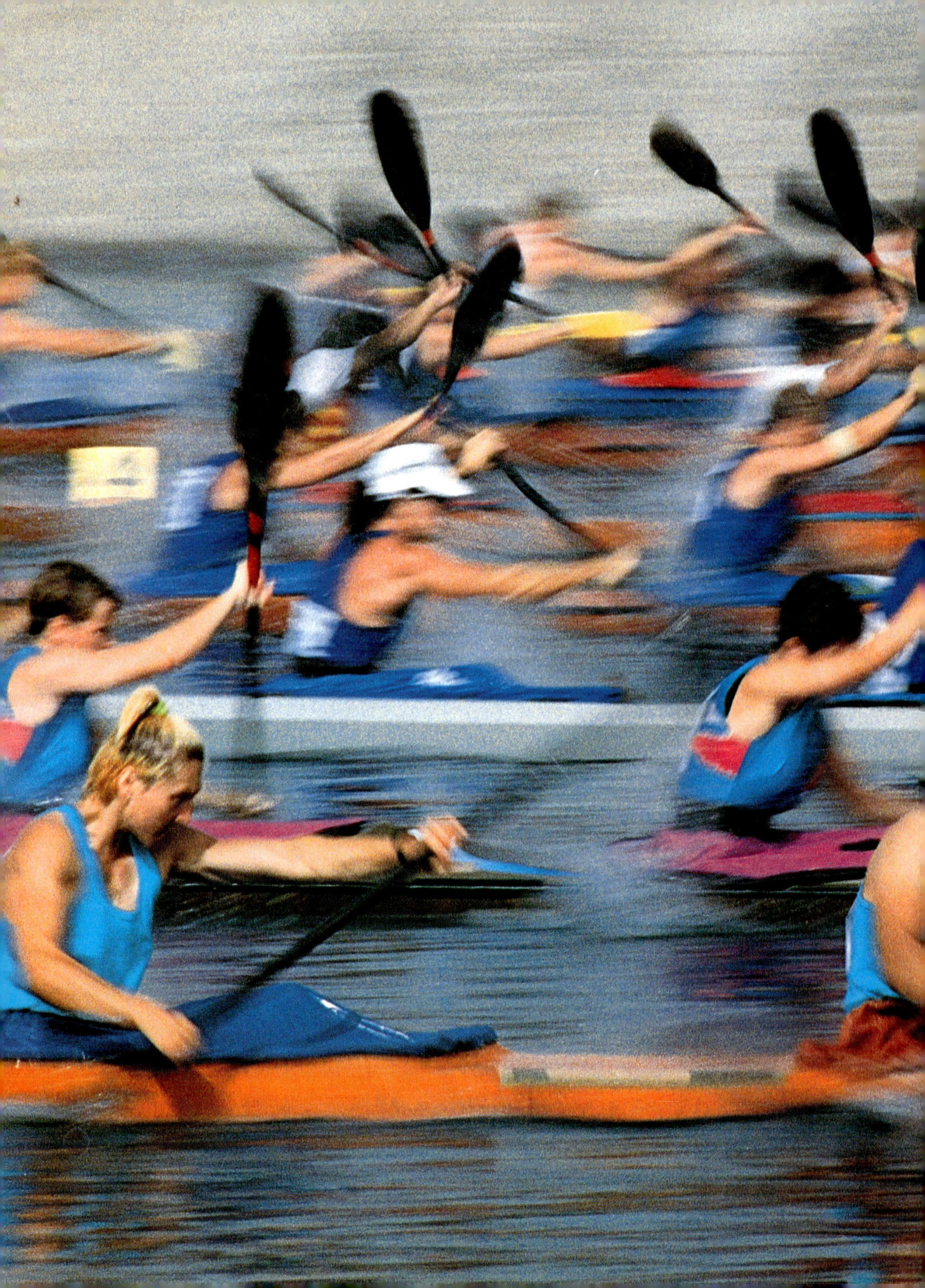

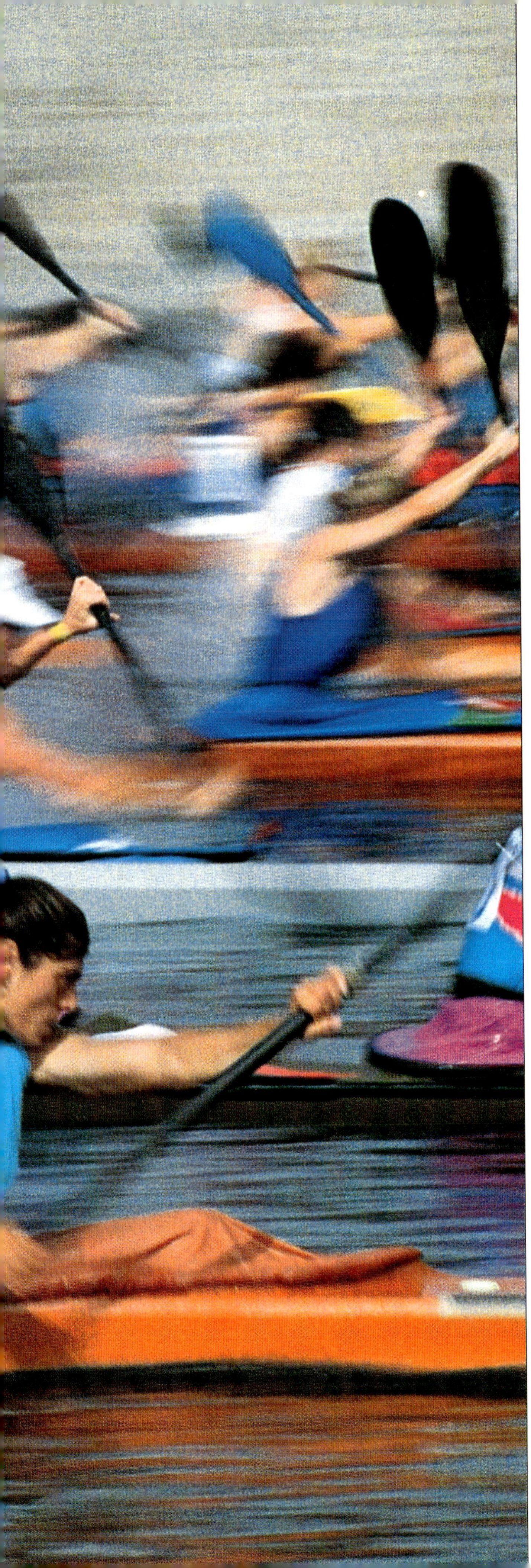

The MOVING BODY

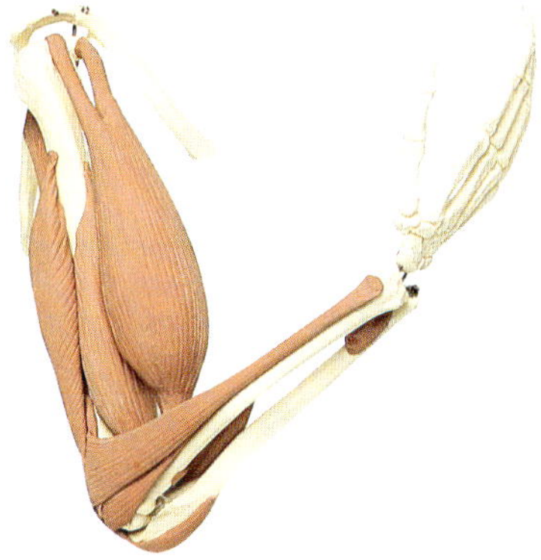

Teaming up
Many body muscles are arranged in pairs. In the arm (above), one muscle makes the elbow bend, while its partner makes it straighten. Even simple body movements rely on large teams of muscles. The canoeists (left) use more than 50 muscles in each arm, together with dozens more muscles in the chest and abdomen, to propel their boat.

THE HUMAN BODY IS MOVED by muscles. There are about 640 skeletal (body-moving) muscles, most of which are attached to the bones of your skeleton. Muscles can only pull, not push. They pull on the bones to shift them into new positions. Controlled in teams by your brain and nerves, muscles enable you to perform a huge range of movements—running and jumping, pulling and pushing, bending in half, and guiding thread through the eye of a needle.

MUSCLES AND MOVEMENT

MUSCLES ARE RESPONSIBLE FOR all of the body's movements, from kicking a ball and writing a letter to squeezing digested food through the intestines and making the heart beat. The body's biggest single muscle is the huge gluteus maximus in the buttock, which drives your climbing, running, and leaping movements. The smallest muscle is the stapedius in the ear, which looks like a tiny piece of thread. It reduces the vibrations of sounds that are too loud.

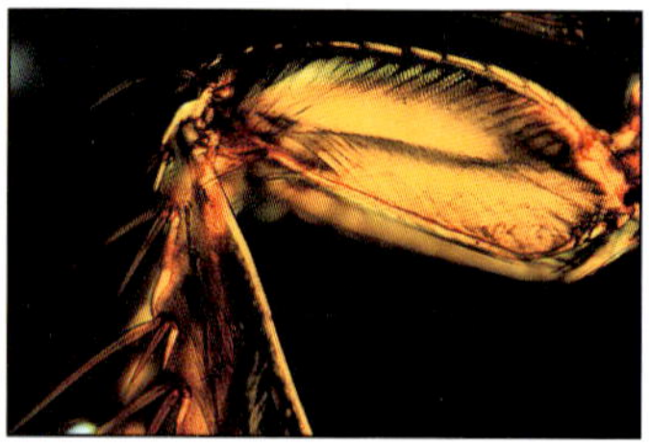

***The leaping flea can jump more** than 100 times its own height. The burst of muscle power in its back legs is boosted by energy stored near the joints in blocks of a special elastic-like substance called resilin.*

Muscle tissue very similar to our own is found in all kinds of animals, from worms and insects to cows and whales. Animal muscle is what we think of as "flesh" or "meat," from the red meat of cattle and pigs to the white meat of poultry and fish. Ancient peoples knew a great deal about the muscle layouts of many different kinds of animal because, like many people now, they consumed animal muscle as food.

Animal spirit

In ancient times, the anatomists of Egypt, Greece, and Rome all studied the shapes of muscles and how they work. Some of the first studies were made by Erasistratus (c.300–250 B.C.), who belonged to the great medical school in Alexandria, Egypt.

Erasistratus recognized that muscles cause movement by becoming shorter and pulling on the body's bones. But he also believed, wrongly, that muscles were made to shorten and bulge out when an invisible "animal spirit" flowed along the nerves to the muscles.

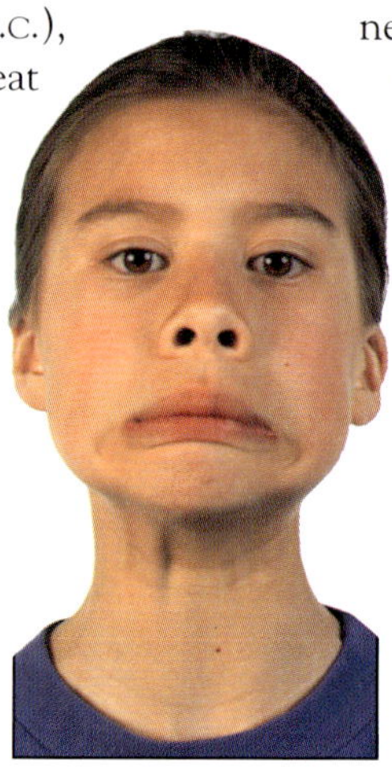

***Facial expressions** are made by the actions of over 40 facial muscles (p.61).*

Myology

Galen (p.13) of ancient Rome made some excellent descriptions of muscles in various animals. In particular, he studied the muscle layouts of the Rhesus monkey—the same animal in which the Rhesus blood system was discovered earlier this century (p.102). Galen noted how a typical muscle's wide, fleshy main part, the body or belly, is attached to a bone at either end by a strong cordlike part known as a tendon or sinew.

During the Renaissance period, myology (the study of muscles) progressed significantly. Leonardo da Vinci (1452–1519) and Andreas Vesalius (p.22) both drew in great detail the 640 or so individual muscles in the body. (We do not all have exactly the same number of muscles. In certain people some muscles—such as the platysma in the neck—may be much reduced in size or even absent.)

It was not just Renaissance anatomists who looked at the design of muscles in great detail. Renaissance artists studied muscles too, so that they could draw and paint the body's bulges and ripples as accurately as possible.

The way that muscles work has been studied by engineers as well as by scientists and artists. Engineers wanted to copy the way that muscles work in teams (p.60), so that they could apply the same principles to machines.

Most muscles are arranged in opposing pairs around the body. This is because a muscle can only pull—it cannot push. One muscle or set of muscles pulls part of the body one way, and an opposing muscle or set pulls it back again.

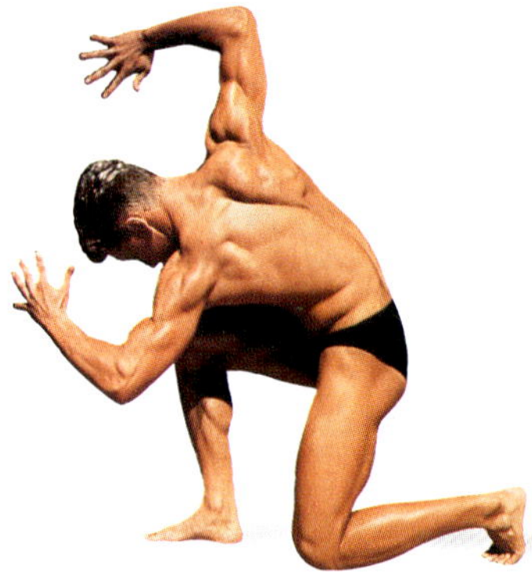

***The bulging muscles visible just** under the skin are only the outermost of three or four layers of skeletal muscles.*

Working in these so-called antagonistic pairs (p.62), muscles can produce a huge range of movements.

Inside muscles

By the 1600's scientists understood the body's muscle layout in detail. But people still had little idea of how the insides of each individual muscle work.

With the invention of the microscope, there was a great deal of progress. Niels Stensen (1638–86) from Copenhagen, Denmark, was a physician, anatomist, geologist, and later a bishop. In 1664 he described how at a microscopic level a muscle is made of hundreds of tiny muscle fibers (p.181). Stensen realized that different combinations of these fibers contract (shorten) and then relax as the body makes different movements. The greater the number of fibers that shorten, the more the whole muscle contracts. When the fibers relax, the whole muscle relaxes too.

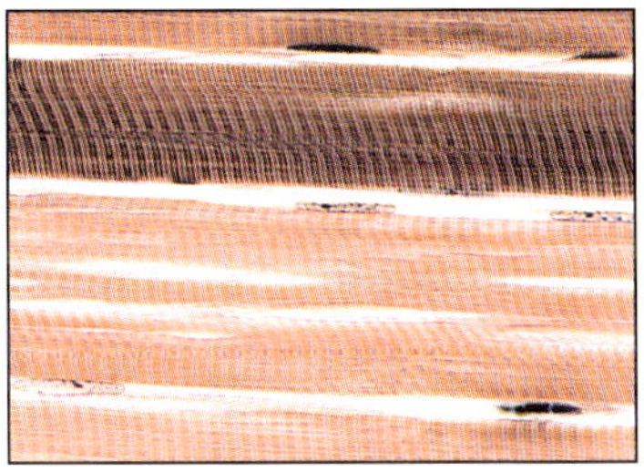

***The faint vertical stripes in these** rodlike muscle cells give skeletal muscle (p.58) the alternative names of "striped" or "striated" muscle.*

Muscle contraction

From the time of Erasistratus, it was thought that muscles increased in volume when they contracted. But in the 17th century this notion was shown to be wrong. In a famous experiment the Dutch microscope expert Jan Swammerdam (1637–80) immersed the leg muscle of a frog in a measuring bath of water. When the muscle was stimulated to contract by pinching the nerve connected to it, the water level stayed the same. This showed that contraction does not change the volume of a muscle, but is instead a result of changes within the muscle fibers.

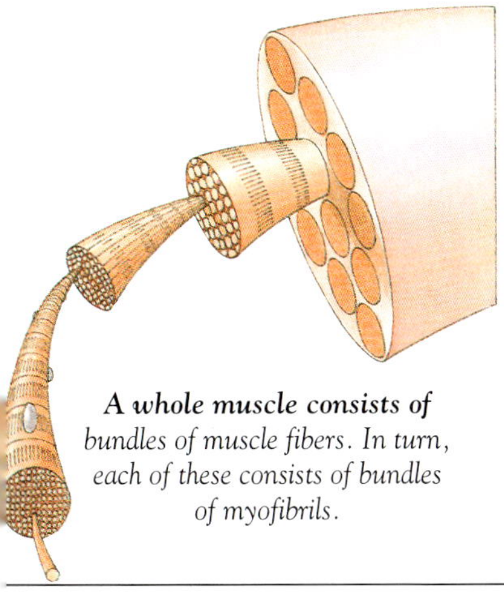

***A whole muscle consists of** bundles of muscle fibers. In turn, each of these consists of bundles of myofibrils.*

A muscle fiber, which is thinner than a hair, can be up to 1 ft (30 cm) long in a large muscle. Yet it is a single giant cell (pp.26–27). Each muscle fiber is made of collections of even thinner fibers called myofibrils. These consist of long strands of two proteins, actin and myosin. When the muscle is stimulated, the actin pulls the myosin along past it, like a line of people tugging on a rope. This slide-past mechanism makes the myofibril shorten, causing the muscle fiber to contract, and the whole muscle becomes shorter.

Energy and control

In the 17th century physiologists discovered that muscles use the sugar glucose as their main source of energy. The glucose energy is released by cellular respiration (pp.70–71), using oxygen, which is brought to the cells by blood. When a muscle is active, blood vessels to it and within it widen to increase the blood supply.

Another 17th century discovery was that muscles are controlled by the nerves, called motor nerves (p.118), connecting them to the brain.

Types of muscle

The microscope shows that there are three types of muscle (p.59). Each type has a different function and is made of a different kind of tissue (p.185).

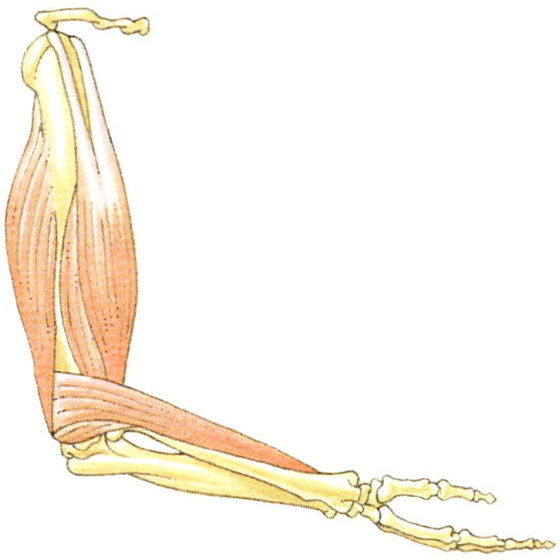

***To lower your hand, the triceps** (p.59) in the back of your upper arm contracts and straightens the elbow, aided by gravity.*

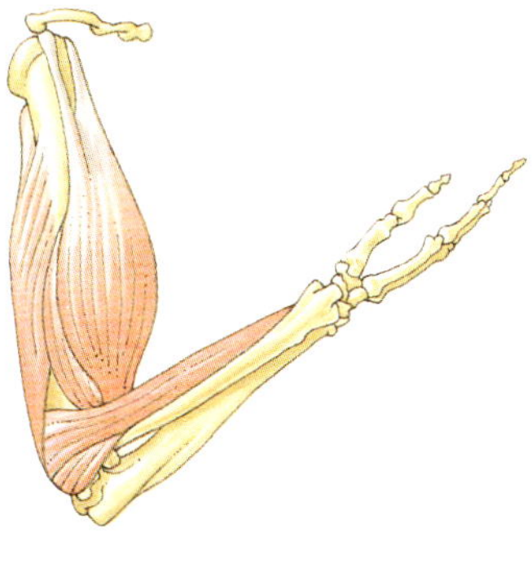

***To raise your hand, the biceps** in the front of your upper arm contracts and pulls up the bones of your forearm.*

Muscles attached to the bones are called skeletal muscles. The cells of these muscles are arranged in parallel bundles, and within these bundles each cell has a striped pattern. Skeletal muscle is therefore also called striped or striated muscle. As we can control the actions of our own skeletal muscles, they are known as voluntary muscles too.

The muscle layers of internal organs, such as the stomach and the intestines, are a second type of muscle called smooth muscle. This muscle type contracts more slowly than skeletal muscle, but uses much less energy. It is responsible for automatic (autonomic) muscle actions such as peristalsis (p.89).

The walls of the heart are the third type of muscle, called cardiac muscle. This muscle continuously sends blood pulsing around the whole body. Because you cannot consciously control the actions of smooth and cardiac muscles, these types are also known as involuntary muscles.

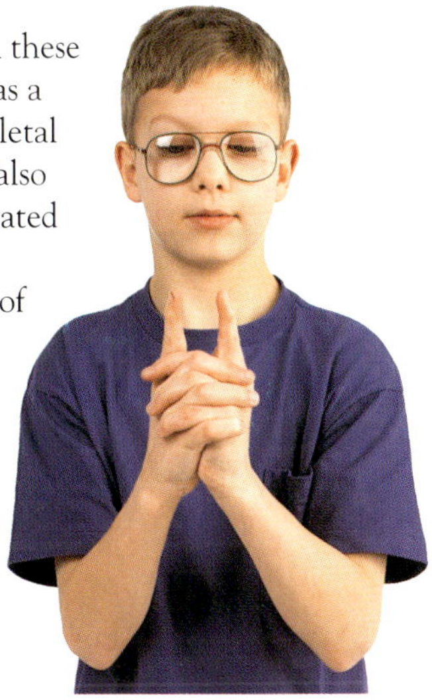

***See how your forefingers move** mysteriously and return to their relaxed state, unless you hold the muscles that work them under tension (p.58).*

Muscles

ABOUT TWO-FIFTHS of your body weight is muscle. There are three types of muscle: skeletal, smooth, and cardiac (opposite). Most of the muscles shown on the following pages are skeletal muscles. Skeletal muscles are designed to contract (get shorter). By doing so, they pull your bones to make you move. They are also known as voluntary muscles, since you can control them voluntarily (at will), unlike the involuntary muscles in parts such as the stomach. Muscles are controlled by electrical signals from the brain. The more signals that arrive, the more the muscle contracts, until it reaches its minimum length—about three-fifths of its relaxed length.

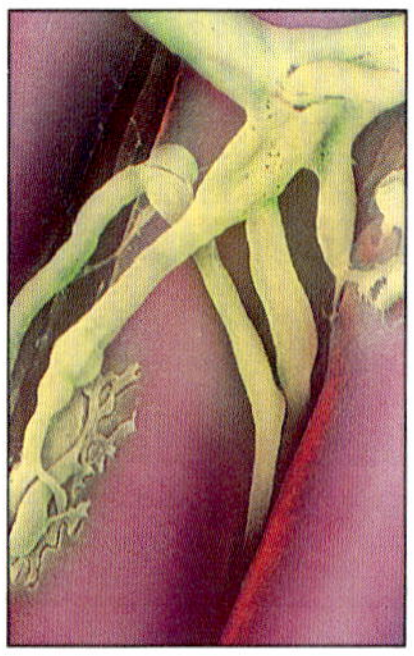

Nerve to muscle
This microscope photograph shows muscle fibers as huge pink rods. The yellow fingerlike parts are the end branches of a nerve. They form a structure called a motor end plate. This is where nerve signals pass from the nerve into the muscle.

Achilles' heel

In ancient Greek mythology, Achilles was a hero of the siege of Troy. When he was a baby, his mother dipped him in the magical River Styx to make him invulnerable. But Achilles was slain when an arrow pierced his one weak point—the heel where his mother had held him. The large tendon in the heel is named the Achilles tendon (opposite) after the myth.

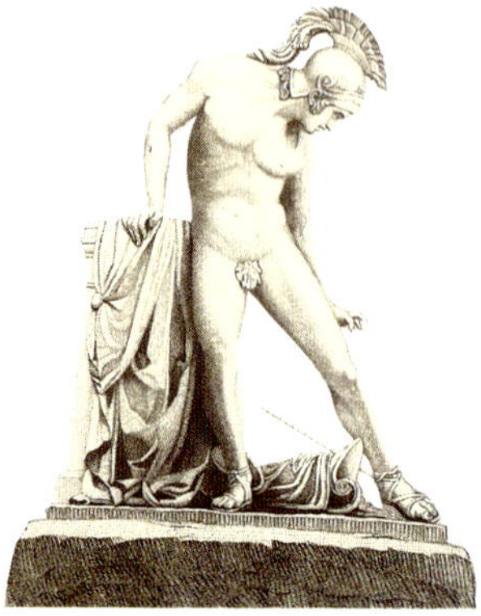

The Greek hero Achilles
This engraving shows the fatal arrow piercing Achilles' heel.

EXPERIMENT

Relaxing fingers

When they are not active, muscles and tendons have natural relaxed positions, in which they use minimal energy. In the resting hand, for example, the fingers are slightly bent under tension from the muscles and tendons. Show this by clasping your hands with your fingers interlocked. Hold your forefingers straight and parallel. Do your forefingers stay parallel when you let your muscles relax, or do they move together?

Moving fingers
Hold your forefingers up like this and see what happens when you relax your muscles.

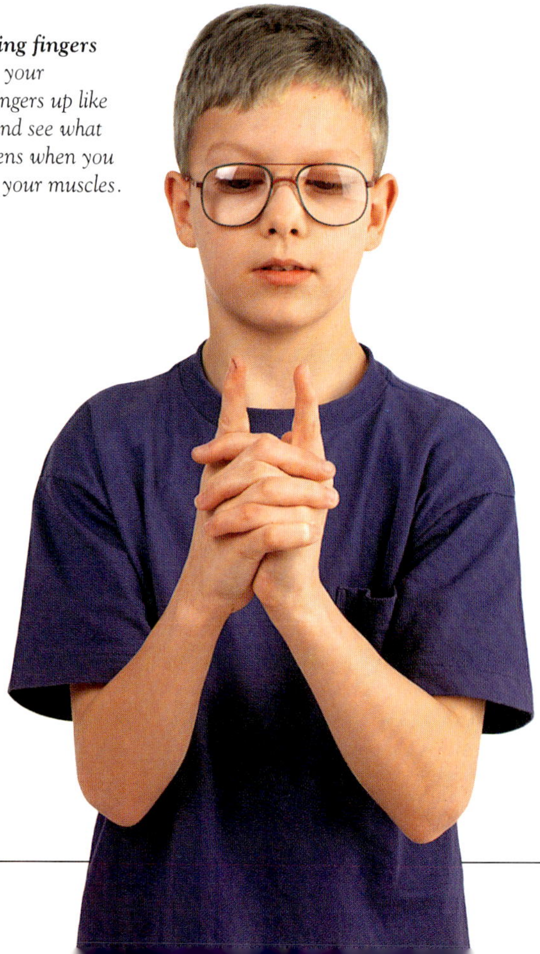

EXPERIMENT

Tightening tendons

A typical muscle has a wide fleshy part, called the body or belly, which shortens when you move. The narrow, ropelike ends of the muscle, called tendons, anchor the muscle to bones. As you move parts of your body, you should feel the tendons tightening as they pull on the bones. Feel how they stand out under your skin, like taut ropes.

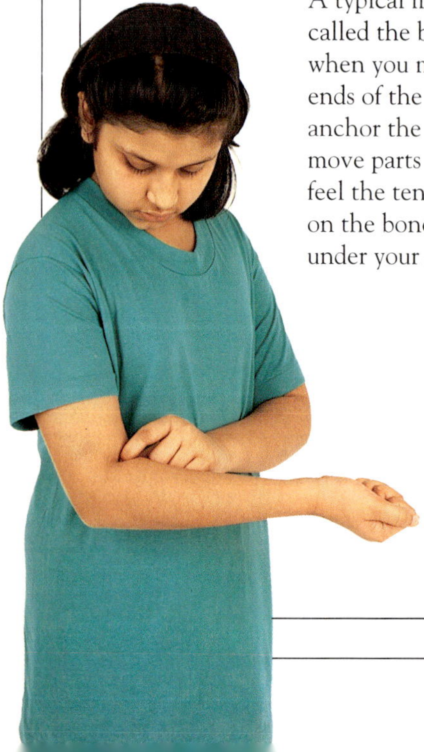

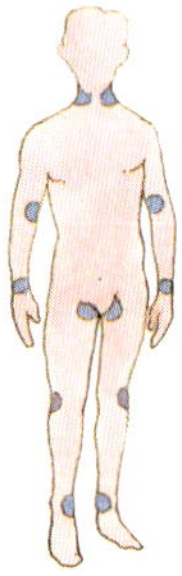

Tendon points
Tendons show up particularly well in the elbows, neck, and other areas shaded in gray. As you tighten your muscles, feel for their taut tendons under your skin.

Muscle maps

These charts show the main muscles at the front and back of your body. However, the muscles shown here are only the superficial muscles—those just under the skin. Beneath them is a middle layer and under that a deep layer. Most muscles have Latin names derived from the movements they produce or the names of nearby bones.

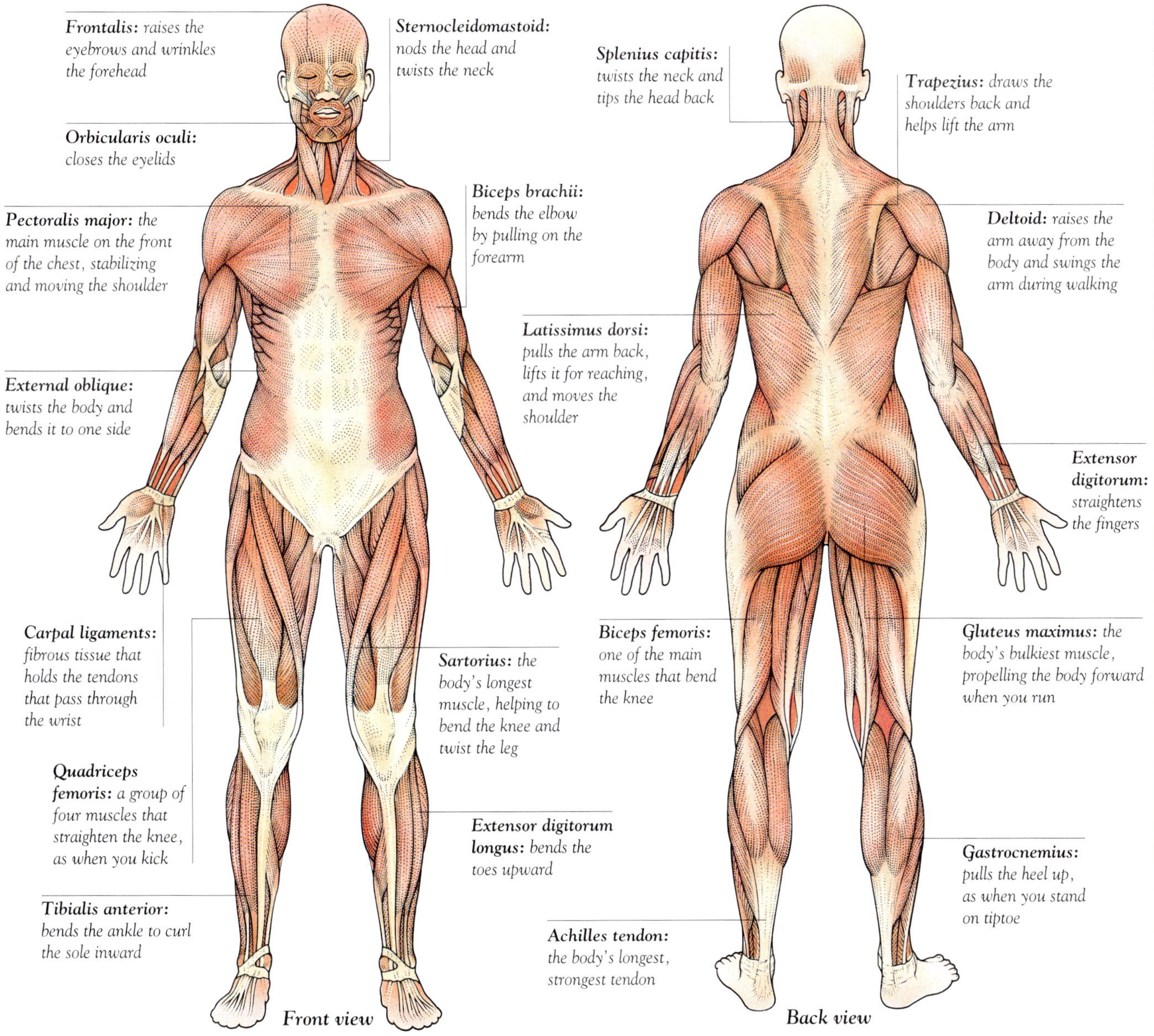

Types of muscle

When magnified, the three types of muscle tissue (p.57) look different. Skeletal muscle cells are rodlike and line up parallel to each other. Smooth muscle cells are thinner and spindlelike. Cardiac muscle has Y-shaped interwoven cells.

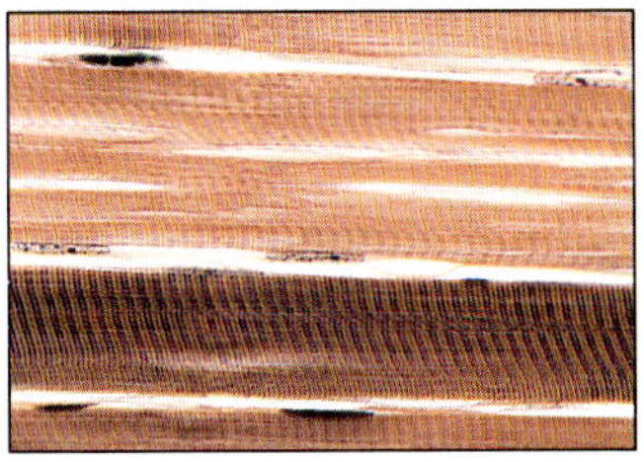

Skeletal (voluntary)
Found throughout the body. It can contract powerfully, but tires easily.

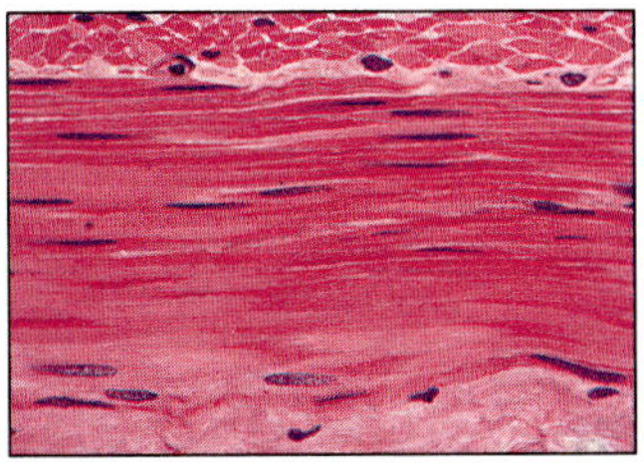

Smooth (involuntary)
Found in internal organs. It can stay contracted for long periods.

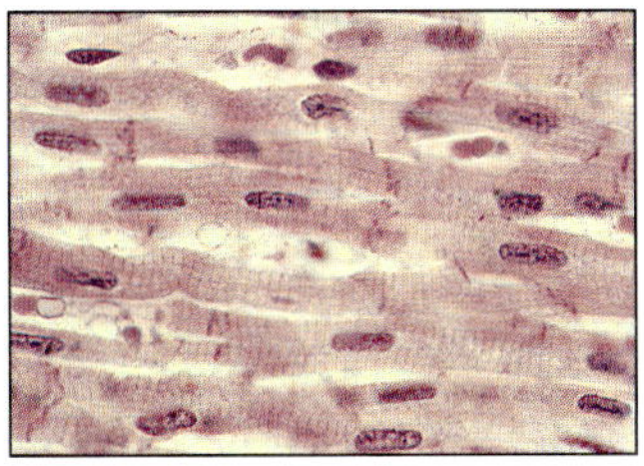

Cardiac (involuntary)
Found in the heart. It contracts every second or faster, yet never tires.

Muscle teams

HOLD YOUR ARM straight out to the side, then bend your elbow. You will feel your biceps, the main muscle on the front of your upper arm, tense as it contracts and pulls on your forearm. But a single muscle hardly ever works on its own. As you bend your elbow, the other muscles in your shoulder, upper arm, and forearm adjust to cope with the new positions of the arm bones. Some of these muscles contract, since they have to take up the strain, while others relax, as the strain has been shifted away from them. Whole teams of muscles around the body adjust and shift even for small movements of one body part. You make most of these minor changes almost without thinking. Your brain learned how to control muscle teams, and how to keep your balance and posture, during the first years of your life.

EXPERIMENT

The stuck finger

Each of your fingers has its own tendons attached to the finger-pulling muscles in your forearm. On the back of the hand there is an "intertendon connection" linking the tendons that run to the middle finger and the ring (fourth) finger. Curl up your middle finger on a tabletop, stretch out your other fingers, and see how this intertendon connection makes your ring finger completely immovable.

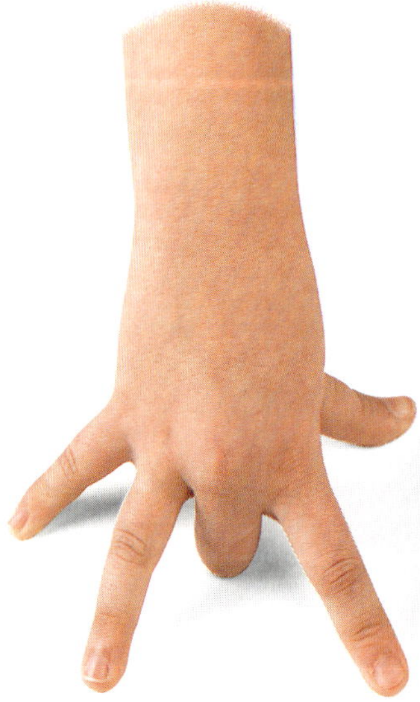

Trying to lift your ring finger
Place your hand fingertips down on a table, with your middle finger curled under. Try to lift your other fingers, one by one. You will be able to lift all of your fingers—except the ring finger.

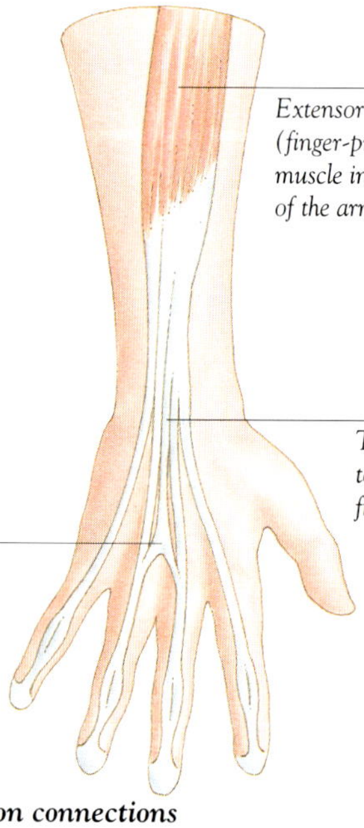

Tendon connections
Tendons to the forefinger and middle finger are not linked, but those to the middle finger and ring finger have an intertendon connection. This restricts their ability to move on their own.

EXPERIMENT

Muscle links

In some body parts, one muscle can cause several movements, because the muscle is linked by different tendons to several bones. An example is the muscle in your forearm that curls your fingers. Bend your middle finger, and see how your other fingers curl up too.

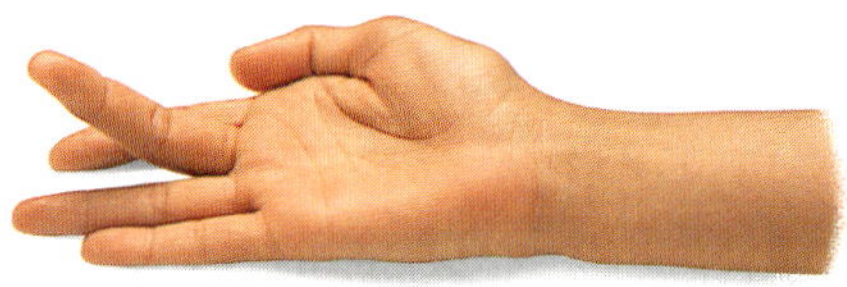

1 PLACE YOUR HAND palm up, flat on a table. Raise your middle finger slowly, keeping it as straight as possible.

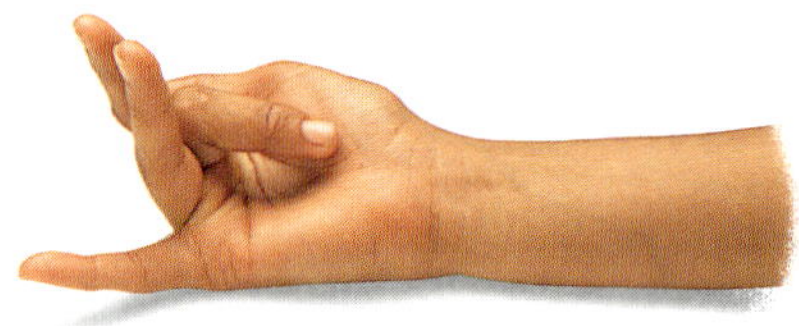

2 WHAT HAPPENS to your ring (fourth) finger? Keep raising the middle finger. Does your forefinger move?

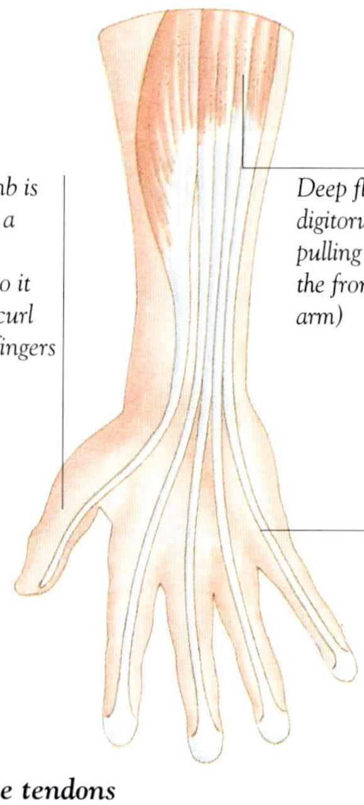

Multiple tendons
The finger-pulling muscle has four main tendons. Each is attached to a finger bone. As the muscle shortens to pull on the middle finger, it also pulls on the other three fingers and lifts them too.

Face muscles

Many of the muscles in the face are attached not to bones, but to each other, or to the skin. We use these muscles to make the huge variety of facial expressions that convey our thoughts, moods, and emotions. We also use these muscles for such activities as eating, speaking, and blinking.

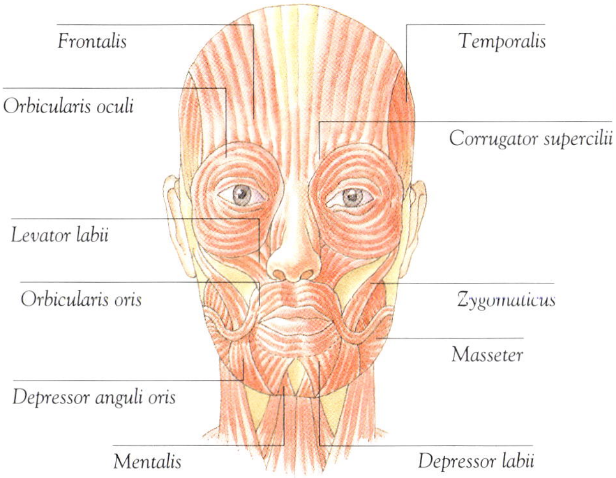

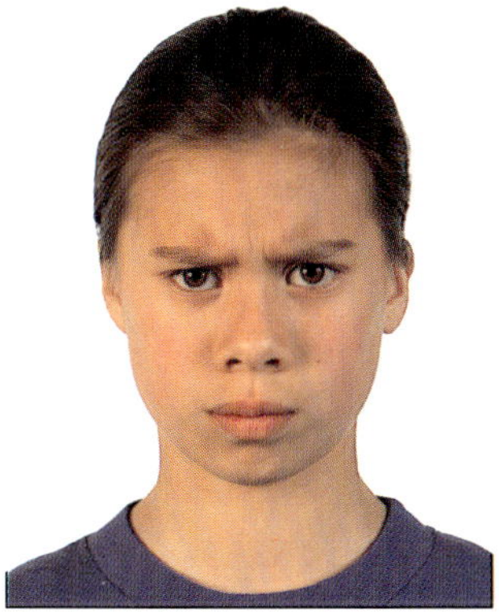

Disapproval
Corrugator supercilii wrinkles the brow in a frown.

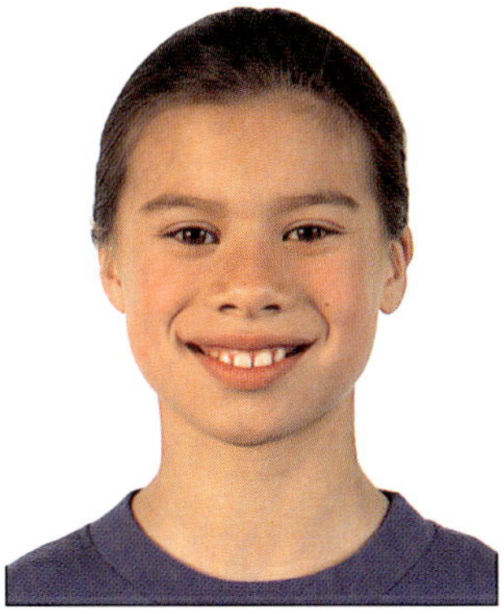

Happiness
Zygomaticus pulls the mouth corners up and out in a smile.

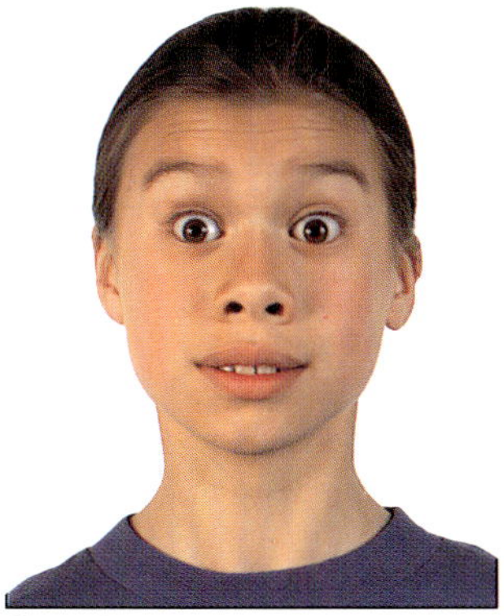

Surprise
Frontalis raises the eyebrows and exposes more of the eyes.

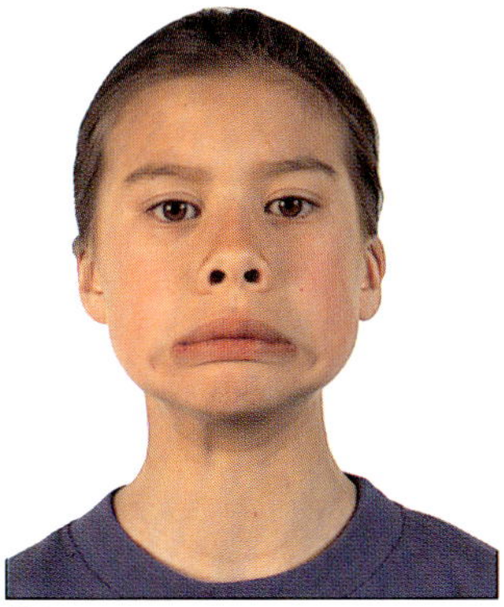

Disgust
Depressor anguli oris lowers and widens the corners of the mouth.

EXPERIMENT

Changing muscle teams

See how the muscle teams in your body change and are replaced by other teams as you move. Choose a movement—such as taking a drink of water—and do it slowly, stage by stage. Feel for the tensed muscles and their taut tendons at each step. Which muscles are involved at each of the stages?

YOU WILL NEED

- *cup of water*

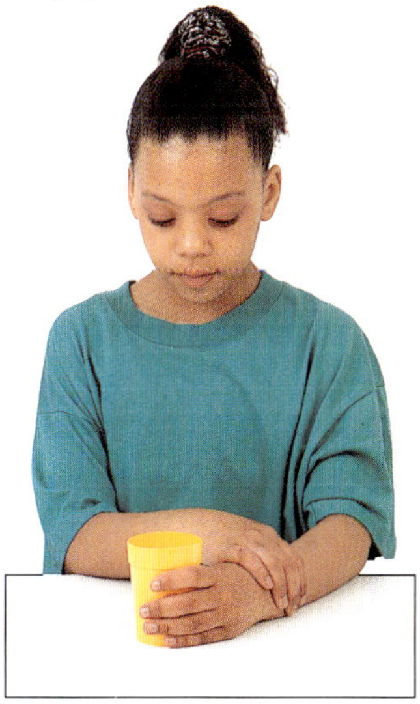

1 PUT YOUR forearm on the table, and grip a cup. Feel the muscles and tendons on the inside of your forearm and wrist, bending your fingers.

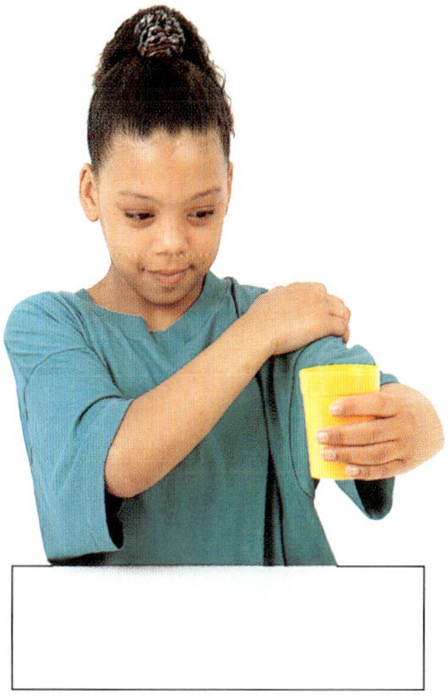

2 SLOWLY RAISE your arm. Press gently around your shoulder to feel muscles such as the deltoid and trapezius, which help to move the arm.

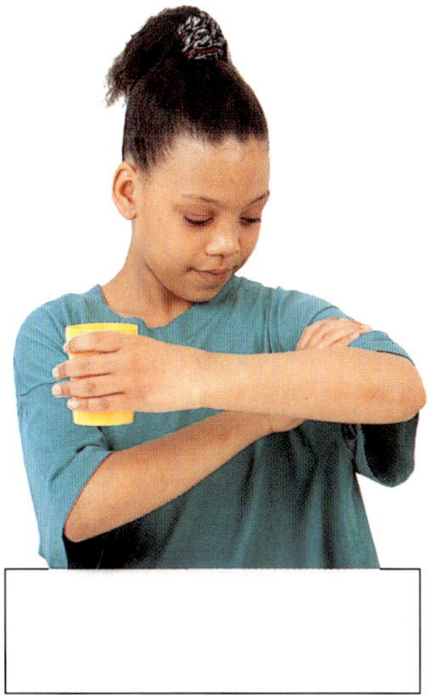

3 BEND YOUR elbow to bring the cup near your mouth. Feel the biceps, the main elbow-flexing muscle, on the front of your upper arm.

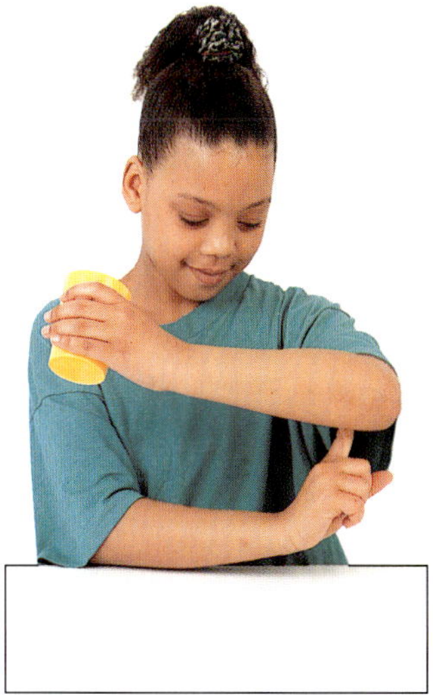

4 TWIST YOUR forearm and wrist to tilt the cup, as if to drink. See how the muscle on the inside of your elbow tightens as you tilt the cup.

Muscle pairs

AN INDIVIDUAL muscle moves its part of the body by contracting (getting shorter) and pulling on the bone that it is attached to. To let the whole body push, pull, and make all its other movements, muscles are usually arranged in pairs, one on each side of a bone. This means that the bone can be pulled in one direction or the other. Muscles that produce opposing pulling forces in this way are called antagonistic pairs.

EXPERIMENT

Making a model of an arm

Adult help is advised for this experiment

In an antagonistic pair of muscles, one muscle pulls a bone in one direction. The other muscle is sited on the other side of the bone. When this muscle contracts, it pulls the bone the other way. As this happens, the first muscle relaxes and is passively stretched. You can make a model of an arm with an antagonistic pair of muscles—the biceps and the triceps—in its upper part. One of these muscles contracts to bend the elbow; the other contracts to straighten it. Working alternately, they can make your arm wave its hand. You can stick "bones" made of poster board to your model arm to make it look more realistic.

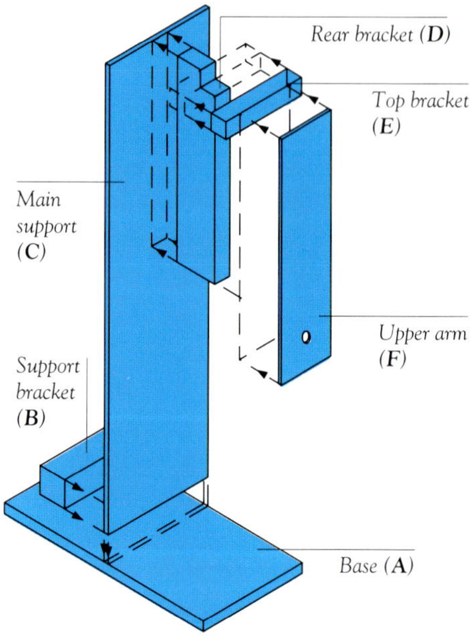

Arm stand
This is an exploded view of parts for the stand. Bolt the lower arm (G—see below) to the upper arm (F) with the washers, so that it can move up and down easily.

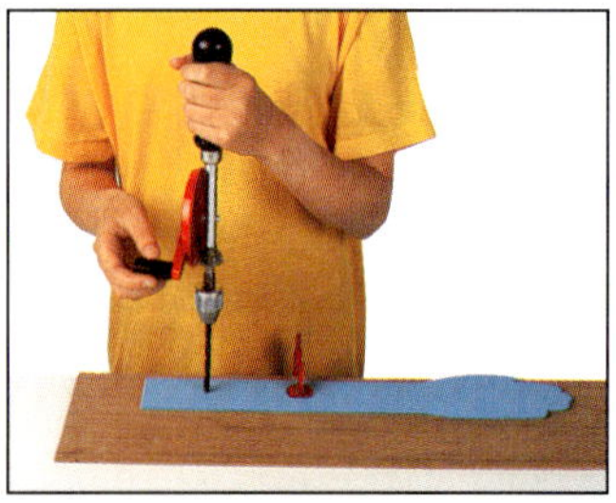

1 CLAMP THE lower arm (G) to the drilling board. With adult help, carefully drill a hole on the center line, $2\frac{1}{4}$ in (6 cm) from its elbow end. The bolt will pass through this hole.

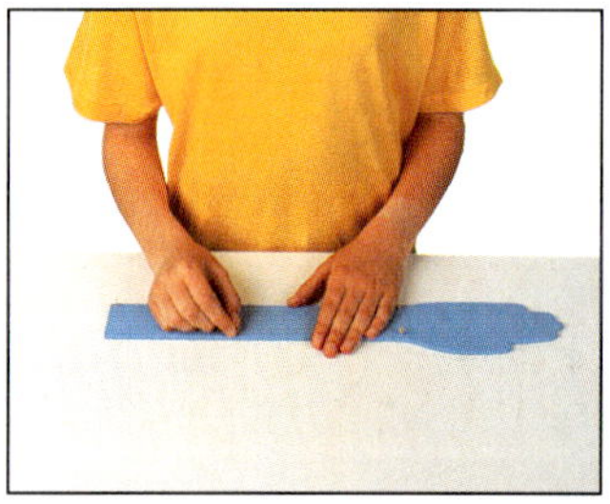

2 SCREW IN the four small eyes: one on each side of the wrist, where hand and arm join; one at the outside corner of the elbow; and one 5 in (12 cm) from the elbow on the inside.

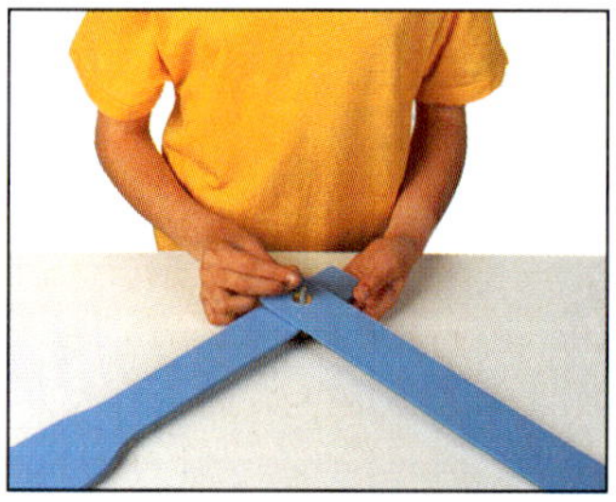

3 DRILL A hole in the upper arm (F), on the center line, $1\frac{1}{2}$ in (3 cm) from the elbow end. Bolt G and F together, with washers under the bolt head and nut, and between the arm parts.

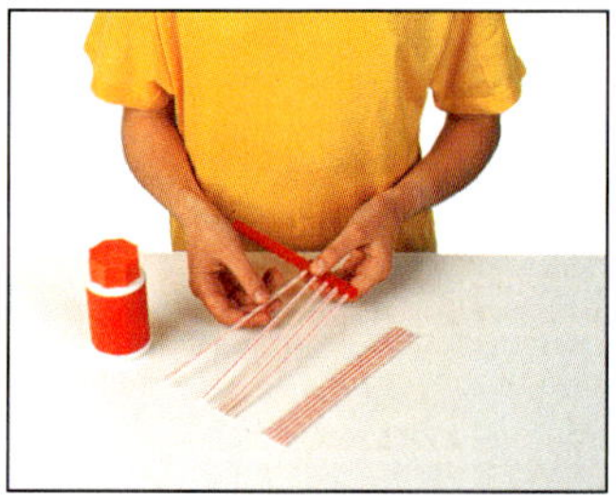

4 GLUE THE ends of the straws into the holes in a strip of corrugated plastic. Space the straws out, so that you use about 12 to 15 straws along the 8-in (20-cm) length of the strip.

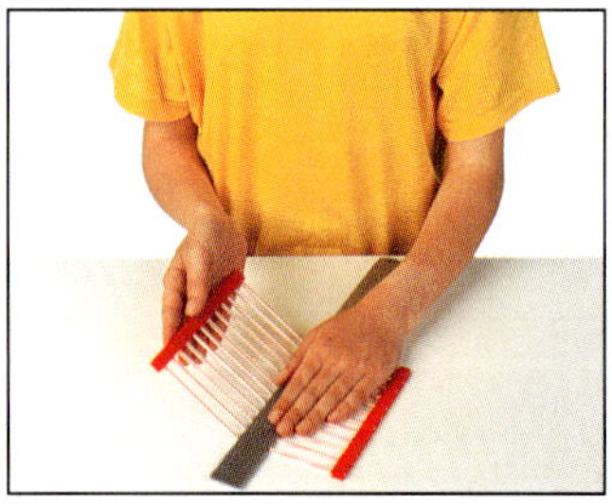

5 GLUE THE other ends of the straws into another corrugated strip. Let dry. Then, with the metal ruler, press on the straws halfway along and crease them, so that they will bend easily.

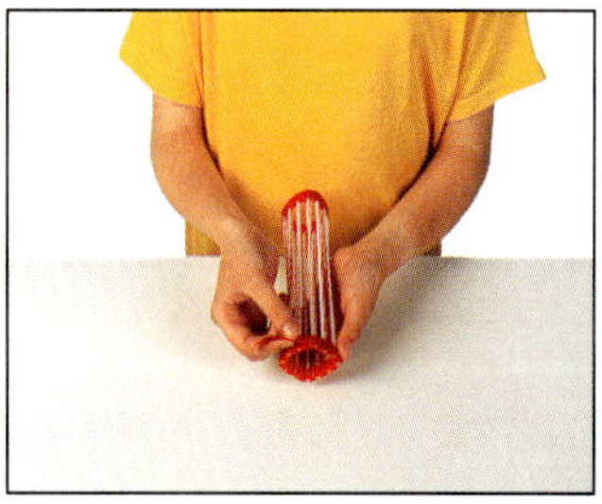

6 ROLL THE strips and straws to make a cylinder-shaped cage, and tape with duct tape. Make sure the creases let the straws bend outward when the ends of the cage are pushed together.

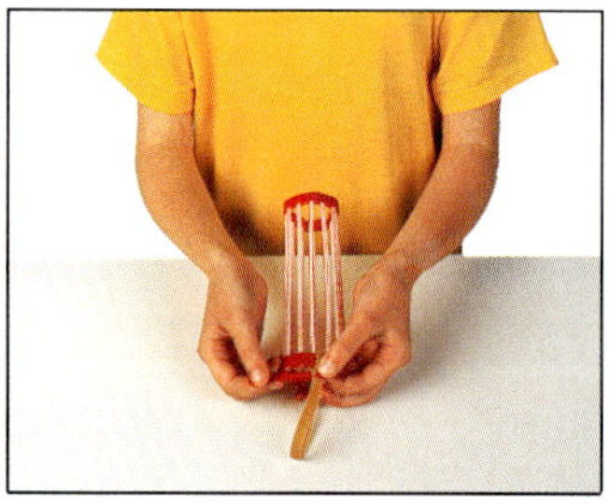

7 CUT A rubber band. Loop one end around a corrugated strip, and tape it down. Loop and tape the other end of the rubber band to the opposite side of the same corrugated-strip circle.

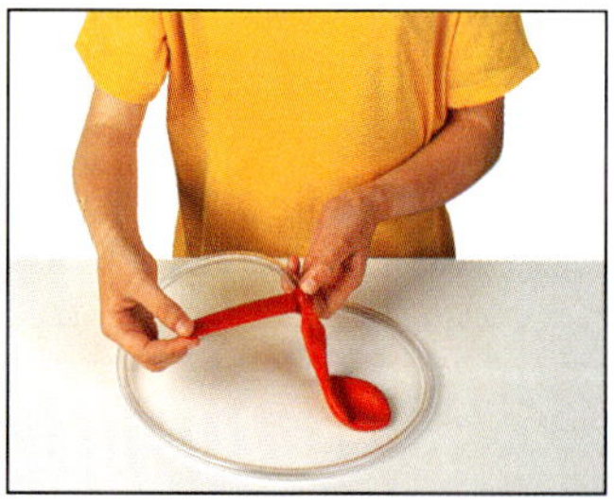

8 REPEAT STEPS 4–7 to make a second straw cage. Now cut the plastic tube in half. Tape the mouth of a balloon very firmly to one end of each piece of tube, making sure the seal is airtight.

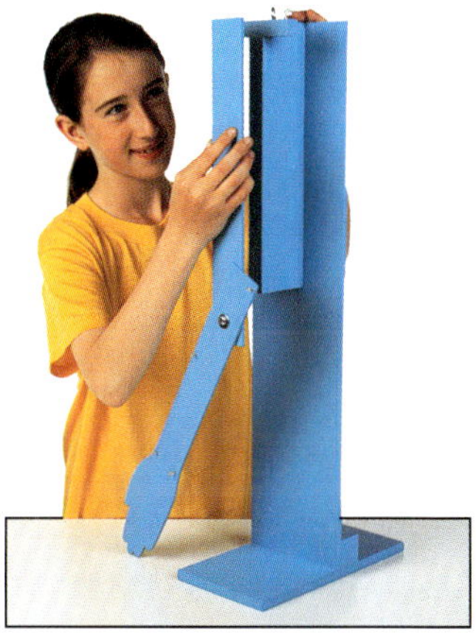

9 ASSEMBLE THE arm stand (opposite) with the double-sided tape. Drill two holes in the top of the rear bracket (**D**), and screw in the large eyes. Stick the whole arm (**F** and **G**) to the top and rear brackets (**E** and **D**) with the double-sided tape, making sure the hand of **G** has its thumb uppermost.

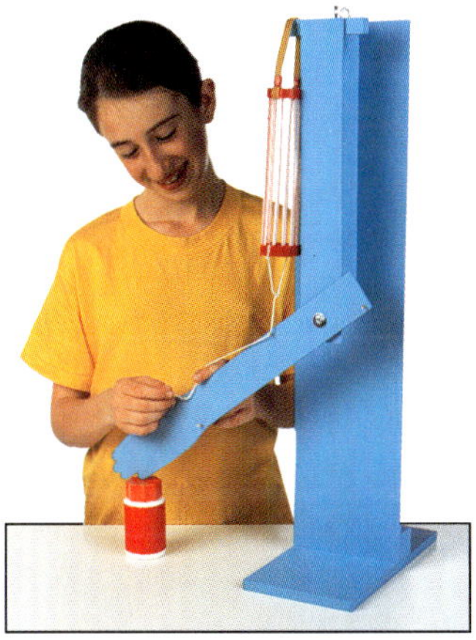

10 HANG ONE straw cage on the left end of the top bracket (**E**), and secure it with a pushpin. Tie a loop of string around the lower corrugated strip. With the hand propped up, tie a piece of string to this loop, thread it through the eye on the inside elbow, and tie it to the eye on the upper wrist.

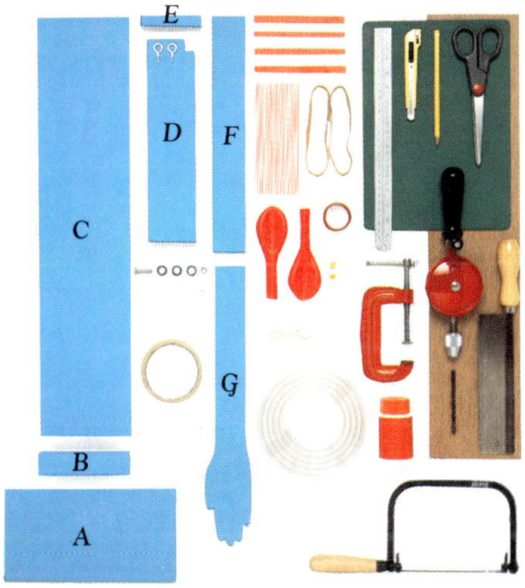

YOU WILL NEED

• pieces of plywood—for **A**, *10 in x 5 in x $\frac{1}{2}$ in (25 cm x 12 cm x 1 cm); for* **B**, *5 in x $1\frac{1}{2}$ in x $1\frac{1}{2}$ in (12 cm x 3 cm x 3 cm); for* **C**, *24 in x 5 in x $\frac{1}{8}$ in (60 cm x 12 cm x 0.5 cm); for* **D**, *12 in x 3 in x $\frac{1}{2}$ in (30 cm x 8 cm x 1 cm) with a $\frac{1}{2}$-in (1-cm) notch; for* **E**, *4 in x $\frac{1}{2}$ in x $\frac{1}{2}$ in (10 cm x 1 cm x 1 cm); for* **F** *(upper arm), 13 in x 2 in x $\frac{1}{4}$ in (33 cm x 5 cm x 0.5 cm); for* **G** *(lower arm), 16 in x 3 in x $\frac{1}{8}$ in (40 cm x 8 cm x 0.5 cm) with hand shape • 2 large screw eyes • 4 small screw eyes • bolt $1\frac{1}{2}$ in (3 cm) long and $\frac{3}{16}$ in (5 mm) diameter with 3 washers and a nut • double-sided tape • 4 strips of corrugated plastic 8 in x 1 in (20 cm x 2 cm) • 30 plastic drinking straws • 2 large rubber bands • glue • 2 balloons • duct tape • 2 pushpins • string • 6 ft (2 m) of $\frac{1}{2}$-in (1-cm) diameter plastic tube with 2 plugs to fit (or 2 clamps) • cutting mat • drilling board • drill with $\frac{1}{4}$-in (6-mm) bit • metal ruler • craft knife • pencil • scissors • G-clamp • tenon saw • coping saw*

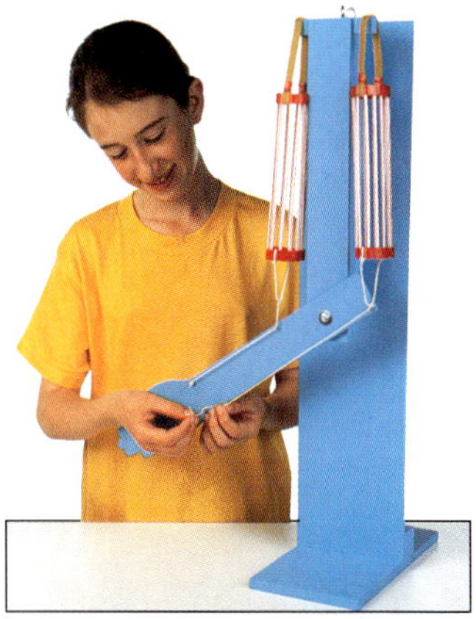

11 PIN THE other cage to the bracket's right end, with a string loop on its lower strip. Tie string to this, thread it through the outside corner eye, adjust its length so there is an equal pull on each cage, and tie to the lower wrist eye.

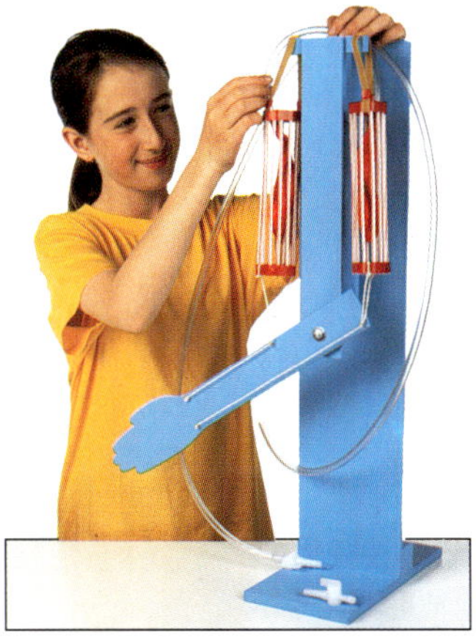

12 DAB SOME glue on all knots, so that they do not unravel. Let dry. Insert a balloon into each cage as a "muscle." Push the attached tubes through the large eyes. Fix a plug or clamp to the free end of each tube.

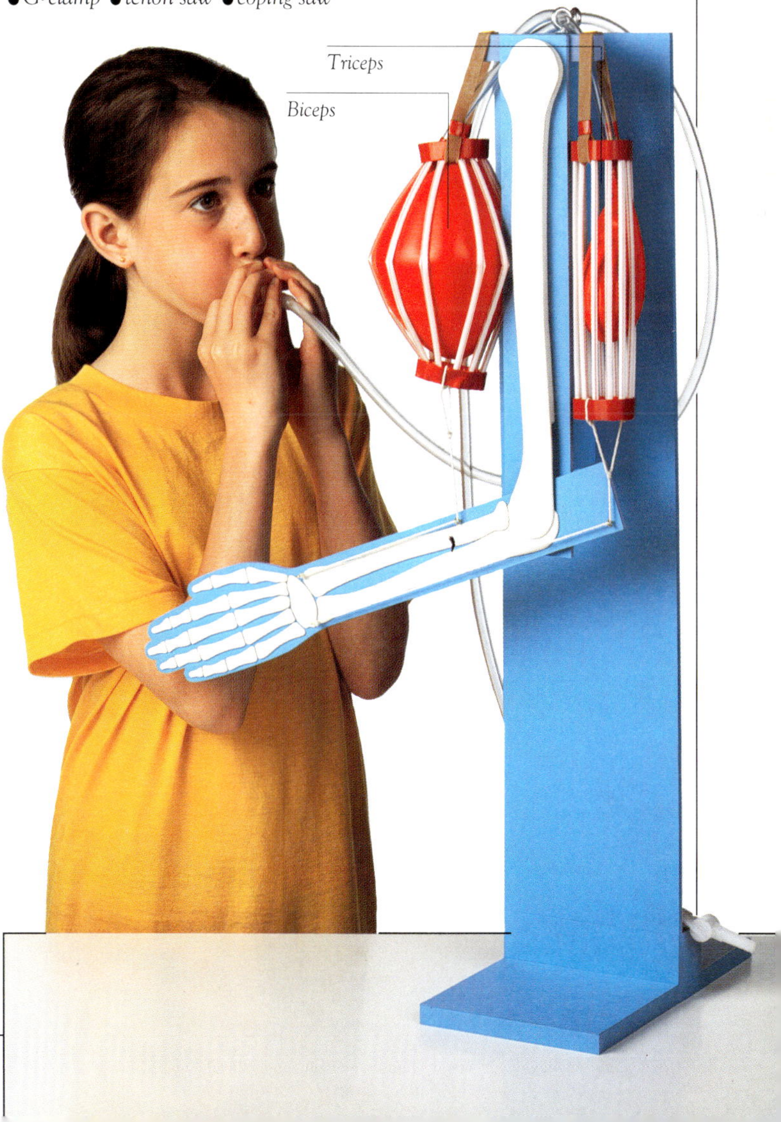

13 YOUR MODEL ARM is now ready. The muscle at the front of the arm is the biceps, that at the back is the triceps. Blow through the tube into the biceps. The inflating balloon shortens the cage, like a contracting muscle. It pulls the strings (the muscle's tendons). These pull on the wooden lower arm, representing the forearm bones (radius and ulna), which pivots at the bolt (the elbow's hinge joint). Make the hand move up with the biceps and down with its antagonistic pair, the triceps. Use the plugs or clamps to hold the muscles in position.

Muscle stamina and strength

YOUR BODY IS LIKE a well-crafted machine. It has moving parts that are perfectly designed for your everyday movements, such as breathing, eating, walking, and running. But, unlike any machine, your body's muscles can adjust themselves, becoming tuned to your regular actions and movements. If a muscle is used more and for longer periods, it becomes larger and more powerful. The blood vessels that supply it widen to bring it more energy-giving food for its activities. Its stamina—how long it works without becoming tired—increases too. In contrast, muscles that are used little become small and weak. Because muscles become accustomed to certain repeated movements, you can trick them into acting in unusual ways (below).

EXPERIMENT
Tired muscles

Finger muscles grip well, but are not designed to have great stamina. Clench your fingers and open them, once a second, for as long as you can. How long can you continue?

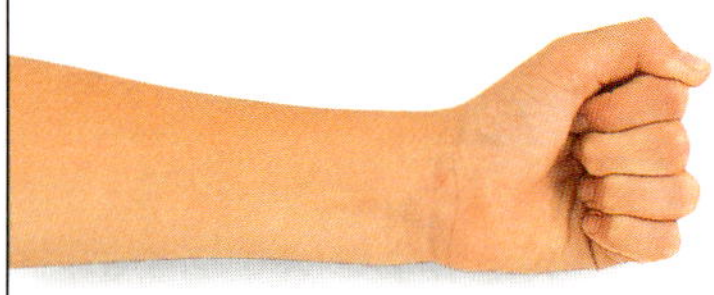

Fingers closed ...

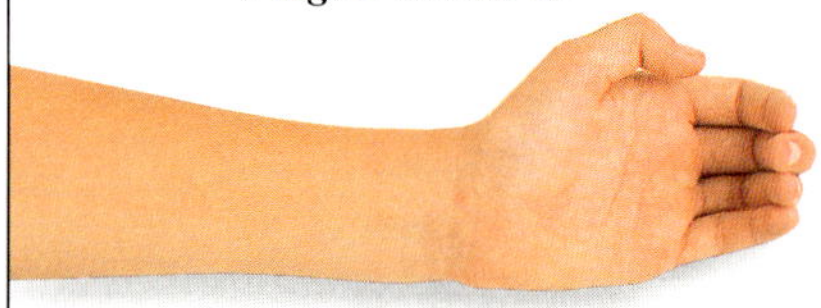

... fingers open, and so on.

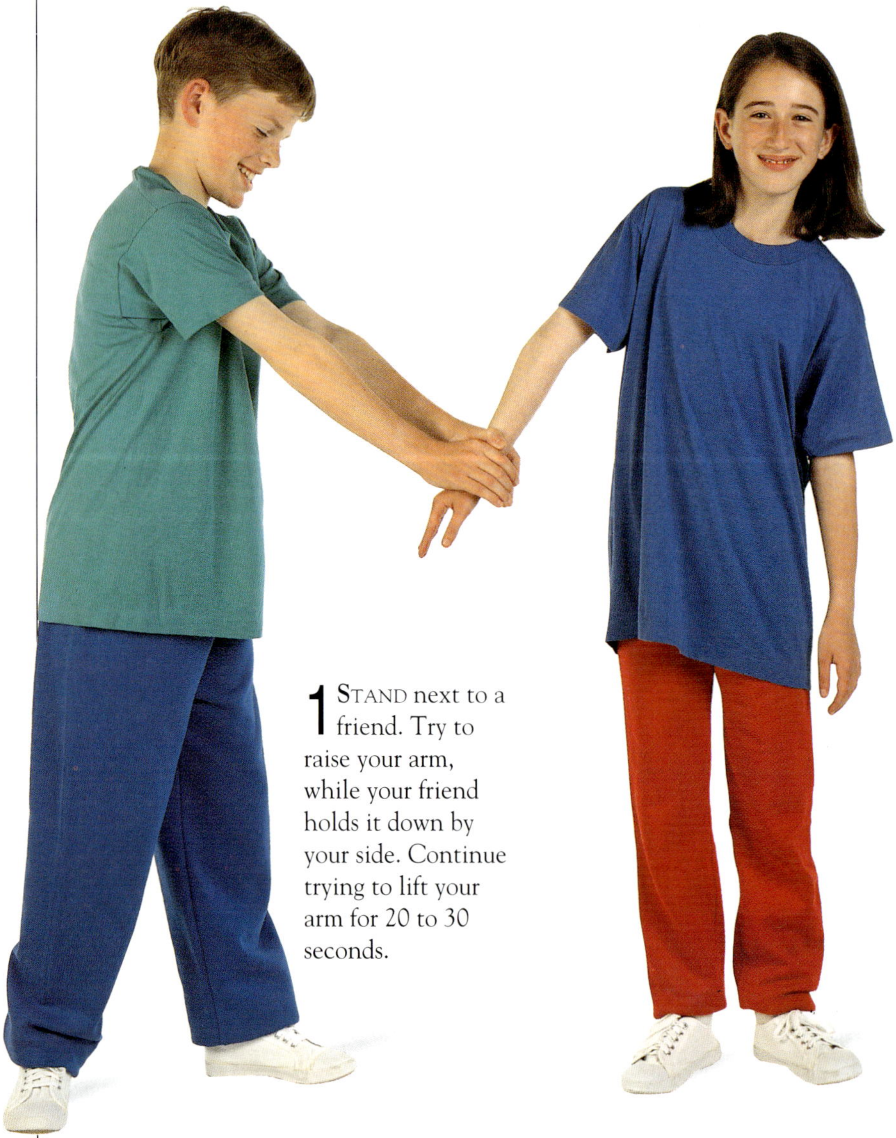

1 STAND next to a friend. Try to raise your arm, while your friend holds it down by your side. Continue trying to lift your arm for 20 to 30 seconds.

EXPERIMENT
Tricking muscles

Sometimes you can trick your muscles. If, when you try to lift your arm, a friend stops you, your brain and muscles soon adapt to this situation. When your friend lets go, the nerves and muscles stay adjusted to the old situation for a few seconds, with strange effects.

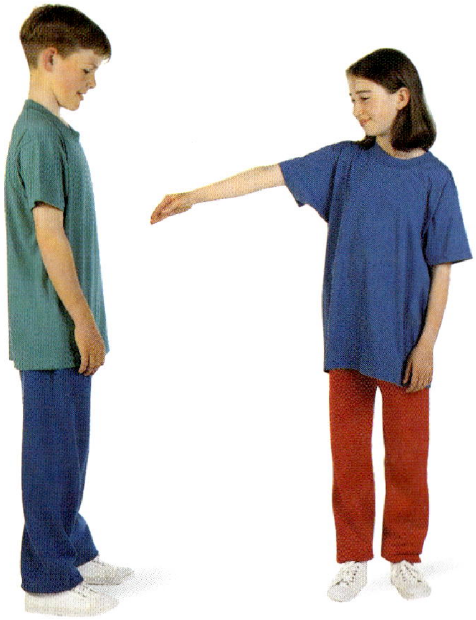

2 ASK YOUR friend to release your arm, and at the same time let it relax. Your arm will try to lift itself. See how it rises upward.

Fast and slow muscles

Some skeletal muscles (p.58) are called fast-twitch muscles and others slow-twitch muscles. The fast-twitch type works rapidly and powerfully. It gives explosive force in sports like weight lifting (below right), but has little staying power. The slow-twitch type contracts slowly, using little energy, so it tires less quickly. It gives stamina in endurance sports, such as long-distance running (below left).

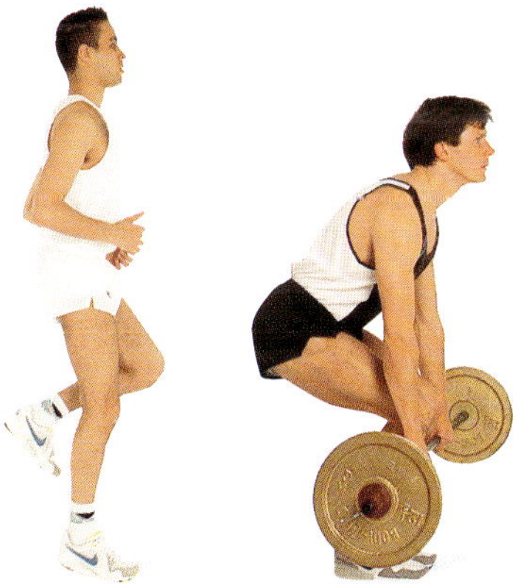

EXPERIMENT

Muscle habits

Habitual movements make the muscles that perform them strong and agile. Tapping your fingers on the table, palm down, is an example of this. Unusual movements, like tapping your fingers palm up, use weak, less coordinated muscles.

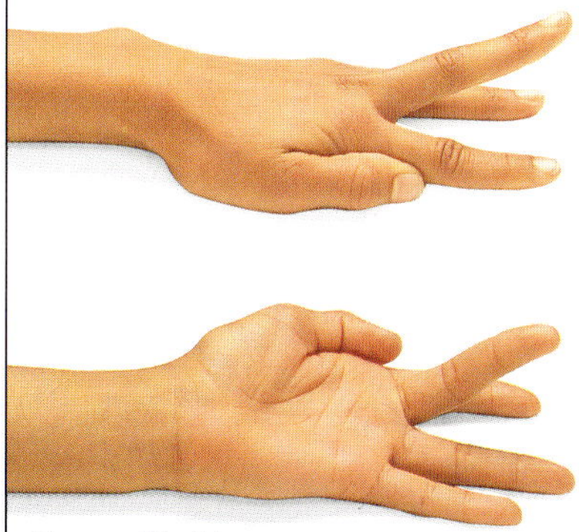

Force of habit
Fingers are more used to bending forward—the position they adopt when relaxed—than to straightening out. So you can probably tap palm down for longer than you can palm up.

EXPERIMENT

Test the strengths of different muscles

Adult help is advised for this experiment

Each team of body muscles has its own special features, to carry out the jobs that it needs to do. Some teams are more powerful than others. You can compare the strengths of the muscle teams in your body using a bathroom scale.

YOU WILL NEED

- *bathroom scale* • *notepad* • *pencil*

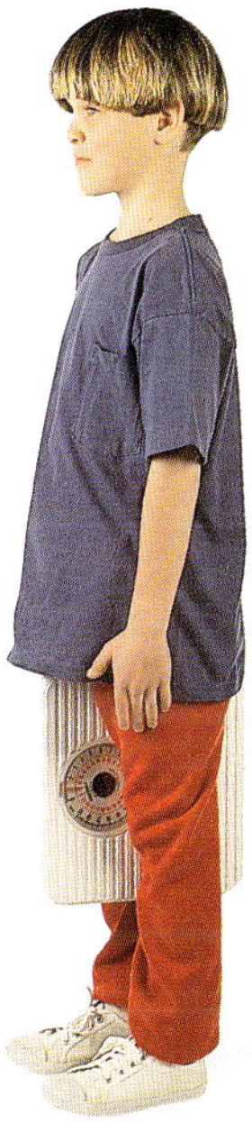

1 HOLD the scale between your knees, and squeeze as hard as you can. This measures the strength of the adductor magnus and other muscles in your inner thighs. Ask a friend to note the highest reading.

2 TRY OTHER positions, such as pressing the scale between your palms or your elbows. Draw an outline of your body, and note the results on the drawing. Which parts of the body squeeze with most power?

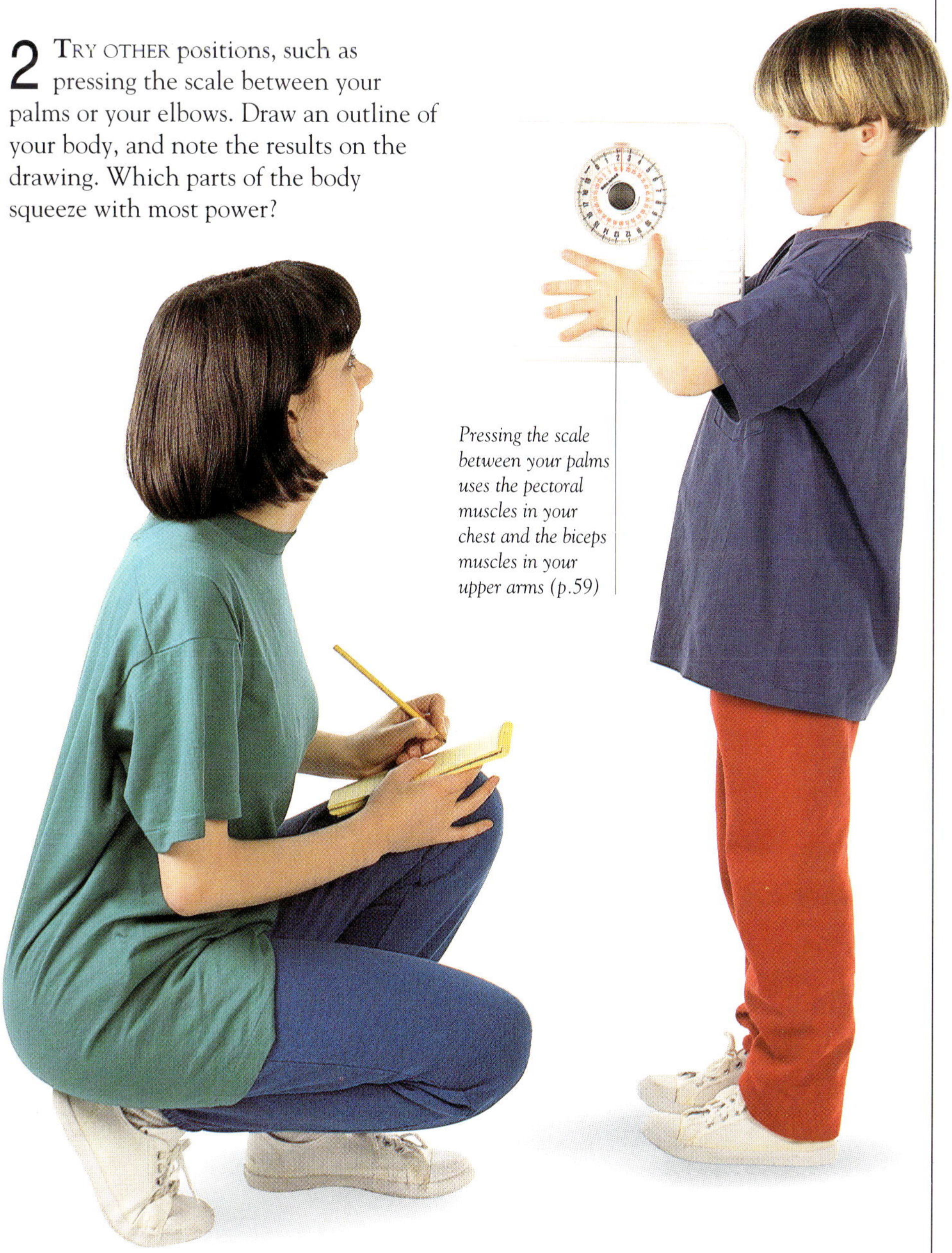

Pressing the scale between your palms uses the pectoral muscles in your chest and the biceps muscles in your upper arms (p.59)

The versatile hand

HOW DID YOU tie your shoelaces this morning? How did you open the pages of this book? How do you carry out hundreds of similar, very precise actions every day? Look at your hand to see why it is such a marvelous device. It combines all of the body structures described so far in this book. The touch-sensitive covering of skin is wrapped around numerous sets of muscles and tendons, joints and ligaments, which are in turn attached to a framework of strong, light bones. The human hand is powerful yet delicate, adaptable yet precise. There is no device in the whole world of animals or of machines that is quite so versatile.

EXPERIMENT

Make a model hand

Adult help is advised for this experiment

When you grip, long muscles on the inside of your forearm contract. They pull their tendons (p.58), which are attached to the jointed sets of bones in your fingers. The tendons and muscles are kept in place by ligaments and other fibrous tissue. Make a model hand to show, in a simplified way, how your own hand works.

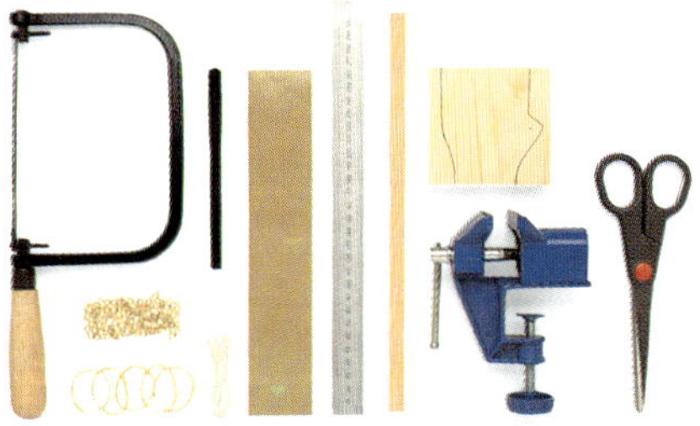

YOU WILL NEED

- *coping saw* • *about 80 small metal screw eyes* • *5 rubber bands* • *pen* • *string* • *carpet tape* • *ruler* • *wood strip 12 in x ½ in x ½ in (30 cm x 12 mm x 12 mm)* • *wood block 4 in x 4 in x ½ in (10 cm x 10 cm x 12 mm)* • *vise* • *scissors*

EXPERIMENT

Precise work

Bones, joints, and muscles in your arm and hand are smaller and finer the farther down your arm they are—from your shoulder to your fingertips. So the movements you can achieve with the fingertips are more precise than those with the shoulder.

YOU WILL NEED

- *felt-tip pen* • *paper* • *ribbon*

Robot "hands"

Engineers have tried for years to build machines that mimic the human hand. But none of these devices has come close to our range of movements. It is hard for scientists to match the control systems of the body. Your eyes and the hand's muscles and skin give your brain sophisticated feedback about your hand's position.

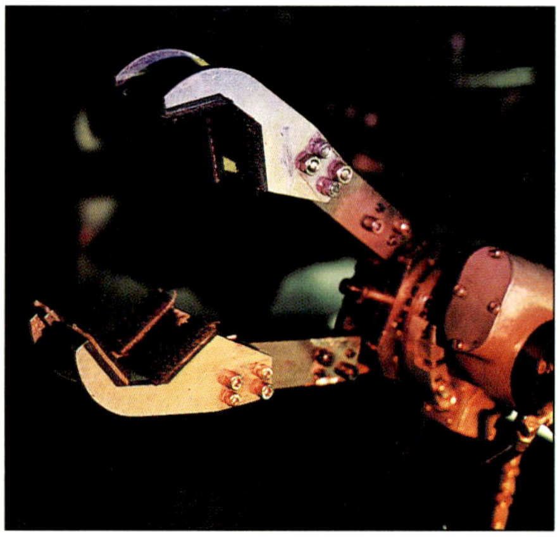

Extra hands

Robot machines on assembly lines carry out certain simple, repetitive tasks in a tireless fashion. But a robot welder-arm cannot spray paint, and a robot suction-grab cannot tighten screws. Each device is designed to do only one or a few of the multiple tasks that our hands can do.

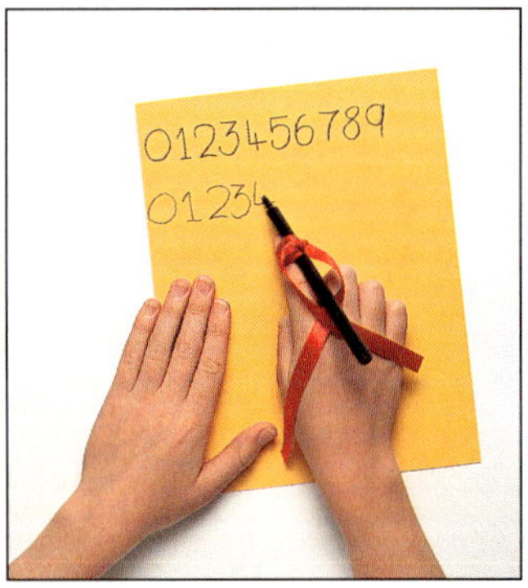

1 WRITE THE numbers 1 to 9 on the paper in the usual way. Then ask a friend to tie the pen to the middle section of your forefinger. Try again —it is still not too difficult.

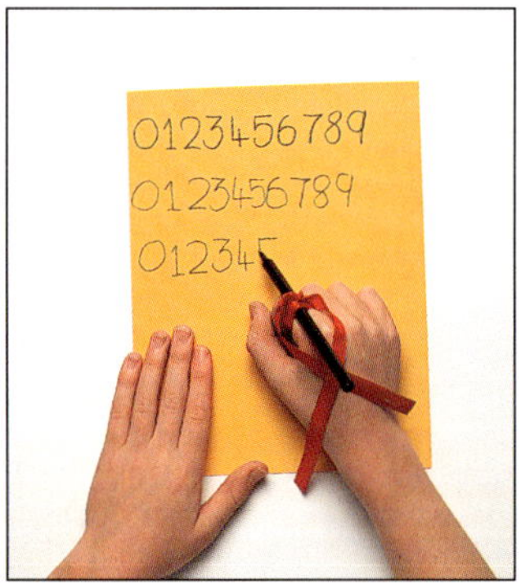

2 USE ONE less joint by tying the pen to the base section of your forefinger, and write 1 to 9 again. The bigger bone, joint, and less practiced muscles make it awkward.

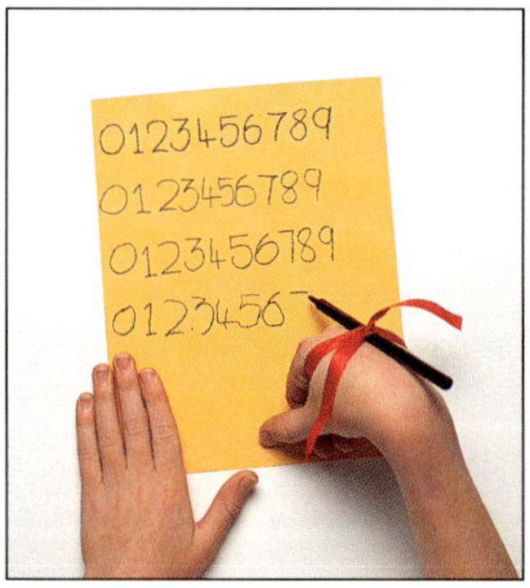

3 ASK YOUR friend to tie the pen to the back of your hand. Now you are using only your shoulder, elbow, and wrist. Is neat writing more difficult?

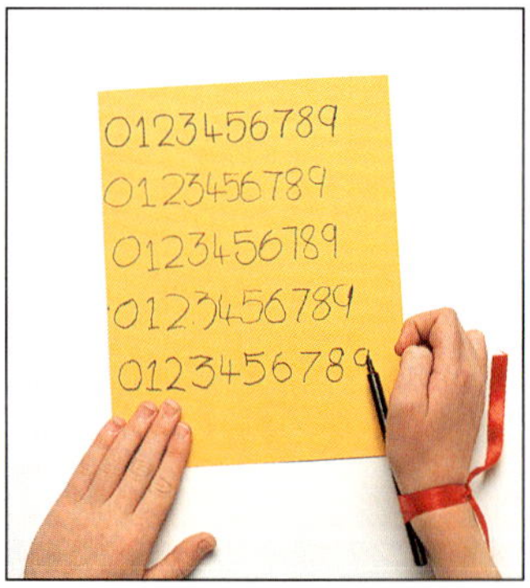

4 ASK YOUR friend to tie the pen to the inside of your wrist. Now you can use only your shoulder and elbow. These are big joints, not designed for precision.

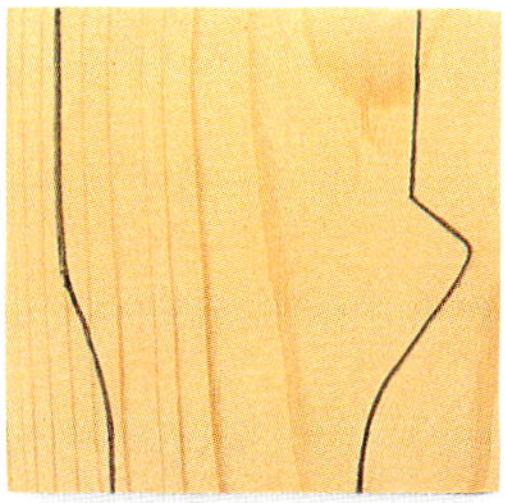

1 DRAW A palm shape on the wood block. The palm top should be about 2½ in (6.5 cm) wide. Ask an adult to cut out the shape, holding the wood in a vise. Next, study your fingers. Is each of their sections the same length?

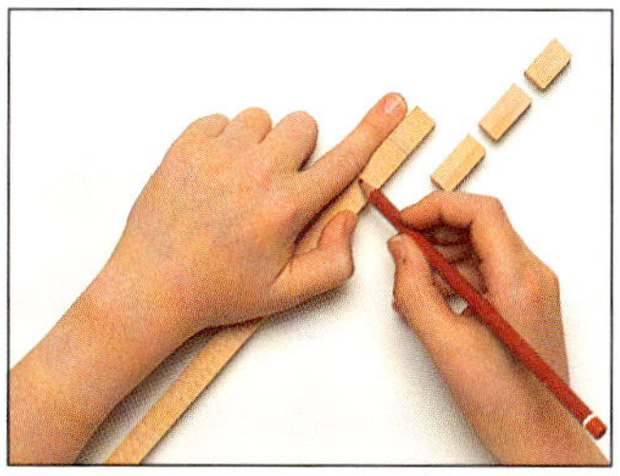

2 LAY YOUR fingers in turn against the side of the wood strip. Mark the length of each finger and thumb section on the strip. Ask an adult to cut off the 14 pieces you have marked (3 for each finger, 2 for the thumb).

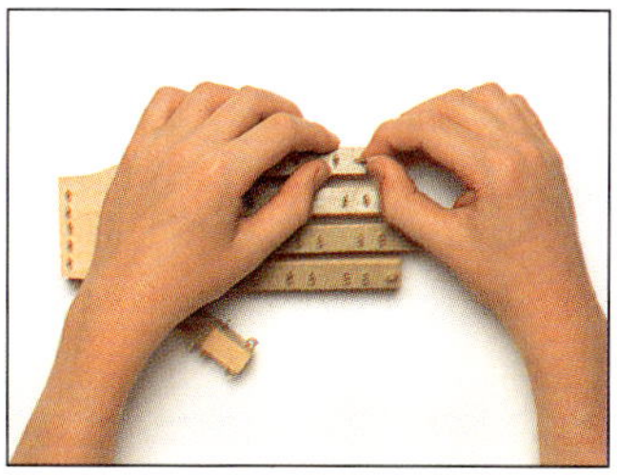

3 TAPE THE pieces together on one side (call this the front), and attach them to the block. Attach an eye to each fingertip and to each side of each knuckle. Fix five eyes in the wrist too. The thumb is slightly different (below left).

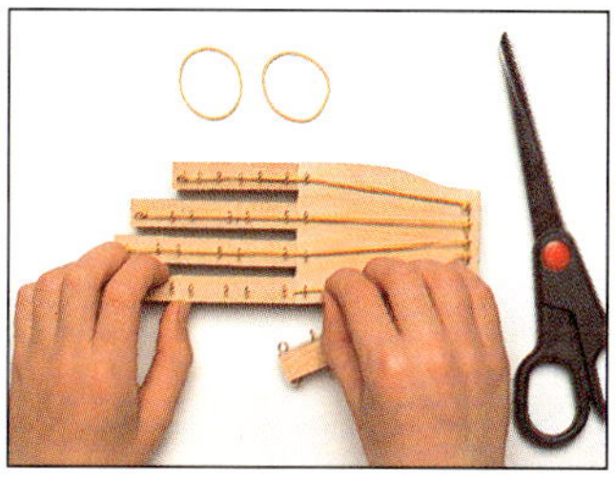

4 FLIP THE hand. Fix eyes in the same pattern (but only four at the wrist). Snip the rubber bands. Tie each to a fingertip eye, and thread it through the others. Tie it at the wrist with slight tension. For the thumb, see below left.

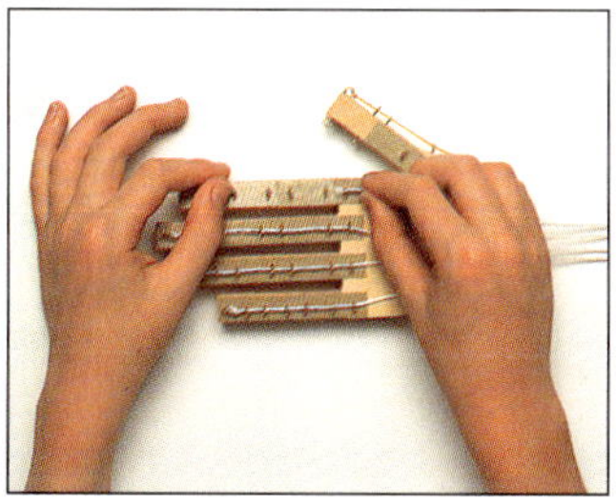

5 FLIP THE hand, so that it is front-up again. Tie a length of string to a fingertip eye, and thread it through the other eyes, including those in the wrist. Leave some string free below the wrist. Repeat for all fingers. For the thumb, see below.

6 YOUR "HAND" is now ready. Hold the block with one hand and all of the strings with the other. When you pull the strings, you mimic the action of the tendons that connect the muscles in your forearm to the ends of your fingers (p.60). The strings run through the screw eyes, which represent loops of ligament and fibrous material in the wrist and knuckles. The rubber bands give the "hand" tension, like the muscles on the back of the hand. The "thumb" twists inward to give a realistic grabbing action. Can you make your model hand drum its fingers on a table?

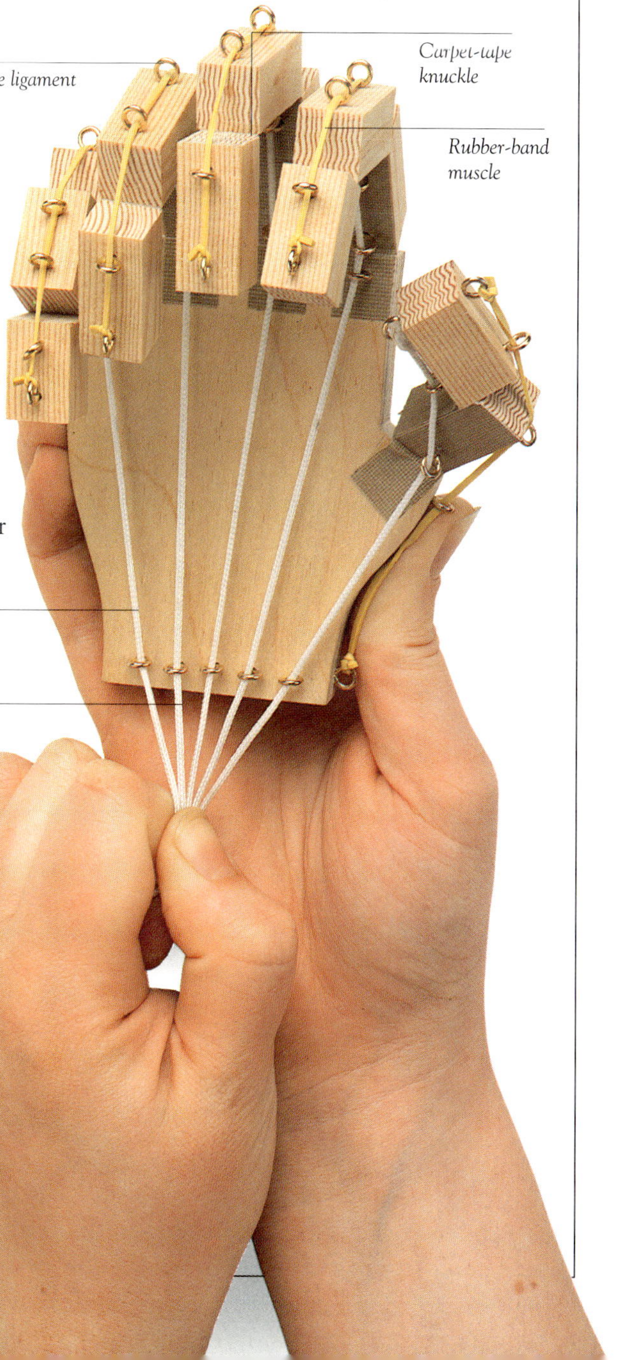

Twisting thumb

Tape the knuckle between the upper and lower thumb sections on the inside. But for the knuckle between lower thumb section and block, tape at the front. Fix four eyes in the sides of the upper thumb section, one on the outside below the knuckle between upper and lower sections, one on the front of the lower section, and two on the side of the block. Feed the thumb's rubber band from the fingertip eye down the outside of the block. Feed the string through the eyes on the inside of the upper section, then through the eye on the front of the lower section, and then through the one free wrist eye.

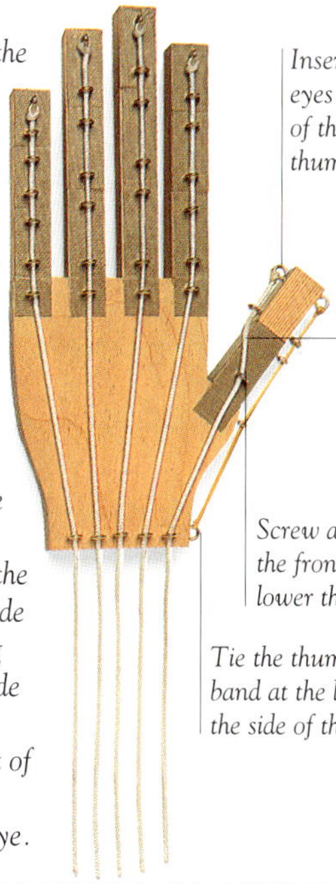

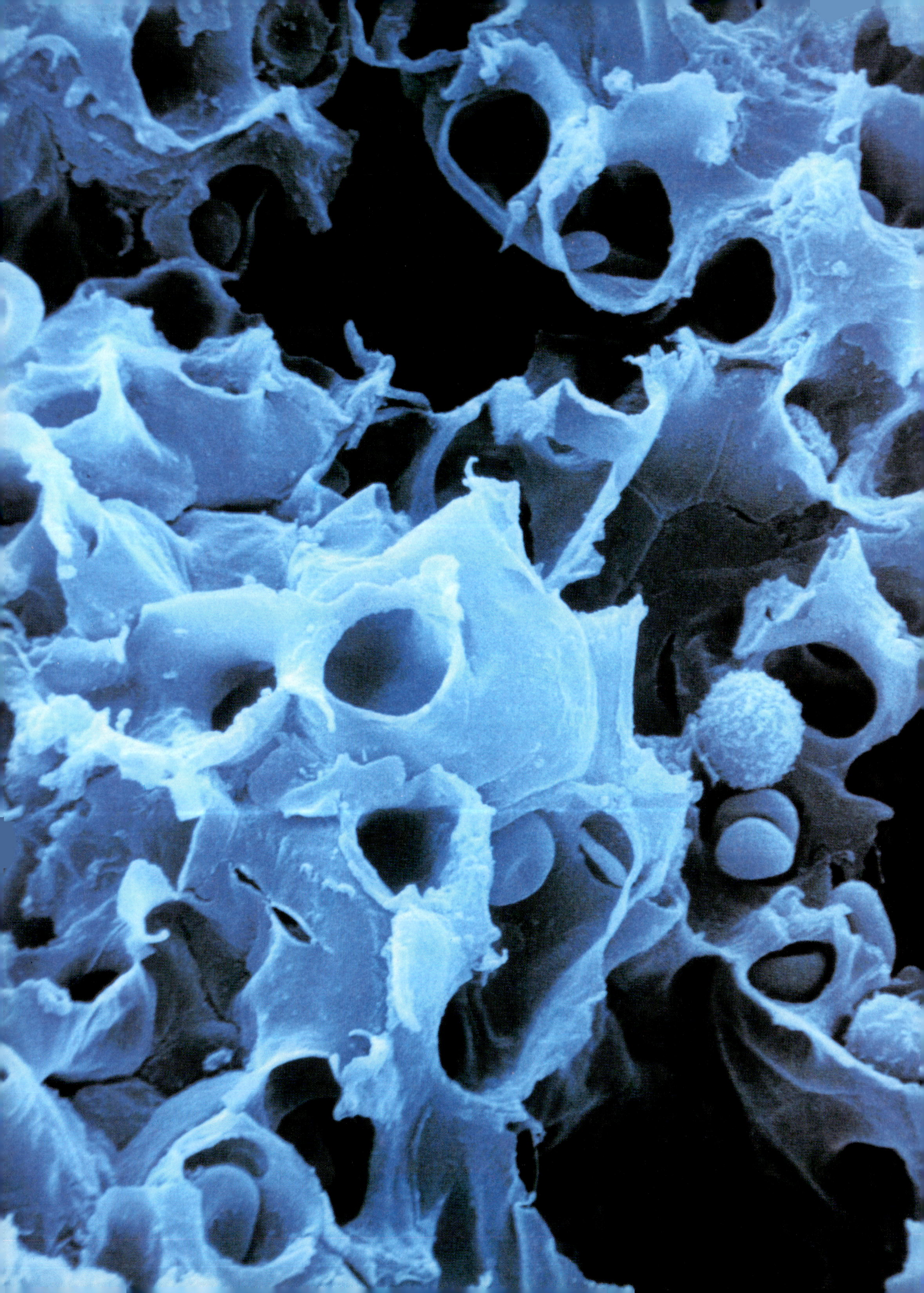

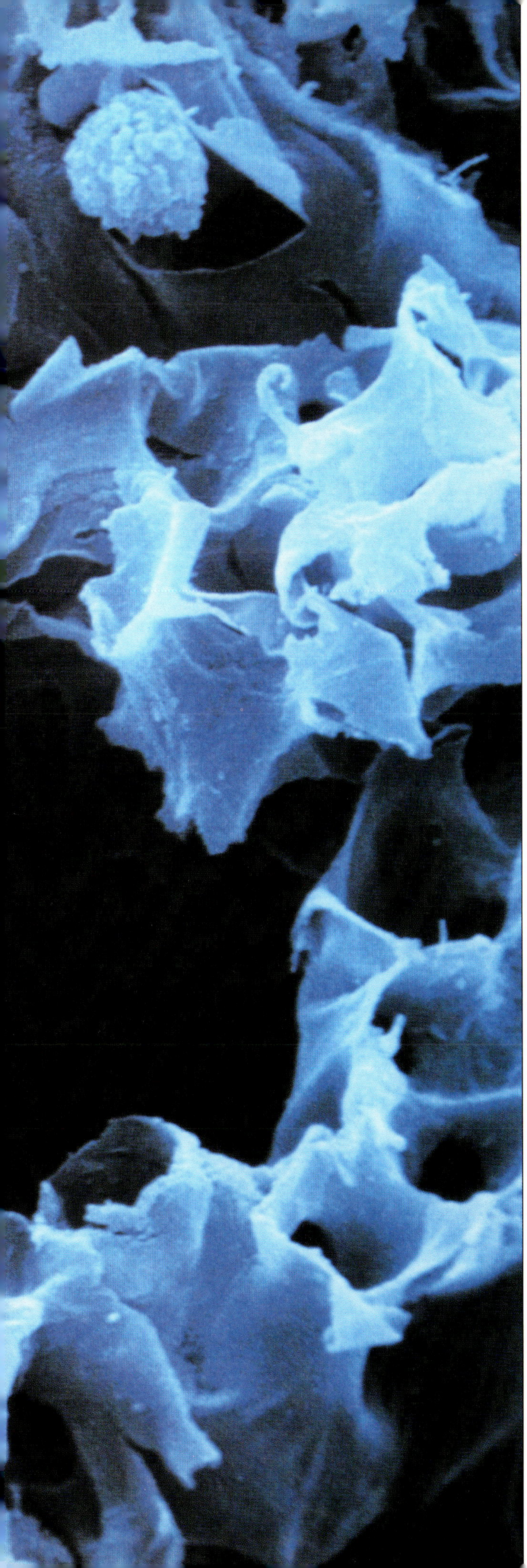

The OXYGEN SUPPLY

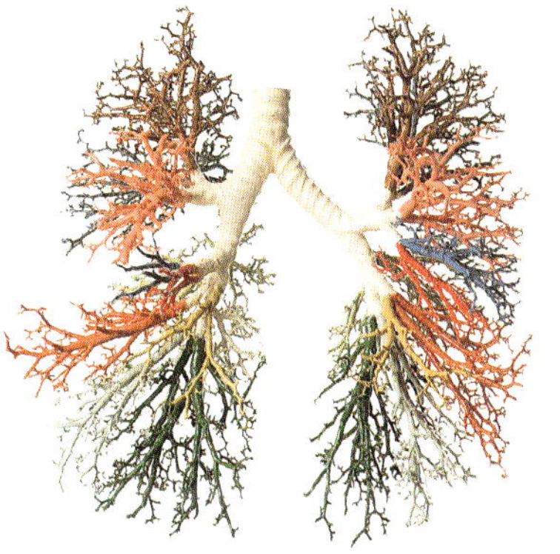

Air travel
A branching system of air tubes known as bronchi (above) carries air deep into the spongy honeycomb of the lungs. The bronchi become narrower and turn into bronchioles. Bronchioles themselves end in microscopic air bags called alveoli. Through a microscope, alveoli appear as cavelike holes (left). The "fluffy balls" are white blood cells, scavenging for bits of dust or germs.

LIFE DEPENDS ON OXYGEN. This substance plays a vital role in the chemical reactions inside every body cell, releasing energy from food to drive life processes. The parts of the body designed to obtain continuing supplies of oxygen—the nose, airways, lungs, and breathing muscles—are collectively known as the respiratory system. In the lungs fresh air is brought into almost direct contact with blood, so that the oxygen in the air can easily pass into the blood and be carried to every body part.

THE LUNGS AND BREATHING

THE BODY CAN STORE many of the substances it needs. For example, the liver holds reserves of vitamins, the bones store minerals, and body fat acts as an energy stockpile. But the body cannot store more than a few minutes' worth of its essential supply of oxygen, so it must continually take in fresh supplies. It does this by a process called respiration. The two lungs are the organs that obtain oxygen from the air and pass it to the blood, and the blood distributes oxygen to cells around the body.

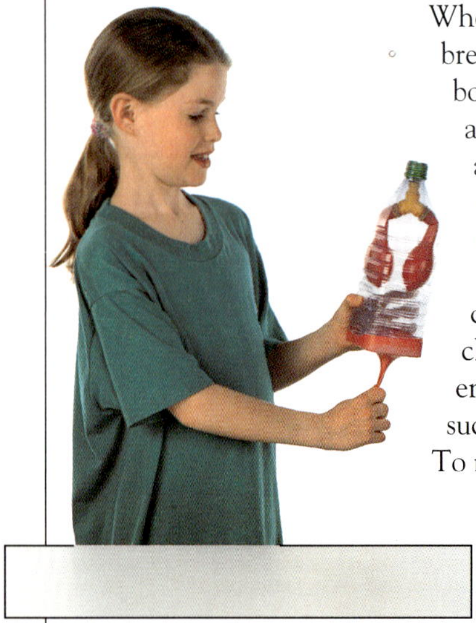

The lungs are filled with air as the chest expands. You can show this with balloon "lungs" in a plastic-bottle "chest" (p.72).

The word "respiration" actually has two meanings.

In one sense the word is another term for "breathing." When you respire, you breathe in and out. Your body takes in fresh air, absorbs oxygen from it, adds carbon dioxide to it, and then expels this now-stale air.

The other meaning is concerned with cell chemistry. A cell needs energy from substances such as the sugar glucose. To release this energy in a form that the cell can use easily, the glucose must be broken up by a series of chemical reactions. Oxygen is a vital ingredient in these chemical reactions, and carbon dioxide is a waste product of them. The process of obtaining energy by these chemical reactions is called cellular respiration.

Cellular respiration is found in almost all living things, from amoebas and worms to trees and mushrooms. They all need oxygen to survive. Only a few microbes, called anaerobic bacteria, do not need oxygen. They live in places, such as the mud at the bottom of the oceans, where no oxygen is available.

Early anatomists did not know about cellular respiration. This was partly because it is essentially a chemical process and cannot be observed with the naked eye. It was also because the central substance in the respiratory process, the gas oxygen, is invisible. There was little progress in our knowledge of how the lungs work until the 17th century, when the microscope was invented, and chemistry began to advance as a science.

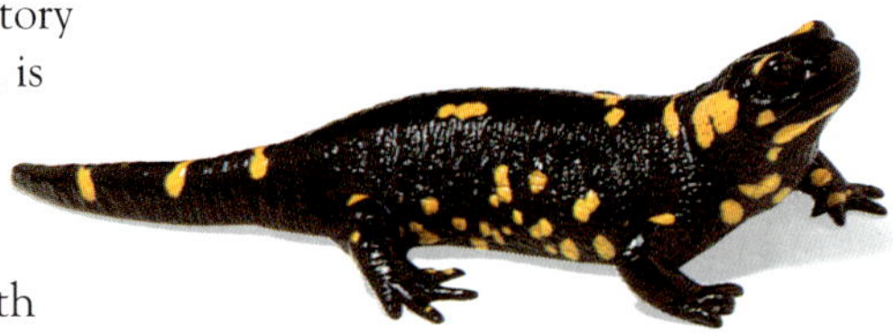

***Amphibians such as salamanders** can take in oxygen through their moist skin, as well as through their lungs.*

The pneuma

The great philosophers of ancient Greece, such as Plato (c.428–c.347 B.C.) and Aristotle (384–322 B.C.), believed that life was based on a type of fire, a "vital flame" that burned within the heart. Nourishment from food supposedly built up the flame, while breathing brought in air to damp it down and keep it from burning out of control. These philosophers thought that if the flame went out, the body became cold and life ended.

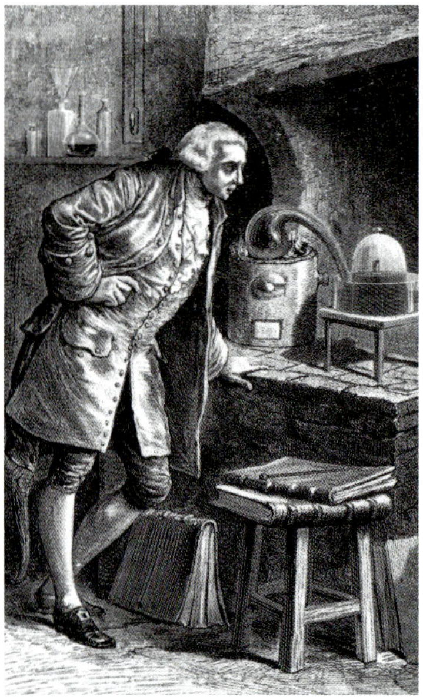

***The Father of Chemistry,** Antoine Lavoisier, carried out many experiments on the gases in air. He first gave the name "oxygen" to the part of air that supports life.*

Galen (p.13) of ancient Rome also had strong views on the roles of the airways and lungs. He believed that a mysterious substance in air, the pneuma (p.94), passed into the mouth, down the throat, and through the trachea (windpipe) into the branching, treelike system of airways deep inside the lungs. He thought that the pneuma then passed into the blood vessels around the airways and traveled to the heart. There the pneuma "vitalized" the blood, bringing life and taking away waste substances.

Although Galen's notion of the pneuma has now been proved wrong, his descriptions of the routes taken by air in the respiratory system paved the way for later discoveries.

Dogs and frogs

In 1660 the Italian microscopist Marcello Malpighi (p.104) described how lungs work at a microscopic level—in this case, in a dog. In the following years, he found out more about lung structure. The big airways, the bronchi, divide many times, to become smaller bronchioles, and then even smaller, when they are called terminal bronchioles. Each of these terminal bronchioles ends in a group of tiny air sacs, called alveoli. There are more than 600 million alveoli in a pair of human lungs (p.72).

When he studied a frog's lungs, Malpighi saw the tiny blood vessels, called capillaries, that pass close to the alveoli. However, the function of this meeting of the alveoli and capillaries was not understood until the 18th century.

Breathing and fire

The British scientists Robert Boyle (1627–91) and Robert Hooke (p.26) were interested in the nature of air. Boyle and Hooke found that all animals need to breathe fresh air to stay alive. This may seem obvious today, but at the time it was a very important discovery.

Another British scientist, Joseph Priestley (1733–1804),

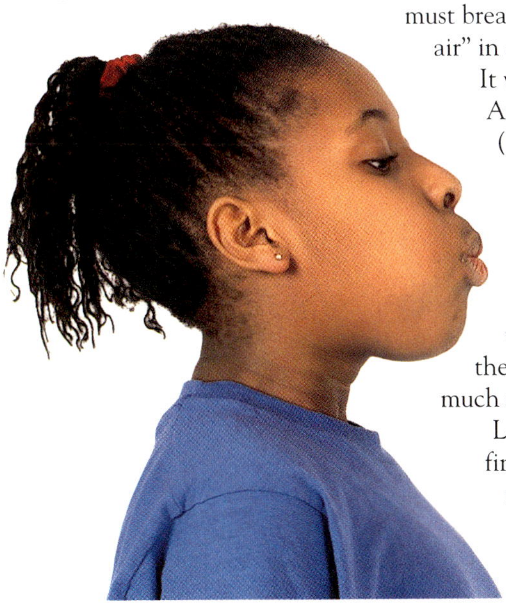

To breathe out, your lungs spring back *from their large, inflated size to their normal smaller volume, like a balloon deflating. To blow hard, your abdominal muscles squeeze to give added push.*

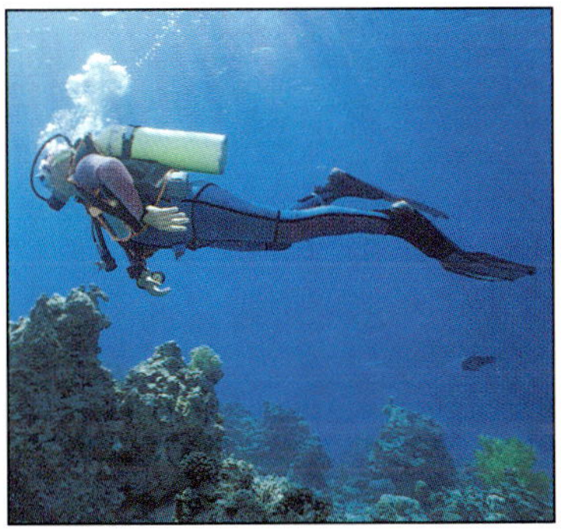

Fish and other water creatures *take in oxygen dissolved in water through their gills. Air breathers like us need oxygen in its gas form. So divers must carry air tanks.*

placed a burning candle in a sealed jar with normal air. Priestley knew that this air contained a gas, which he called "dephlogisticated air." (This gas later came to be known as oxygen.) He also placed a second burning candle in a jar with air from which he had removed this gas. He found that the first candle burned for some time, whereas the second went out almost immediately. Priestley also carried out experiments on animals and discovered that they must breathe "dephlogisticated air" in order to survive.

It was the French chemist Antoine Lavoisier (1743–94) who named this vital gas "oxygen." He realized that the body uses oxygen and produces carbon dioxide in the same way as a fire, although the process in the body is much slower.

Lavoisier's discoveries finally made clear the reason for the internal design of the lungs. Blood flowing through the capillaries that pass next to the alveoli comes very close to the air inside the alveoli. So the oxygen in breathed-in air travels the short distance from the alveoli to the blood. Once in the blood, the oxygen is delivered all around the body so that cellular respiration can take place. Carbon dioxide is carried in the other direction—from the blood to the air in the lungs, and it is then breathed out.

If the alveoli in human lungs were spread out flat, they would cover a surface as large as a tennis court. This huge surface area (p.185) within the lungs ensures that enough oxygen can be absorbed, from the alveoli into the blood, to keep the body working efficiently.

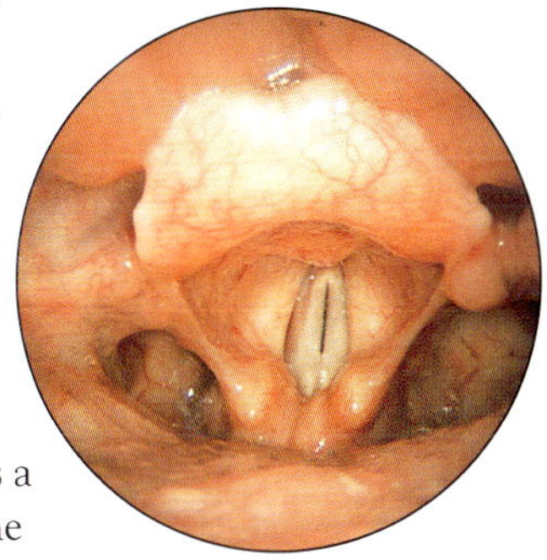

This view down the throat *shows closed vocal cords. The cords are vibrated by air passing between them, making sounds.*

Speech

Vocal communication is a useful "by-product" of the respiratory system. Air flowing in and out of the lungs along the trachea passes between two tough pearl-pink ridges in the larynx (voice box). These are the vocal cords.

The air flow makes the cords vibrate, which produces sounds. Stretching the cords by varying amounts produces vibrations of varying pitch (high or low sound). If the cords are stretched tight, they vibrate faster and produce a high pitch. If they are loose, the pitch is low. Sounds are louder when air flows faster and in greater amounts over the vocal cords.

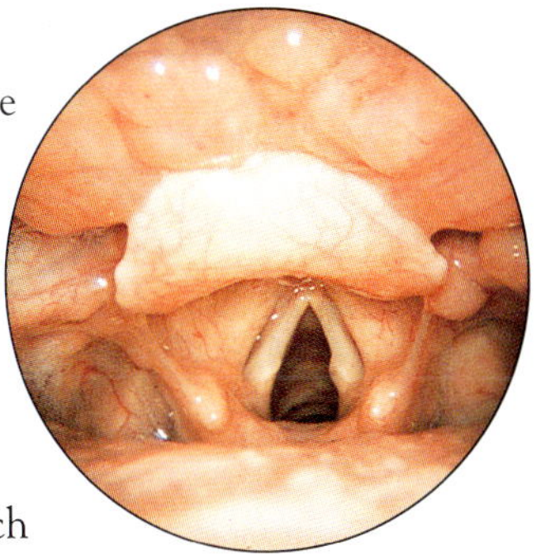

When breathing is normal, *the vocal cords are apart, so there is usually no sound.*

As you speak, these sounds are altered by the positions of your tongue, teeth, cheeks, and lips. The result is the immense range of words, whispers, shouts, screams, laughs, and other kinds of sound we use to communicate.

The respiratory system

THE RESPIRATORY SYSTEM gets oxygen from the air into the blood via the lungs. It consists of the nose, throat, trachea (windpipe), and lungs. As you inhale (breathe in) you draw in fresh air. As you exhale (breathe out) you expel stale air from the lungs. Deep in the lungs, in air pockets called alveoli, the air is brought into very close contact with blood passing through tiny blood vessels. This process allows oxygen, which is vital for cellular respiration (p.70), to pass from the lungs into the blood. It also allows the waste product carbon dioxide to pass from the blood to the lungs, and then out into the air. If carbon dioxide were allowed to accumulate in the body, it would be poisonous. Listen to your own breathing, and see how your chest movements suck in and blow out air.

EXPERIMENT

Model lungs

Adult help is advised for this experiment

When you inhale, muscles cause the chest to expand (opposite), making the lungs do the same. When this happens, air is sucked into the lungs. Make a model to demonstrate this.

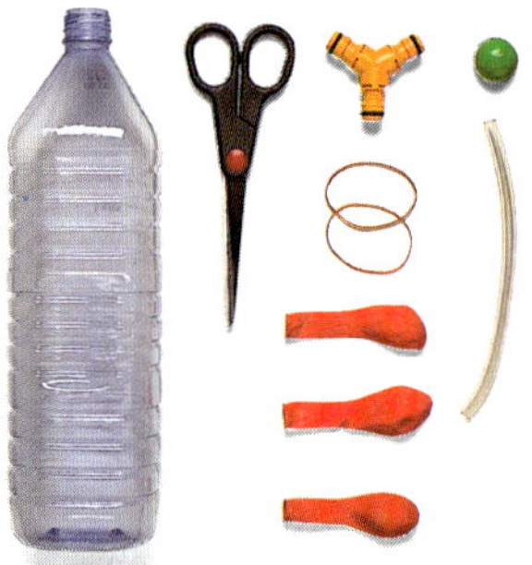

YOU WILL NEED

- *large clear-plastic bottle*
- *three-way hose connector*
- *modeling clay*
- *2 rubber bands*
- *plastic tube*
- *3 small balloons*
- *scissors*

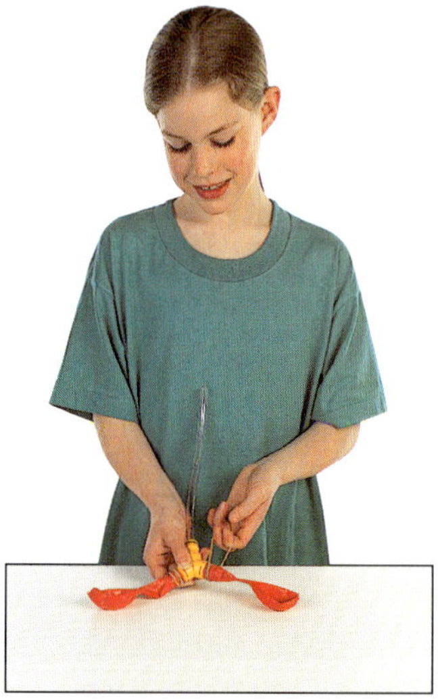

1 PUSH THE plastic tube into one opening of the hose connector. Use modeling clay, if necessary, to make an airtight seal. Fix the balloons tightly onto the other openings with rubber bands, making sure that the joins between the connector and the balloons are airtight.

Inside the chest

Air passes to and from the lungs through the trachea (windpipe). The top of the trachea opens into the pharynx (throat). The lower end divides into two main bronchi (air tubes), one of which enters each lung. The bronchi branch again and again inside the lung, becoming smaller and smaller until they are as thin as hairs. Now called terminal bronchioles, they end at the microscopic, bubble-shaped alveoli. There are about 300 million alveoli in each lung. Each alveolus is surrounded by capillaries (p.179). Oxygen in the air inside the alveolus passes the short distance to the blood in the capillary, and the blood carries it around the body.

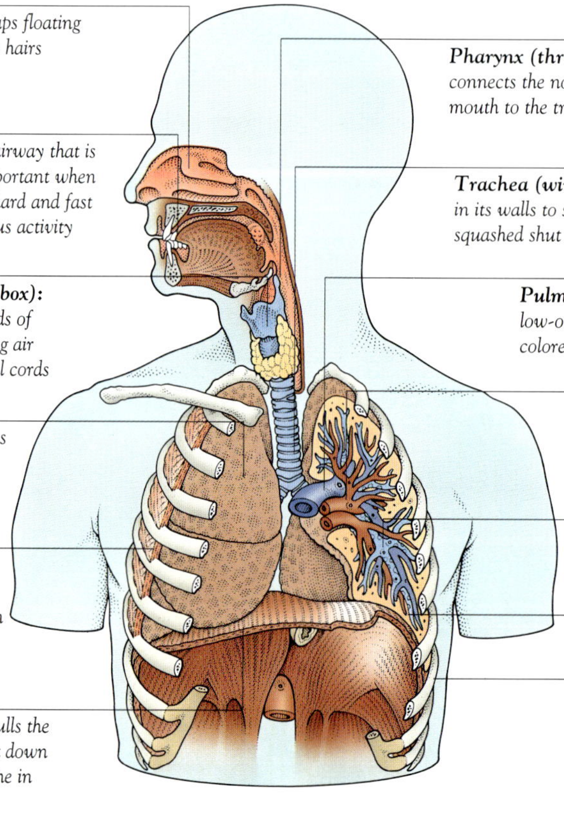

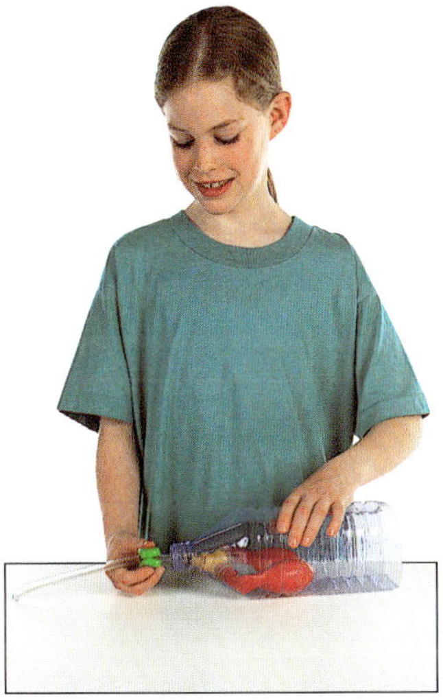

2 Carefully cut off the bottom 1 in (2.5 cm) from the bottle, using the scissors. Make sure the cut edge of the bottle is smooth. Place the balloons and connector inside. Seal the plastic tube into the neck of the bottle with the modeling clay to make an airtight fit.

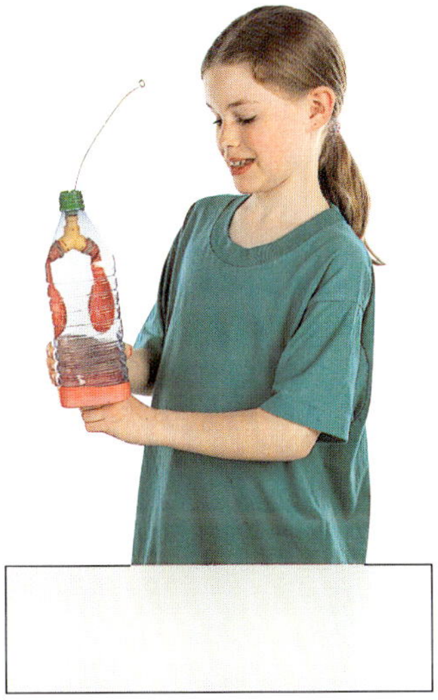

3 Tie a knot in the neck of the third balloon. Then carefully cut it in half, crossways. Gently stretch the knotted part of the balloon over the lower end of the bottle, and pull it around the sides. Make the balloon as taut as you can—like a drum skin. Now hold it by its knot.

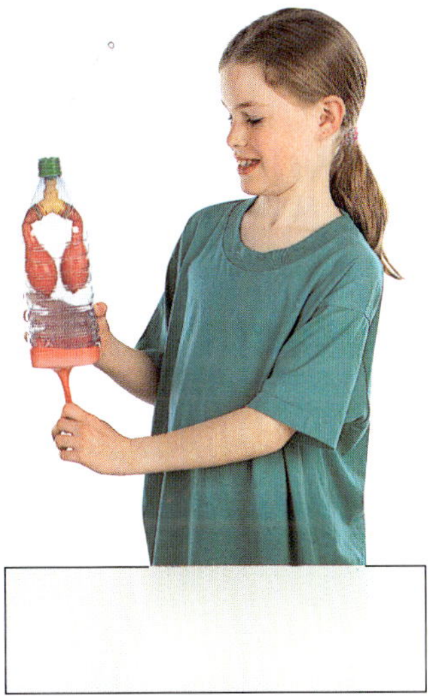

4 The lower balloon represents the diaphragm, the main breathing muscle (right). Pull it down, as though you were inhaling. This lowers the air pressure in the bottle. Air from outside rushes in and makes the two balloons expand, just like the real lungs in your chest.

Breathing

When you inhale, the lungs become bigger and draw in air. When you exhale, the lungs spring back to their smaller size.

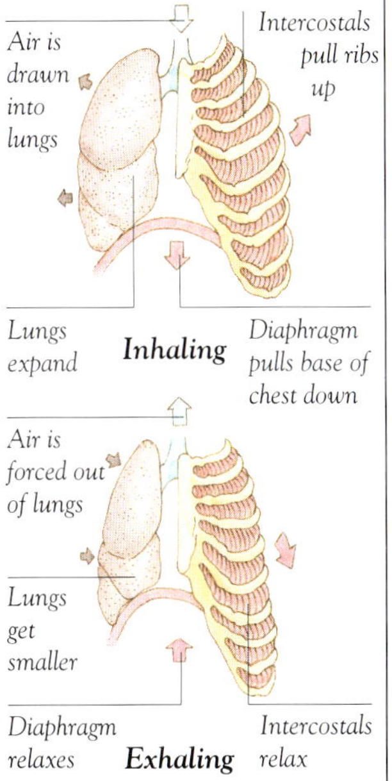

EXPERIMENT

Lung surface

Adult help is advised for this experiment

The millions of alveoli in a lung expose its insides to air. They make the lung's surface area (p.185) much greater than if the lung were one hollow chamber, so the lungs can absorb lots of oxygen. Make "alveoli" out of poster board.

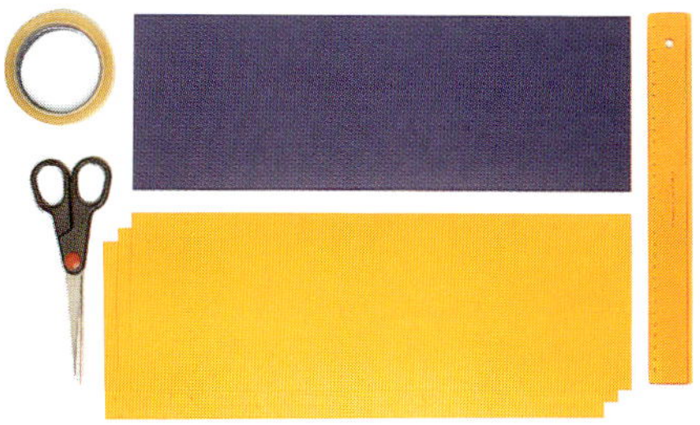

You Will Need

- *cellophane tape* • *scissors* • *thin sheet of blue poster board 18 in x 6 in (45 cm x 15 cm)*
- *lots of thin sheets of yellow poster board* • *ruler*

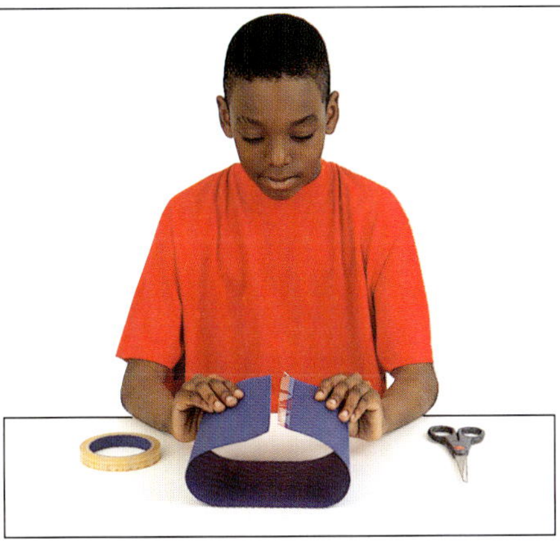

1 Bend the large blue sheet into a cylinder. Tape its edges. This represents the outside of a lung. Now you are ready to make tubes representing the alveoli for the inside of the "lung."

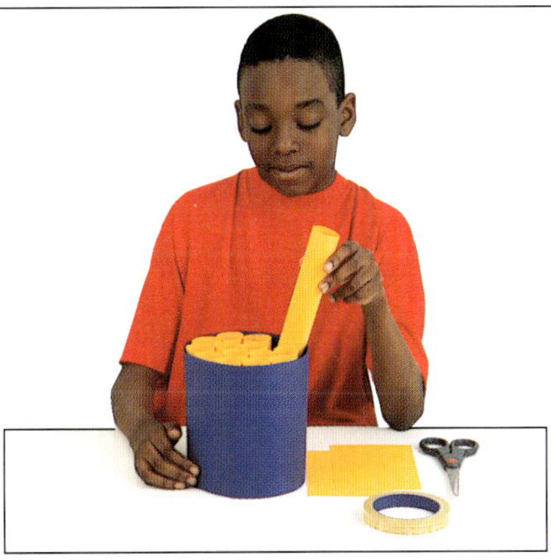

2 Cut the yellow sheets into pieces 6 in x 4 in (15 cm x 10 cm). Roll into tubes, to represent alveoli, and tape their edges. Place the tubes inside the large blue "lung" until it is full.

3 Now unravel the alveoli tubes, and spread them out flat. You have increased the surface area of your "lung" greatly by adding just a few alveoli tubes. Imagine how great the oxygen-absorbing surface area of a real lung is, with millions of alveoli packed inside.

Breathing in and out

NEXT TIME YOU are outside on a dry winter morning, exhale (breathe out) slowly. Your breath looks like steam from a kettle. Exhaled air contains more water vapor than the air you inhale (breathe in). Its moistness comes from moisture in the lining of the respiratory system. In cold air the vapor condenses (turns into tiny water droplets). In warm air the vapor does not condense, but it is still there. Exhaled air is different from inhaled air in other ways. Because it has been in the body, it is warm. And it contains less oxygen, as well as more waste carbon dioxide, than breathed-in air.

EXPERIMENT

Using up oxygen

Adult help is advised for this experiment

Accurate measurements show that the normal air you inhale contains about 21 percent oxygen, but the air that you exhale has only 17 percent oxygen. The missing 4 percent is used by the body to help it stay alive and work properly. Show how breathing removes oxygen from the air by exposing a candle flame to a jar of fresh air and then to a jar of exhaled air. A candle flame only burns in air that contains enough oxygen. For this experiment, you must use a large heat-proof jar and a short, wide candle that will not topple over. Make sure you wear the oven mitts, because the jar will become hot.

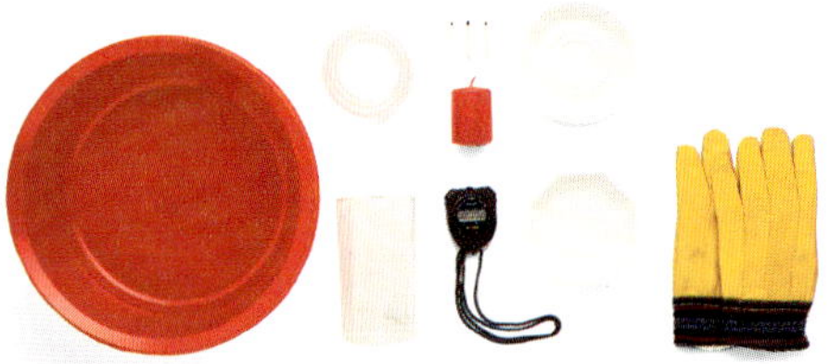

YOU WILL NEED

• *bowl* • *water* • *stopwatch* • *plastic tube* • *large heat-proof jar* • *matches* • *short, wide candle* • *saucers* • *oven mitts*

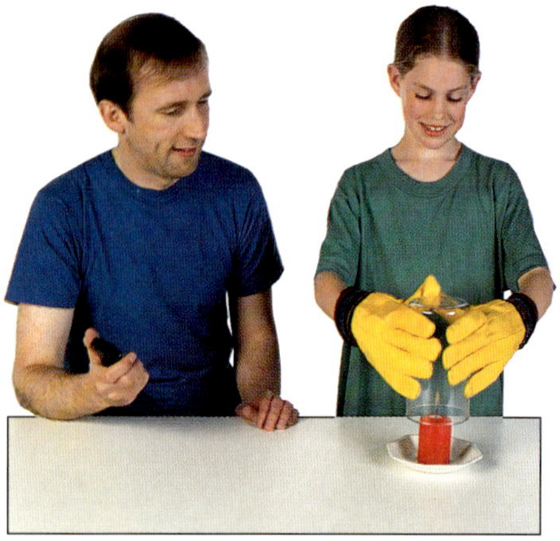

1 LIGHT THE CANDLE. Put on the oven mitts and carefully cover the candle with the jar so that the mouth of the jar rests fully on the saucer. Time how long the flame burns before it goes out (uses up all of the oxygen in the jar). Now fill the jar and bowl with water.

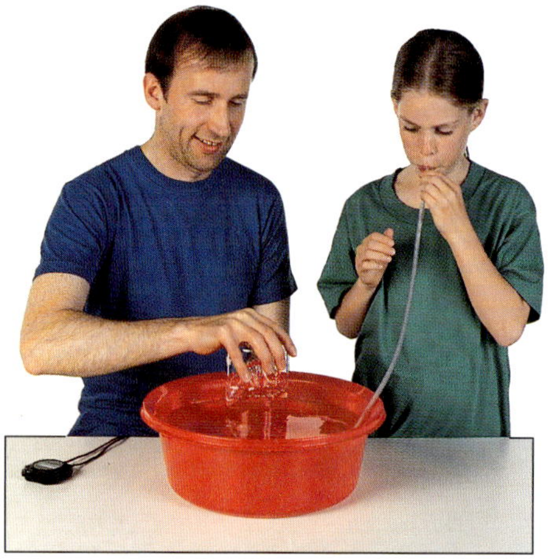

2 TIP THE JAR upside down in the bowl of water. Put the end of the tube under its rim. Inhale, wait a few seconds, then put the tube to your mouth and exhale down it into the jar. Steady the jar with your hand. Repeat until the jar is full of exhaled air.

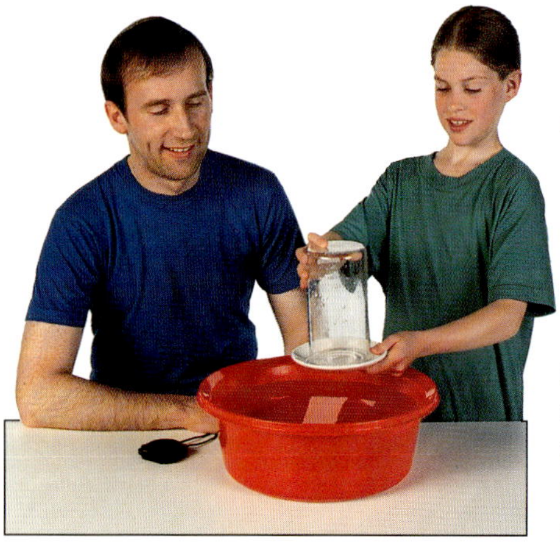

3 DO THIS STEP quickly. Lift out the jar, keeping it upside down. Cover the mouth of the jar with the second saucer, so your breath is trapped inside.

4 LIGHT THE CANDLE, and put on the oven mitts again. Quickly remove the second saucer and place the jar over the lit candle. How long does the flame burn in exhaled air? Does this air have more oxygen than normal air or less? *Caution: Remember that the jar will become hot.*

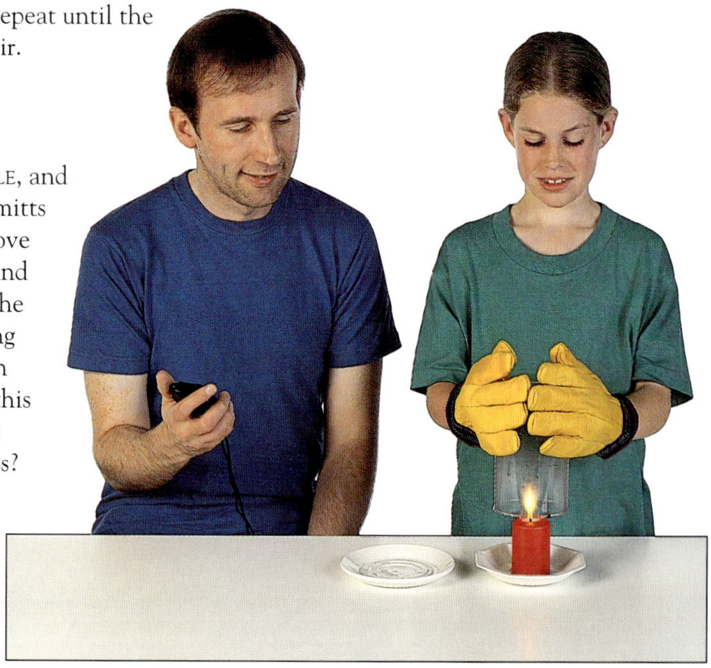

EXPERIMENT

Moist breath

The air that you breathe out contains water vapor. Show this by turning the vapor back into liquid water on the surface of a mirror.

You Will Need

- *small plastic-edged mirror*

Condensing breath

Put the mirror in the fridge for an hour. Wipe it, hold it in front of your mouth, and breathe on it. The vapor in your breath condenses as a fog of droplets on the cold mirror surface.

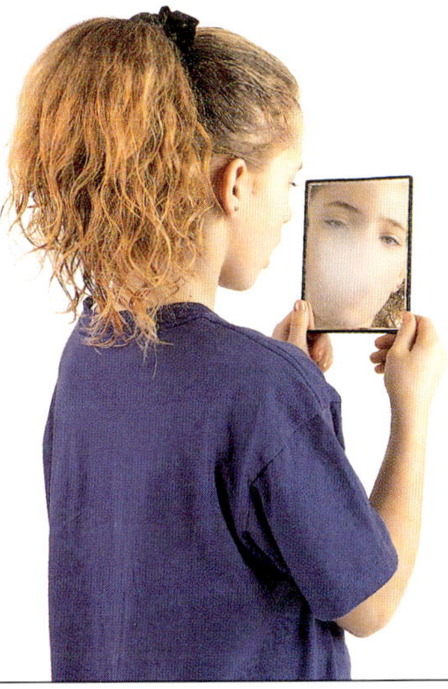

Altered breathing

Breathing muscles respond automatically to everyday hazards. If your diaphragm is irritated, you may hiccup; if there is too little oxygen in your blood, you may yawn; and if dirt finds its way into your air passages, you may cough or sneeze.

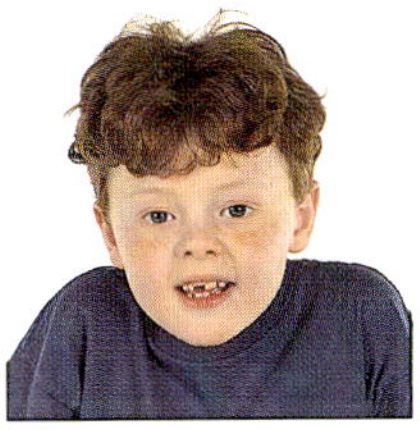

Hiccups
In normal breathing, the diaphragm muscle at the base of your chest (p.72) works smoothly. But if you eat or drink too much, your stomach stretches and irritates the diaphragm, which contracts jerkily. As a result, you hiccup.

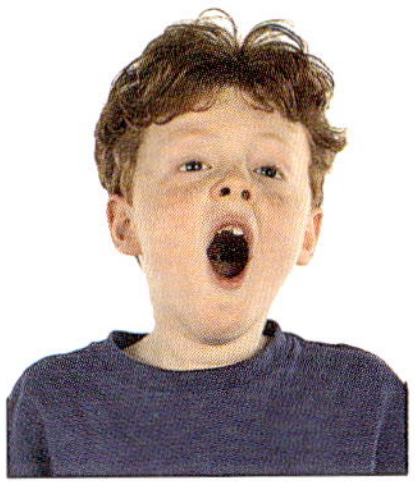

Yawns
If you breathe slowly at rest, the lungs do not get rid of enough carbon dioxide, and it builds up in the blood. So the brain triggers an extra-deep breath, called a yawn. This "blows off" the excess carbon dioxide and brings in more oxygen.

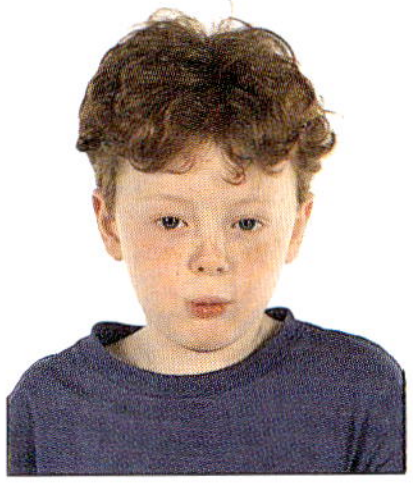

Coughs
A cough gets rid of mucus and dirt in the trachea (p.72) or the air passages to the lungs. You breathe in deeply, close the top of the trachea, build up lung pressure, and let out the air with an explosive rush that rattles the vocal cords.

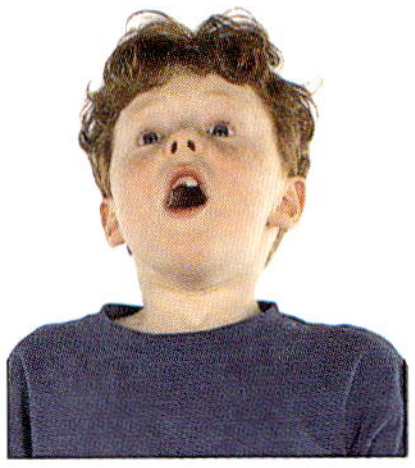

Sneezes
Sometimes mucus or dirt irritates the linings of the air spaces in your nose. So you take a deep breath, and blast the air through your nose at more than 100 miles per hour (160 km per hour) to blow out the irritation.

EXPERIMENT

Breath temperature

Adult help is advised for this experiment

Exhaled air carries heat from the warm inner core of your body—from the vital organs such as your heart. In this experiment you use a thermometer to find out how much warmer exhaled air is, compared to the air around you. *Caution: If the thermometer cracks, do not touch it. Get help from an adult.*

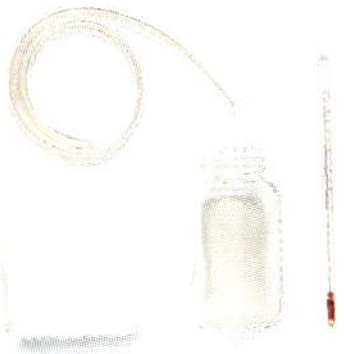

You Will Need

- *plastic tube* • *cotton*
- *small jar* • *standard scientific thermometer*

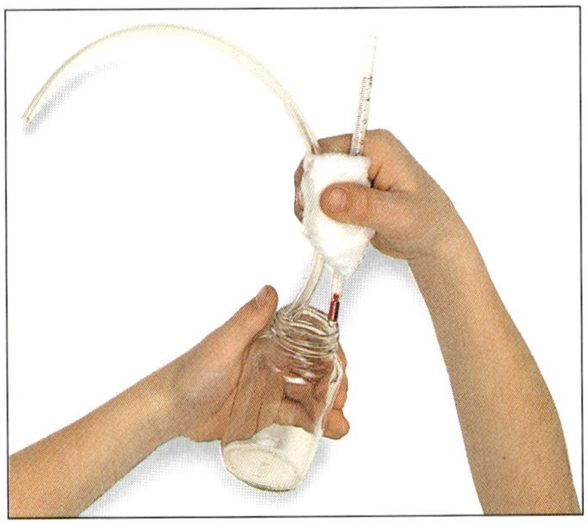

1 Put the tube and the bulb end of the thermometer carefully into the jar. Pack the cotton in the neck of the jar quite firmly, making sure that the thermometer is held securely.

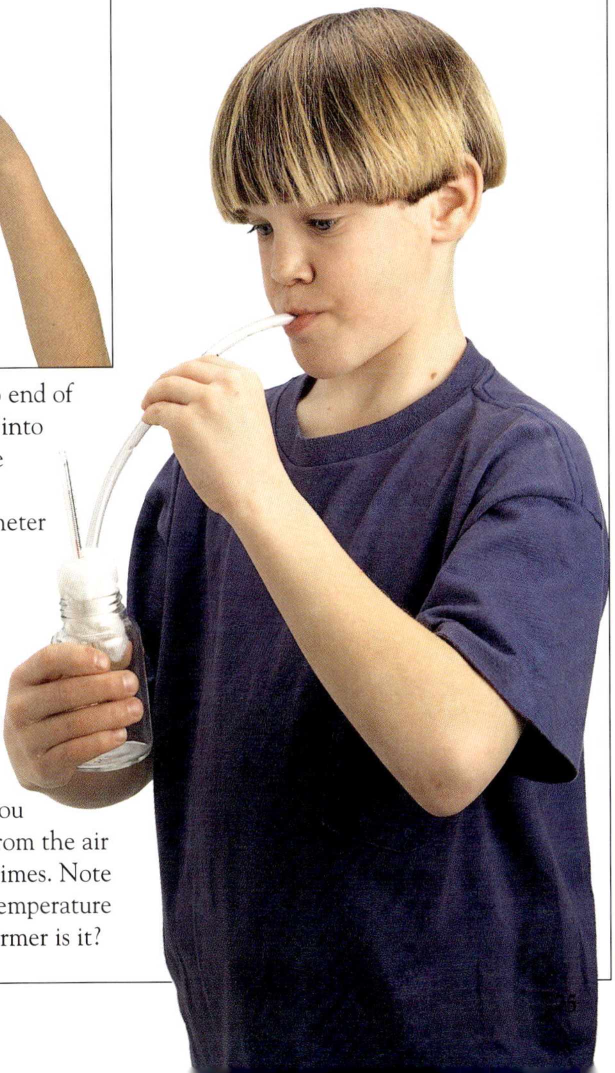

2 Put the other end of the tube in your mouth, and breathe in deeply. Then breathe out away from the tube. Do this 10 times, and note the temperature. This is the temperature of the air you breathe in. Then breathe in from the air and out through the tube 10 times. Note the temperature. This is the temperature of your breath. How much warmer is it?

Lung power

WHEN YOU EXERCISE or play a sport, you sometimes find yourself breathless and panting. This is because your hard-working muscles need more oxygen and energy-rich nutrients to fuel their movements. The heart rate increases so that more of the oxygen and energy carried in the blood can reach the muscles. You breathe faster and deeper to get the extra oxygen from the air into your blood. With regular exercise, your breathing muscles and lungs become better at taking in more air, more quickly. Breathing rate and lung power are two good indicators of fitness and health.

EXPERIMENT

Fast breaths

To measure your breathing rate, see how many breaths you take in 1 minute. The rate depends mainly on how active you have just been. Sit still for 5 minutes and measure the rate. Then do 2 minutes of vigorous exercise, such as running in place. Check your breathing rate every minute after this. How long does it take to return to the resting rate? *Caution: If you feel dizzy or sick when exercising, stop at once and rest.*

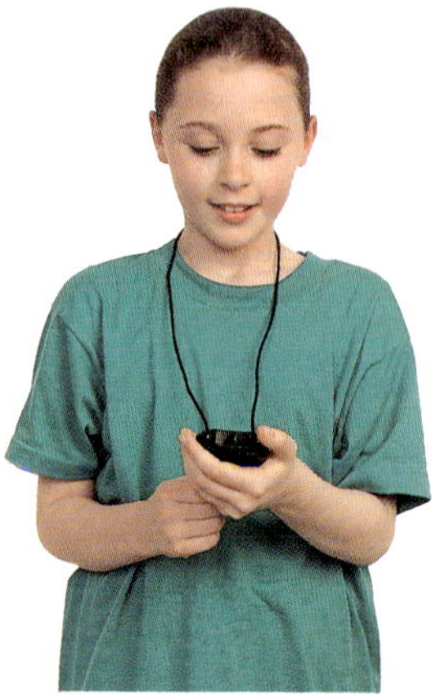

Counting and timing
Breathing in and then out again counts as one breath. To time the number of times you breathe in 1 minute, use a stopwatch.

EXPERIMENT

Blowing power

Adult help is advised for this experiment

This experiment tests lung power—how hard you can blow and for how long. Make a fan-shaped engine that pulls a car up a ramp to see how much lung power you have. *Caution: If you feel dizzy or sick, stop blowing at once and rest.*

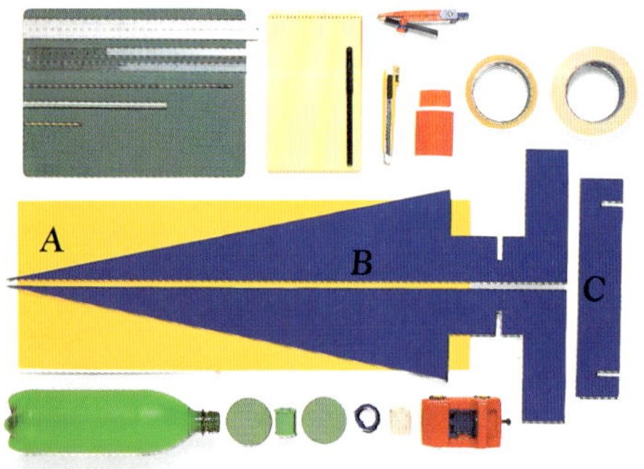

YOU WILL NEED

• *cutting mat* • *ruler* • *cutting edge* • *drinking straw* • *1-ft (30-cm) of stiff wire* • *compass* • *toothpick* • *cellophane tape* • *double-sided tape* • *craft knife* • *glue* • *foamboard—for the ramp top, 24 in* x *8 in (60 cm* x *20 cm), shaped as* **A**; *for the ramp sides, 2 pieces 30 in* x *7 in (75 cm* x *18 cm), shaped as* **B**; *for the ramp crosspiece, 11 in* x *2½ in (28 cm* x *7 cm), shaped as* **C** • *scissors* • *plastic bottle* • *small poster-board disks* • *spool* • *thread* • *large cork* • *toy car* • *notepad* • *pen* • *drill*

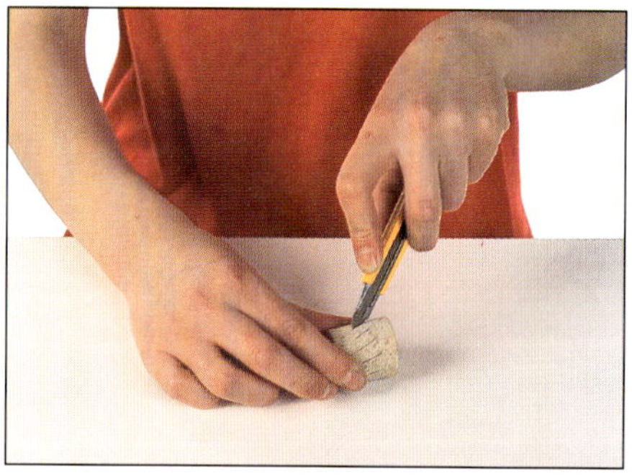

1 CUT 12 SLOTS around the cork. Be sure to cut away from the hand that holds the cork. Make the slots slightly angled and equally spaced. Ask an adult to drill a hole—the right size for the straw to fit tightly—through the cork.

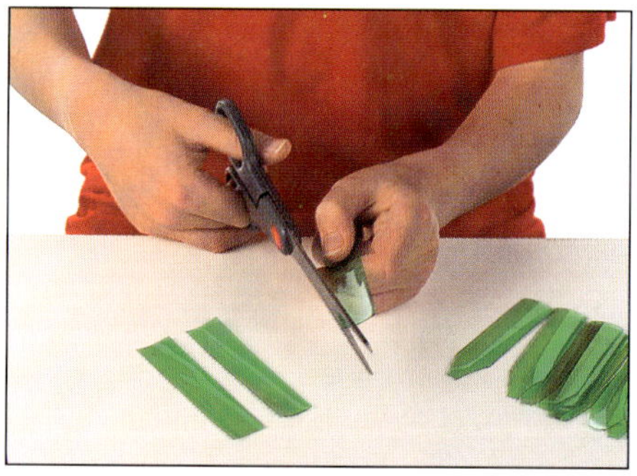

2 CAREFULLY CUT 12 vertical strips from the bottle, each about 4 in x 1 in (10 cm x 2 cm). Trim the ends of the strips into V shapes. Push these into the cork's slots. Make sure that the curves in the strips all face in the same direction.

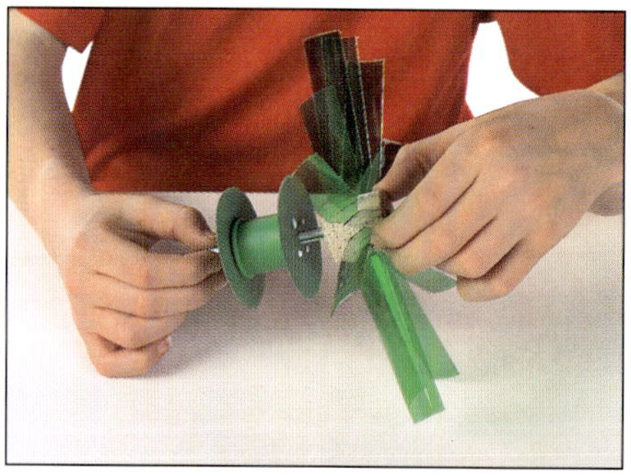

3 CUT SINGLE holes in the centers of the foamboard disks. Slide one disk onto the straw, followed by the spool, then the other disk, and finally the cork. Glue these parts together so that no part moves on its own. This is the engine.

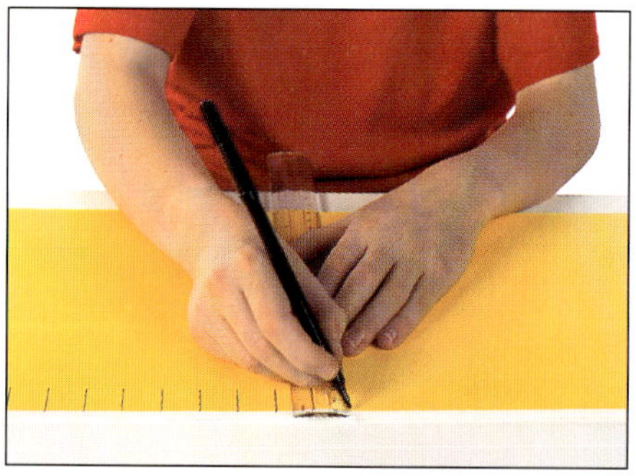

4 DRAW MARKER lines at regular intervals—say 1 in (2 cm)—along one edge of the ramp top. Number each marker, beginning with number 1 at the lower end of the ramp. This is the lung-power scale.

EXPERIMENT

Deep breaths

To breathe in very deeply, your rib and chest muscles pull your ribs up and out (p.73). Your whole chest gets bigger and sucks in more air than with an average breath. Measure this chest expansion using a flexible measuring tape. Compare results with your friends. How much your chest expands is one indication of your lung efficiency. In athletes, chest expansion is usually greater than normal.

Breathing out
A friend holds the tape around the widest part of your chest, usually just above the lowest of your ribs. Breathe out as far as you can. Your friend quickly takes the measurement around your chest.

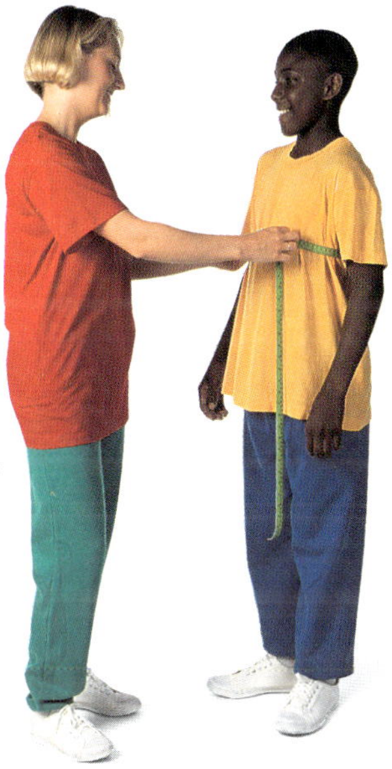

Breathing in
Take the deepest breath that you can. The friend now measures around your fully expanded chest. The difference between the two measurements gives your chest expansion.

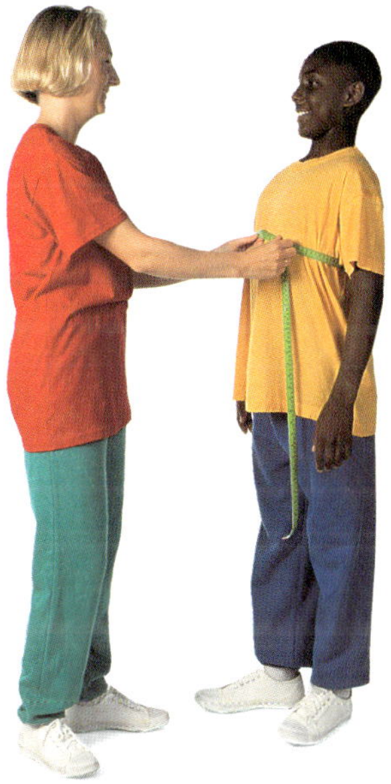

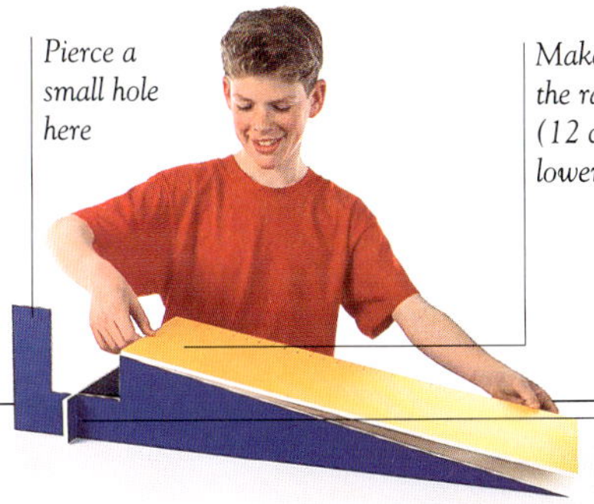

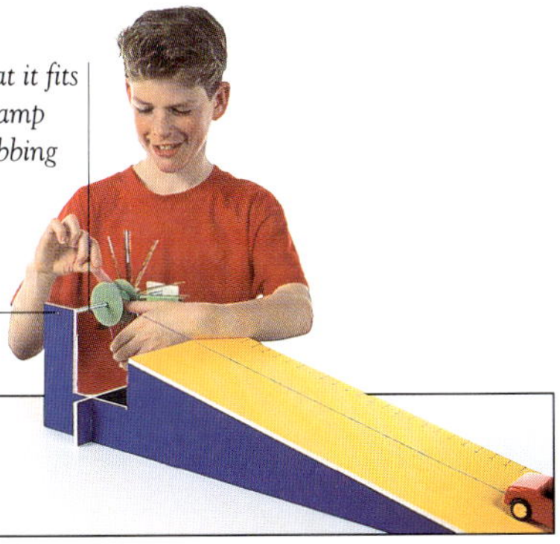

5 JOIN THE sides and the crosspiece (**B** and **C** opposite) by the slits you have cut into the foamboard. Glue or tape the ramp top (**A**) to the top edges of the ramp sides. Use the toothpick to pierce a small hole in the upper part of each ramp side.

6 HOLD THE engine in place, and push the wire through the hole that you have pierced in one ramp side, along the inside of the straw, and then out and through the other hole. Check that the engine spins freely. Tape one end of the thread to the toy car. Cut the thread to the length of the ramp, and tape the other end firmly to the spool.

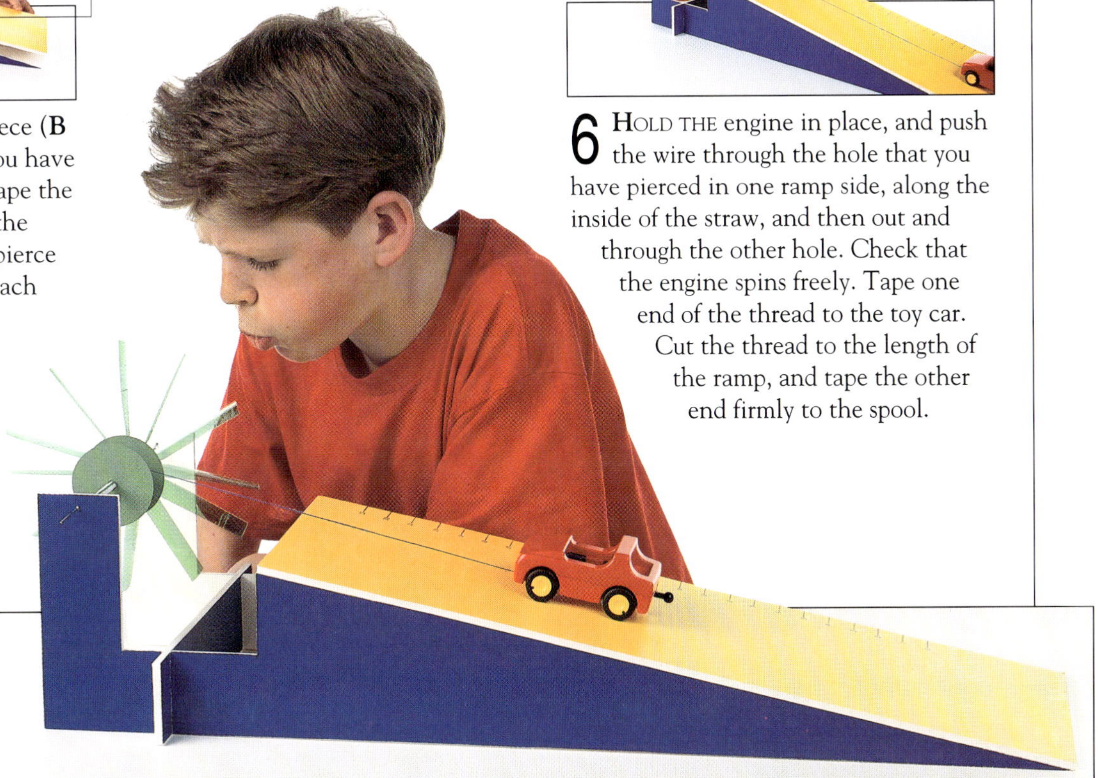

7 TAKE A DEEP breath, and from 2 in (5 cm) away, blow hard and steadily at the engine until your air runs out. Get a friend to see how far the car has traveled up the ramp. Practice aiming your breath. (If the car moves too easily or not easily enough, try a heavier or lighter one.) Now test the lung power of your friends. *Remember to stop at once if anyone feels dizzy or sick.*

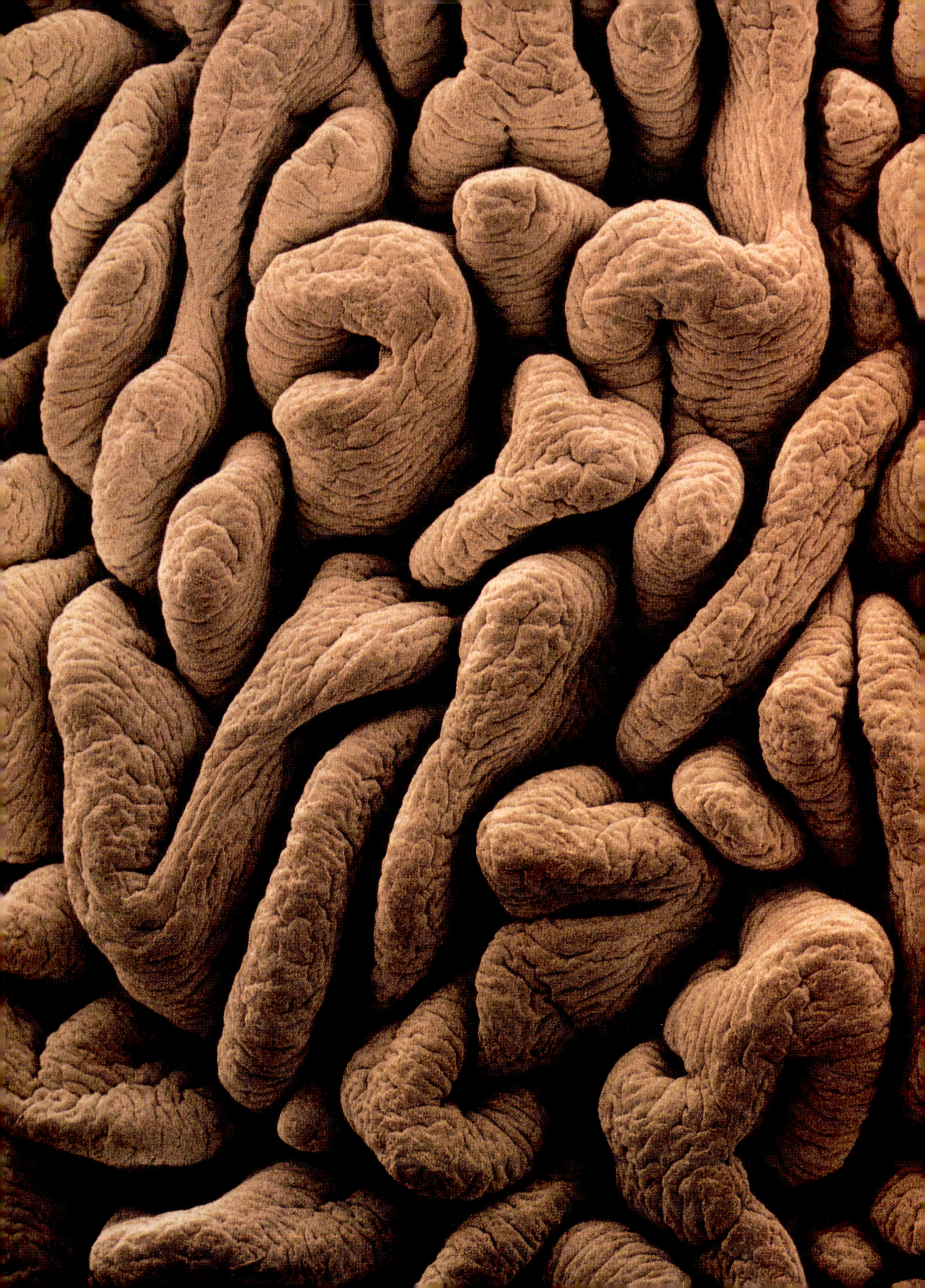

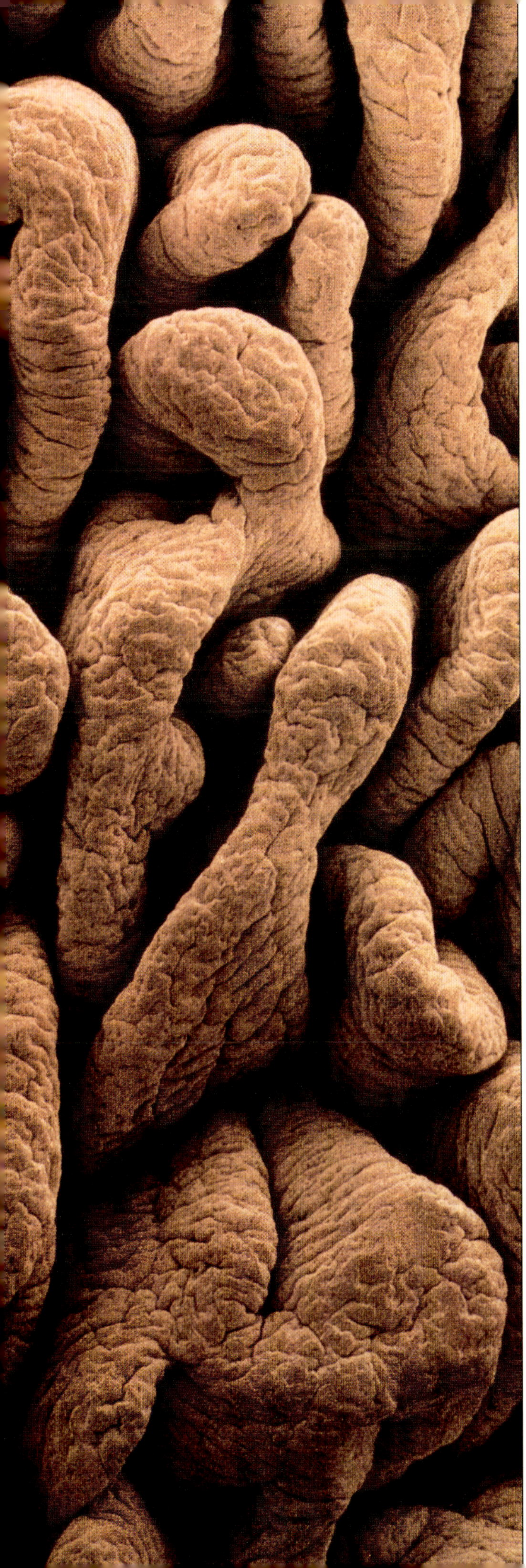

FUELING the BODY

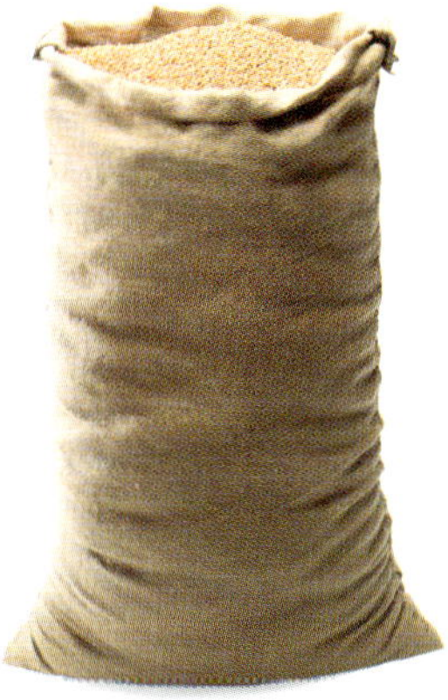

An absorbing business
Even seemingly simple foods usually contain a variety of nourishing substances. Wheat (above), for example, contains starch, fiber, vitamins, and minerals. These are absorbed into the body in the small intestine, which has many tiny folds and fingers known as villi (left).

ALL MACHINES, FROM A flashlight to a jet plane, need energy to make them run. That energy comes from fuel. The body "machine" is no exception. Its fuel is food, which contains energy to drive life processes and raw materials for body growth and maintenance. Food gets into the body through the digestive system, which includes the stomach, intestines, liver, and pancreas. Their task is to break down and process food into simple parts, small enough to be absorbed by the cells of the body.

EATING AND DIGESTION

THE OLD SAYING IS VERY TRUE: "You are what you eat." Your body is built up from the food you take in. The conversion of food into body substances takes place in two stages. Stage one involves eating (getting food to the stomach) and digestion (breaking it down into subunits). The subunits are absorbed by the body and distributed to cells. Stage two takes place in the cells, where the subunits are reassembled to make body parts. Food also provides energy to carry out these processes.

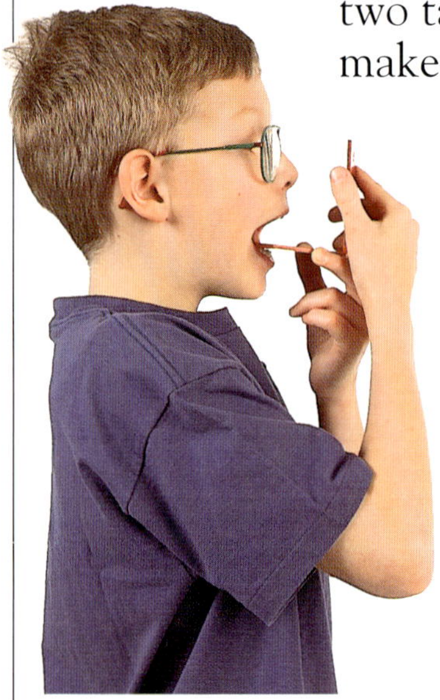

***Your teeth have different shapes** for different jobs. You can use mirrors to study the shapes of your own teeth (p.86).*

To an observer, the digestive system might seem one of the easier body systems to understand. Food goes in one end. Parts of it come out the other end, usually in a changed form. The early anatomists opened the body and traced a long tube through it. They called this tube the digestive tract. They found that the digestive tract is wide at some points, such as the stomach and the large intestine, and narrow at others, such as the esophagus and the small intestine.

However, there was little interest in the study of digestion for many centuries. Galen of ancient Rome (p.13) realized that nutrients in food are absorbed by the intestines and that they go mainly to the liver, along a blood vessel called the hepatic portal vein. However, Galen wrongly believed that the liver converted the digested food into blood and that it gave the blood "animal spirit." In fact blood is not made out of digested food. It is simply a liquid carrier, which transports nutrients from digested food around the whole of the body.

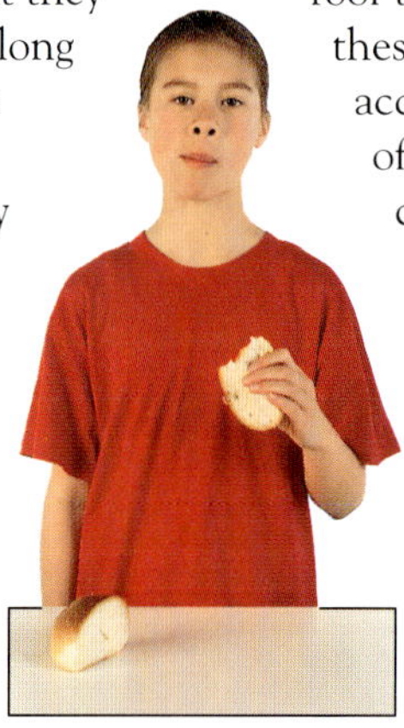

***Chewing mixes food** with saliva, beginning the breakdown of food substances (p.90).*

Food bricks

Not until the 19th century was the chemistry of the digestive process understood in detail. We now know that digestion starts when the food is bitten off and chewed by the teeth in the mouth. It continues in the stomach, and is completed in the small and large intestines.

There are two main reasons why we eat. First, food is fuel for our bodies, providing the energy for living. Second, food provides the nutrients that are the "spare parts" required for the body's growth, maintenance, and repair processes.

The whole process of digestion is like dismantling a building brick by brick—including the doors, windows, flooring, and roof tiles—and then putting these parts back together according to another set of plans, to make a completely different building. In this comparison, the first building is your food, while the second building is your body tissue.

Food groups

To stay healthy, a body needs enough of the right kinds of food. This means eating a range of foods that provide a good balance of the main dietary components.

The first group of components is proteins (p.15). These are the main body-building nutrients. Proteins form the bulk of the structures in every body cell, including parts of the cell membranes (p.28). The tough keratin in the upper skin, the fibers of collagen in the lower skin and in bones, the actin and myosin in muscles, and the hemoglobin in red blood cells are all proteins. The dozens of different enzymes in the body that help to digest food (opposite) are also proteins.

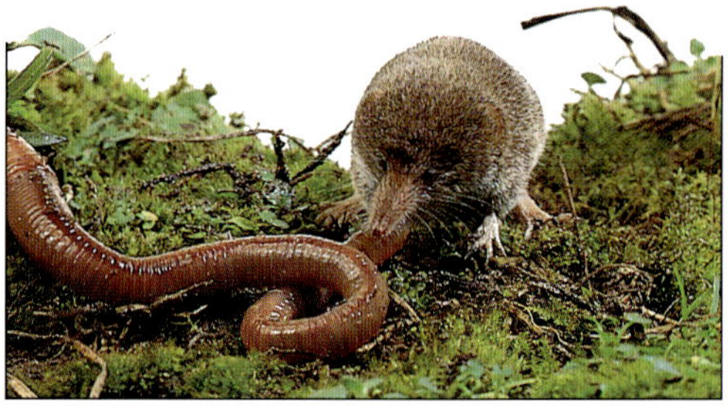

***The tiny shrew, the smallest of mammals,** uses so much energy that it must eat its own weight in food every day.*

The second dietary group is carbohydrates (p.15), which are the main energy-containing nutrients. In most foods, these take the form of starches. In the body, carbohydrates are mostly broken down into their subunit sugars such as glucose.

The third group is lipids (fats and oils, p.15). They are made mostly of subunits formed from fatty acids. Lipids provide structural building blocks for cells, and they also contain

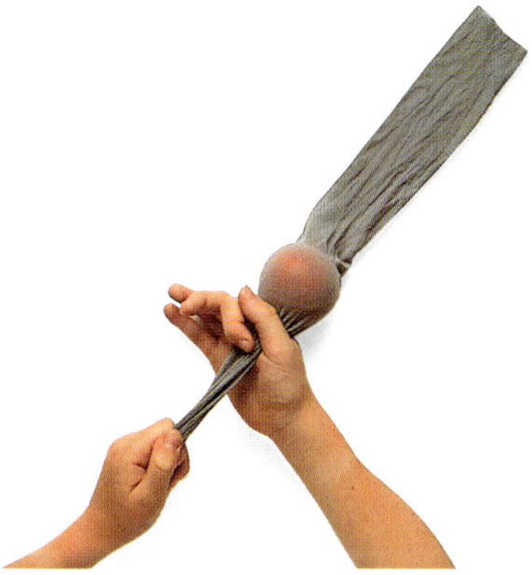

With a ball and a stocking, *demonstrate how waves of muscle contraction propel lumps of food through the digestive tract (p.85).*

energy. Together with proteins, they form the membrane around each cell, and the membranes of the organelles within the cells. The body's stores of fat are also a long-term reservoir of energy. This can be used if the body runs low on the short-term energy that it gets from sugars. In addition, the myelin sheaths around the axons of many nerve cells (p.119) are made from lipids.

The fourth dietary group is vitamins. Compared with the quantities of proteins, carbohydrates, and lipids that the body requires, the amount of vitamins that it needs is very small. Vitamins take part in many chemical processes inside body cells. The body can make some vitamins of its own, such as vitamin D, which is produced in the skin by the action of sunlight. However, it must take in ready-made supplies of other vitamins in food.

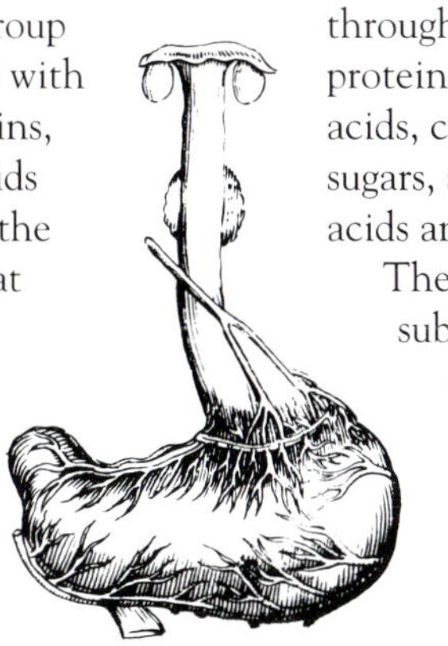

The stomach does not only *digest food. It can also absorb certain substances, such as sugars and alcohol, directly into its network of blood vessels.*

Fifth are minerals (p.15). These contribute mainly to the structural upkeep of cells. Calcium is an important mineral for strong bones and teeth. Iron is essential for hemoglobin (p.95). And sodium in the nerves is vital for the nerve signals that constantly flash around the body.

The sixth dietary component is fiber (roughage). This is found only in plant foods, especially fresh fruit and vegetables, unrefined flour, and legumes such as lentils. Fiber is made up of huge molecules of cellulose, which the body cannot break down or absorb. So it passes right through the digestive tract and is expelled in feces. Fiber helps the digestive process because it gives food "bulk" and allows the intestines to massage the food on its way, providing enough time for thorough digestion.

Subunits

The huge molecules of carbohydrates, proteins, and lipids are too big to pass through the lining of the intestines and become absorbed into the body. Digestion breaks these large food substances into their subunits, so they are small enough to pass through. With digestion, proteins are split into amino acids, carbohydrates into sugars, and lipids into fatty acids and other subunits.

The nutrients and subunits are carried around the body in both blood and lymph (p.182) and supplied to the cells. In each cell, the nutrients are used according to the cell's needs—perhaps to provide energy or to make new substances.

Enzymes

The chemical splitting of food substances into subunits is aided by enzymes. These are special proteins that control the rate of chemical changes but are not changed themselves. Digestive enzymes are made by the salivary glands, stomach, pancreas, and small intestine. Hundreds of other types of enzyme are found all over the body, regulating cell chemistry. In digestion, enzyme action is particularly intense in the stomach.

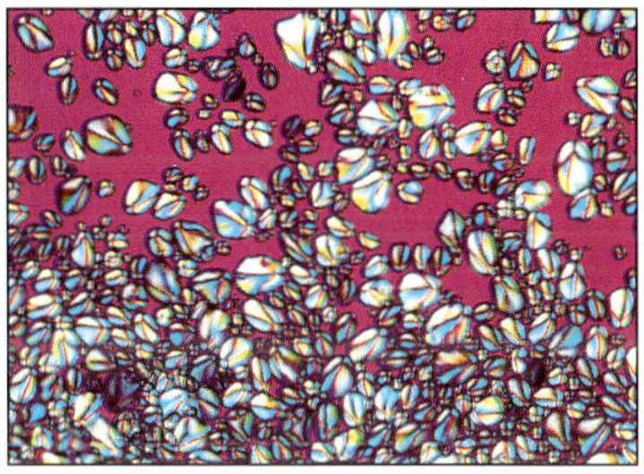

Grains of potato starch, shown in *this microscope photograph, are massive lumps of molecules that are broken down by digestion into sugar subunits.*

By-products

In addition to enzymes, the stomach lining makes hydrochloric acid. This eats away at the food and helps to kill germs that have entered the body in food. To stop itself from being digested by its own enzymes and acid, the stomach lining produces a thick layer of slimy mucus.

As the stomach contents ooze into the small intestine, they meet more enzymes—from the intestine lining and in juices made by the pancreas. The pancreatic juices also contain an alkali. This counteracts the stomach acid, so that it does not harm the rest of the digestive tract.

These by-products of digestion, together with undigested food leftovers, move through the large intestine, where minerals and water are removed and recycled by the body. Finally the remains are expelled from the body as feces.

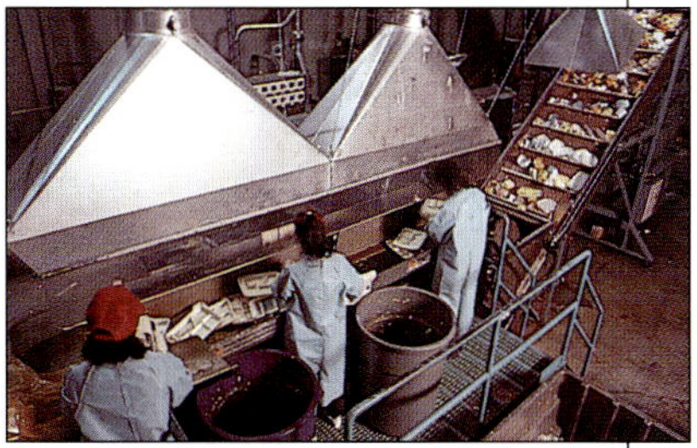

Like this recycling factory, the *large intestine reabsorbs into the body valuable leftovers of the digestive process, such as minerals from the digestive juices and water.*

Diet and energy

JUST AS WE put gasoline in a car or wood on a fire, so we must put food into our bodies. Food contains energy that drives the body's many chemical processes. But it differs from such fuels as gas or wood in one very important way. Food contains not only energy but also the raw materials needed for the body's growth, maintenance, and repair. It is as if you put gas into a car's tank and then watched the car change the gas into replacement bearings, nuts and bolts, and new tires for itself! To carry out its maintenance and repair processes, the body needs a selection of nutrients, such as proteins, carbohydrates, fats and oils, minerals, and vitamins (pp.80–81). It must get these from food. Your diet (the food and drink you take in) should contain enough of each type of nutrient, as well as a good balance of them.

Energy units and equivalents

Like fuels such as coal, food contains energy in chemical form. How does the energy content in food compare with that of other fuels? The modern international unit for energy is the joule (J). A meal of chicken with salad in a roll, a container of fruit yogurt, and an orange totals about 2,300 kJ (1 kJ, or kilojoule = 1,000 J). This equals the energy in a lump of a coal about half the size of the yogurt container. Another energy unit is the calorie (cal). But 1 cal, like 1 J, is a small unit, so the more common measure is the kilocalorie, also called kcal or Cal (with a capital "C"), which is 1,000 cals. To convert calories to joules, 1 cal = 4.2 J, and 1 kcal (1 Cal) = 4.2 kJ. The number of kcals or kJ in food products is often indicated on their packaging.

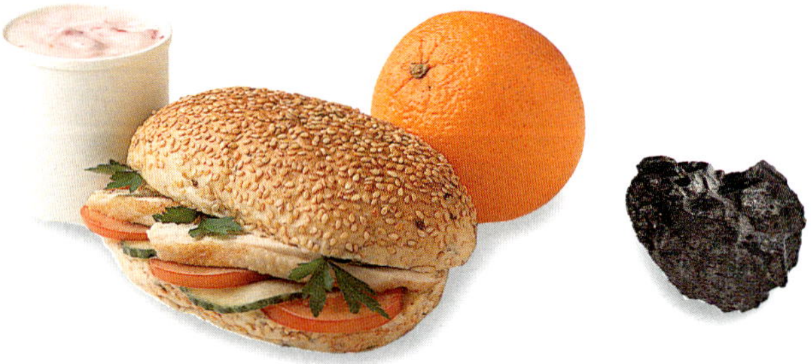

Picnic lunch
This meal, which gives 2,300 kJ of energy, weighs 19 oz (530 g). Most of the energy is in the bread and chicken.

Coal comparison
When it is burned, this piece of coal gives the same amount of energy as the meal, but it weighs only 3 oz (80 g).

EXPERIMENT

Energy in a peanut

This is an adult demonstration and should not be attempted by children

Measure the energy content of a peanut by making your own simple calorimeter (heat-measuring device) with a tin can. Compare the peanut's energy to that of an ordinary type of fuel, wood.

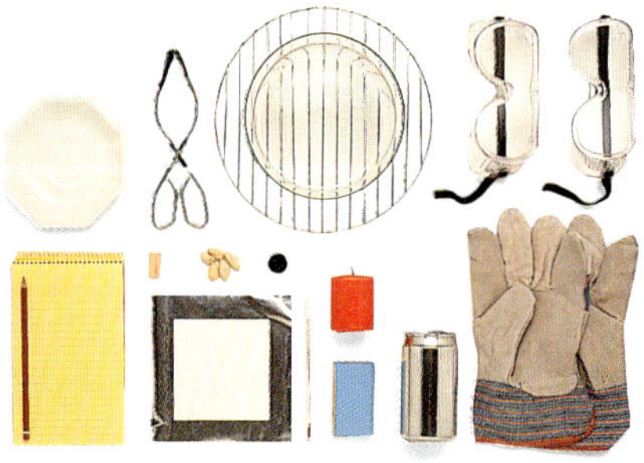

YOU WILL NEED

- *saucer* • *short, wide candle* • *notepad* • *pencil* • *metal tongs* • *wire cooling rack* • *bowl of water* • *fresh (uncooked) peanuts* • *piece of wood of the same weight as a peanut* • *ceramic tile wrapped in aluminum foil* • *standard scientific thermometer* • *matches* • *metal soft-drink can* • *goggles* • *oven mitts*

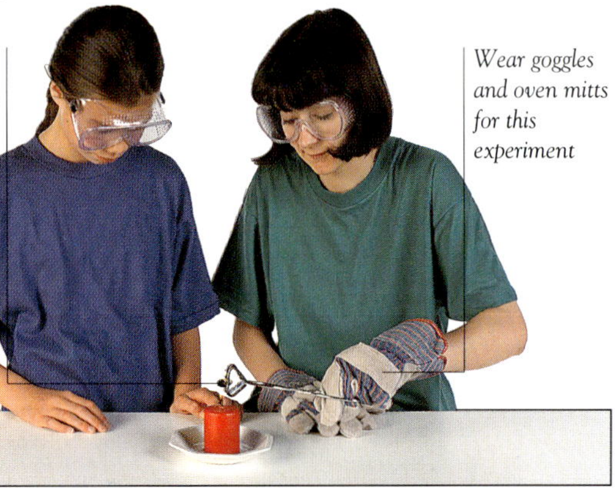

Peanuts burn well for this experiment, as they have a high oil content and so are packed with energy

Wear goggles and oven mitts for this experiment

1 FILL HALF the can with water, and place it on the rack. Hold a peanut in a candle flame with the tongs.

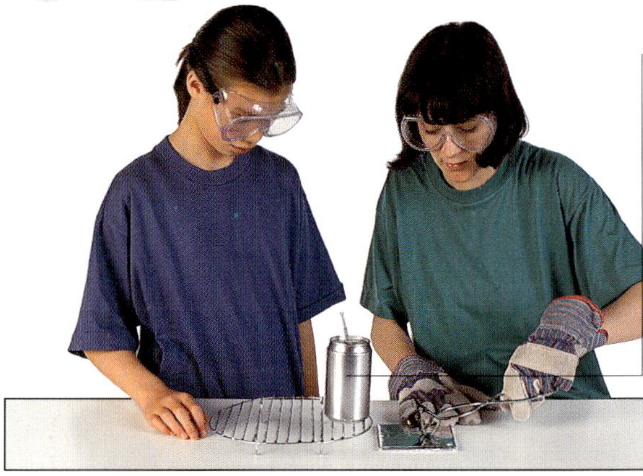

Check the temperature of the water before you heat it with the peanut

2 AS THE PEANUT catches fire, place it on the foil-covered tile. Slide the tile under the can on the wire rack.

Your energy needs

Even when you sleep, your body uses energy to keep warm and make your heart beat. The more active you are, the more energy your muscles use. The blood brings energy to the muscles in the form of glucose (a sugar). Your daily energy needs depend on various factors, such as your age and lifestyle.

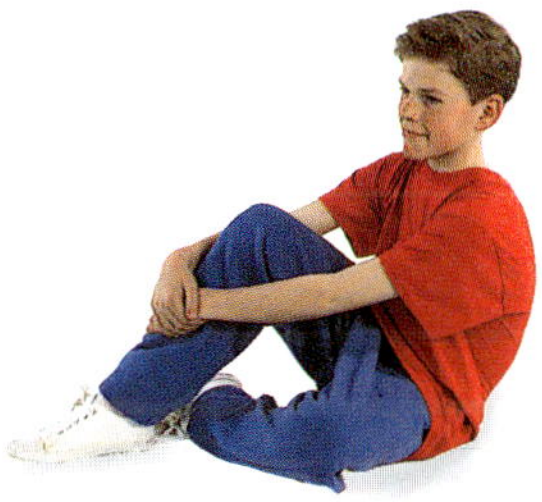

At rest
Basic energy use is about 3–4 kJ per minute for a 12-year-old.

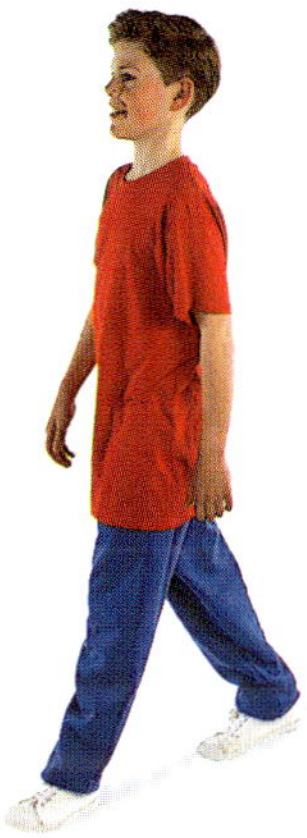

Mild activity
Brisk walking raises the energy use rate to 10–15 kJ per minute.

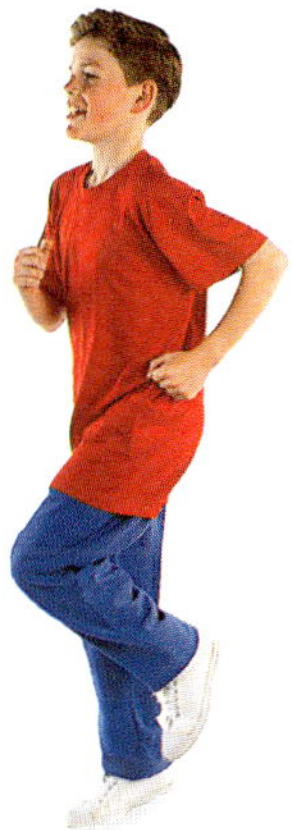

Strenuous activity
When jogging or playing sports, the body uses 30–40 kJ per minute.

Energy and nutrients

Each type of food has a typical energy value. But energy alone is not always desirable. You could run all day on the energy in chocolate bars. But chocolate is made almost solely of high-energy sugar, with few other nutrients.

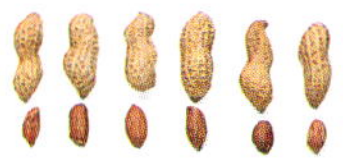

Nuts
Nuts are high in fats, carbohydrates, and proteins. Nearly 2 oz (50 g) of peanuts contain 1,200 kJ.

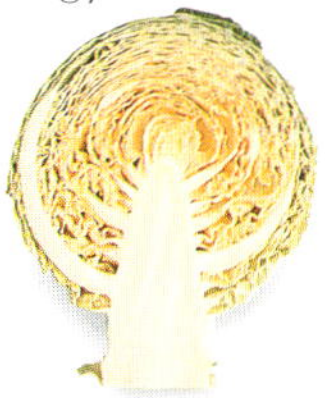

Vegetables
Leafy vegetables are high in fiber, minerals, and vitamins, but low in energy. A cabbage leaf contains 25 kJ.

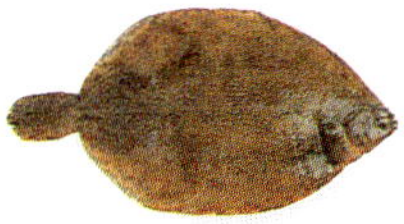

Fish
Fish is rich in protein, but has few carbohydrates. A portion gives up to 1,000 kJ.

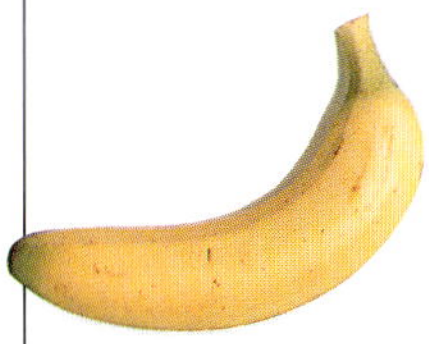

Fruits
These contain fiber, vitamins, and some carbohydrates. Bananas have more energy than most fruits, at 250 kJ.

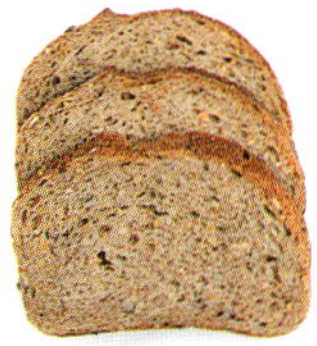

Breads
These starchy, high-carbohydrate foods are packed with energy for their weight, about 250 kJ per slice.

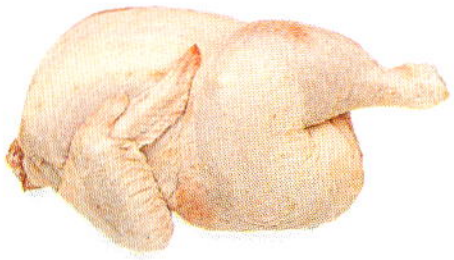

Meats
Like fish, meat is high in protein. A chicken leg gives 600 kJ, and a serving of steak 1,700 kJ.

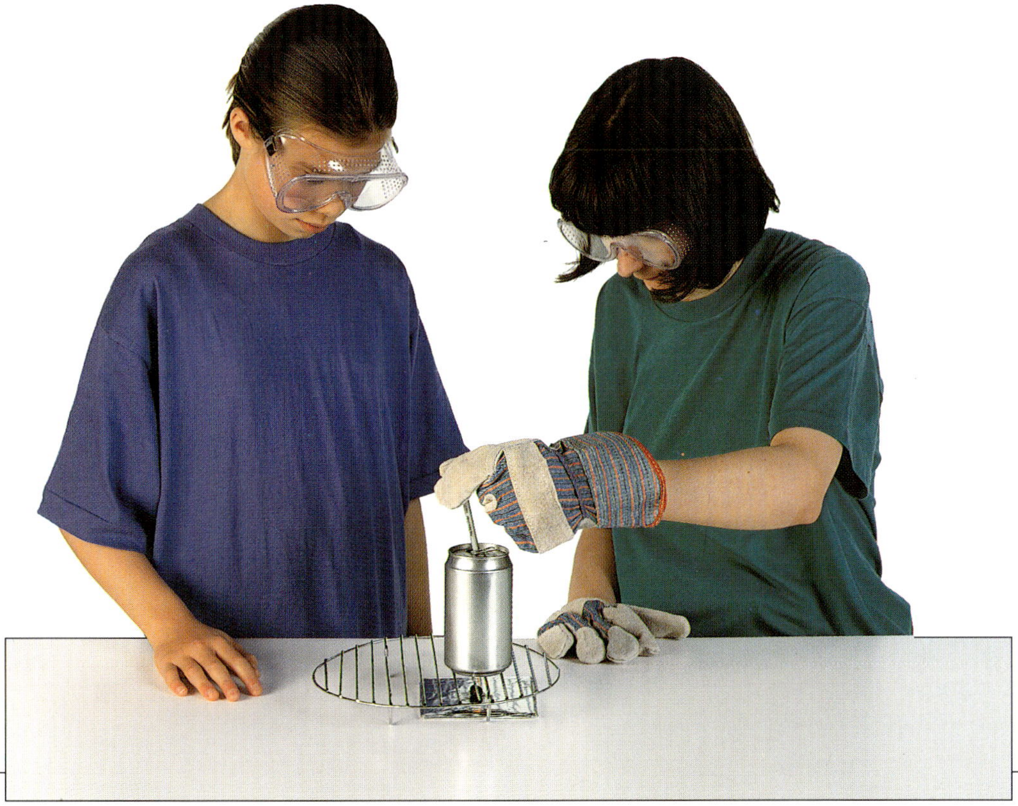

3 KEEP TWISTING the peanut with the tongs to make sure it burns all over. The peanut's chemical energy converts to heat energy, which warms the water. Keep your eye on the thermometer scale, and make a note of its highest reading. Now repeat the process with the wood. Before burning the wood, cool the tongs in water. Add fresh water up to the same level in the can as before, and make sure that the water is the same temperature as at the start of the first test. Check that the burned peanut and wood are cold before you dispose of them. Which fuel gives the highest thermometer reading, indicating that it contains the most energy?

The digestive system

WHEN YOU SWALLOW FOOD, it enters a long tube, called the digestive tract (gut). This tract has several main sections—the mouth, pharynx (throat), esophagus, stomach, and intestines—each of which has a special role in digestion. When food reaches the small intestine, it passes through the intestine lining into the body. This process is called absorption. The lining of the small intestine has thousands of tiny finger- or tongue-shaped parts called villi, which are themselves covered by thousands of microvilli (opposite). The villi absorb digested food into the blood, to be distributed to the body tissues. The digestive system as a whole also includes the pancreas, liver, and gall bladder (opposite), which make and distribute different digestive juices.

The digestive tract

The basic parts of the digestive system are common to all but the smallest, simplest animals. Food enters at the mouth and is swallowed through the pharynx. However, there are differences between the digestive systems of humans and of animals like the worm shown here. Unlike humans, worms do not have teeth, so their digestive tube includes a muscular chamber called a gizzard, which crushes and mashes the food. Also, worms eat bulk food that is low in nutrients. They store this in a chamber called a crop, which expands to hold as much food as possible.

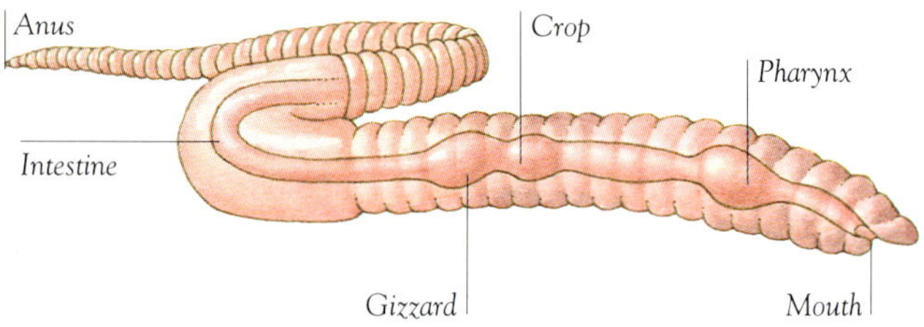

The worm's digestive tract
The basic design of the digestive tract and the specialized parts of the system that carry out particular jobs can be seen clearly in a relatively simple creature such as the earthworm. Its intestine is not looped and folded as in the human body, but is a straight tube.

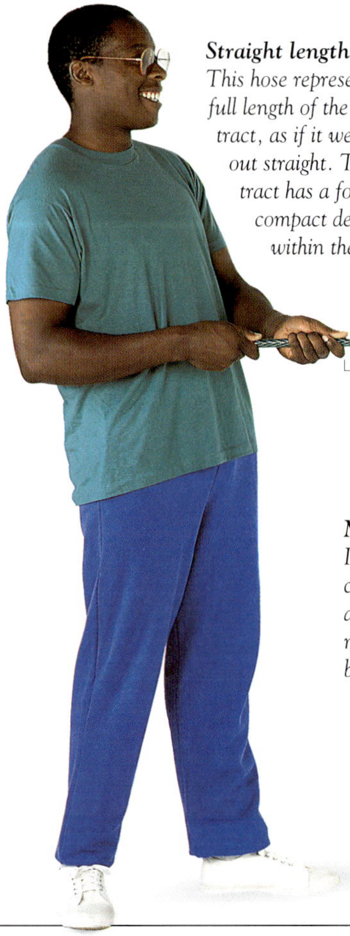

Straight length
This hose represents the full length of the digestive tract, as if it were pulled out straight. The real tract has a folded, compact design within the body.

The digestive journey

A piece of food that disappears into a child's mouth is starting a journey that is about 20 ft (6.5 m) long. The typical length of each region of the digestive tract is shown below. Exactly how long digestion takes depends on the types and amounts of food that you have eaten. Foods with plenty of carbohydrates are digested faster than those containing large amounts of fats. Also, like most body processes, digestion tends to be slightly slower during the night. The approximate amount of time that has passed by the end of each stage of digestion is shown on the clocks below.

Mouth (3 in/8 cm)
It takes a few seconds to chew a mouthful of food and mix it with saliva, to make an easy-to-swallow bolus (p.88).

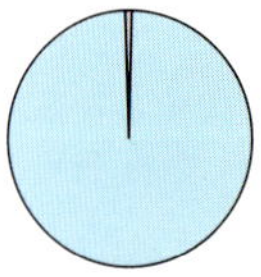

Eating: for 5 to 30 seconds

Pharynx and esophagus (10 in/25 cm)
The back of the tongue pushes food down the pharynx, and waves of muscle action thrust it through the esophagus.

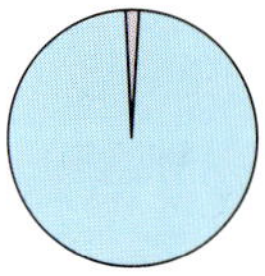

Swallowing: for 10 seconds

Stomach (6 in/15 cm)
The stomach expands during the meal to hold all of the food that it receives. About 2 to 3 hours after eating, semidigested foods are passed from the stomach on to the intestines.

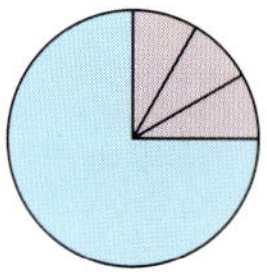

In the stomach: for 3 hours

Parts of the system

Each section of the digestive system has its own role. The esophagus is a transfer tube; the stomach is a food squasher and chemical bath; the small intestine finishes food breakdown and carries out absorption; and the large intestine recycles body substances by absorbing water, minerals, and other useful items into the body. The appendix is a mysterious, finger-size part that seems to lack a major function. It may be an evolutionary remnant from our distant ancestors.

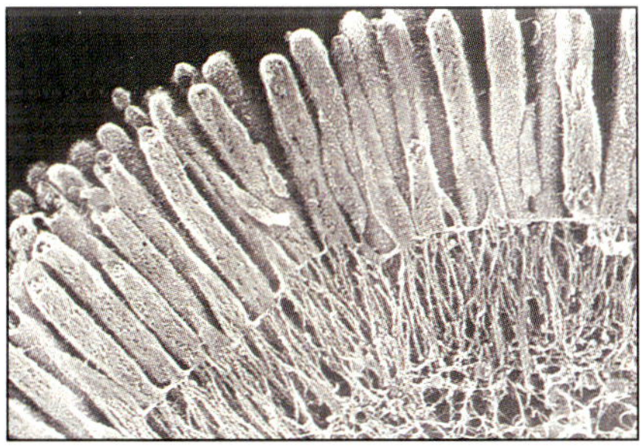

Huge surface area of microvilli
Microvilli like these cover the tiny villi in the small intestine. The villi and microvilli create a huge surface area—10 times greater than your whole skin area—for absorbing food.

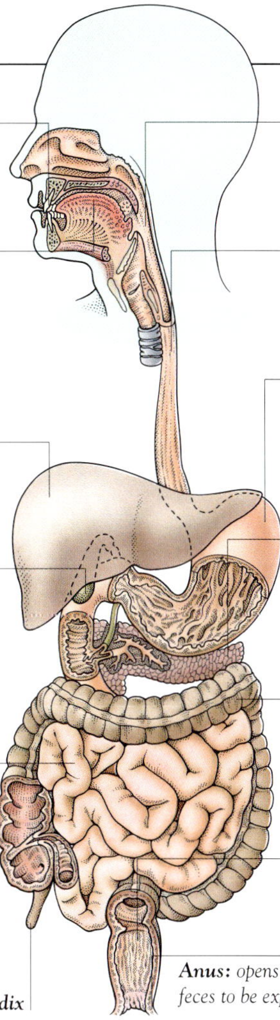

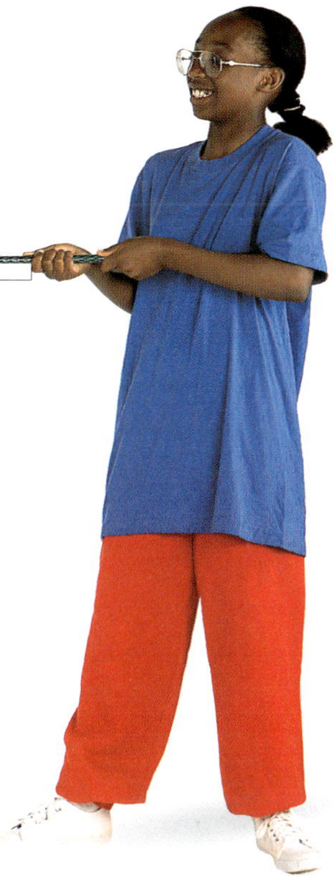

Small intestine (13 to 16 ft/4 to 5 m)
Some 6 hours after eating, the partly digested food is like a thick milk shake. It oozes along the three parts of the small intestine: from the duodenum to the jejunum and then to the ileum.

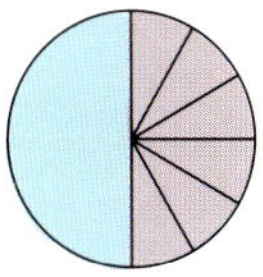

In the small intestine: for 3 hours

Large intestine (4 ft/1.2 m)
Water and minerals are absorbed into the body by the colon. Feces (solid wastes) accumulate in the last part of the large intestine, the rectum, where they remain until a convenient moment, when they exit through the anus.

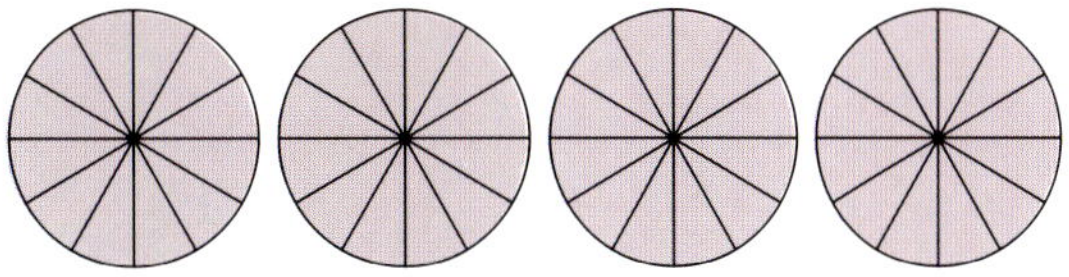

In the large intestine: for up to 2 days

Teeth

TEETH ARE THE FIRST STOP for the fuel entering your body. They have several jobs. First, they bite and chop mouth-size lumps out of large food items, like bread or an apple. The chisel-shaped front teeth, called incisors, do this best. The pointed canine teeth just beside them may tear and rip at the food. The teeth then squash, crush, and chew the food into a pulp. They mix it with saliva into a soft, squishy lump—ready to swallow. The broad, flat-topped rear teeth, the premolars and molars, are best at doing this. They are near the hinge of the jaw joint, where the powerful jaw-closing muscles allow them to exert tremendous pressure.

Your second set of teeth—32 adult (permanent) teeth—is designed to last from childhood into old age. These teeth are covered by white or yellow enamel, the hardest substance in your body. Enamel can stand years of physical wear as the teeth bite and chew hard foods. But it may be worn down in a chemical way. If old food and bacteria build up in the mouth, they can decay the enamel, cause toothache, and destroy the whole tooth.

EXPERIMENT

Look at your teeth

Study your teeth using small mirrors. How many do you have?

YOU WILL NEED

- *2 small plastic-edged mirrors*

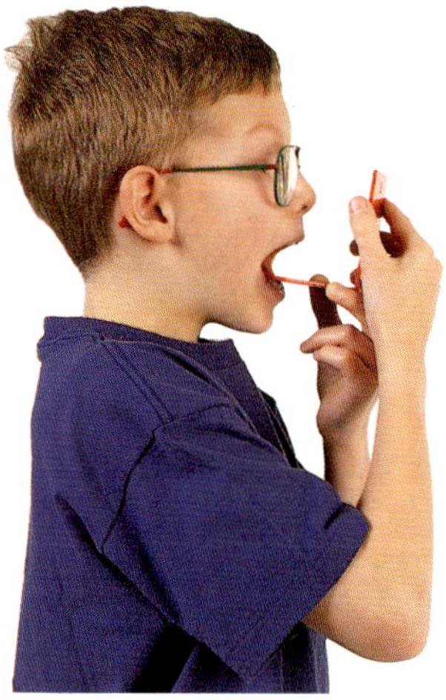

Getting a good view
For your lower teeth, open your mouth wide, and angle the mirror to reflect them. For the upper set, hold one mirror just inside your mouth, facing upward. Adjust the second mirror to reflect the teeth in the first one.

How teeth grow

You are born with all the teeth you will ever have. At birth they are tiny tooth buds, deep inside the jawbone. As you grow, your teeth grow too. Your initial teeth enlarge and appear through the gums between the ages of 6 months and 3 years. They are called milk or deciduous teeth, and there are 20 in the full set. Milk teeth start to fall out when you are about 6 years old. By the age of 20, most people have all of their adult teeth. There are 32 in total, although not all of these appear in everybody. Some adults never grow their back four molars, which are called wisdom teeth.

Teeth at birth (milk teeth in gray)

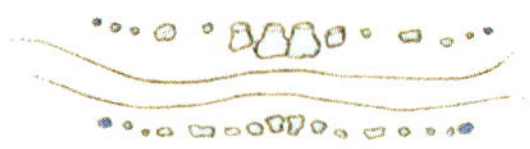

Teeth at 3 years (adult teeth in blue)

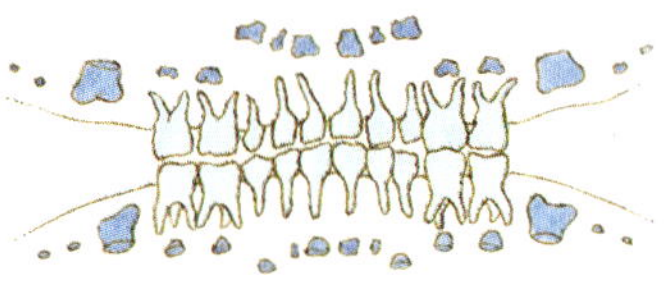

Teeth at 9 years

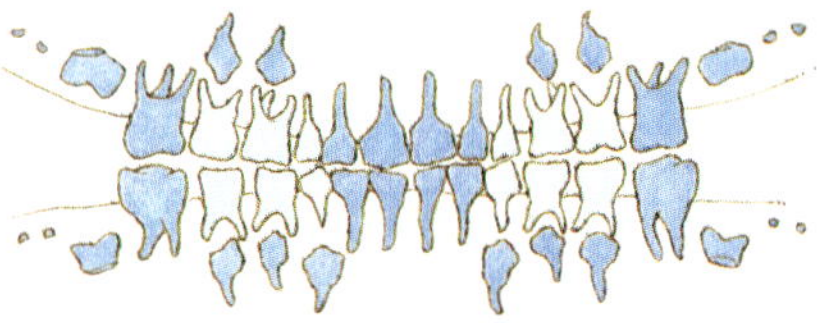

Full set of adult teeth (with the right-hand side of the mouth separated into tooth types)

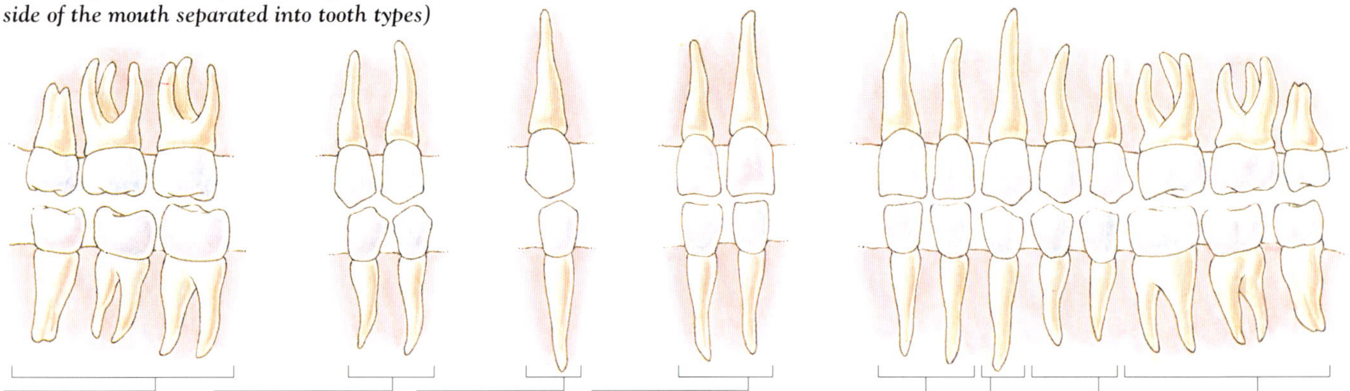

3 pairs of molars chew and crush

2 pairs of premolars chew and cut

1 pair of canines rip and tear

2 pairs of incisors cut and chop

Incisors

Canines

Premolars

Molars

Inside a tooth

This cutaway diagram shows the main parts of a human molar. The outer layer is enamel, which resists years of wear. Under it is dentine, which is softer than enamel. The pulp cavity in the center of the tooth is filled with blood vessels and nerves. (Blood vessels are shown in one root of the tooth and nerves in the other, but in reality all roots have both.) The roots of the tooth are fixed into their sockets in the jawbone by cementum, a kind of living glue. The soft gum covers the jawbone.

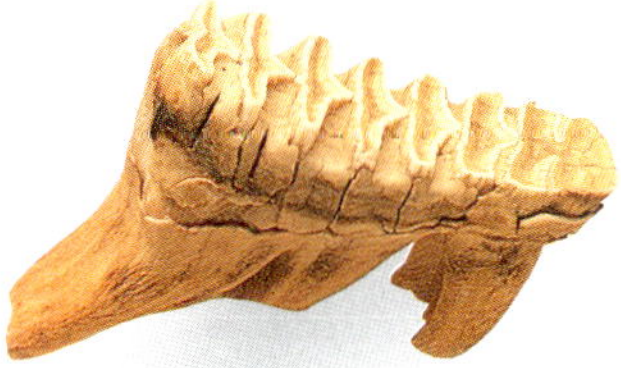

Specialized teeth
Animal teeth are designed to chew particular types of food. An elephant molar is as big as a fist and has sharp ridges for munching plants.

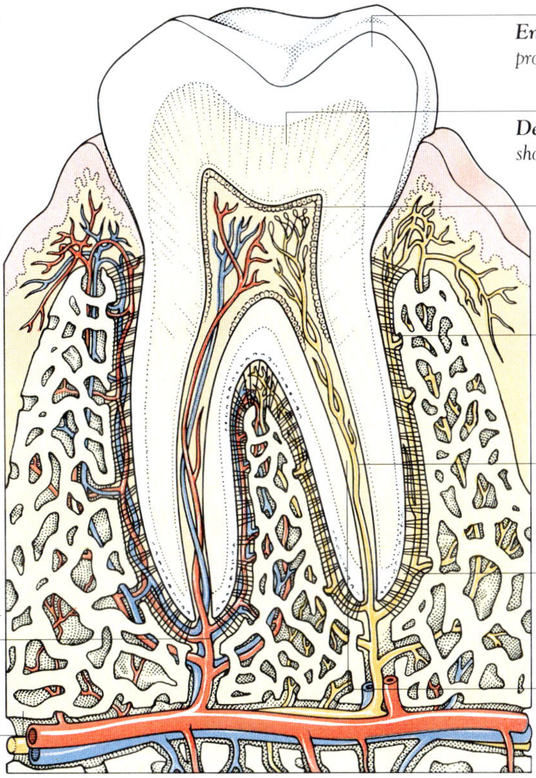

Plaque on teeth

Teeth are good places for bacteria to grow. The bacteria feed on leftover particles of food, and they make waste products, such as acids, which then attack the teeth. On uncleaned teeth the dead bacteria, their wastes, old food, and saliva build up into a sticky, tooth-decaying layer called dental plaque.

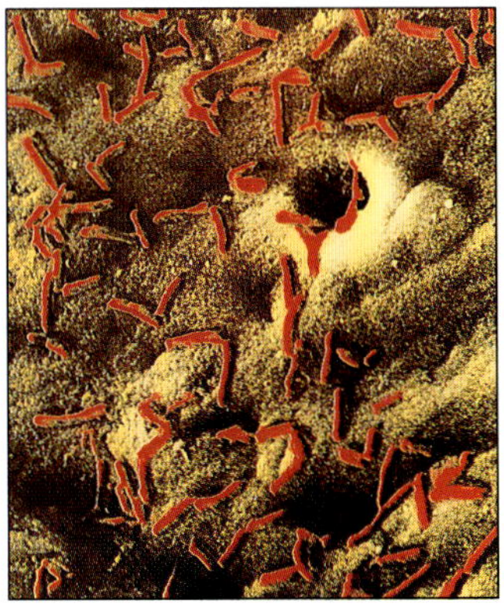

Microscopic attackers
Rod-shaped bacteria find food on the smooth surface of teeth.

EXPERIMENT

How clean are your teeth?

Disclosing tablets show whether your teeth are clean or not, by coloring plaque and bits of old food. Use the tablets to check how effective your tooth cleaning is, and see if you can improve it.

You Will Need

- *disclosing tablets (from a dentist or pharmacist)*
- *toothbrush and toothpaste*
- *mirror*
- *water to rinse*

Using disclosing tablets
Follow the instructions on the tablet package. Look at your mouth in the mirror. Can you see the colored patches where plaque and old food lurk? Brush your teeth well, then try the tablets again. How much plaque remains?

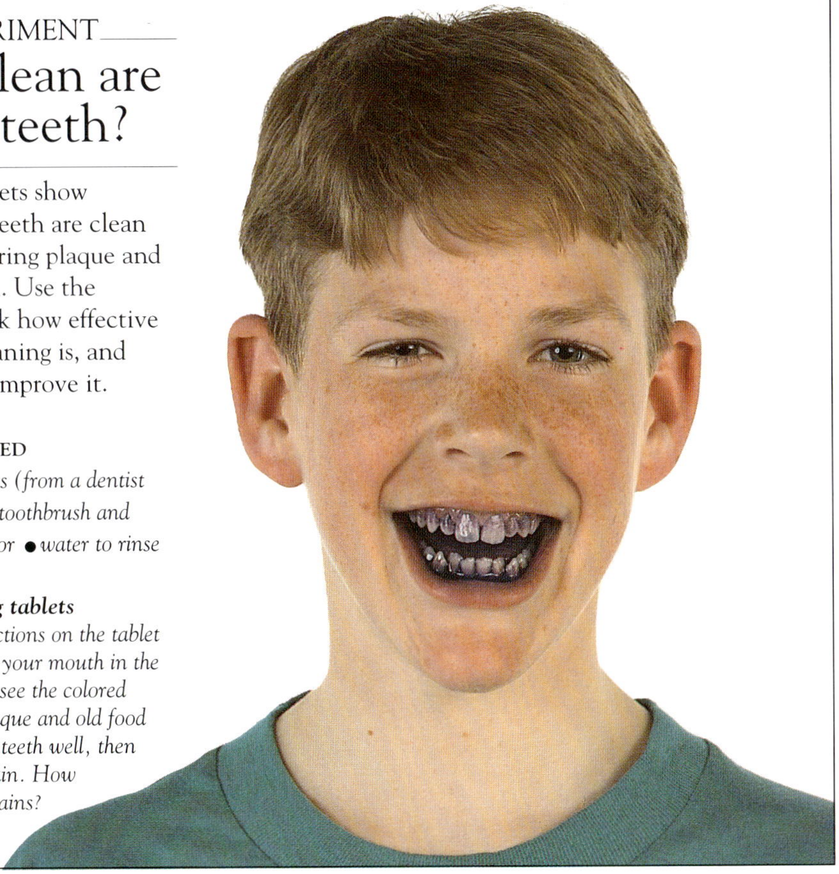

Chewing and swallowing

ONCE YOU HAVE bitten off a piece of food, using your sharp front teeth, the second stage in the digestive process is to chew it, using your big, broad back teeth (p.86). Chewing crushes and mashes the food, mixing it with watery saliva (spit). The saliva comes from three pairs of salivary glands—one pair at the back of the mouth close to each ear, one pair under each side of the lower jaw, and one pair under the tongue. Saliva is mainly water, which turns foods into a pulp. This makes it easier to carry out the third stage of digestion, swallowing the food down the esophagus, the muscular tube that connects the throat with the stomach.

EXPERIMENT

Mouth-watering food

As soon as you put food in your mouth, or even just smell it, your salivary glands release saliva. You can feel the saliva collecting in your mouth as the sensation we call mouth-watering. Study this by encouraging salivation with strong-tasting juice from fresh fruit. Does it matter where on the tongue you drop the fruit juice?

YOU WILL NEED

- *dropper*
- *strong-tasting fruit juice such as lemon or lime*

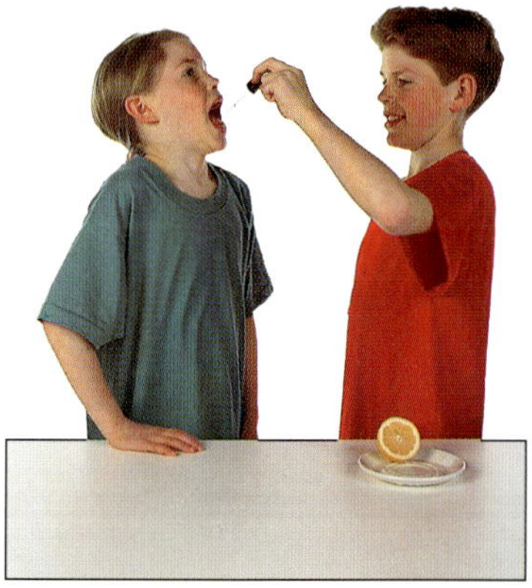

Using the dropper
Collect some fruit juice in the dropper. Carefully place a few drops on different parts of your tongue, and feel the saliva flow.

EXPERIMENT

Chewing and leverage

Adult help is advised for this experiment

Next time you eat an apple, feel how your mouth and teeth work. After you bite off a mouthful, your lips seal to prevent food from falling out, and your tongue moves the food around. The main chewing power comes from your premolar and molar teeth. They are nearest to the hinge joint (p.52) of your jaw, where the leverage is greatest, as this experiment shows.

YOU WILL NEED

- *sheet of medium or thick poster board*
- *strong scissors*

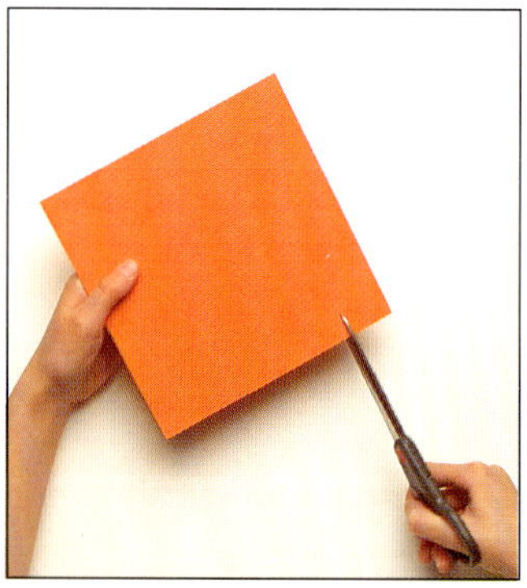

1 TRY TO cut the poster board with the scissors' tips, which are farthest from the fulcrum (p.51). This is like chewing with your front teeth. Feel the pressure you need to slice the poster board.

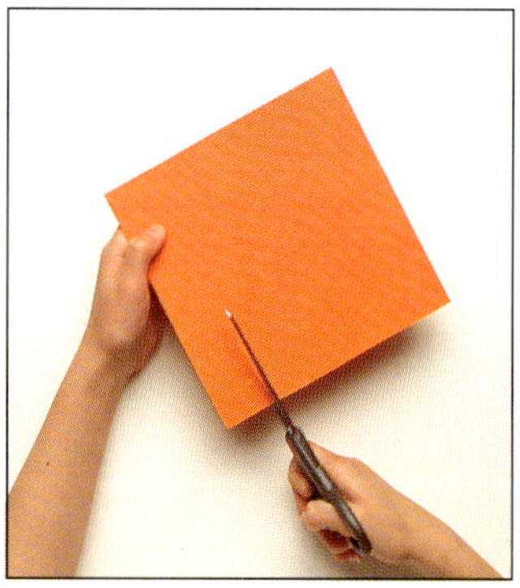

2 CUT THE same poster board with the part of the scissors nearest the fulcrum. You have more leverage here, and cutting should be easier. This is like crushing food with your back teeth.

Swallowing

When you swallow, a small lump of food, called a bolus, passes from your mouth, through your pharynx, into the upper esophagus. You can control only the first part of this process. When the bolus reaches the back of the pharynx, reflex actions seal off the trachea (windpipe) by closing a flap, the epiglottis. This stops food from going the wrong way. Peristalsis (opposite) takes over to force food through the esophagus.

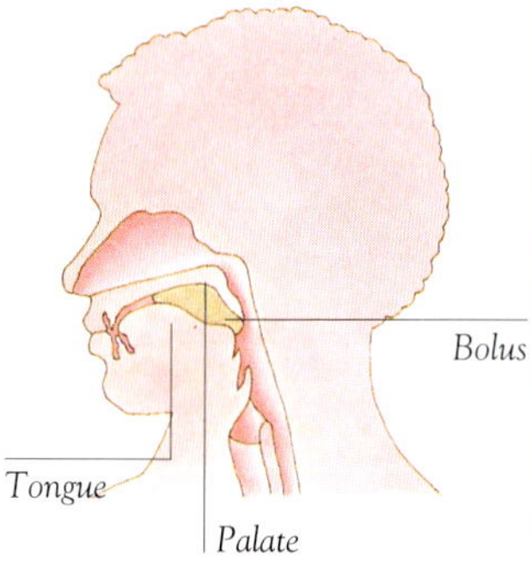

1. To the back of the mouth
The tongue feels for and shapes a suitable-size lump of food and pushes it to the back of the mouth.

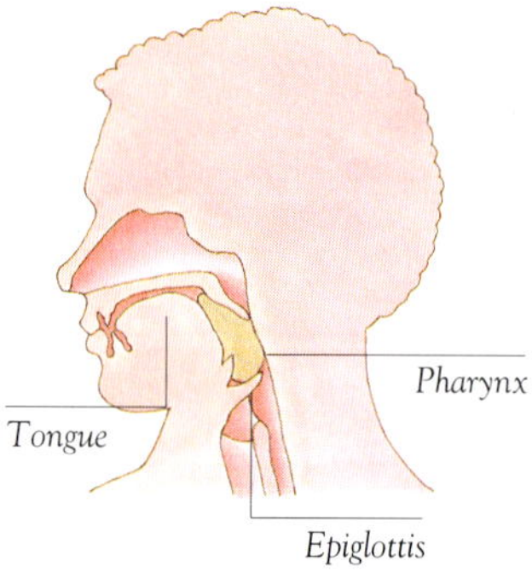

2. Through the pharynx
As the back of the tongue lifts and pushes back, the food is squeezed into the upper part of the pharynx.

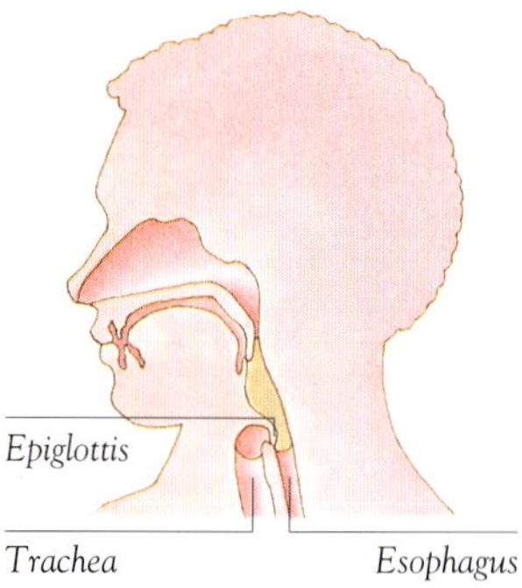

3. Into the esophagus
The epiglottis covers the trachea, the food slides into the top of the esophagus, and peristalsis begins.

EXPERIMENT

Peristalsis

Food is pushed through the esophagus and intestine tubes by a process called peristalsis. In this process two layers of smooth muscle (p.59) in the tube wall—one circular layer and another lying lengthwise—contract and relax in a coordinated wave.

You Will Need

- *small ball such as a tennis ball or baseball*
- *old stocking, long sock, or the like*

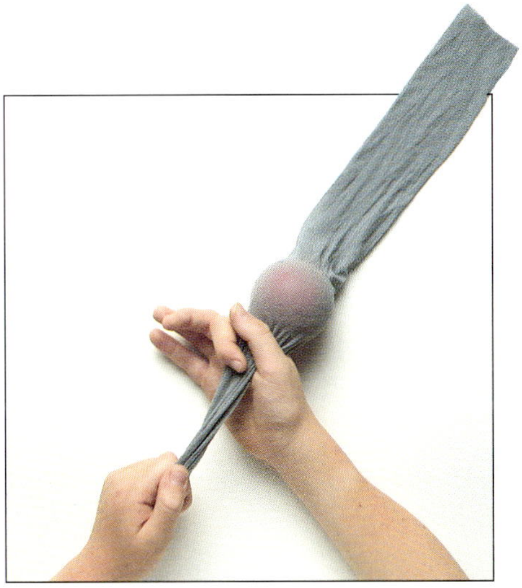

1 To show the principle of peristalsis, imagine that the stocking is the esophagus and the ball is a just-swallowed lump of food. Place the ball in the stocking, and make a small ring with your fingers, as shown, to represent the circular layer of smooth muscle.

2 Hold the end of the stocking firmly with your other hand. Squeeze and push the ball so that it slides along in the stocking. In swallowing, muscles in the esophagus wall contract, massaging food along in a similar way (below).

Moving food

Peristaltic waves of muscle contraction travel along the esophagus at a speed of 1–2 in (2.5–5 cm) each second. As the esophagus is about 10 in (25 cm) long, it takes several seconds for the food to reach the stomach.

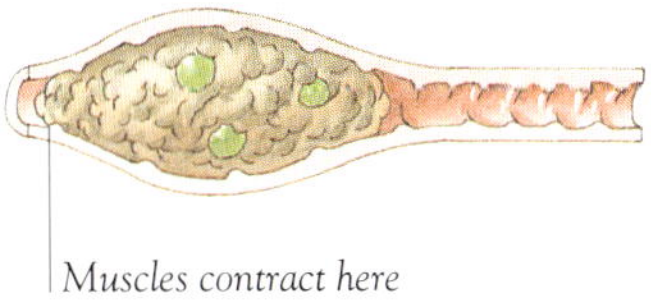

1. Upper esophagus
The lump of food is set in motion by a wave of peristaltic muscle contraction behind it.

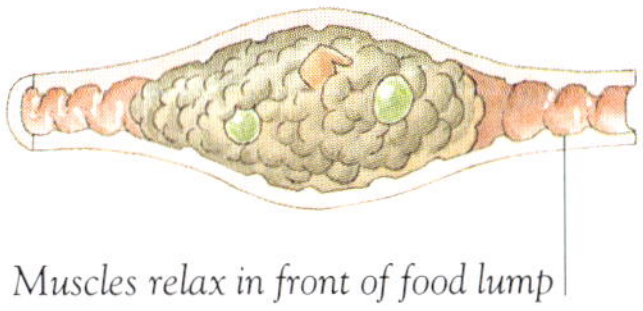

2. On the move
The muscles in the wall just in front of the food relax, so the lump can slide forward more easily.

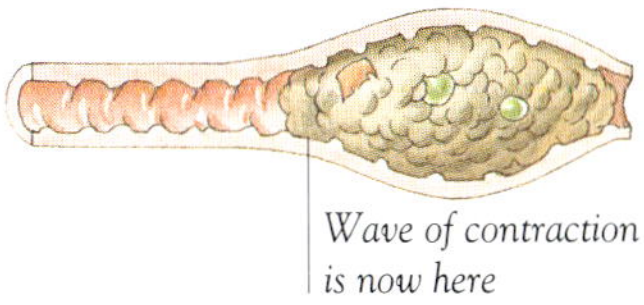

3. Toward the stomach
The peristaltic wave moves along the esophagus. Subsequent waves push along any food left behind.

EXPERIMENT

Feel how you swallow

Swallow slowly, and feel the movements in your neck. When you swallow, the epiglottis forms a tight seal over the trachea (opposite). As it does so, you can feel the "Adam's apple"—part of your larynx (voice box)—rise up to get out of its way.

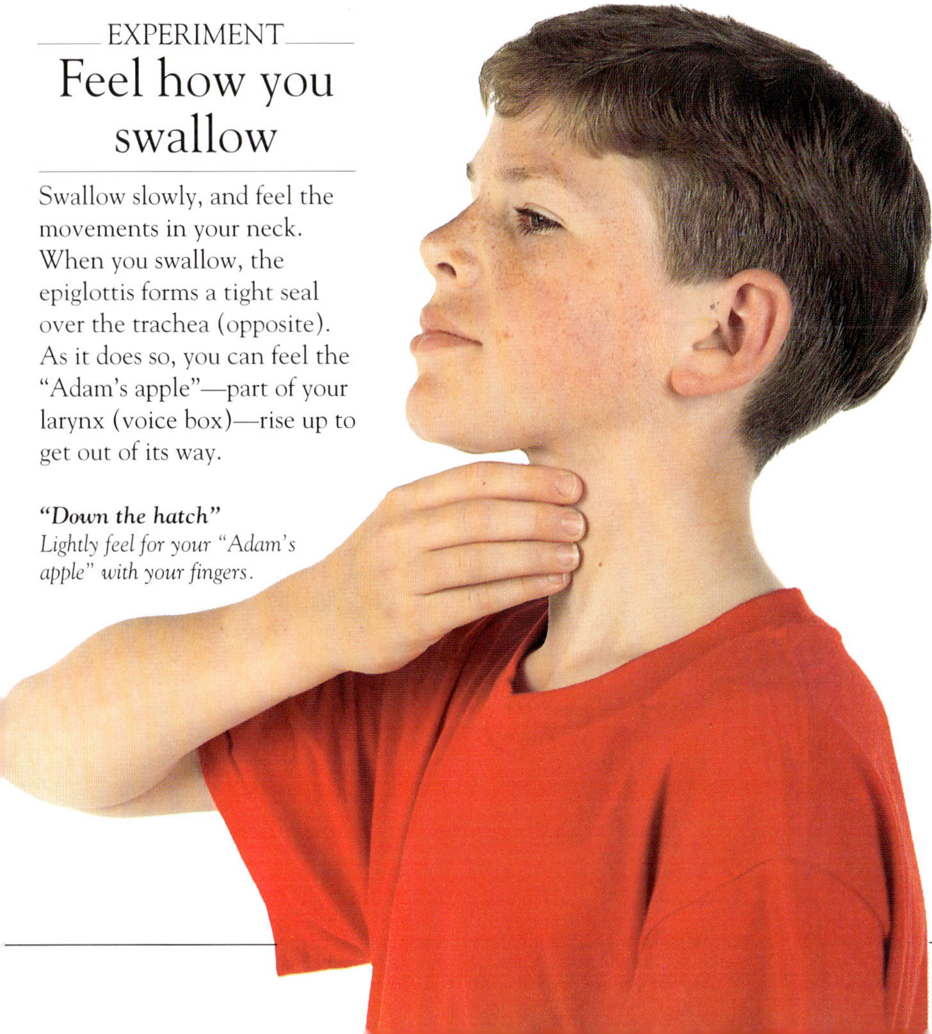

"Down the hatch"
Lightly feel for your "Adam's apple" with your fingers.

Swallowing upward

When you swallow, food does not "fall" through your esophagus under the force of gravity. The esophagus is normally pressed almost flat by the internal pressure in the chest. This is why you need peristalsis to push food into the stomach. The movements are so strong that they can force food and drink upward. So you could swallow food while standing on your head! But do not try this—you might choke.

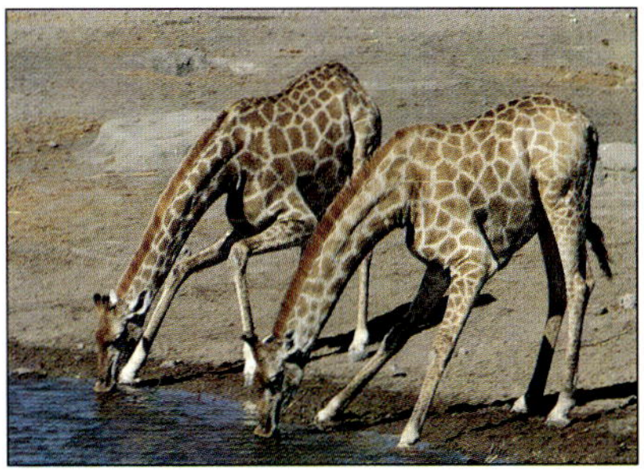

Drinking upward
When tall animals like giraffes bend down to drink, they use muscles in their throat and esophagus to swallow the water upward.

Digestion

FOOD CONTAINS MOLECULES of many different nutrients (pp.80–81). The main ones are proteins, carbohydrates (starches and sugars), and fats and oils (also known as lipids). Most of these molecules are too big to pass through the lining of the small intestine, which is the main area where food is absorbed into the body itself. Digestion is a combination of physical and chemical processes that break the big molecules into small ones. Teeth cut and mash the food (pp.86–87). Then the stomach churns and squashes it. The salivary glands, stomach, small intestine, and pancreas make body substances called enzymes, which attack the chemicals in the nutrient molecules and speed their breakdown. There are different digestive enzymes for each type of nutrient. For example, proteases split proteins into amino acids, the building blocks that they were constructed from. In addition, the stomach lining makes strong hydrochloric acid to dissolve the food. This "acid bath" also helps to kill germs found in food.

EXPERIMENT

Listen to digestion

Digestion of food in your intestines produces gases that bubble along and make gurgling noises. Record them using a tape recorder and microphone. Play this back at high volume. Where on your abdomen are they loudest?

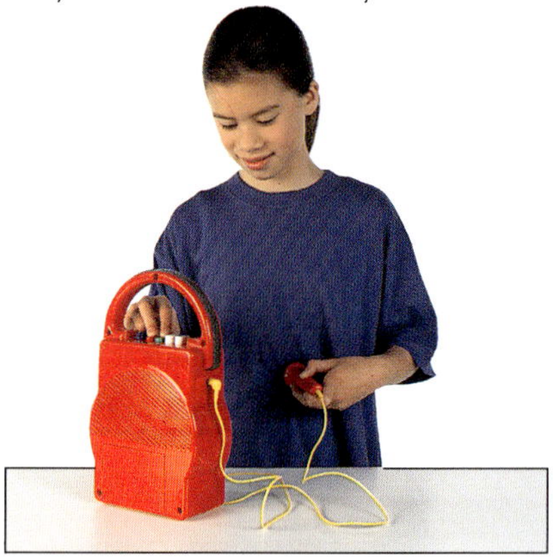

Recording the gurgles
If the tape recorder has a recording level, turn it up to maximum. Hold the microphone still, so that it does not scrape on your skin or clothes. Record about 1 minute each time.

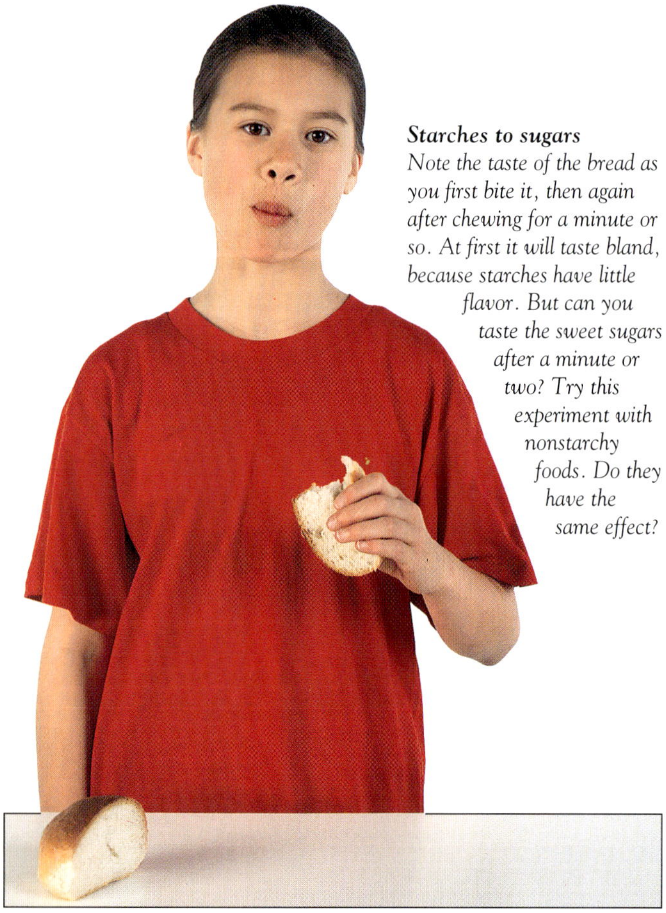

Starches to sugars
Note the taste of the bread as you first bite it, then again after chewing for a minute or so. At first it will taste bland, because starches have little flavor. But can you taste the sweet sugars after a minute or two? Try this experiment with nonstarchy foods. Do they have the same effect?

EXPERIMENT

Digesting starches

You start to digest starches in food while the food is still in your mouth. Saliva has an enzyme, amylase, that splits big starch molecules into smaller sugar ones. You can taste this for yourself by chewing a starchy food such as bread. Try other starchy foods and compare results.

YOU WILL NEED

- *slice of bread, cooked potato, spoon of cooked rice, or similar starchy food*

How enzymes attack starches

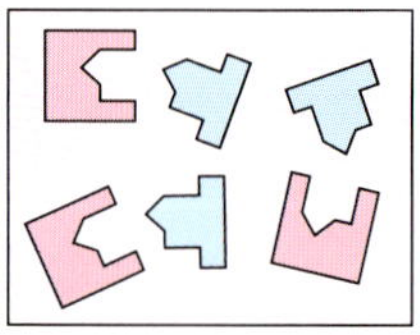

At first
Starch molecules in the bread (blue) and the molecules of the amylase enzyme (pink) are separate. Their shapes have been simplified for clarity.

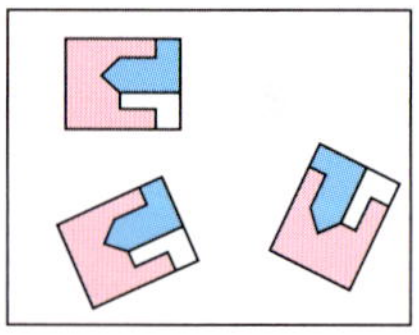

After a short time
Starch and enzyme fit together like a lock and key. The enzyme begins to break the starch molecule into smaller sugar ones (light and dark blue).

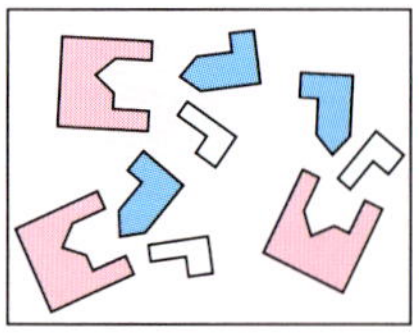

Later
The enzyme detaches, leaving the starch split into different types of sugar molecule. The enzyme is now ready to repeat this action on other starch molecules.

EXPERIMENT

Digesting proteins

Like the human body, some laundry detergents contain enzymes. These split big molecules into smaller ones, to remove stains such as egg or tomato from cloth. In this experiment you use washing powder to break down the protein parts of the pigment that makes tomatoes red, destroying the pigment color. Check the label of the washing detergent to make sure that the detergent includes enzymes.

You Will Need

• 2 glasses • warm water • rubber gloves • laundry detergent containing enzymes • ordinary laundry detergent • scraps of cotton material • tomato ketchup with no artificial coloring

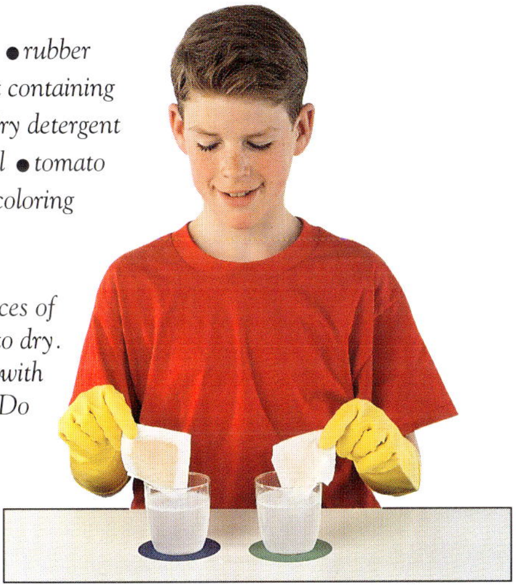

Splitting the proteins
Smear ketchup on two pieces of cotton material. Allow it to dry. Mix one of the detergents with warm water in one glass. Do the same with the other detergent in the other glass. Lay a piece of cotton in each glass. Which tomato color fades first?

EXPERIMENT

Digesting fats

Fats and oils are awkward to digest. Their molecules do not dissolve in water. Instead, they clump into blobs, which makes it difficult for enzymes to work on them. Fats and oils must be emulsified (broken into tiny droplets), so that their molecules are more exposed to the enzymes. In the body, fats and oils are emulsified in the small intestine by bile fluids (p.179). You can imitate this digestive action with dishwashing liquid.

You Will Need

• 2 glasses • warm water • dishwashing liquid • cooking oil • tablespoon • teaspoon

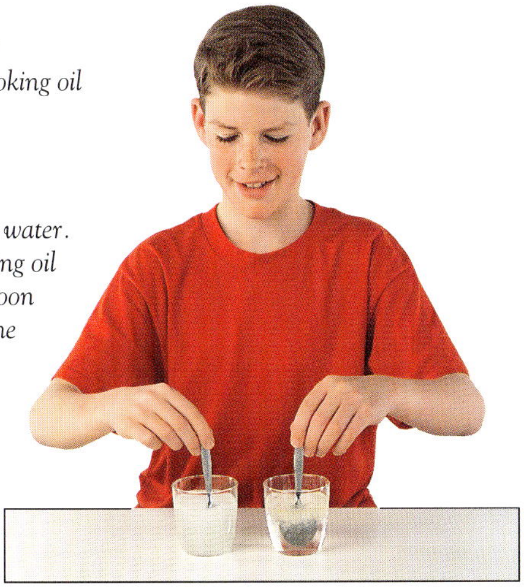

Breaking up the oil
Fill the glasses with warm water. Add a tablespoon of cooking oil to each. Now add a teaspoon of dishwashing liquid to one glass. Stir both. The dishwashing liquid emulsifies the oil, forming a milky fluid of tiny oil drops in water. Does the oil in the other glass change?

■ DISCOVERY ■

Captain William Beaumont

U.S. Army surgeon William Beaumont (1785–1853) had a unique opportunity to study digestion in action. In June 1822 he attended a patient, Alexis St. Martin, who had been accidentally shot in the stomach. The wound healed, but left a hole leading right into the stomach. St. Martin had to plug this with a bandage to stop the contents from leaking out. With the cooperation of the patient, Beaumont watched the stomach's movements and did tests on the foods and stomach juices. He discovered and published many facts about digestion—for example, the fact that the stomach produces a strong acid.

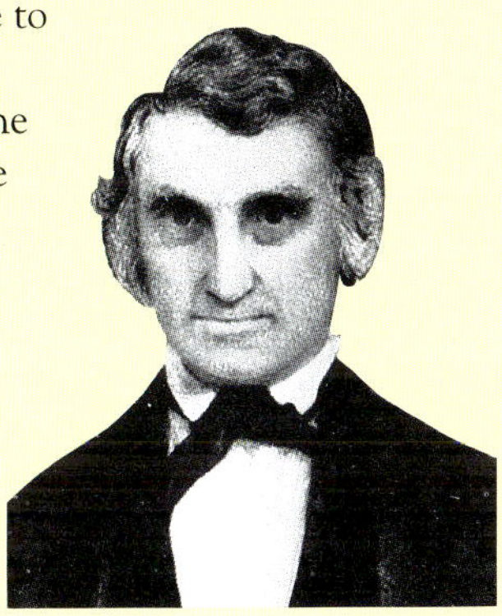

Intestine images

Modern X-ray techniques allow doctors to see the stomach and intestines in great detail. One technique involves swallowing barium sulphate, a substance that shows up clearly on X-rays. The barium "meal" spreads through the digestive tract, making the shape of the tract appear on X-rays. This use of barium allows blockages and other problems to be identified.

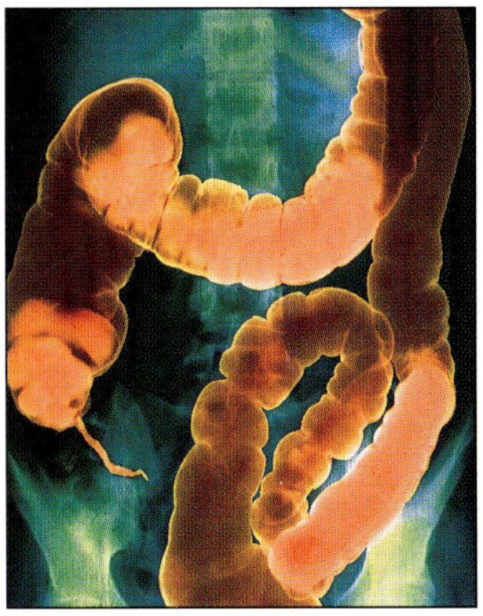

Colored colon
This X-ray shows the colon containing barium.

How emulsifiers attack fats and oils

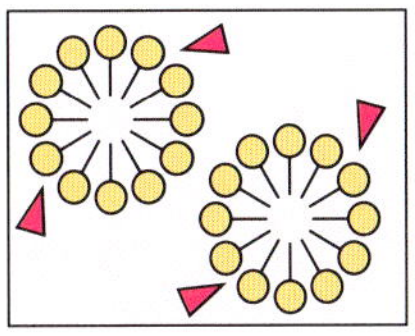

At first
Oil molecules have a "head" (yellow) and a "tail," and they clump together in blobs. The emulsifiers (red) begin to attack the oil molecules.

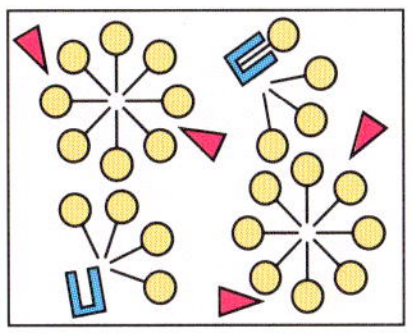

After a short time
The emulsifiers split the oil blobs and turn them into smaller droplets. In the body this exposes the oil to lipase (fat-splitting) enzymes (blue).

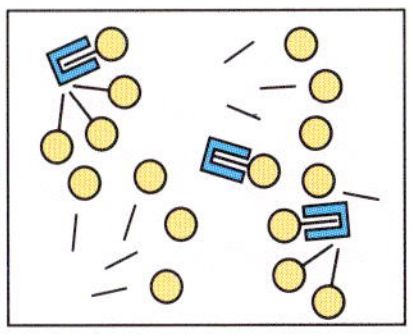

Later
The lipase enzymes can now get to work on the oil molecules, breaking the heads from the tails, and allowing further digestion to occur.

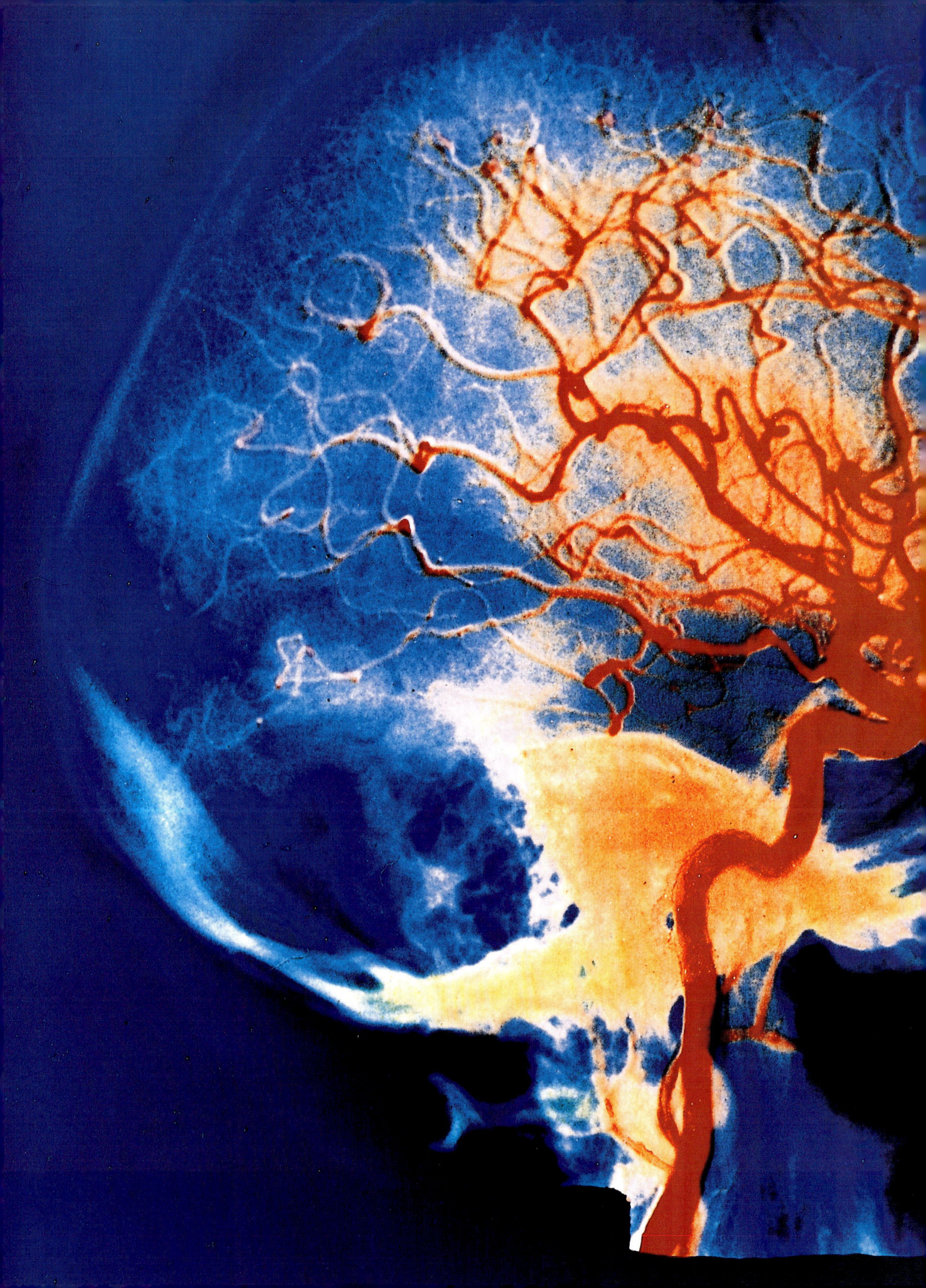

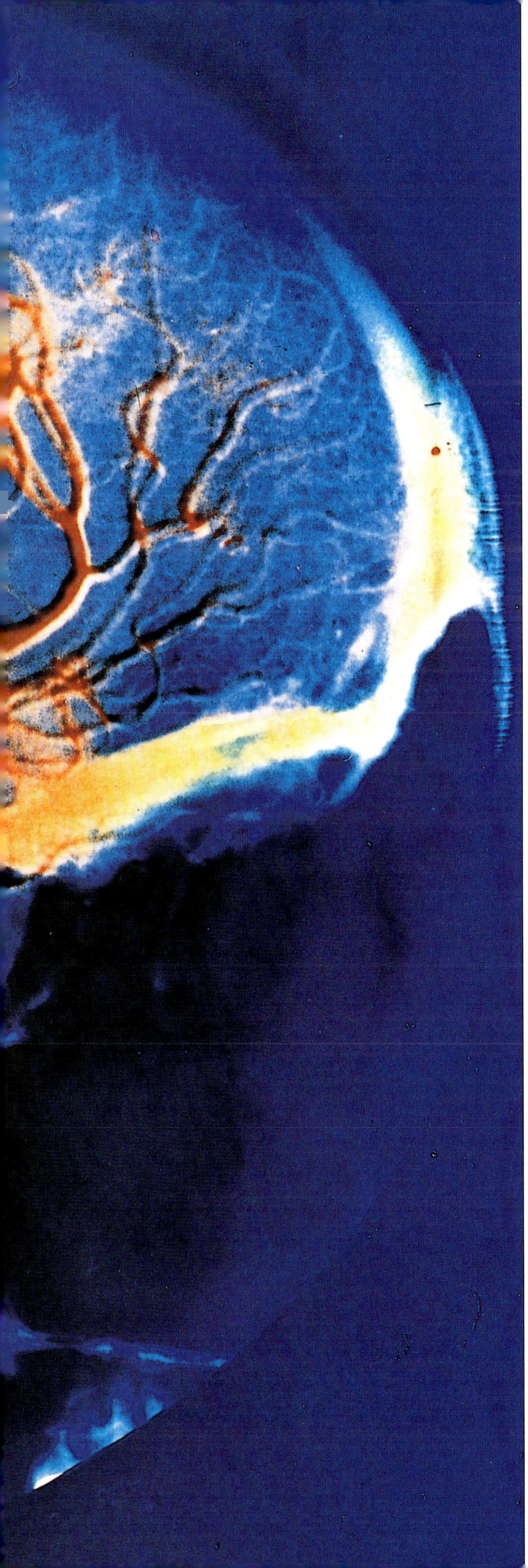

TRANSPORT and MAINTENANCE

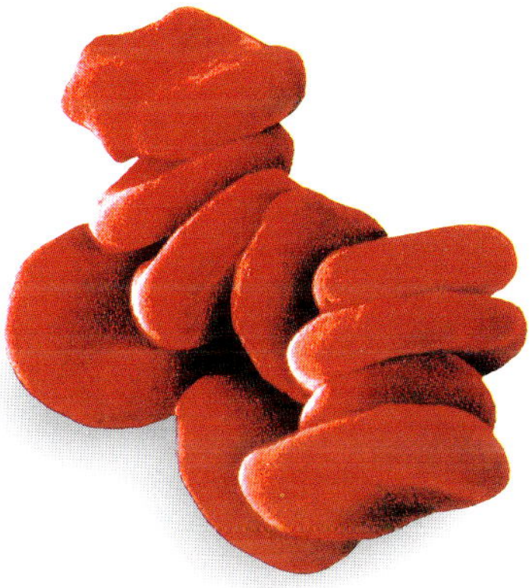

Red for go
Blood's red color is due to the oxygen-carrying substance known as hemoglobin. Nearly 300 million molecules of hemoglobin cram into each doughnut-shaped red blood cell (above). Billions of red cells hurtle through the body's blood vessels, which are shown in this special X-ray of the head and brain (left).

WITHOUT ITS NETWORK OF roads, railways, and waterways, a country could not function. Your body has its own network—the blood vessels of the circulatory system. Through them flows red blood, pumped nonstop by the heart. Blood carries innumerable substances from one part of the body to another. It also distributes nutrients and collects wastes, in the never-ending task of keeping every body part fueled and serviced.

THE CIRCULATORY SYSTEM

IT IS ESTIMATED THAT if all the blood vessels in the body's transport system were laid end to end, the total length would be more than 60,000 miles (100,000 km). In reality the blood vessels form an immense branching network. They fan out from the heart and eventually converge back there. The shortest return trip that blood makes from the heart—to the heart's own muscle—takes only a few seconds. The longest—to the toes—takes over a minute.

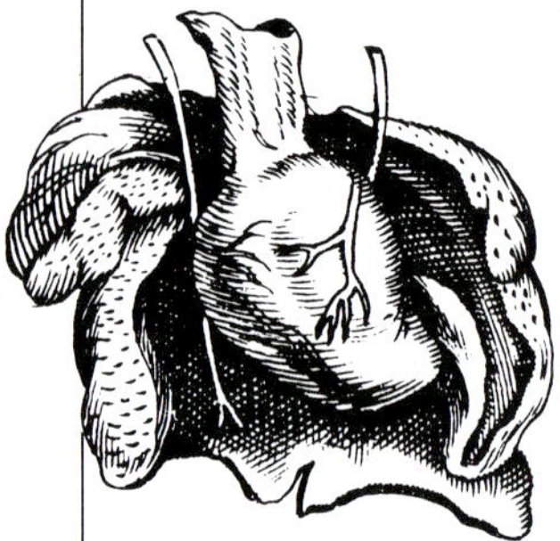

***The heart lies** between the two lungs, almost in the center of the chest. It is tilted slightly to the left side.*

The first people to investigate the body did not know of the circulatory system. They did not realize that the heart pumps blood around and around the circular network of blood vessels, carrying oxygen and nutrients to all the cells and collecting wastes. They did notice, however, that when a person feels deep emotions, such as fear or anger, the heart produces strong physical sensations, such as heavy pounding or skipping a beat. This led to the belief that emotions were based in the heart. We now know that it is not the heart but the brain that is the center of emotions. The brain sends signals to the heart, by way of nerve messages and hormones (p.106), to make the heart beat harder and faster in certain situations. As a result, more blood is supplied to the muscle. This is particularly important in reactions such as the "fight or flight" response (p.105).

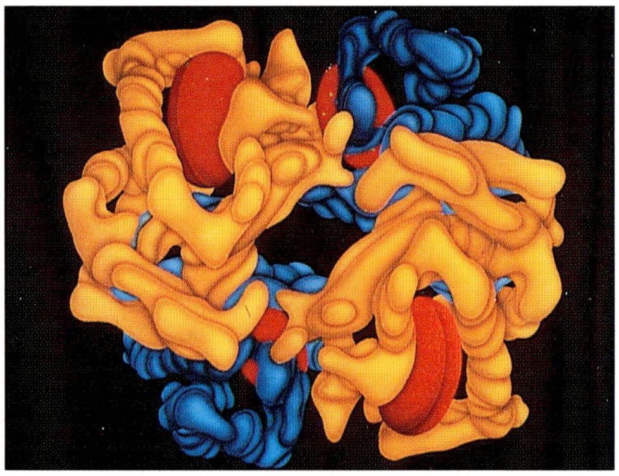

***This computer model of a hemoglobin molecule** shows proteins in yellow and blue, and heme pigments as red disks. Oxygen molecules link with each disk. In this way oxygen is carried around the body in the blood.*

Ebb and flow

The role of the blood as the body's main transport fluid has long been accepted. But how and where blood flows was not understood until the 17th century. Before the invention of the microscope, anatomists believed that blood ebbed and flowed to and from the heart.

In reality blood moves through the vessels in one direction—from arteries to capillaries to veins. Arteries branch out many times, finally becoming tiny vessels called capillaries, whose walls may be only one cell thick. These capillaries then join together to make small veins, which merge to form larger veins.

The arteries carry blood away from the heart. They have muscular, elastic walls, which expand to cope with the high-pressure surge of blood from each heartbeat (p.100). The veins return blood to the heart. They have thinner and slacker walls because the blood that oozes sluggishly through them is under almost no pressure.

Early anatomists believed that only veins carried blood, and that arteries had another purpose. This was a natural assumption, because after death, when the heart stops, blood is quickly squeezed out of the arteries by their muscular walls and drained into the veins. So each time an anatomist examined the arteries of a corpse, they were found empty.

Four humors

Hippocrates (c.460–c.377 B.C.) of ancient Greece, the Father of Medicine, believed, like many of his colleagues, that the body was made of four substances called humors—blood, yellow bile, phlegm (mucus), and black bile. He thought that if the humors lost their natural balance, people would become ill.

It was thought that a mysterious life force, the pneuma (p.70), "vitalized" humors into action. Galen of ancient Rome (p.13) believed wrongly that blood seeped from one of the heart's ventricles to the other through tiny pores in the septum—the dividing wall of the heart. He thought that at this point it mixed with the pneuma from the

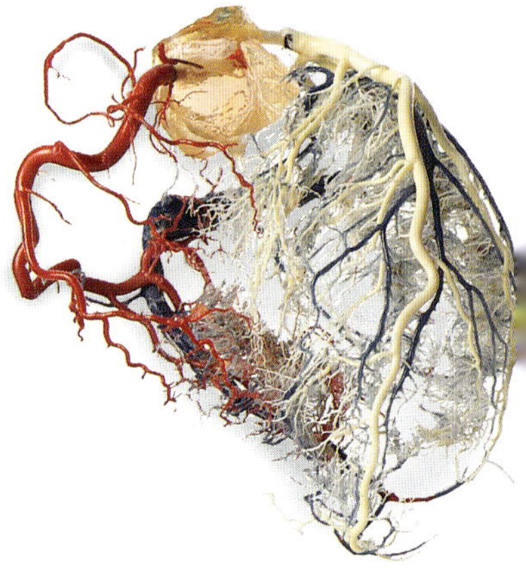

***This is a resin cast of the coronary** vessels, which supply the heart muscle (not shown) with blood.*

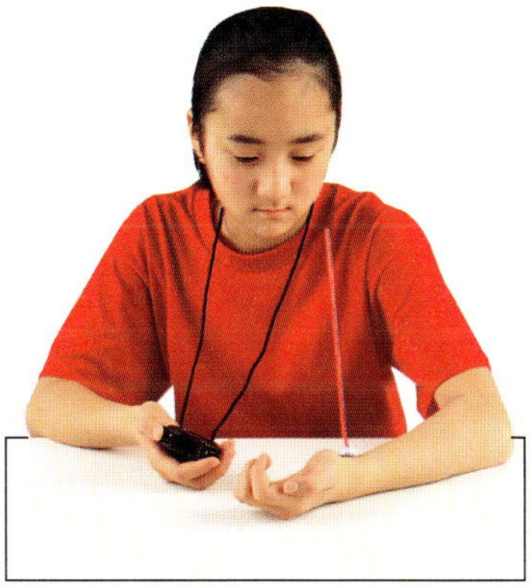

Where arteries come near the skin, you can feel your pulse—pressure surges of blood from the heart. Count the beats to find your heart rate (p.101).

air to create a "vital spirit" that flowed along the arteries.

Many of Galen's theories were accepted right up to the time of the Renaissance. In their anatomical studies both Leonardo da Vinci (1452–1519) and Andreas Vesalius (p.22) drew pores in the heart's septum.

Harvey's discovery

By the late 16th century scientists had still not worked out the way that the heart pumped blood. Several Italian anatomists made important advances but could not work out an overall system. Realdo Columbus (1516–59) suggested correctly that there is a separate system of blood vessels to the lungs in addition to the supply to the whole body. Hieronymus Fabricius (1537–1619) studied one-way valves in the main veins, but he thought that their function was to slow down the blood flow.

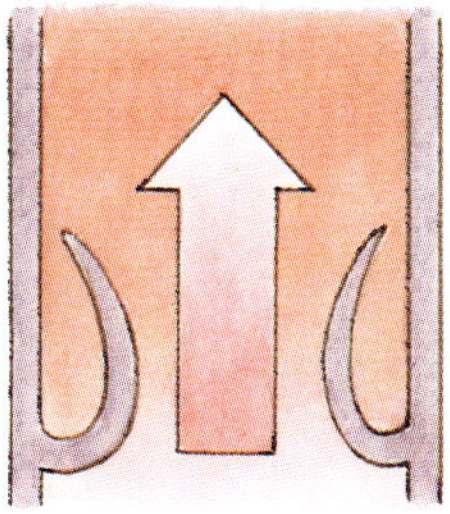

Blood flowing the right way pushes open the flaps of valves in the heart and main veins.

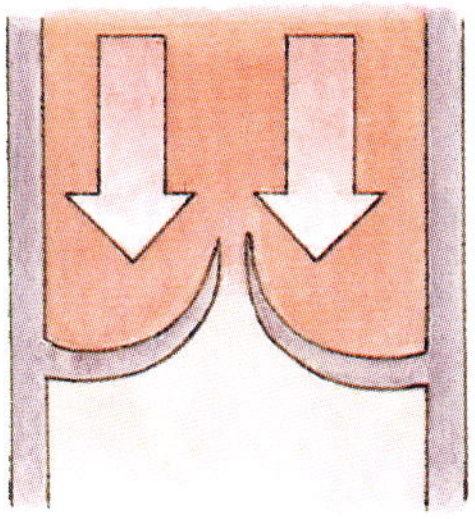

After each heartbeat, the valves are pressed shut, preventing blood from flowing backward.

Andrea Cesalpino (1519–1603) came close to realizing that blood travels around the body, rather than swishing to and fro within the blood vessels. He even used the word "circulation." But Cesalpino thought that blood flowed from the heart along both the arteries and the veins.

In 1628 a student of Fabricius, the English physician William Harvey (p.96), proposed that the function of the heart is to pump blood in a continuous circuit through the system of vessels. Once this discovery had been made, it became obvious that the valves in the heart (p.98) and veins (p.96) are to keep blood flowing in one direction only.

Although Harvey understood that blood flows in one direction only, he did not know how it passes from the arteries to the veins. The answer was found by Marcello Malpighi (p.104), who discovered connecting capillaries through his microscope.

Two pumps

We now know that the heart is two separate pumps (p.98). The right pump sends low-oxygen blood along the pulmonary artery to the lungs. There the blood gets rid of carbon dioxide and picks up oxygen. The oxygen-rich blood returns to the heart's left pump via the pulmonary vein. This pump then sends the blood along the aorta (main artery) and other arteries, out to the whole body. The blood delivers its oxygen to the body's cells, collects carbon dioxide, and returns along the main veins to the heart's right pump again.

The one-way valves in the heart sometimes become stiff and leaky, allowing a backflow of blood. Surgeons can then replace them with artificial ones.

Red blood

The heart is muscle. Like any other muscle, it needs a blood supply to provide it with oxygen and nutrients. So the heart has a system of blood vessels that bring it oxygen. These blood vessels are called coronary arteries and veins, because they surround and permeate the upper heart muscle like a crown (*corona* in Latin).

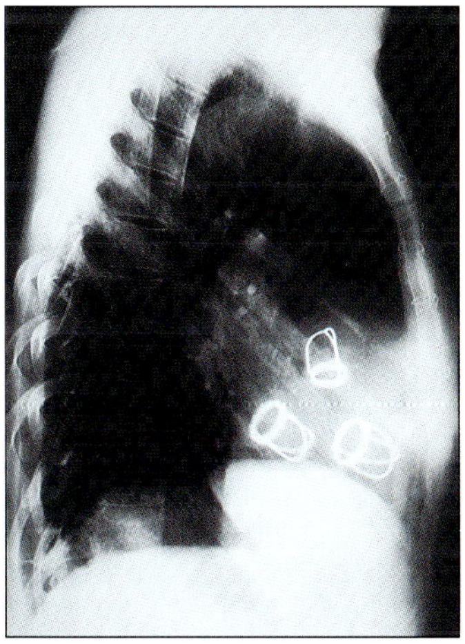

An X-ray image reveals three artificial heart valves. They show up clearly because they are made of dense metal.

By the 1860's physiologists discovered that the red cells in blood are packed with a protein called hemoglobin. This protein links easily with oxygen, with the result that it carries oxygen around the circulatory system. In the lungs, where a lot of oxygen is available, hemoglobin becomes bright red. In lower-oxygen surroundings in the body tissues, hemoglobin releases its oxygen and becomes darker in color.

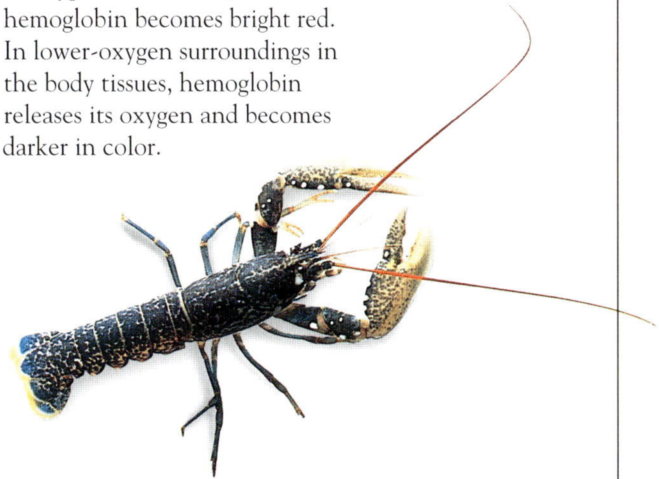

Not all blood is red. A lobster's blood is blue, because it contains copper-based hemocyanin instead of iron-based hemoglobin.

Circulation

BLOOD FLOWS around and around through vessels. This is called circulation. From the heart's left side blood passes into the aorta (main artery), then into other arteries. Each artery branches 15 or 20 times, becoming smaller and smaller. The smallest arteries lead into a network of minute capillaries. The thin walls of these capillaries allow oxygen and nutrients to diffuse (p.27) through them from the blood into the body tissues. In due course, the capillaries join other capillaries, eventually forming veins. These take blood back to the heart's right side. This side pumps it to the lungs to collect more oxygen, and from there it returns to the heart's left side. Blood thus makes a double circuit: around the body (systemic circulation), then to the lungs and back (pulmonary circulation).

■ DISCOVERY ■

William Harvey

Since ancient times, there have been many explanations for the roles of the heart and blood vessels. One theory was that blood ebbed and flowed in the vessels, like the tide. The English physician William Harvey (1578–1657) did many experiments on blood flow. In 1628 he published the results in his book *De Motu Cordis et Sanguinis* ("On the Motion of the Heart and Blood"). He showed that blood flows around the body in a circular route, pumped by the heart.

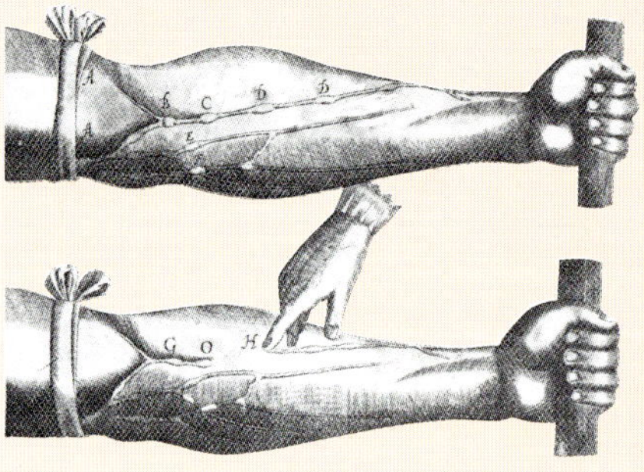

Studying veins
These illustrations from Harvey's book show how blood flows along veins back to the heart and how valves in the veins stop blood from flowing the wrong way (below).

EXPERIMENT

Blood flow and gravity

Adult help is advised for this experiment

In some parts of the body, blood has to flow against gravity. To see the effect of this, hold one arm up high and one down by your side for a minute. Then compare hands.

Contrast in color
From the hand held high, blood drains easily to the heart, speeded by the force of gravity. In the lower hand, blood struggles to rise against gravity. The blood collects in this hand, making it darker.

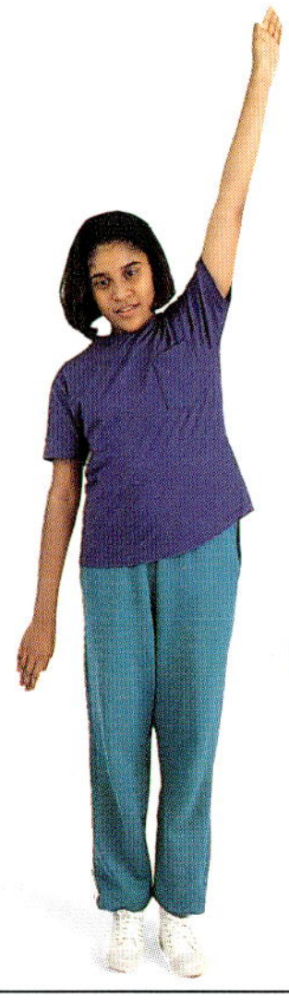

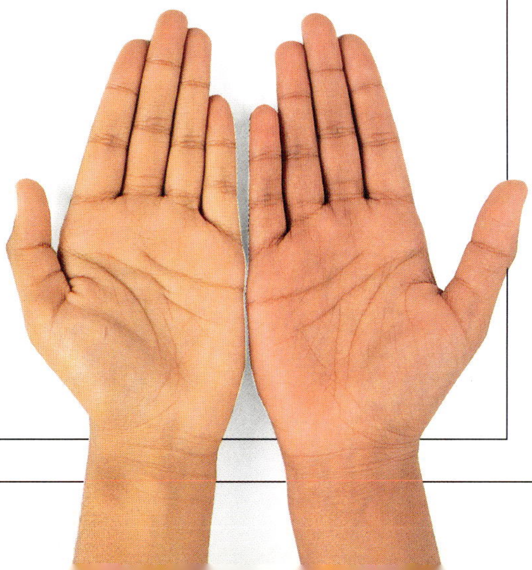

EXPERIMENT

Vein valves

Adult help is advised for this experiment

William Harvey realized that vein valves (p.95) stop blood from flowing backward. You can re-create a version of one of Harvey's experiments. Before starting, ask an adult with prominent veins on his or her hands to let one hand hang low for a minute, so that its veins stand out.

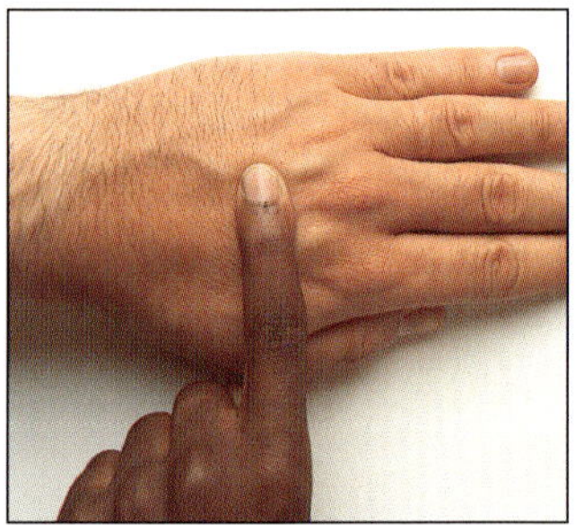

1 NOW ASK the adult to put his or her hand on a table, palm down. Find an unbranched vein on the back of the hand, and firmly but gently place your finger on it.

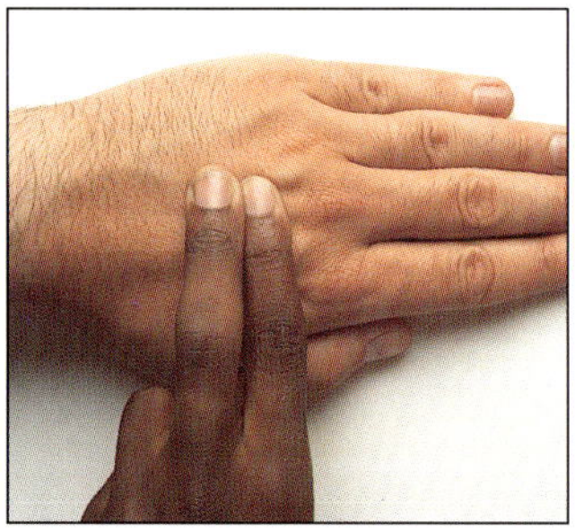

2 PLACE A second finger next to your first finger, then stroke the vein in the direction of blood flow—toward the heart. This empties the vein of blood.

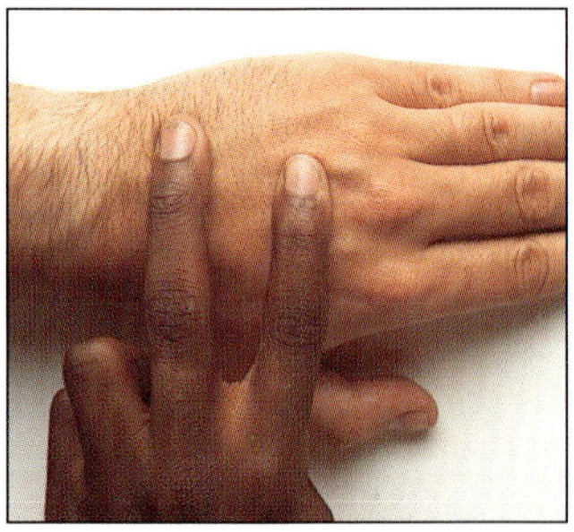

3 NOW LIFT your second finger. The vein should not refill. The vein's valve stops the blood from flowing backward. Lift your first finger to allow more blood to arrive.

Arteries and veins

Arteries carry blood away from the heart, and veins carry blood toward the heart. Most arteries contain bright red, high-oxygen blood (red in the illustration below). But the pulmonary arteries, which run from the heart to the lungs, contain dark reddish-blue blood, which is low in oxygen and needs new supplies. Most veins contain blood that is low in oxygen (blue in the illustration), except for the pulmonary veins, from the lungs to the heart, which contain oxygen-rich blood. At any instant, three-fourths of your blood is in veins, one-fifth in arteries, and one-twentieth in capillaries.

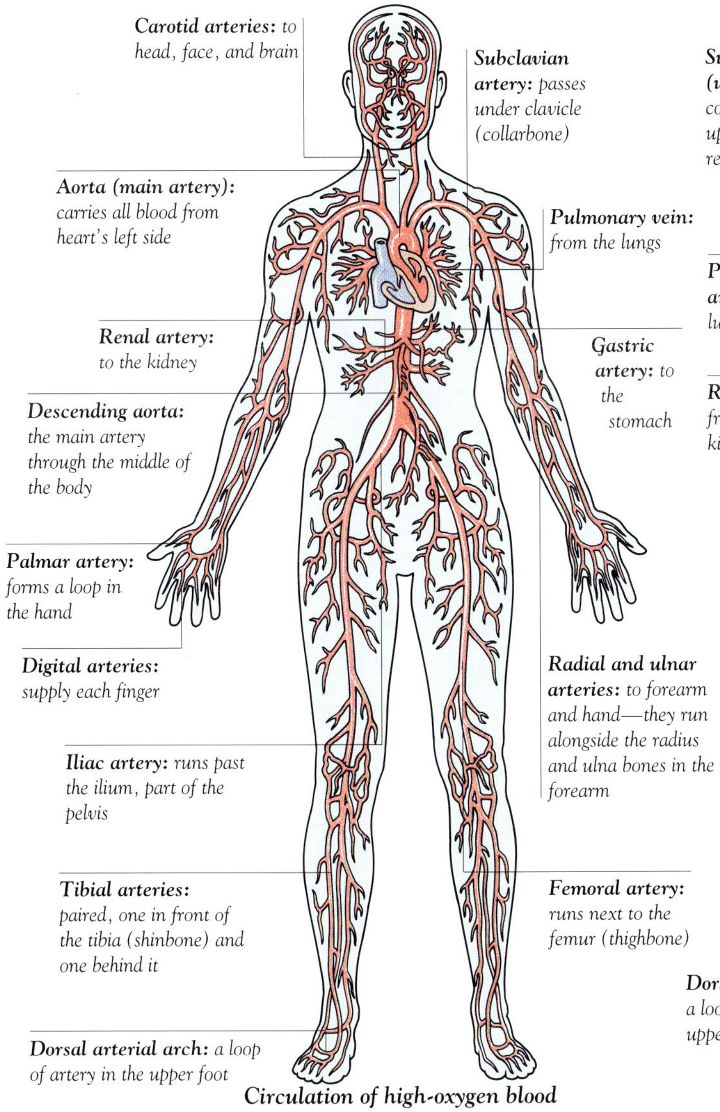

Circulation of high-oxygen blood

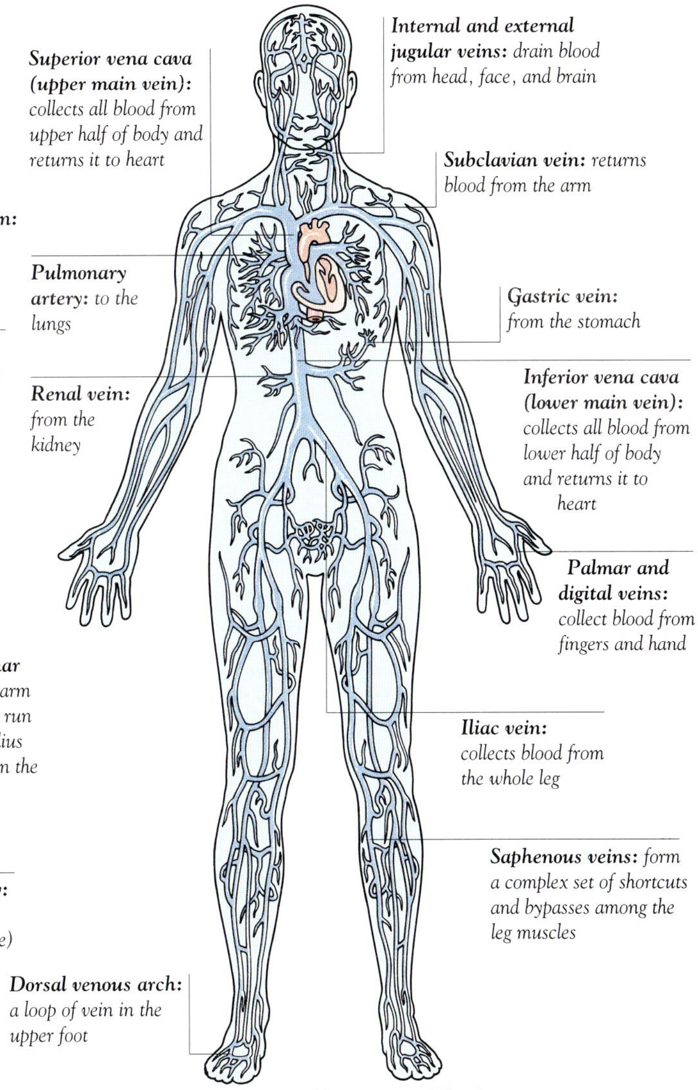

Circulation of low-oxygen blood

Blood vessel structure

Each of the three major types of blood vessel is designed for a specific job. An artery has a thick, muscular wall to cope with the high-pressure surges of blood from the heart. A capillary has a wall only one cell thick. Oxygen and nutrients can easily diffuse through these cells to the surrounding tissues. A vein has a loose, slack wall, since the blood in it is under very little pressure.

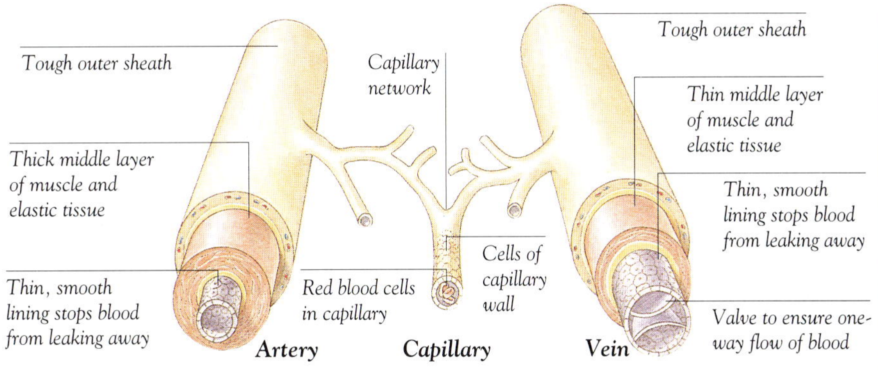

The heart

AT ONE TIME people thought that the heart was the seat of love, desire, courage, and bravery. Today we know that these feelings are based in the brain. The heart is simply a bag of muscle that—about once every second—squeezes itself to send blood flowing through the body's network of blood vessels. The heart has two pumps, working side by side. The left one sends blood out along arteries to the whole body, from head to toes. This blood gives up oxygen (p.71) and returns along veins to the right pump. From here it is sent on a much shorter trip— to the lungs to gather more oxygen. Two special features make the heart incredibly hardworking and versatile. The first is the muscle in the heart's walls. It is called cardiac muscle, and unlike normal muscle, it never tires. The second is the heart's ability to change its pumping speed and force to match the body's needs. Nerve signals from the brain (p.118) and hormones in the blood (p.106) help to control these changes.

The EKG

This wavy line is part of an EKG (electrocardiogram). It shows a pattern of tiny electrical signals. These signals pass through the heart as it pumps. They are detected by metal sensors placed on the skin, and the line is shown on a monitor. This EKG section shows the signals from one complete heartbeat. Doctors study EKG's to see if a heart is healthy.

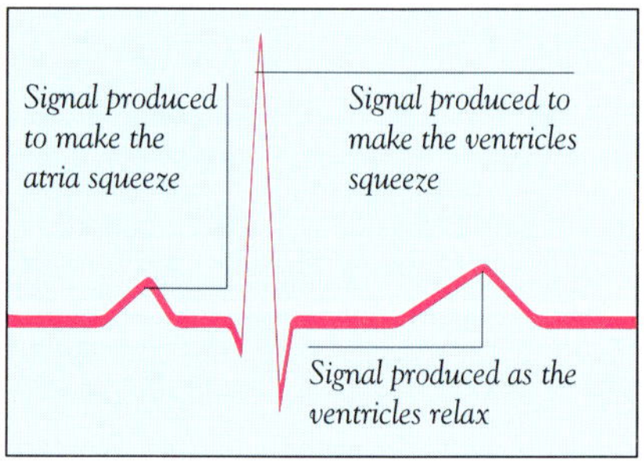

Inside the heart

Look inside the heart, and you see its two pumps side by side. Each pump has a small upper chamber known as the atrium (plural: atria). Blood flows into this from the vena cava (main vein) or the pulmonary vein. Below the atrium is a larger chamber, the ventricle. This provides the heart's main pumping power. The cardiac muscle of the ventricles squeezes hard during each heartbeat, forcing the blood inside them into the aorta (main artery) or the pulmonary artery. From there the blood is distributed around the body and to the lungs. Blood is kept flowing the right way through the heart by four one-way valves. On the right of the heart (the left side in the illustration) is the tricuspid valve, and on the left is the mitral valve. When the ventricles squeeze, blood presses on the flaps of these valves and closes them. This means that the blood cannot flow back into the atria. The other two valves are the aortic and pulmonary valves at the entrances to the arteries. After the ventricles have squeezed the blood out into the arteries, these valves close to stop it flowing back into the ventricles.

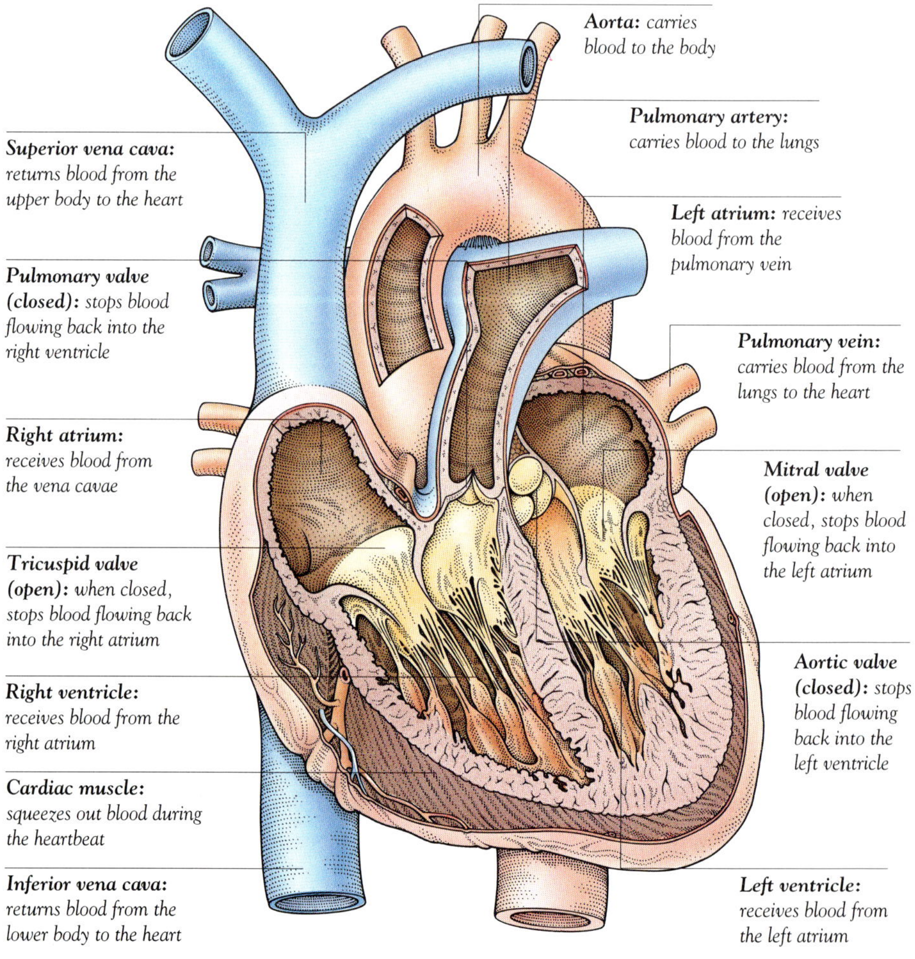

The heartbeat

A heartbeat can be shown in three stages, though in reality these stages merge into each other and into the next beat. When the body is resting, each ventricle pumps out about an eighth of a pint (70 milliliters) of blood with each beat. When the body is active, the muscles need extra oxygen and nutrients from the blood. So the heart pumps harder and faster to keep up the supply.

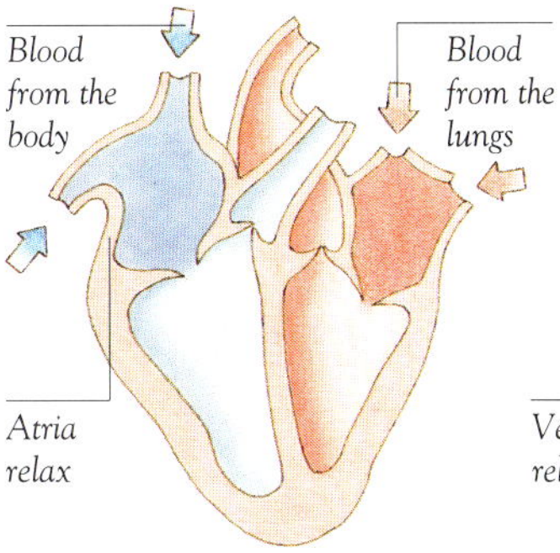

Atria fill
The aortic and pulmonary valves are shut. The right atrium fills with low-oxygen blood (blue) from the body, and the left atrium with high-oxygen blood (red) from the lungs.

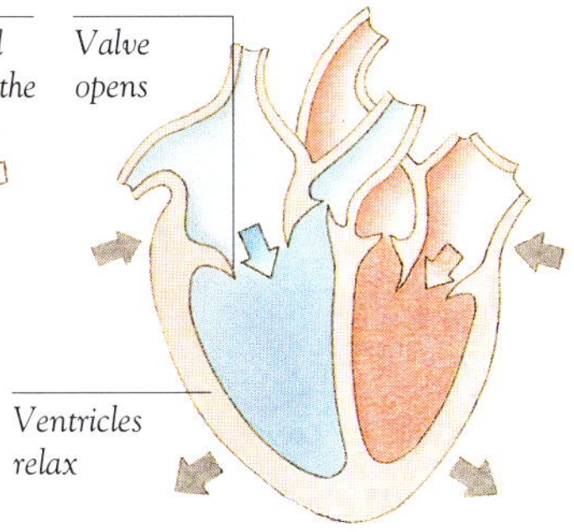

Ventricles fill
The muscles in the walls of the atria squeeze gently. Blood flows from each atrium into the ventricle below, through the one-way valves. The ventricle walls bulge.

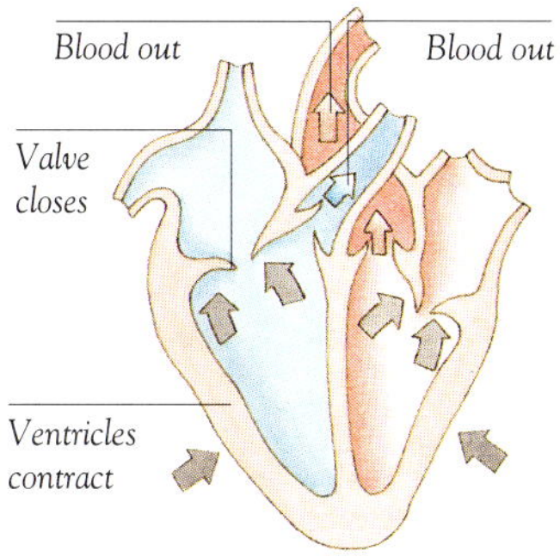

Ventricles empty
The ventricles contract. The mitral and tricuspid valves close, and blood is ejected into the arteries. Then the aortic and pulmonary valves close.

EXPERIMENT

Hearing the heart

Adult help is advised for this experiment

Each time the heart pumps, both pairs of valves close suddenly with a snap-shut sound. Doctors use a device called a stethoscope to listen to this sound. Make your own stethoscope to listen to your heart, and find out how exercise changes your heart rate. *Caution: If you feel dizzy or sick when exercising, stop at once and rest.*

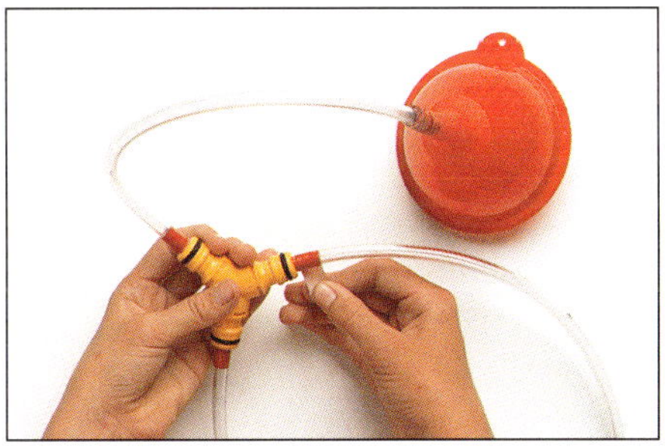

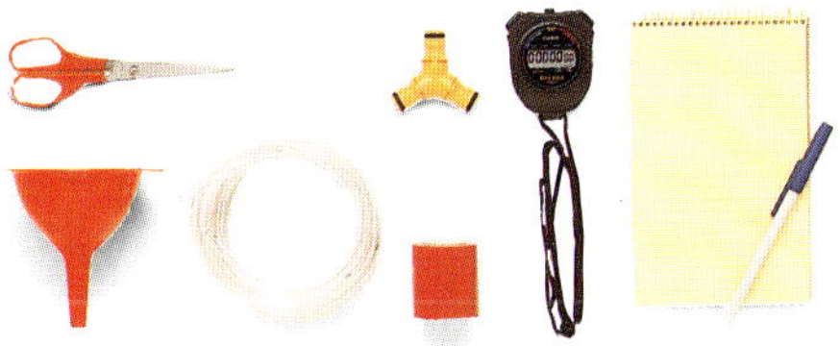

YOU WILL NEED

• scissors • small plastic funnel • plastic tubing • three-way hose connector • cellophane tape • stopwatch • notepad • pen

1 CAREFULLY CUT three lengths of tubing, each about 1 ft (30 cm) long. Tape the funnel to the end of one of the tubes. Push the other end of this tube and one end of each of the other tubes into the hose connector. Use tape to make sure that they fit snugly.

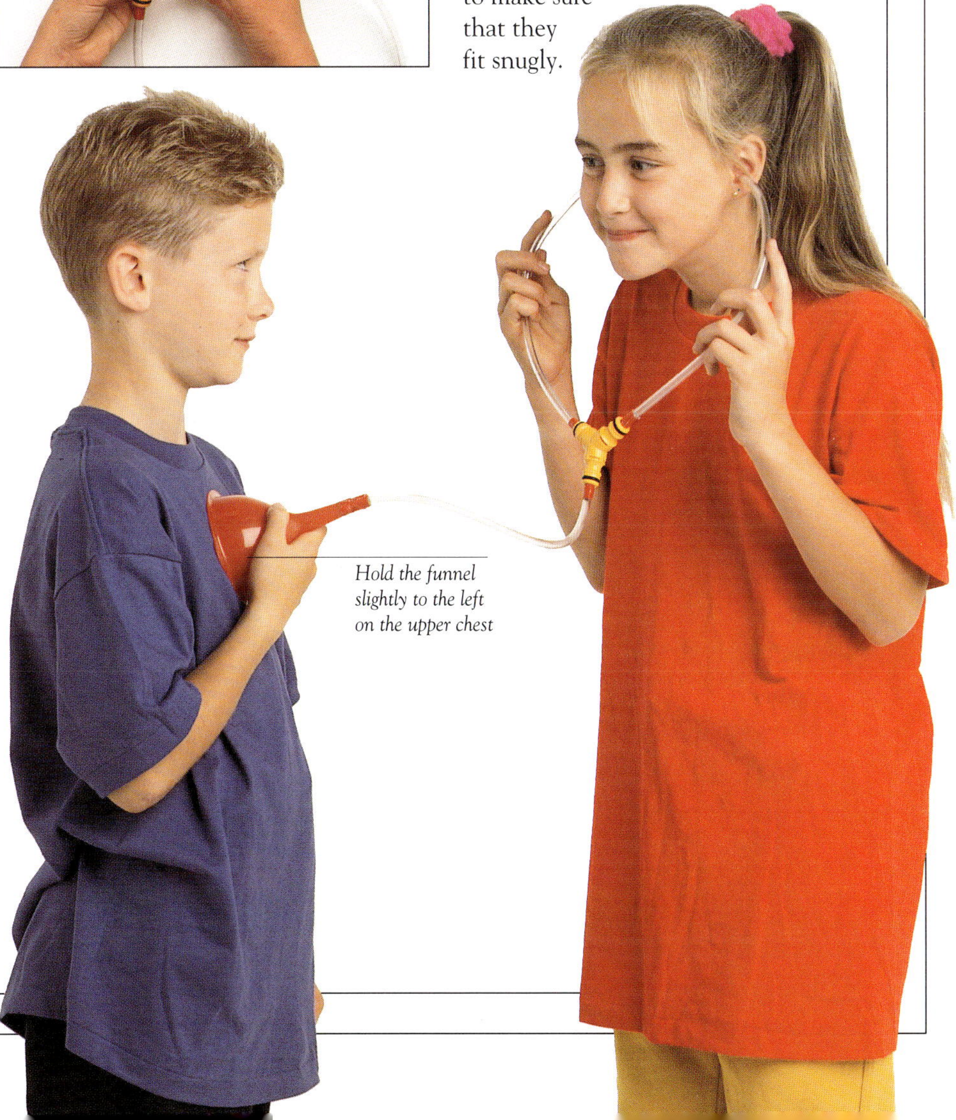

Hold the funnel slightly to the left on the upper chest

2 ASK A FRIEND to do something active, such as running, for 1 minute. Now ask your friend to hold the funnel over his or her chest (as right), and hold the tube ends to your ears. (Do not push them in.) Count the number of heartbeats in 1 minute. This is the heart rate. Now ask your friend to run around for 2 minutes. Count and note the rate again. Is it faster and louder after more exercise?

The heartbeat

EACH POWERFUL heartbeat sends a high-pressure surge of blood, like a miniature tidal wave, racing into the elastic-walled arteries. As the surge travels out through the body, it loses force and becomes lost in the vast network of microscopic capillaries—only to be followed, a second or less later, by another surge of pressure from the next heartbeat. You can feel these pressure surges—your pulse—at various places in the body. Your pulse can be most easily felt where an artery lies near the surface of the body, such as at the inside of the wrist. The pulse rate is the same as the heart rate, and it allows a convenient check on how hard and how quickly your heart is pumping.

EXPERIMENT

The pulsing leg

If you sit with your legs crossed in a certain position, the bulging surges of blood through the arteries in the upper leg make it rock slightly on the lower one. This turns your leg into a pulse meter that measures your heart rate.

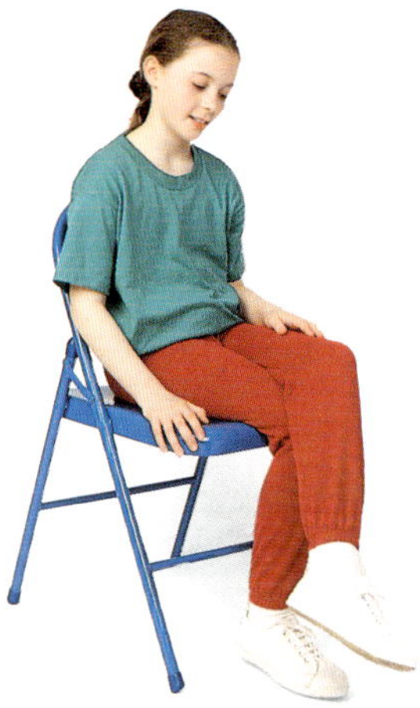

The leg pulse meter
Sit upright in a chair. Cross your legs so that the knobby part of the knee of the lower leg fits snugly into the hollow behind the knee of the upper leg. Relax and let your muscles loosen. Your upper leg should kick up very slightly with each heartbeat, as a pressure bulge passes through the large popliteal artery inside the back of the knee. Experiment by shifting your legs to different positions. The movement may be very small, but you should be able to notice it.

EXPERIMENT

Hardworking heart

When you are at rest, each heartbeat sends about ⅓ pint (150 ml) of blood into the arteries. In an average adult, this happens between 60 and 80 times each minute. See how hard the heart works by getting your hand and arm to work at the same rate as your heart.

YOU WILL NEED

- *plastic beaker that holds about ⅓ pint (150 ml)* • *2 bowls* • *water* • *stopwatch*

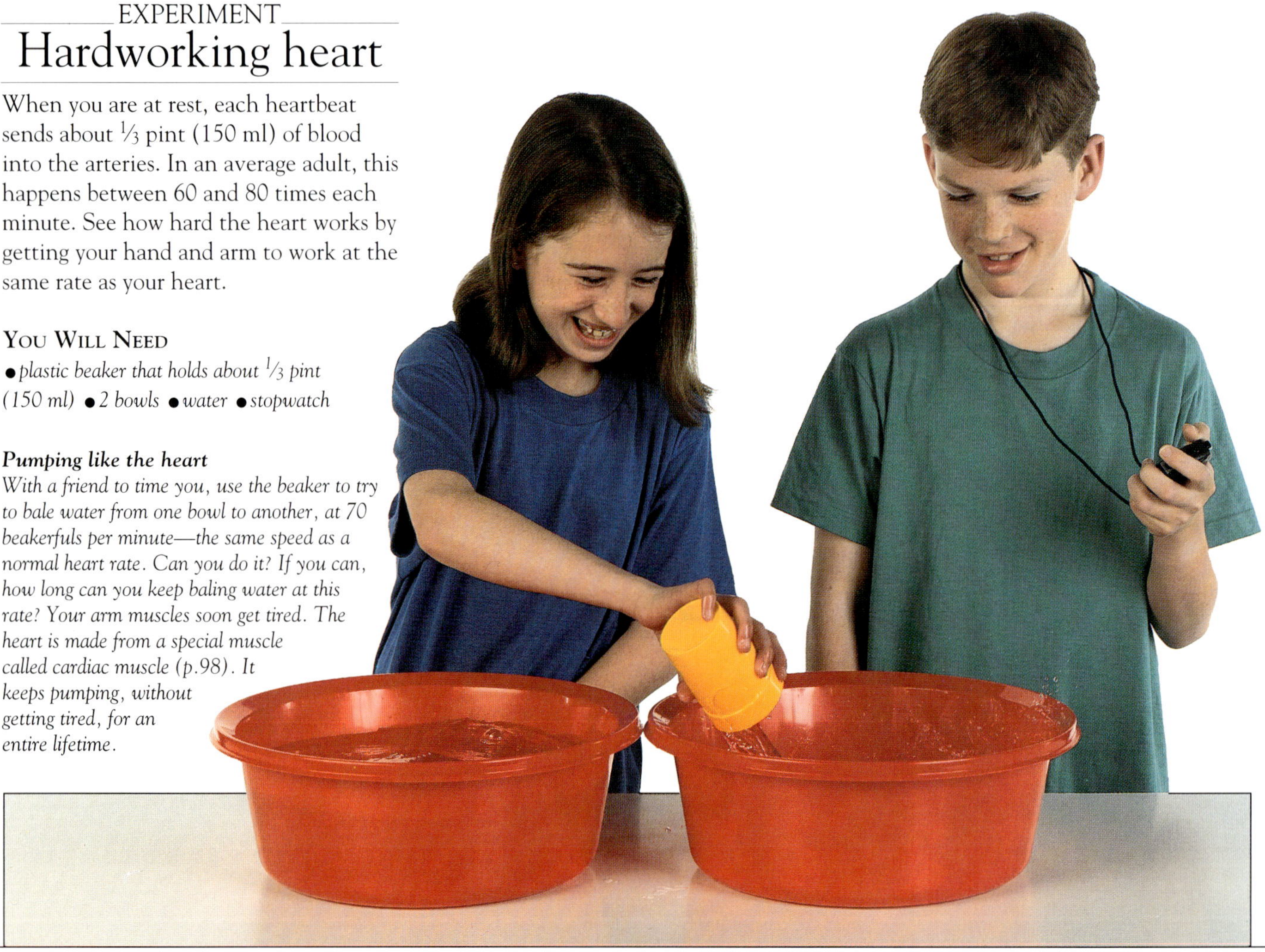

Pumping like the heart
With a friend to time you, use the beaker to try to bale water from one bowl to another, at 70 beakerfuls per minute—the same speed as a normal heart rate. Can you do it? If you can, how long can you keep baling water at this rate? Your arm muscles soon get tired. The heart is made from a special muscle called cardiac muscle (p.98). It keeps pumping, without getting tired, for an entire lifetime.

EXPERIMENT

Seeing your pulse

At a medical checkup, the doctor will probably take your pulse. Your pulse rate gives a rough guide to the general health of your heart and body. You can take your pulse in the standard way at the radial artery (below) in the wrist (as in Step 1, right). But in this experiment you can actually see your pulse by making a simple visual pulse meter with a drinking straw and a piece of plastic putty or modeling clay.

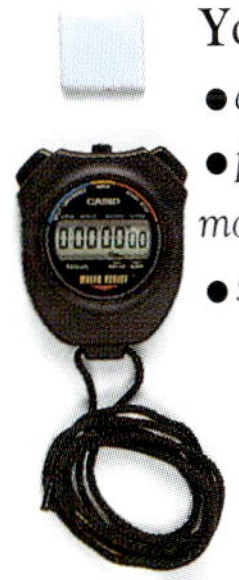

You Will Need

- *drinking straw*
- *plastic putty or tacky modeling clay*
- *stopwatch*

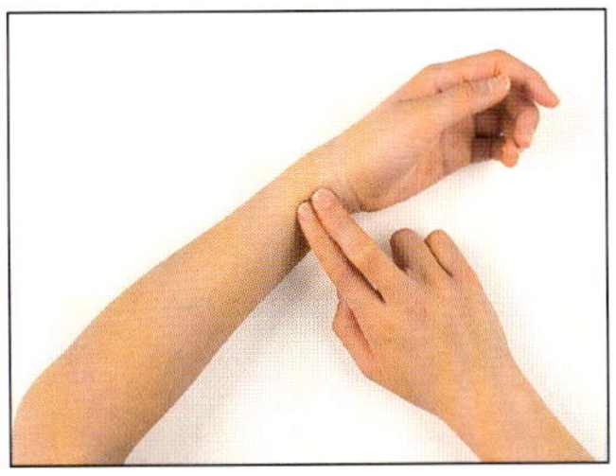

1 Feel with your fingertips on the inside of your wrist, below your thumb, until you detect pulsations. Do not use the tip of your thumb, as that has its own pulse, which you may feel instead.

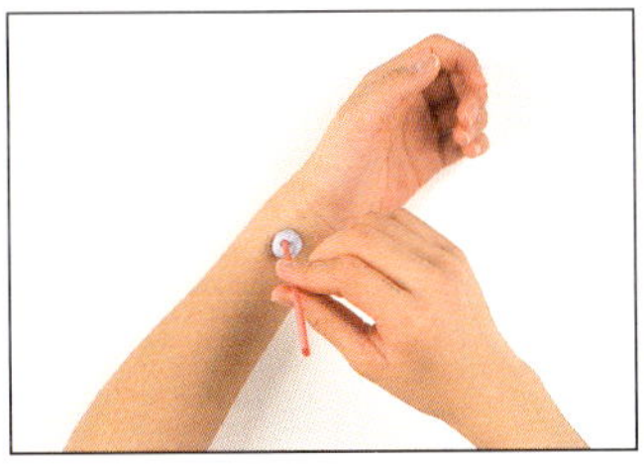

2 Place a blob of plastic putty at the place where you can feel the pulsations most strongly. Carefully push one end of the drinking straw into this blob so that it sticks upright from your wrist.

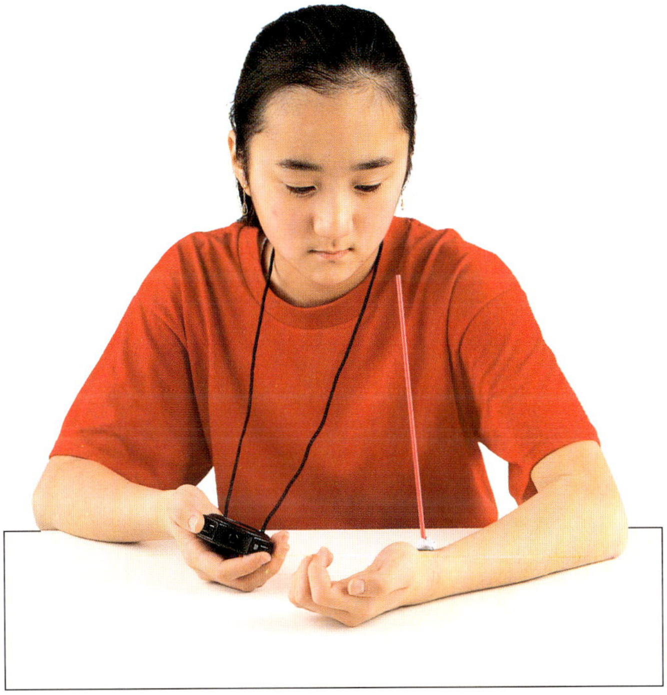

3 Let your arm lie flat on a table. The straw should twitch slightly to and fro, as the surge of blood produced by each heartbeat passes through your wrist into your hand, making the radial artery bulge. Measure your pulse rate by counting the number of times the straw rocks in 1 minute. The average resting pulse rate of humans varies with age. It is about 130 to 140 at birth, 110 to 120 at 1 year of age, 90 to 100 by 3 years, 80 to 90 by 10 years, and 60 to 80 in adults.

Animal heart rates

In general, big mammals have hearts that beat more slowly than smaller ones. Humans are relatively large mammals, and therefore we have correspondingly slow heartbeats. This difference is partly due to the size of the heart. The huge heart of an elephant could not beat at the same rate as the mouse heart because the heart muscle is too bulky and heavy.

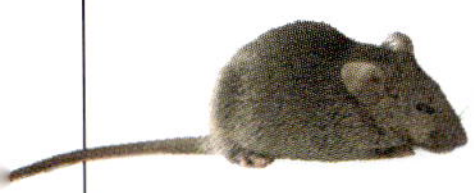

Mouse
This tiny mammal's pulse rate is over 500 beats per minute.

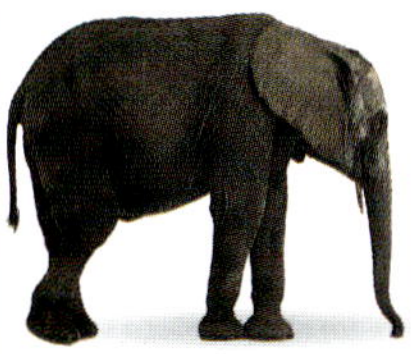

Elephant
This huge mammal has a resting pulse rate of 20 to 30 beats per minute.

Pulse points

The throbbing pressure bulges of the pulse travel through all of the body's arteries. The wrists are not the only places where you can feel them, but they are usually the most convenient. The radial artery lies just below the skin and directly above the wrist bones, so the bones make a firm base on which to press the artery. There are several other sites where the pulse can usually be felt clearly, especially after you have been exercising. An especially important site is the carotid artery in the neck, which carries blood to the head and brain.

Around the body
Try to find your pulse at each of these places. Do not press too hard on the body parts when feeling for it.

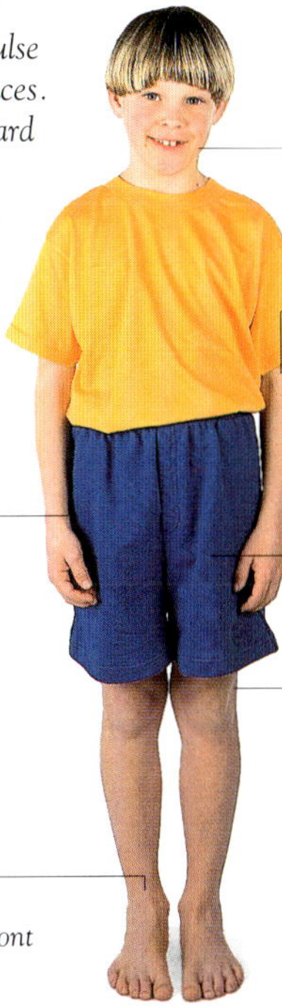

Blood

BLOOD IS ESSENTIAL TO HUMAN LIFE. As the body's major transport medium, it has numerous roles. Blood carries life-giving oxygen to all body parts and collects carbon dioxide for removal by the lungs (p.71). It also distributes vitamins, nutrients, and energy-rich sugars from digested food, and picks up wastes such as urea (p.109) for disposal by the kidneys. Blood is a highway for the white blood cells that fight germs. It also carries hormones, the chemical messengers that stimulate and coordinate body processes (p.106). It evens out the temperature in the different parts of the body by taking heat from busy parts, such as the heart and active muscles, to warm the less active, cooler parts and the extremities (p.113). Blood protects the body by clotting at the site of a wound to prevent any leakage of body fluids. It then hardens into a scab to help the injury heal.

■ DISCOVERY ■

Karl Landsteiner

For centuries people tried to transfuse (transfer) blood from humans—and animals—into people with blood diseases or who had lost blood through injury. Most of these patients died. The Austrian physician Karl Landsteiner (1868–1943) discovered why in 1900—one person's red blood cells agglutinate (clump together) on contact with blood from certain other people. This agglutination blocks the blood vessels. Landsteiner worked out that there must be a number of types of blood, which we call blood groups. His work led to the discovery of the ABO system (below left) in 1909. Landsteiner and others went on to find several other ways in which a person's blood can differ from another person's, such as the Rhesus system. This system shows the presence or absence of another agglutinating factor—the Rhesus factor—which is passed on in your genes (p.181).

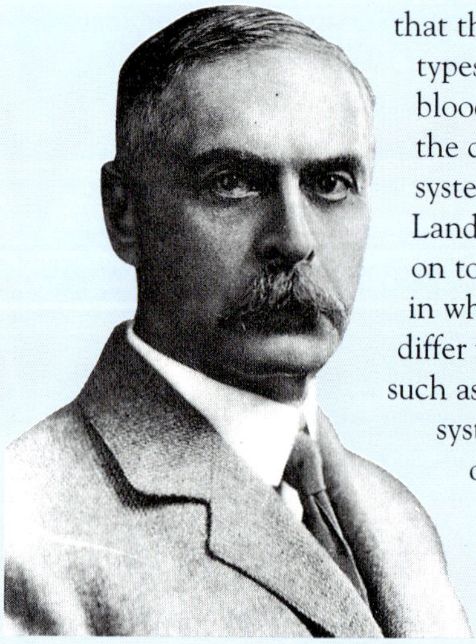

The ABO system

Not everyone's blood is the same. There are a number of different systems for classifying blood. Everybody's blood has a combination of elements from each of these systems. One of these systems is the ABO system. In this system, blood may belong to group A, B, AB, or O. The group you belong to depends on the presence or absence of chemicals called antigens on the surface of your blood cells and chemicals called antibodies in the watery part of your blood (opposite).

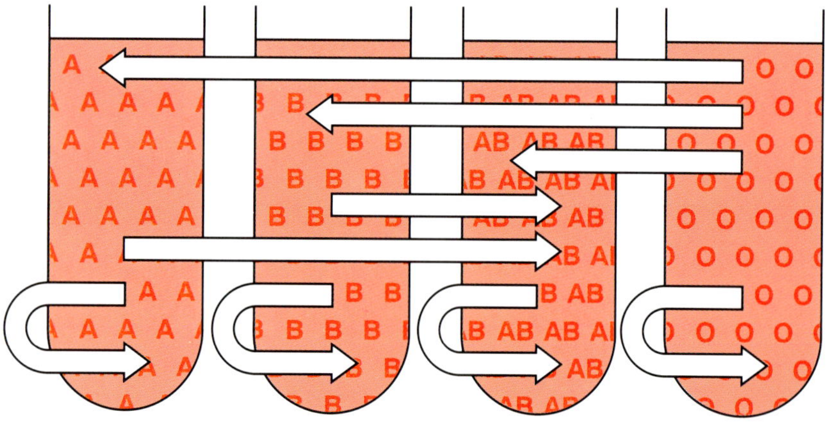

ABO compatibility
In a blood transfusion, donated blood must be of the correct group. These arrows show which groups can safely be donated to, or taken from, which others. Each group is compatible with itself. O blood can be donated to any patient. Patients with AB blood can take from any donor.

Threads of fibrin

When body tissues are damaged, they trigger off a series of reactions in the blood. First, chemicals are released by platelets in the blood. Then these chemicals convert a protein called fibrinogen into microscopic threads of fibrin. These form a sticky mesh that traps blood cells, and in this way the clot builds up (opposite).

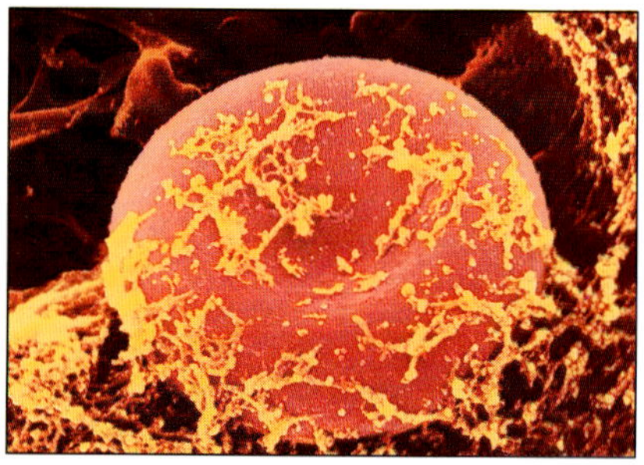

About to clot
This red blood cell is becoming trapped in threads of fibrin, as a clot begins to form.

What is in blood?

More than half of blood is a pale yellow fluid called plasma. Plasma is over nine-tenths water and contains sugars, nutrients, acids, salts, minerals, and proteins. The rest of blood consists of three types of blood cell—red cells, white cells, and platelets—as shown by an electron microscope (p.24) below.

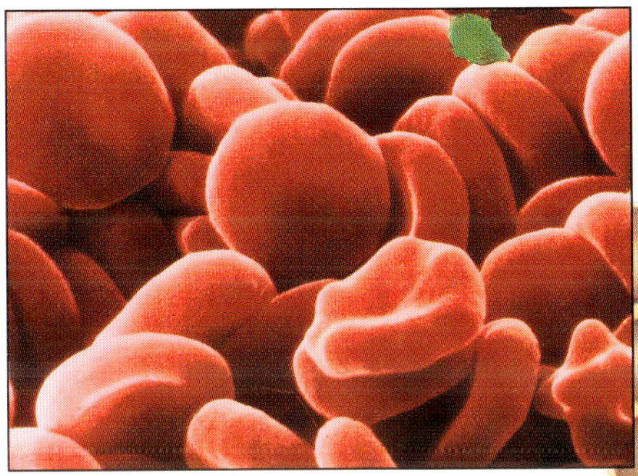

Red blood cells (erythrocytes)
Shaped like tiny doughnuts, they carry oxygen.

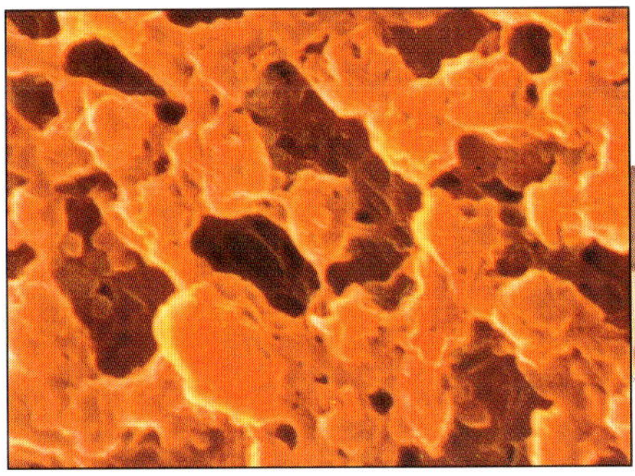

Platelets (thrombocytes)
These cell fragments take part in blood clotting.

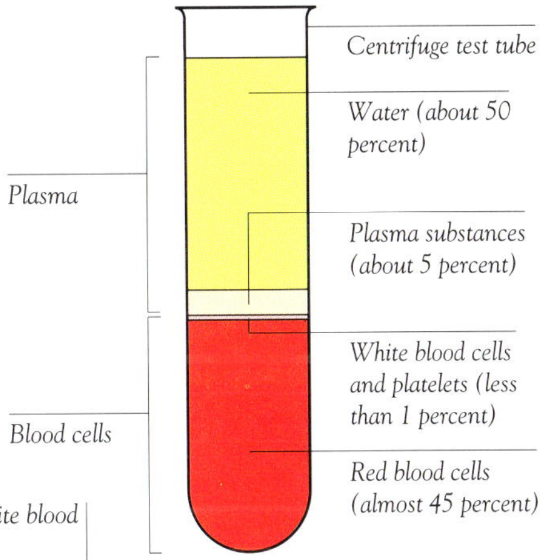

Separated blood
A centrifuge spins things around very quickly—faster than the spin cycle on a washing machine. Blood centrifuged in a test tube separates into layers. The densest (heaviest) portion—red blood cells—is at the bottom. There are 5 million red cells in a pinhead-size drop of blood. Next come the white cells and platelets. There are about 10,000 white cells and 250,000 platelets in the same-size drop. The lightest, watery portion of blood, called plasma, is at the top of the tube.

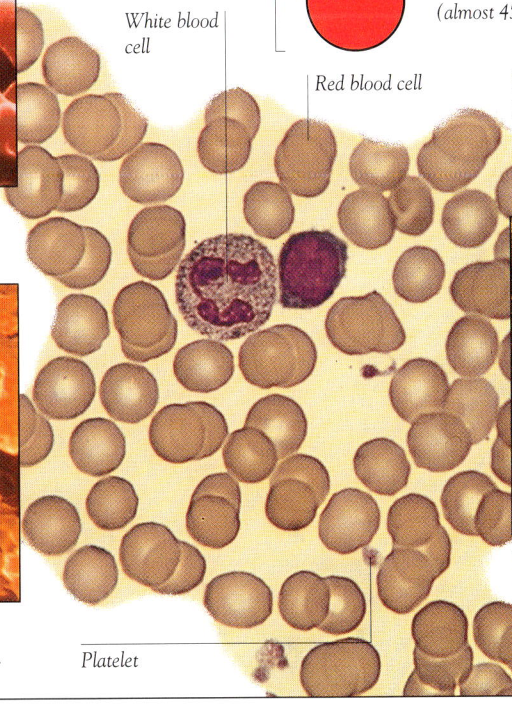

Blood through a light microscope
Here red blood cells, one white cell, and a few platelets are seen through a light microscope rather than an electron microscope.

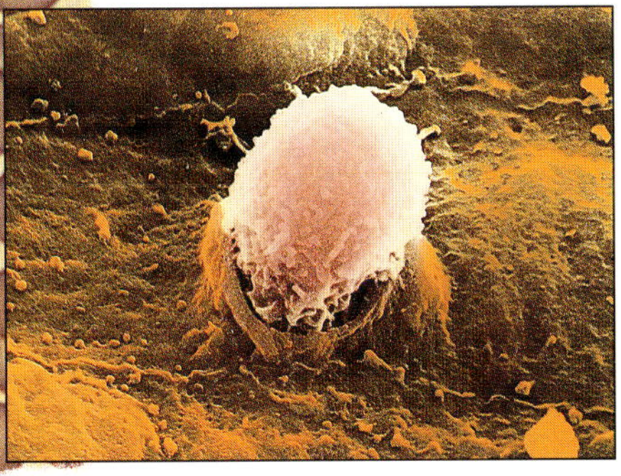

White blood cell (leucocyte)
Most of the many types of white cell fight germs.

Clotting and healing

A sticky lump known as a blood clot forms at the site of tissue damage, such as a cut in the skin. Unless the wound is large and gaping, the clot prevents more blood and other body fluids from leaking out. When the skin is cut, platelets become sticky and clump together at the site. Also, sticky strings of the clotting protein fibrin (opposite) make a tangled net that traps blood cells. Within a few minutes the clot starts to take shape. Gradually it shrinks and hardens, forming a tough scab. This protects the tissues while the cells in them multiply to heal the damage.

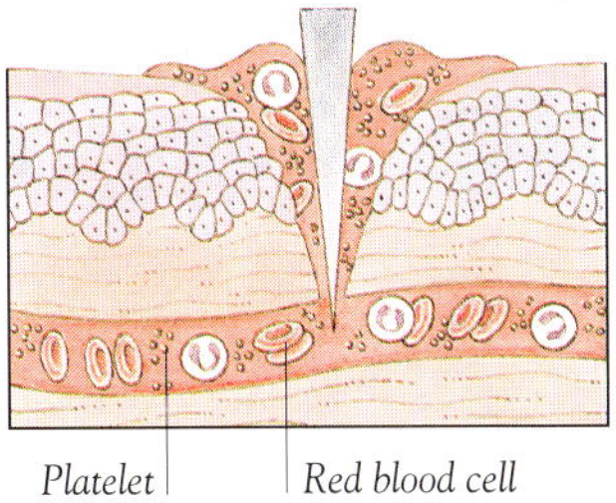

Damage
A sharp pin pricks into the skin and punctures a small blood vessel just under the surface. Blood, under pressure inside the body, oozes from the cut.

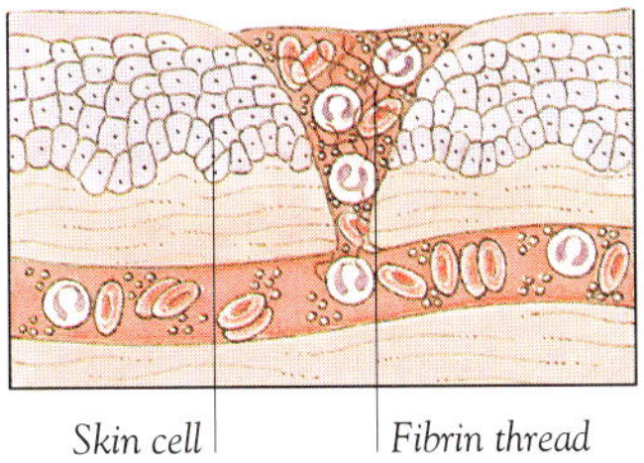

Young clot
Platelets clump together at the site. They release chemicals that turn the protein fibrinogen into fibrin threads, which trap more platelets and other blood cells.

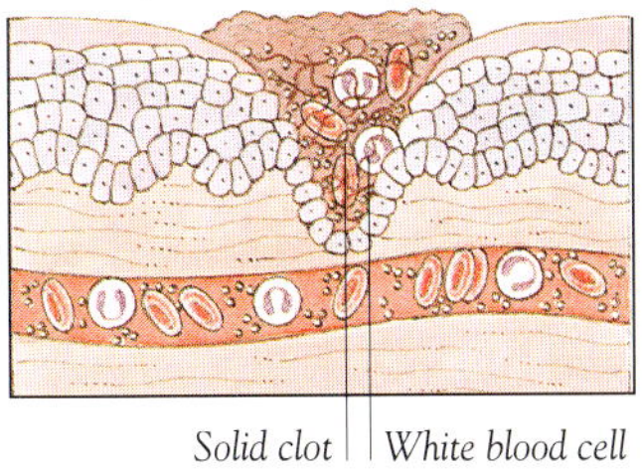

Mature clot
The platelets trigger chemical reactions that make the clot harder and more solid. White blood cells attack invading germs. Skin cells below multiply to repair the cut.

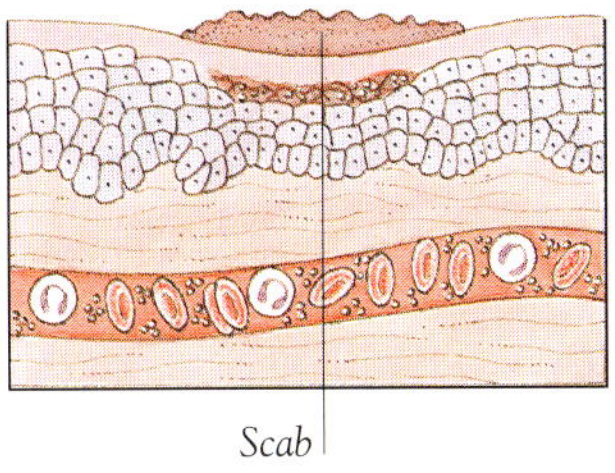

Scab
The clot continues to dry and harden, and becomes a scab. By the time it loosens and falls off, the skin and blood-vessel wall will have healed any damage.

THE INTERNAL ENVIRONMENT

DELICATE MACHINES SUCH AS SUPERCOMPUTERS or medical scanners are kept in conditions that are constantly monitored. If there is a change in the temperature, humidity, or other conditions around these machines, their immensely complex circuits may fail. The same is true of the body. The workings of its fragile cells (pp.24–25) are easily disturbed by changes in temperature, fluid levels, or chemical concentrations. The body must constantly check and adjust its internal conditions.

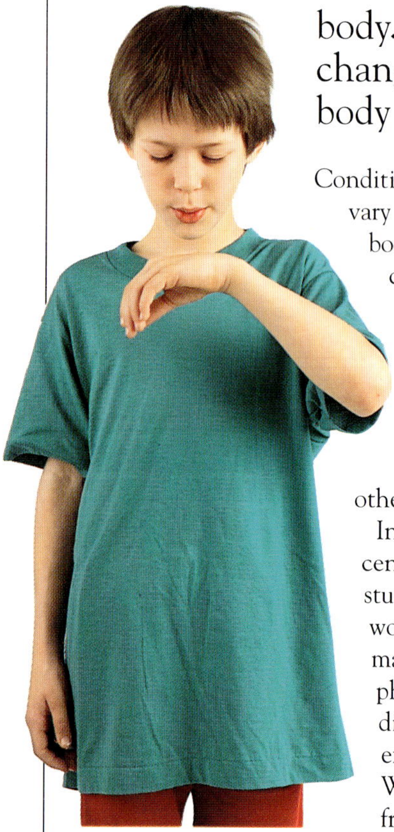

Test the cooling effect *of evaporation from the skin by blowing on a "sweat substitute" (p.112).*

Conditions outside the body can vary enormously. Yet inside the body they remain remarkably constant. The temperature stays at about 98.6°F (37°C), fluid concentrations are kept at certain levels, and so are the amounts of sugars, minerals, and other substances in the blood. In the 18th and 19th centuries, physiology—the study of the way the body works—developed into a major science. But physiologists found it difficult to carry out experiments on cells. When they removed cells from the body and put them in water to work on them, the cells swelled up and died. But gradually scientists found ways of producing fluids with concentrations of chemicals similar to those in the body. In these fluids, they could keep cells alive outside the body.

Homeostasis

In the mid 19th century the French physiologist Claude Bernard (p.110) introduced the idea of "the constancy of the internal environment." He saw that many body processes, such as shivering and sweating (which help adjust the body's temperature), were designed to maintain a steady environment inside the body, so that its cells could work efficiently.

The American physiologist Walter Canon (1871–1945) refined Bernard's theories. He coined the term "homeostasis," from the Greek "to stay the same." Homeostatic mechanisms in the body keep its internal conditions stable.

The kidneys are involved in many homeostatic mechanisms, such as regulating levels of water and minerals in the blood and removing waste substances—particularly urea, which is poisonous if it is allowed to build up. This removal is carried out by the urinary system, which comprises the two kidneys, the bladder, and their connecting tubes (p.108).

The kidneys

The early anatomists knew that the kidneys make urine, but they did not understand how they work. The invention of the microscope changed this. One of the early microscopists was an Italian philosopher-turned-doctor, called Marcello Malpighi (1628–94). He described the tiny structures in the kidneys that are now called Malpighian corpuscles. One corpuscle together with a microtube forms a filtering unit called a nephron (p.108). Blood entering a nephron flows through a knot of capillaries, termed a glomerulus. Water, wastes, and some salts and chemicals are squeezed through the capillary walls into a system of microtubes. From there, water and useful salts and chemicals are taken back into the blood as they are needed. The remaining wastes and excess water flow into collecting tubes in the kidney medulla and then leave the kidneys as urine.

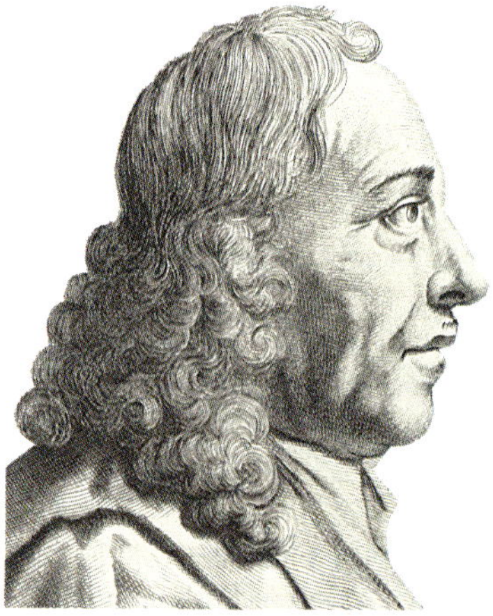

A pioneer in microscopic study, *Marcello Malpighi made important discoveries about the kidneys, lungs, spleen, and other organs. He also studied silkworms and how chicks develop in their eggs.*

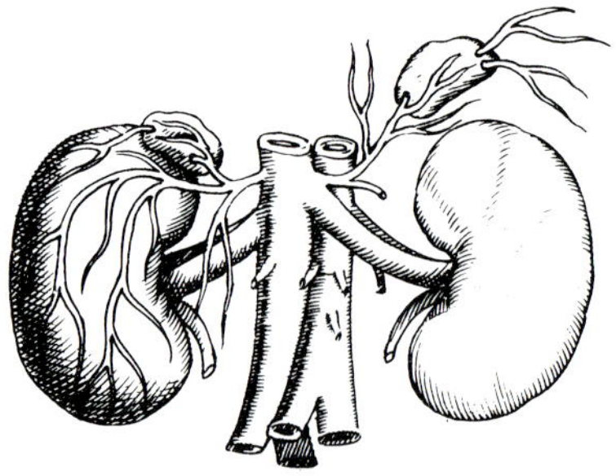

A hormone-making adrenal gland *(p.108) sits on top of each kidney. These glands release hormones directly into the blood.*

Hormones

How are the body's many homeostatic mechanisms controlled? A comparison may help. In the modern world, we can send and receive information

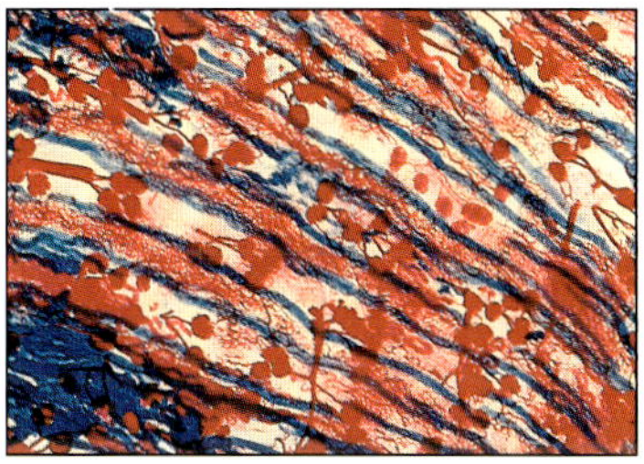

The tiny red blobs in this light microscope picture of a kidney are called glomeruli. They are knots of capillary blood vessels in nephrons (p.108), which filter substances out of the blood.

in different ways. One way is by telephone. The messages are represented by electrical signals that travel along wires. They go from the sender, through a series of exchanges, to the receiver only. Another method is by radio. The radio waves are

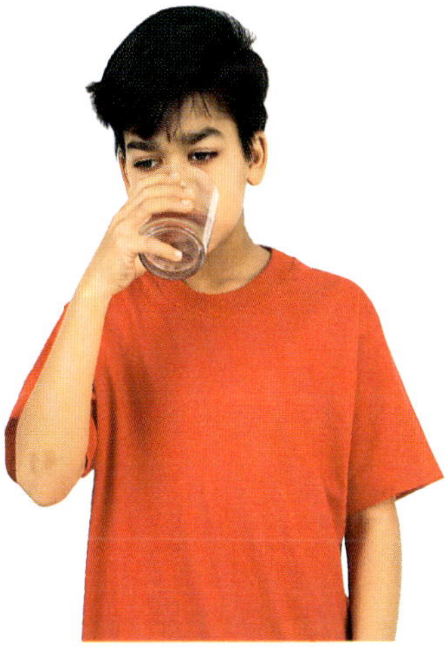

If your brain detects that your blood has become too concentrated, you feel thirsty and hormones are sent to instruct the kidneys to retain water.

produced by a transmitter and broadcast over a wide area. Anyone with a receiving set that is tuned in can pick up the waves.

Similarly, the body has two communications systems. Together they control and coordinate homeostasis. One is the nervous system (pp.118–119). The nerves are "wires," like telephone wires, through which signals go from the sender to the receiver, usually with the brain as the "exchange."

The second system is the endocrine system (pp.106–107). It uses "waves" of body chemicals called hormones, like radio waves. These are produced by hormonal glands, which are "transmitters." There are several types of hormonal gland, such as the adrenal glands on top of the kidneys. Also, certain organs, such as the stomach, pancreas, kidneys, and ovaries and testes (p.23), make hormones as well as carrying out their other roles.

The hormones spread around the whole body, carried by the blood. But they affect only certain parts, the target organs, which, like radio receivers, are "tuned" to detect them.

Early anatomists had seen and described the hormonal glands, but they did not really know how they worked. They could see that these glands do not have tubes leading from them, unlike glands such as the salivary glands, which pour their products along a duct. For centuries, hormonal glands—which gained the alternative name "ductless glands"—were virtually ignored by scientists.

Physiological research gradually showed that chemicals from these glands were transmitted around the body. The true nature of the glands was then understood, and the science of endocrinology (p.106) was established.

Fight or flight

The nervous system controls the actions of the body that take place over a very short period of time—such as speaking or writing. In contrast, the endocrine system controls actions that take place over a long period of time. For example, the hormone thyroxine controls the body's growth. But often the two systems work together.

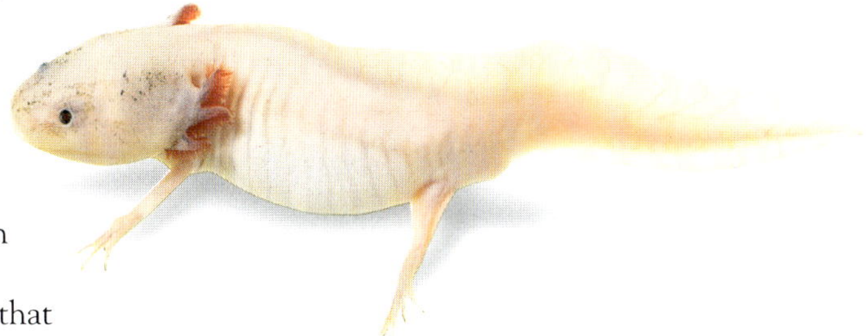

Because of its lack of the hormone thyroxine, the axolotl never grows up. It breeds while it is still a "tadpole."

The "fight or flight" response is a very good example of this. This is the choice of response that you must make if you find yourself threatened—you must face the situation (fight) or avoid it (flight). The hypothalamus in your brain (p.126) alerts several organs and glands through the autonomic nervous system (p.118). Among these are the

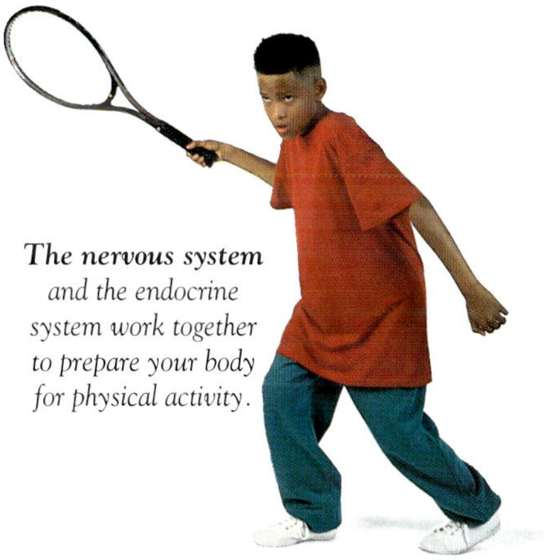

The nervous system and the endocrine system work together to prepare your body for physical activity.

adrenal glands. These release the hormones adrenaline and noradrenaline, which spread through the blood and body tissues to their target organs. As a combined result of nerves and hormones, whether you fight or flee, your heart beats harder and faster, your lungs breathe more rapidly, blood is diverted from your skin and inner organs to your muscles, and your liver releases high-energy glucose to give your body energy. You are ready for action.

Hormones

YOUR BODY HAS two control systems. One is the nervous system (pp.118–119), which sends messages around the body in the form of nerve signals. The other is the endocrine system, which sends messages around the body in the form of chemicals called hormones. Hormones are made in special glands called hormonal glands. Each gland releases its hormone directly into the bloodstream. As the blood carries the hormone through the body, the hormone affects the working of specific body parts, called its target organs. The higher the level of a hormone in the blood, the greater its effect on its target organs. The amounts of hormones released are controlled by the nervous system and by other hormones, mostly produced by the pituitary gland.

■ DISCOVERY ■

Ernest Starling

The study of hormones is called endocrinology. This branch of physiology (the workings of the body) did not begin until the late 19th century. The name "hormone" comes from a Greek term, meaning "to set in motion." It was coined in 1905 by the English scientist Ernest Starling (1866–1927), a professor of physiology in London, England. In 1902 Starling and a colleague, William Bayliss, isolated (separated out) a hormone for the first time. The hormone was secretin, a digestive hormone made by the small intestine. Starling also studied the lymphatic system (p.23) and other body fluids, and the kidneys. A scientific law that predicts the amount of blood pumped out by the heart under various conditions is named after him.

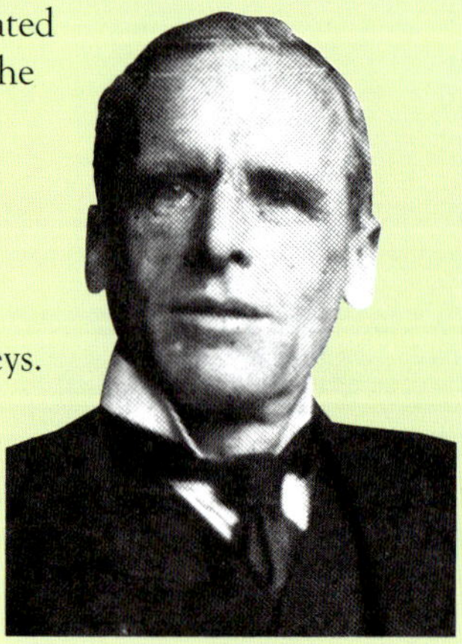

Hormones and glucose

The body needs a relatively constant level of glucose sugar (p.181) in its blood to supply energy to its millions of cells. If the glucose level falls too low, cells run out of energy and die. If the glucose level rises too high, the extra glucose disturbs the working of the kidneys. Follow the arrows in this chart to see how the pancreas (p.85) can release either of two hormones—called insulin and glucagon—to maintain steady levels of glucose in the blood.

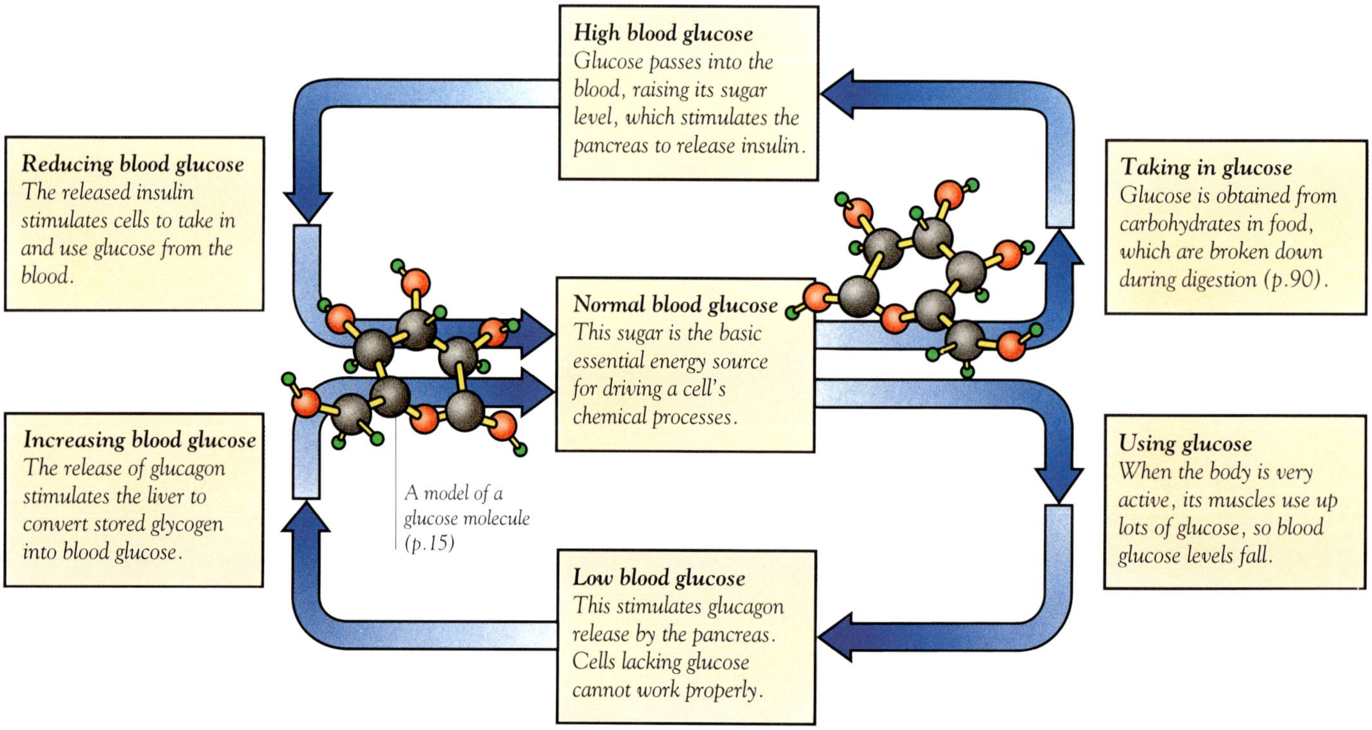

Dual functions

Several body organs make hormones, in addition to their other roles. One example is your pancreas (p.85). It makes insulin and glucagon (opposite). These pass directly into the blood that flows through the pancreas. The pancreas also produces enzymes, which flow along a tube called the pancreatic duct into the small intestine to digest food.

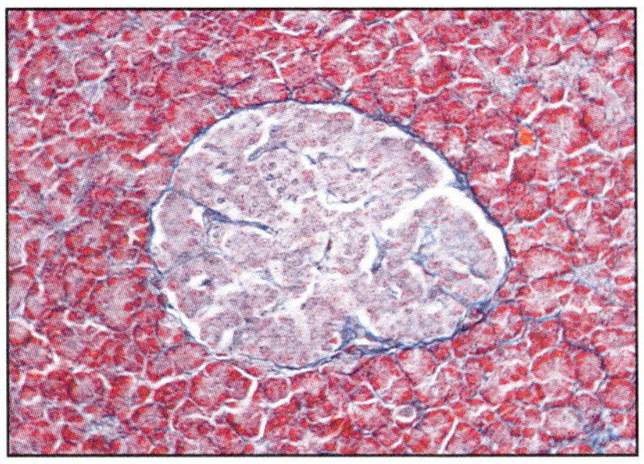

Hormone making in the pancreas
This microscope photograph shows an islet of Langerhans, one of a million hormone-producing knots of cells inside the pancreas.

Long-term control

The nervous system tends to control rapid, short-term body functions, such as muscle movements. The endocrine system is concerned more with the control of slower, long-term processes, such as digestion, fluid balance, the body's mineral levels, and growth and sexual development.

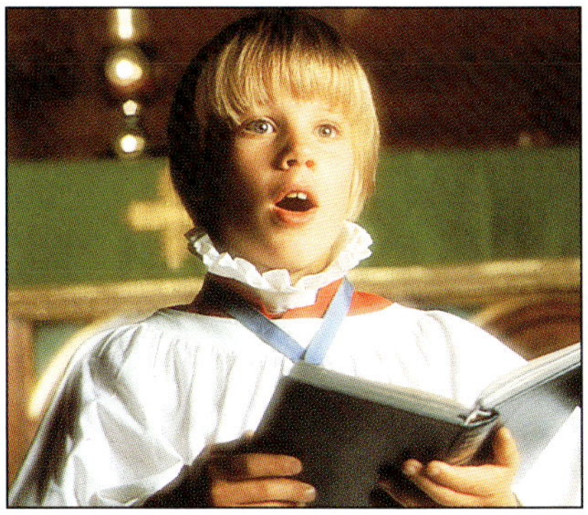

Child to adult
Male voices deepen in adolescence as more of the hormone testosterone is produced. This hormone affects the growth of the vocal cords.

Hormones through a day

We are usually less aware of the actions of the endocrine system than those of the nervous system. But each day dozens of hormones from various hormonal glands and other organs circulate in the blood, regulating and coordinating the activities of their target organs and tissues. The activity of the hormonal glands is mainly controlled by other hormones and by nerves. Most of the hormone-controlling hormones are produced by the pea-size pituitary gland, just beneath the brain. The pituitary gland is the "chief gland" of the endocrine system. It is connected by a short stalk to the hypothalamus (p.126), which monitors levels of hormones and other substances in the blood. The hypothalamus instructs the pituitary gland to release the appropriate hormones into the body. Here are some examples of hormones released during various situations that you might find yourself in—some normal, some less so.

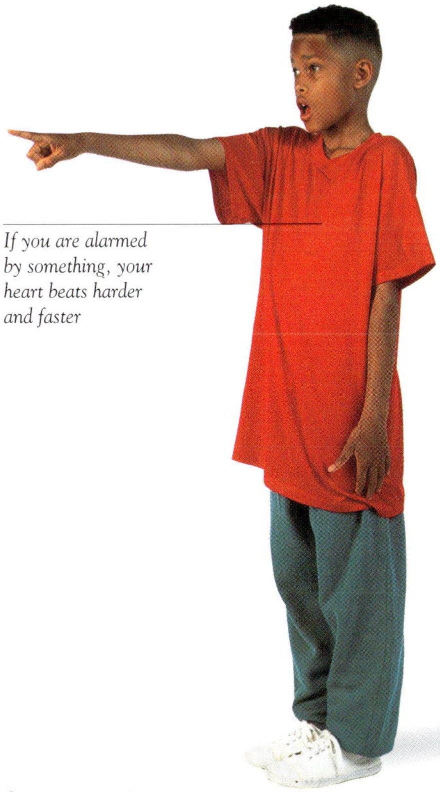

Stress situations
If you are under stress, the adrenal glands, above the kidneys, make adrenaline. This hormone works with the nervous system to raise blood pressure and heart and breathing rates (p.105).

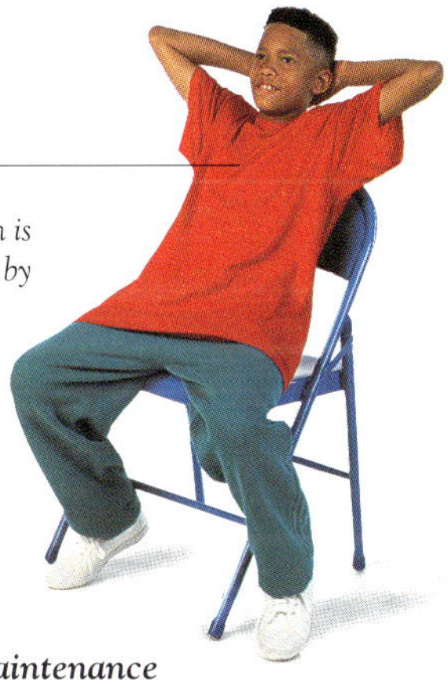

Body maintenance
Even as the body rests, hormones are at work. The kidneys make the hormone erythropoietin, which stimulates the production of new red blood cells at the rate of 2 million each second.

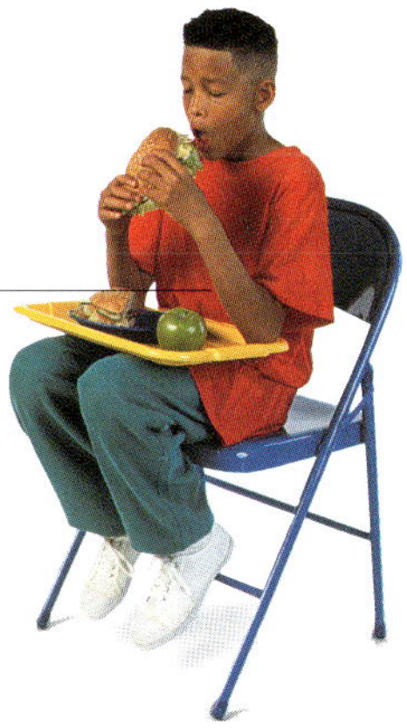

Digestion
As you eat a meal, your stomach stretches. This stretching triggers the release of hormones such as gastrin and secretin, which prepare the stomach, pancreas, and intestines for digestion.

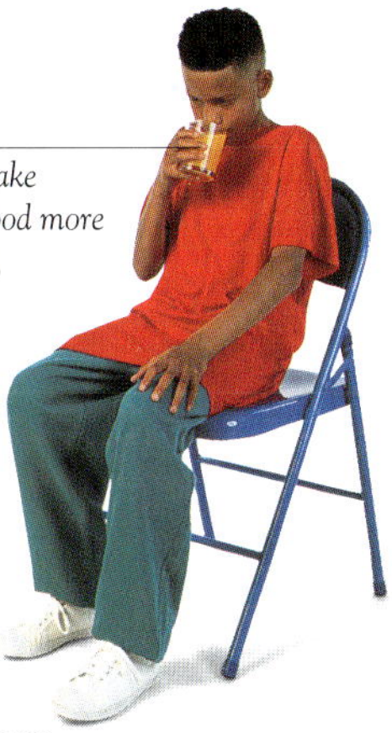

Fluid balance
Another adrenal hormone is aldosterone. When fluid intake is low, it stimulates the kidneys to conserve salts and water. After you have a drink, the level of aldosterone goes down.

Cleaning the blood

A CAR EMITS exhaust fumes. A heating furnace gives off smoke and soot. These are waste products. The body produces wastes, too. Most body wastes are end products of chemical reactions that are carried out in cells (pp.24–25), as the cells build up new substances and break down old ones. Examples of wastes include urea, containing broken-down proteins, and creatinine, produced when muscles contract. These wastes are collected by the blood, the body's main transport fluid. They are filtered and removed from the blood as it flows through the two kidneys in the upper rear abdomen. The filtered wastes and excess water form a fluid, called urine, which is stored in a stretchy bag, the bladder, before being expelled from the body.

EXPERIMENT

Invisible wastes

The body's waste fluid, urine, is mainly water, with a yellowish tinge. It does not look as if it carries dozens of waste substances. It does—but they are in dissolved form. Show this principle using ordinary table salt and water. If the water was removed from urine in a similar way, it would leave a thimbleful of solid wastes daily.

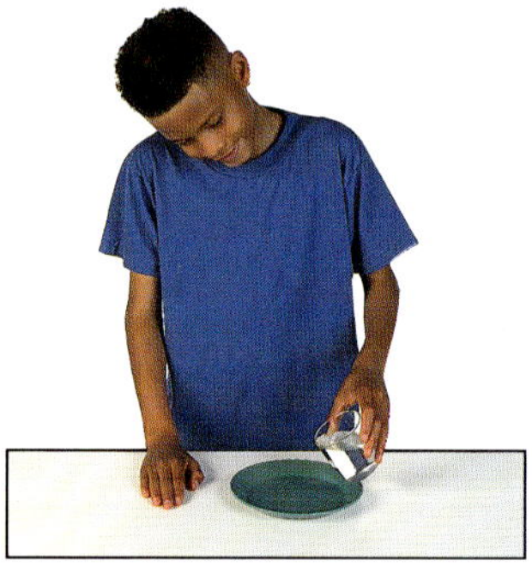

Disappearing salt
Stir 2 tablespoons of salt into a jar of warm water. The salt grains dissolve and disappear. Pour some of this salt solution onto a plate.

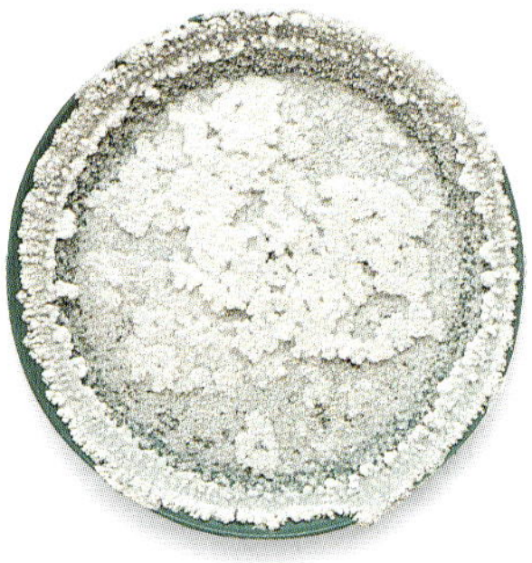

Reappearing salt
Leave the plate in a warm place. Gradually the water evaporates. It leaves behind the salt, which has become visible again.

Urinary system

The kidneys, bladder, and connecting tubes make up the urinary system. The kidneys receive a huge blood flow—up to 440 gallons (2,000 liters) a day. Each kidney has a million tiny filtering units, called nephrons, which extract wastes from blood to form urine. The left kidney in this illustration has been cut away to show its interior.

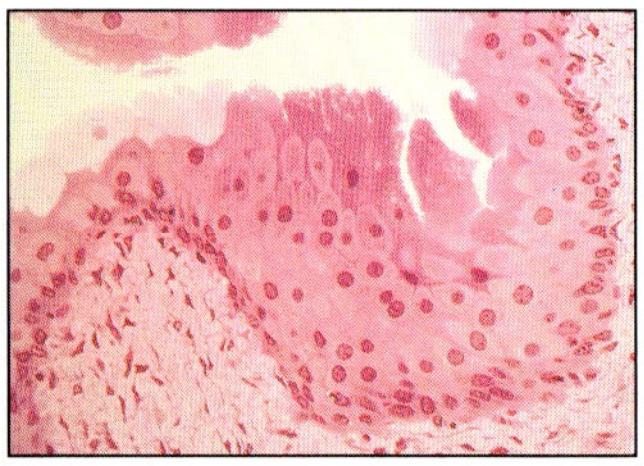

Bladder lining
This microscope photograph shows the lining of the bladder. It is made of a type of tissue (p.185) called transitional epithelium, which is strong and stretchy, and resists the corrosive chemical attack of urine.

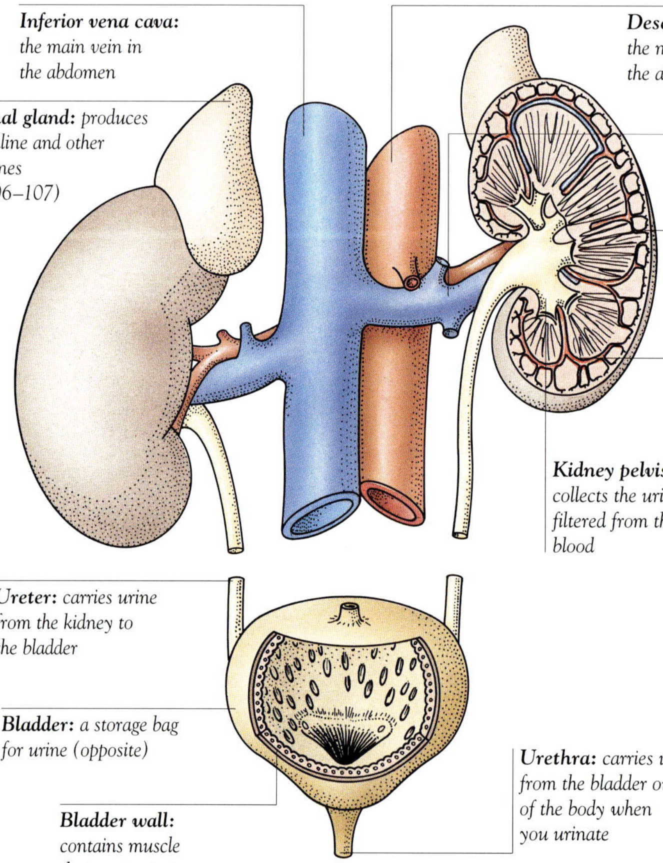

The bladder

The kidneys of an adult produce on average nearly 2 pints (1 liter) of urine each day. The exact amount is controlled by hormones (p.106). These adjust the filtering and water-absorbing rates of the kidneys. If you have plenty to drink, the kidneys produce a lot of dilute urine, so that the excess water is disposed of. If you drink only a small amount, the kidneys do not expel much water in urine, so the urine is more concentrated. From the kidneys, the urine oozes down the ureters into the bladder. The tough, stretchy walls of the bladder can expand to hold up to almost 1 pint (500 ml) of urine. However, the desire to urinate begins when the bladder is about half full.

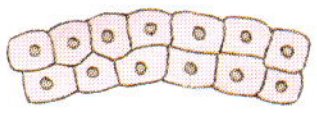

Lining of empty bladder
Cells of the transitional epithelium lining the bladder are tall and rounded.

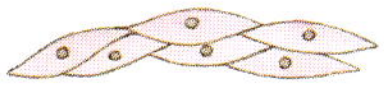

Lining of full bladder
Cells of the transitional epithelium are stretched thin and flat.

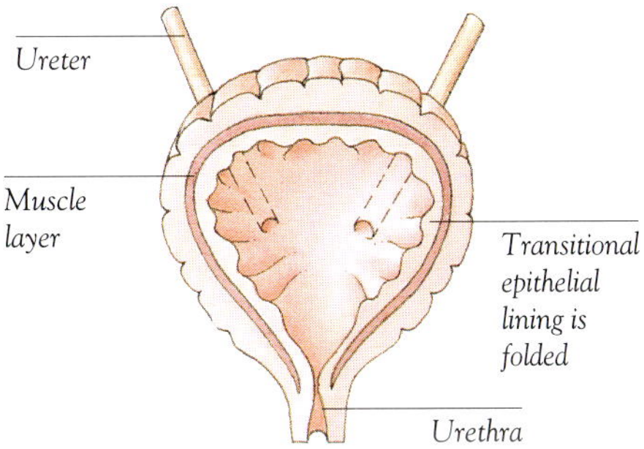

Empty bladder
The multilayered bladder wall thickens and folds up as urine flows away along the urethra. The empty bladder looks like a wrinkled prune.

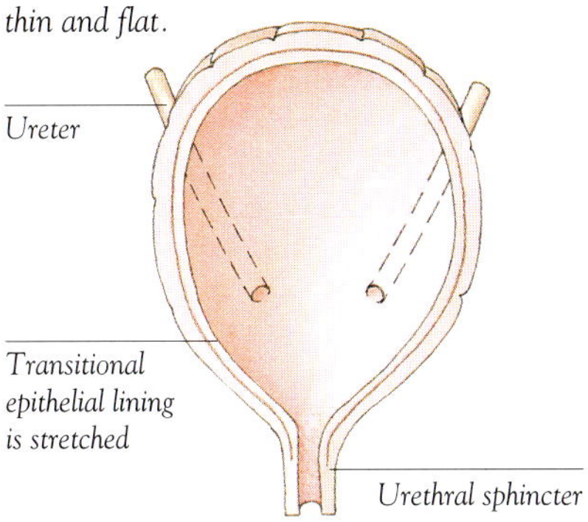

Full bladder
The muscle wall stretches thin as the bladder blows up like a balloon. The urine is held in by a muscular ring, the urethral sphincter.

Filtering and sorting

A series of various-size pores (holes) in the nephron microfilters retain selected chemicals—according to the size, shape, and other features of their molecules—and allow other chemicals through. In the same way, this model kidney has holes that filter out balls of certain sizes only. Red blood cells are big, and so do not pass into the filtering system at all. Urea passes through all filtering stages and ends up in urine. Glucose, salts, and other essential chemicals are first filtered out, in the cortex, but then taken back into the blood in the medulla.

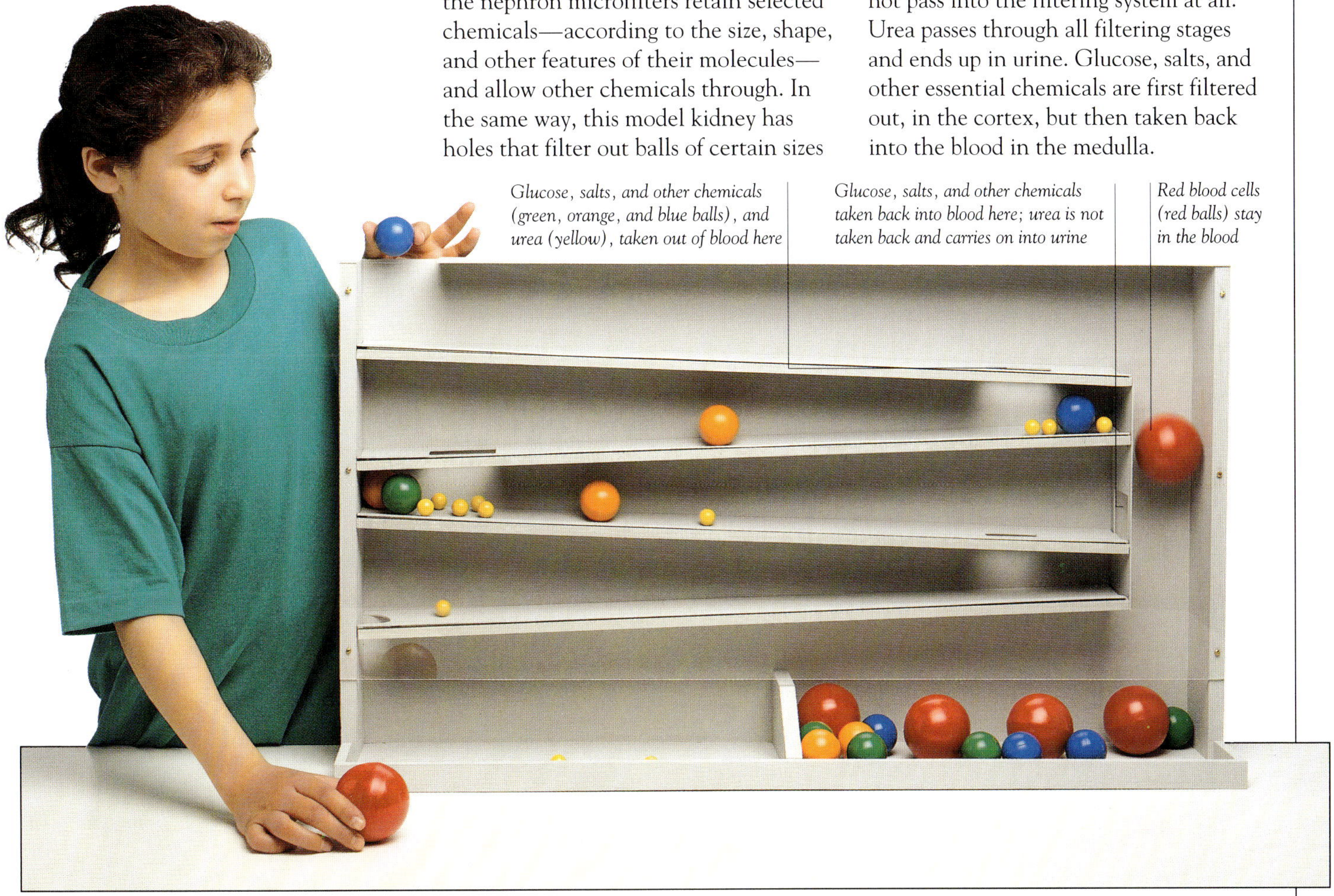

Glucose, salts, and other chemicals (green, orange, and blue balls), and urea (yellow), taken out of blood here

Glucose, salts, and other chemicals taken back into blood here; urea is not taken back and carries on into urine

Red blood cells (red balls) stay in the blood

Balancing body fluids

NOW AND THEN, you may feel that you need a drink. But have you ever been truly thirsty? A lack of body fluid brings on a powerful basic urge to take in water—because water is essential for life. All of the chemistry that takes place in your body occurs in a watery environment. Only when chemicals are dissolved in water are they able to move and react, combine and separate, diffuse and osmose. These reactions and processes take place constantly among the billions of cells in your body. Several body systems (pp.22–23) play a role in making sure that your fluid levels are balanced. These include the urinary and the endocrine systems. It is the job of the brain to detect when blood and other body liquids have become too concentrated, which means that water is running low.

DISCOVERY

Claude Bernard

During the 18th and 19th centuries, chemistry developed into a major science for the first time. Researchers began to delve deep into the chemistry of the body. Some of the most important discoveries were made by the French physician Claude Bernard (1813–78). Instead of simply observing nature, Bernard carried out many experiments, on animals and in test tubes. He suggested that the body has mechanisms that maintain and stabilize its internal conditions—such as fluid balance, nutrient levels, and temperature. This idea led him to the concept of homeostasis, or "the constancy of the internal environment" (p.104). Bernard also made discoveries about the stomach, liver, intestines, pancreas, blood vessels, and curare—a muscle-relaxing drug extracted from a poisonous plant root. In 1865 he wrote the classic *Introduction to the Study of Experimental Medicine*.

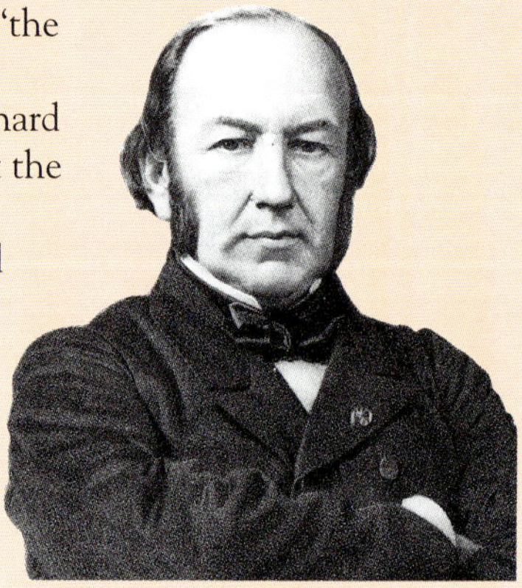

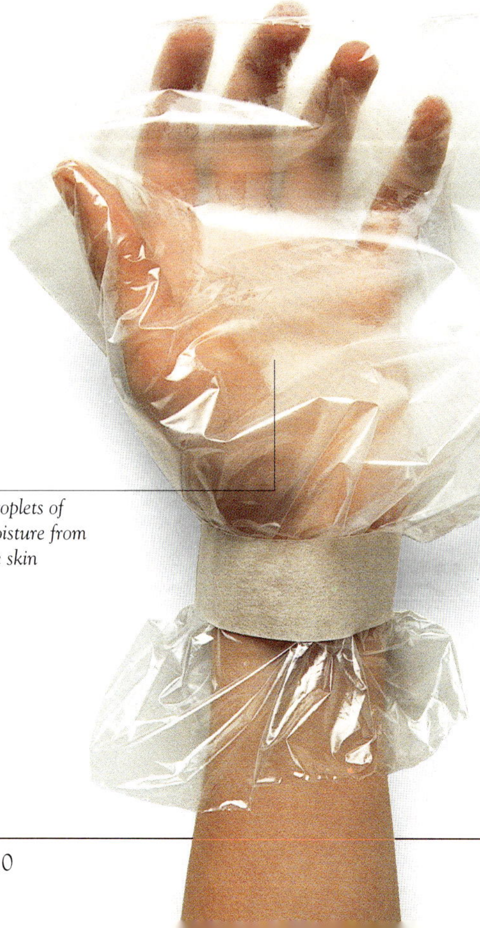

Droplets of moisture from the skin

EXPERIMENT

Always in a sweat

Adult help is advised for this experiment

Although you sweat most when you have been very active in hot conditions, the body loses small amounts of water all the time, as shown by this simple experiment.

YOU WILL NEED

- *clear-plastic bag*
- *cellophane tape*
- *microscope*
- *slide*
- *red dye*

1 PUT YOUR hand in the bag, and tape it loosely to your wrist. Study the bag after 10 to 15 minutes. Can you see tiny, misty drops condensing on the inside of the bag? This is some of the moisture (sweat) that is constantly evaporating from the skin in small amounts. *Caution: Do not tape the bag to your wrist too tightly. Do not leave it on when the experiment is finished.*

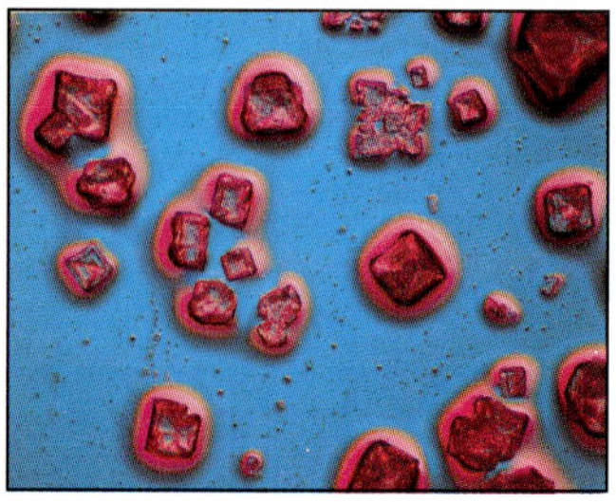

2 REMOVE THE BAG. Smear the slide on your hand to collect moisture. Look through the microscope (p.178) to see crystals of sodium chloride (salt) in the sweat. Dye the crystals red to make details stand out.

Water in and out

Water evaporates from the skin and the lungs. It is also needed to carry dissolved wastes, such as urea (p.108), from the body. This lost water must be replaced by water in drinks and food—especially leafy vegetables and juicy fruits. This chart shows the average daily flow of water in and out of a child's body—although the amounts vary, according to factors such as the surrounding temperature.

In

Metabolic water (made in the body by chemical reactions) $\frac{1}{3}$ pt (150 ml)

Water in food $\frac{2}{3}$ pt (300 ml)

Water in drink $1\frac{2}{3}$ pt (750 ml)

Total $2\frac{1}{2}$ pt (1,200 ml)

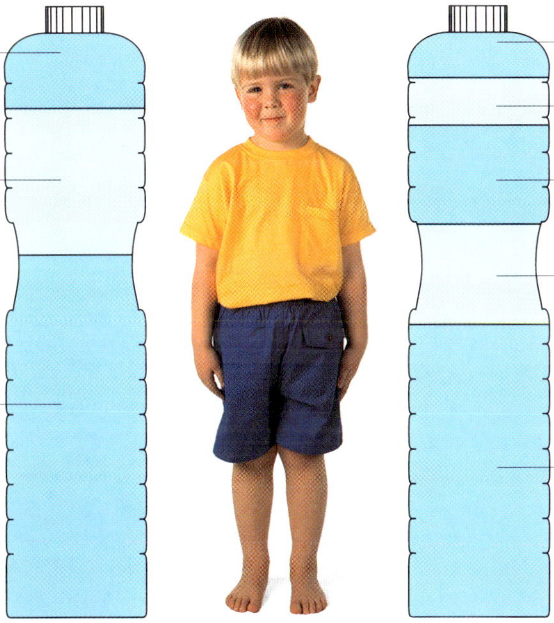

Out

Water in sweat $\frac{1}{5}$ pt (100 ml)

Water in feces $\frac{1}{5}$ pt (100 ml)

Water evaporating from the skin $\frac{2}{5}$ pt (200 ml)

Water evaporating from the lungs and breathing airways $\frac{2}{5}$ pt (200 ml)

Water in urine $1\frac{1}{4}$ pt (600 ml)

Total $2\frac{1}{2}$ pt (1,200 ml)

Survival without water?

Some desert animals never seem to drink. But they do need water. The main reason that they can drink so little is that they expel very little water. The urine that they produce is highly concentrated, and their droppings are dry. Also, desert animals avoid the hot, drying sun by being active only at night. Much of the water that they obtain comes not from drink, but from food, such as moist leaves and seeds, and the juicy bodies of other creatures.

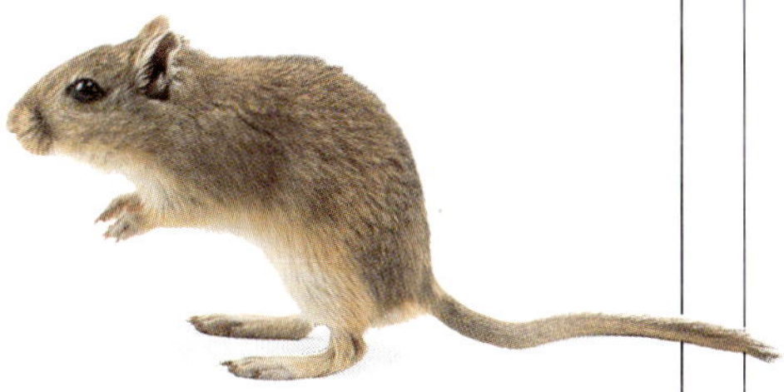

Drought in the desert
The gerbil rarely has to drink. It can survive on the water in seeds and other plant foods.

Why we feel thirsty

The desire to drink, like all conscious urges, comes from the brain. Water flows in and out of cells and around the body, mainly in the blood and also in the lymphatic system. When water levels fall, the concentrations of various substances in the blood rise. If this happens, the part of the brain called the hypothalamus (p.126) triggers the feeling we call thirst, so that we try to obtain more water. The hypothalamus also communicates by hormones (pp.106–107), which instruct the kidneys to retain some of the water that would otherwise be lost as urine. This makes the urine more concentrated, giving it a darker color.

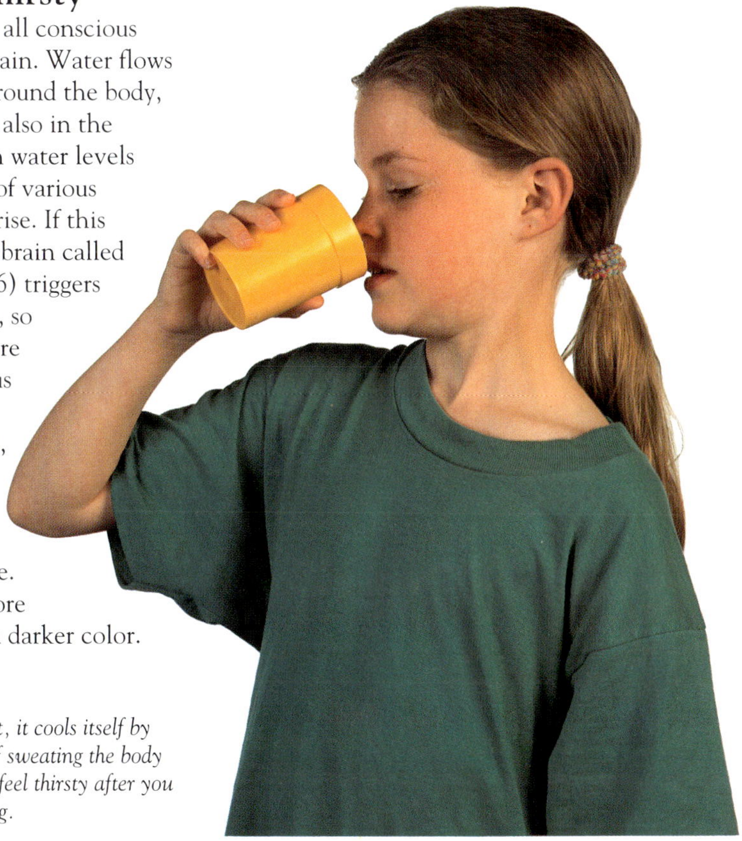

Getting thirsty
When your body becomes hot, it cools itself by sweating more. As a result of sweating the body loses water. This is why you feel thirsty after you have been active and sweating.

Water in the body

About two-thirds of your body weight is water. Two-thirds of this water is inside body cells (intracellular), where it acts as a solvent in which cell chemicals dissolve. It also maintains the shape and size of the cells. The other third of the body's water is outside cells (extracellular).

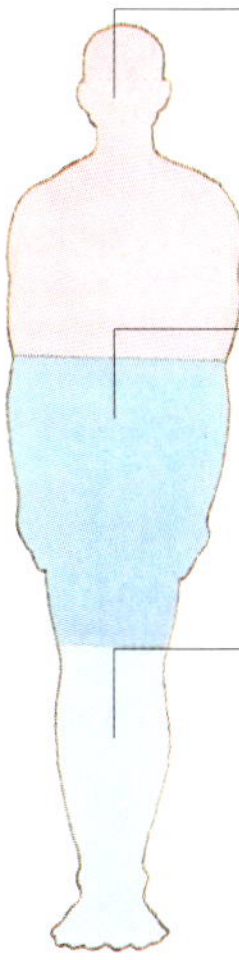

Nonwater substances
These include proteins, fats, and minerals. They make up about one-third of your body weight

Intracellular water
Two-thirds of body water is inside cells. It can pass in and out of the cells by osmosis

Extracellular water
One-third of the water is in blood plasma and lymph, and in the spaces between cells

Body temperature

HAVE YOU BEEN in a small room that is crowded with people? Even if it is cold at first, the room soon begins to warm up. It may become uncomfortably hot. This is because human bodies give off heat, like very slow-burning fires. A fire turns the chemical energy of its fuel, such as coal or wood, into rapidly released heat. To obtain the energy that runs its thousands of chemical processes, the body "burns" its own type of fuel—food. It turns chemical energy in foods into slowly released heat. This warmth helps to keep your body at 98.6°F (37°C), the temperature at which its cells work most efficiently. A whole range of processes prevent your body from becoming too hot or too cold.

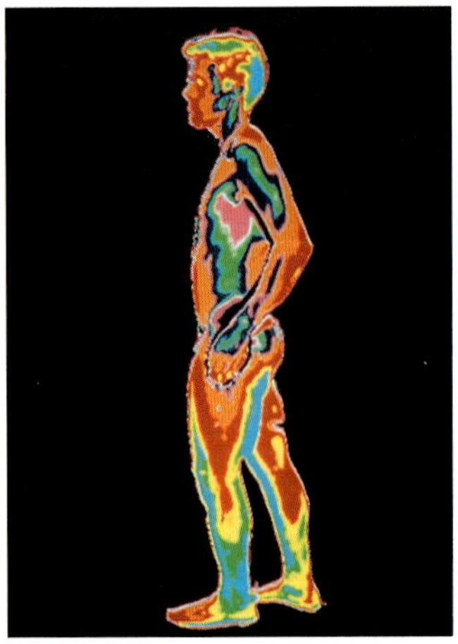

The body's "heat map"
A thermograph is a map of body heat. Here, cool parts are red, warm ones purple and green.

Warm-bloodedness

All mammals, from rabbits to humans, are warm-blooded, maintaining a high body temperature even in cold weather. To keep warm and active in the cold, mammals need lots of food to burn as fuel. The greater our body surface, the more heat we lose from it. Closely related animals that live in different climates may have body features with very different surface areas, to help them adapt to the climate.

Keeping cool

If the body gets too hot, part of the brain called the hypothalamus (p.126) registers this and triggers body-cooling processes such as sweating and flushing.

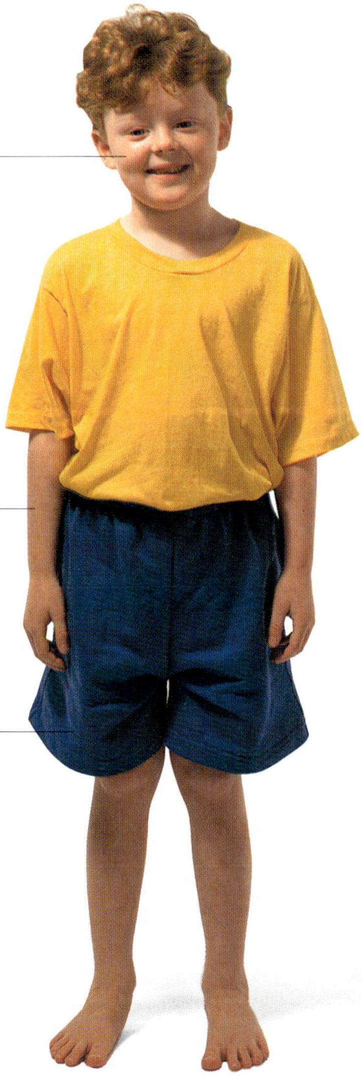

Sweat glands release sweat that oozes onto the skin and cools it by evaporation (left)—this is called perspiration

Blood vessels near the body surface become wider, so that more blood flows through them, giving off more heat—which makes the skin flushed

Loose, light clothing lets air blow past and carry heat away from the body

EXPERIMENT

Cooling sweat

Adult help is advised for this experiment

When a puddle evaporates (turns into vapor), it uses a tiny amount of the sun's heat. Similarly, when sweat evaporates from your skin it draws heat from your body. Show this with rubbing alcohol, a liquid that evaporates faster than water.

YOU WILL NEED

- *rubbing alcohol*
- *cotton balls*

1 POUR A little alcohol on to a cotton ball, and dab the back of your hand.

2 BLOW ON your hand to speed the evaporation. Does the patch feel cool as the alcohol draws warmth from the skin? (Wash your hands afterward.)

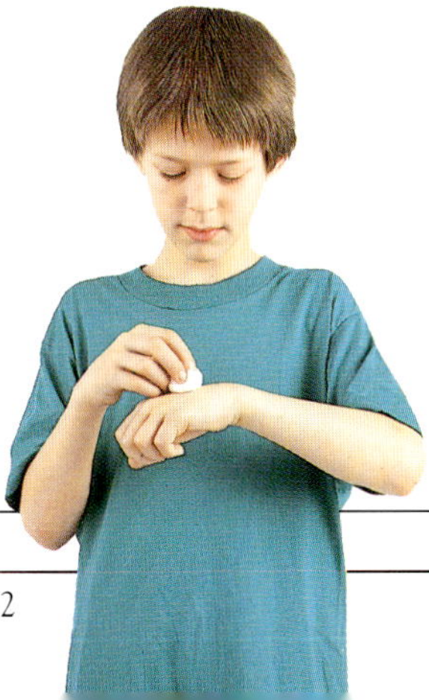

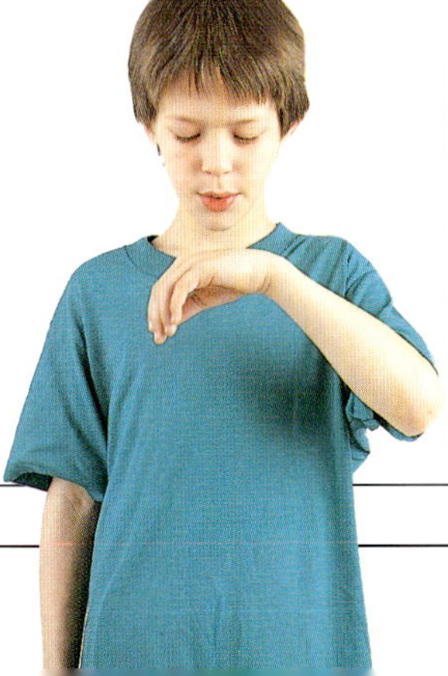

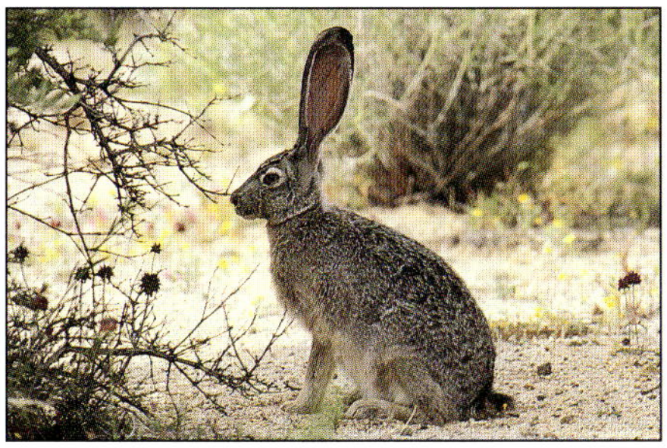

Big ears in hot places
The jackrabbit's huge ears help to get rid of excess body warmth in the hot, dry scrub and grassland.

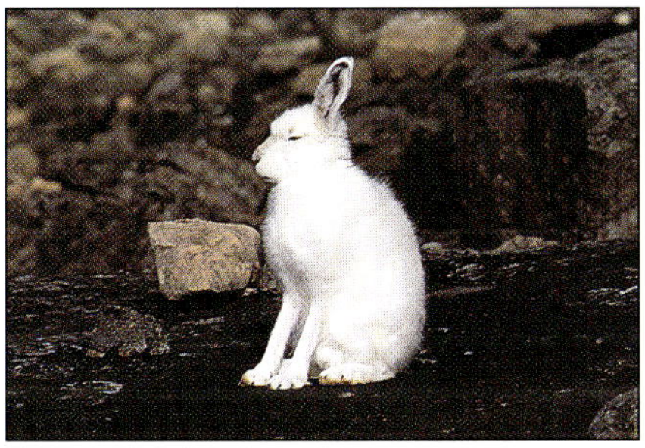

Small ears in cold places
In the icy Arctic, the snowshoe hare has small ears, so there is less area for heat loss.

Keeping warm

In cold conditions, the cooling body processes (opposite) are reversed, to conserve heat. You can help these natural warmth-retaining reactions by putting on thicker clothes. A hat is particularly useful, since up to two-fifths of all heat coming from your body is lost from your head and face.

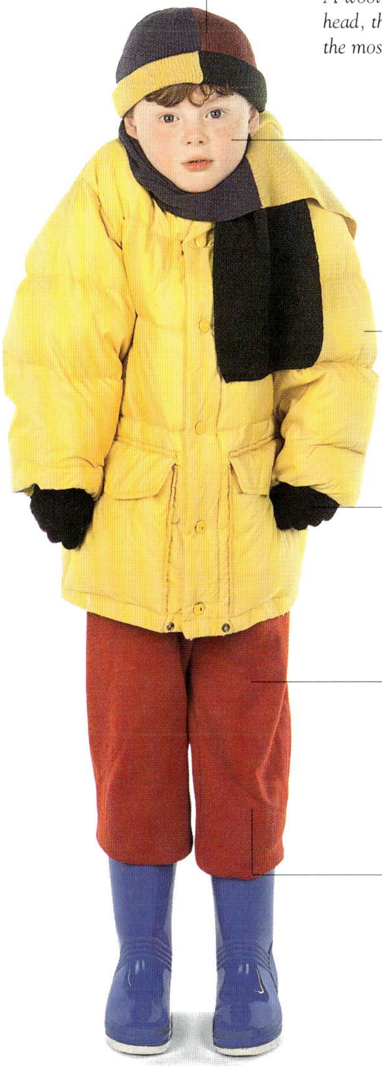

A wool hat prevents heat loss from the head, the part of the body that gives off the most heat

Blood vessels near the body surface become narrower, so that less blood flows through them, giving off less heat—which makes the skin paler

Thick, snug-fitting clothing keeps warm air next to the body and prevents air blowing past and carrying heat away

Gloves prevent heat loss from the hands and fingers, where the body is coolest

Muscles contract and relax in small, quick movements, and as they do this they generate heat—this is called shivering

Sweat glands close down and release hardly any sweat

EXPERIMENT

What's warmest?

Adult help is advised for this experiment

The temperature of the brain, heart, and other vital organs is 98.6°F (37°C). But blood cools as it flows to the extremities, like the fingers and toes. So one part of the body frequently has a different temperature from another. Measure the differences with a thermometer. *Caution: If the thermometer cracks, do not touch it. Get help from an adult.*

You Will Need

- *thermometer*
- *cotton balls*

1 Shake the thermometer so the silver mercury goes into the bulb. Place the thermometer against your finger ends, and hold it in place with cotton for 2 minutes. Read off the temperature shown by the mercury thread.

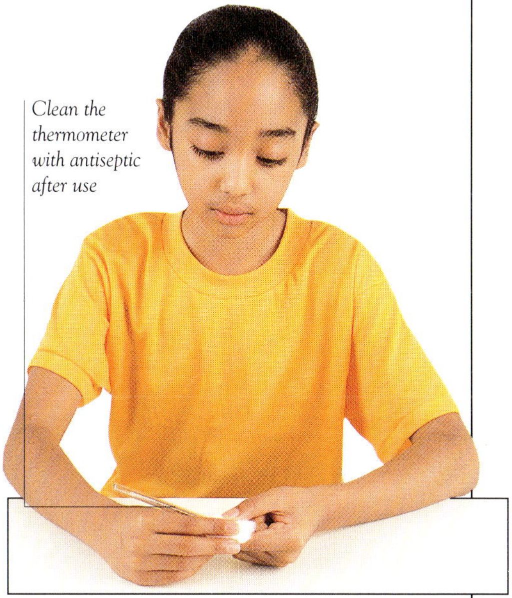

Clean the thermometer with antiseptic after use

2 Shake the thermometer again. Take temperatures in the crook of your elbow, behind your knee, between your toes, and elsewhere on your body. Where is it warmest, and where coolest?

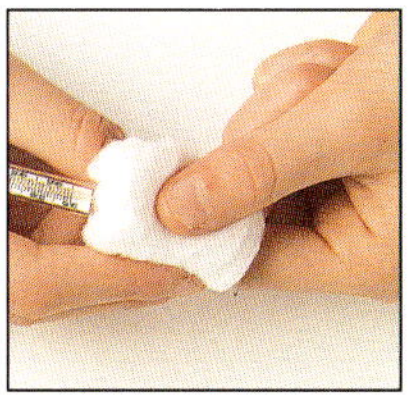

Thermometer use
Hold the bulb in cotton so that heat from the fingers holding the thermometer does not affect the results.

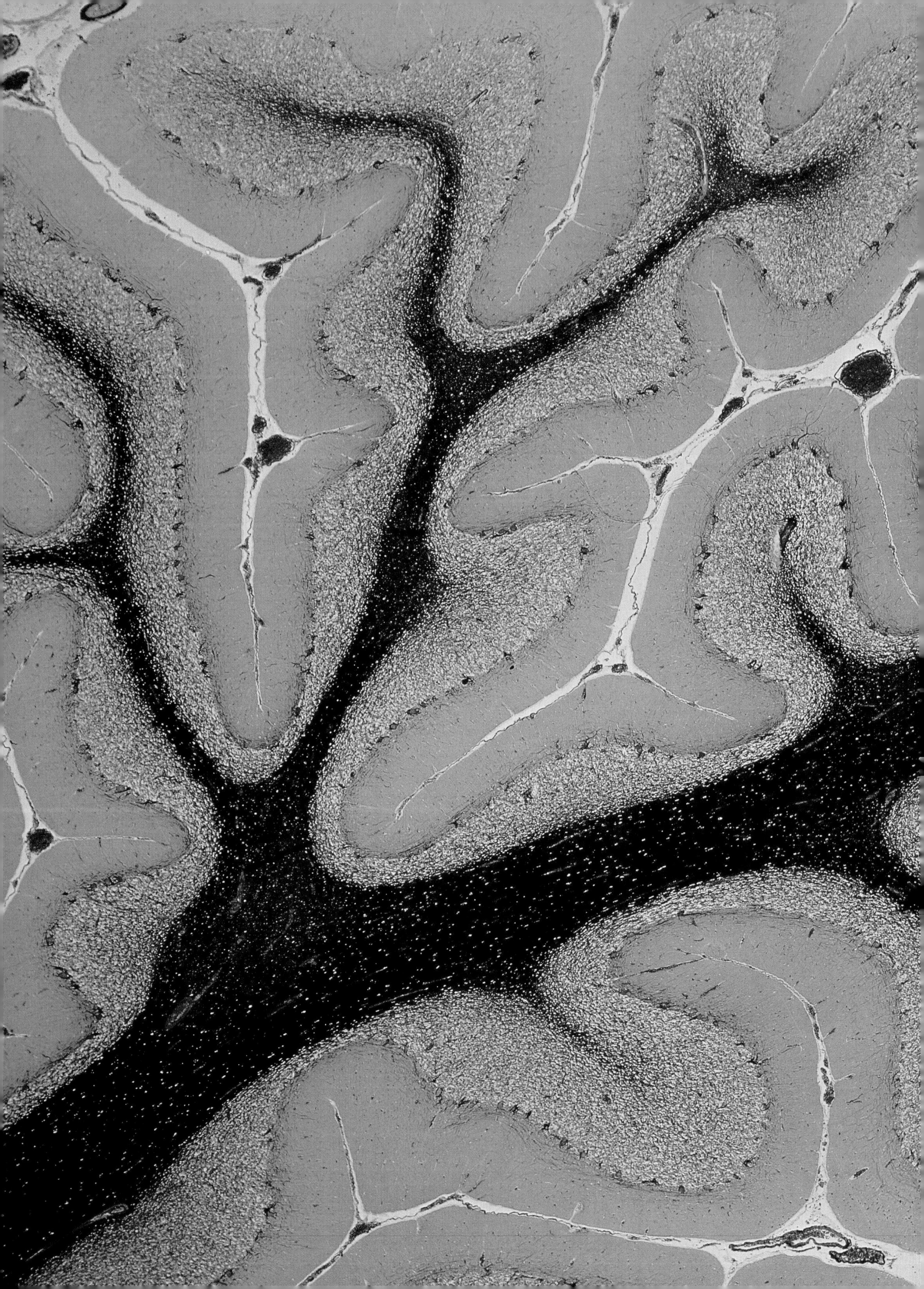

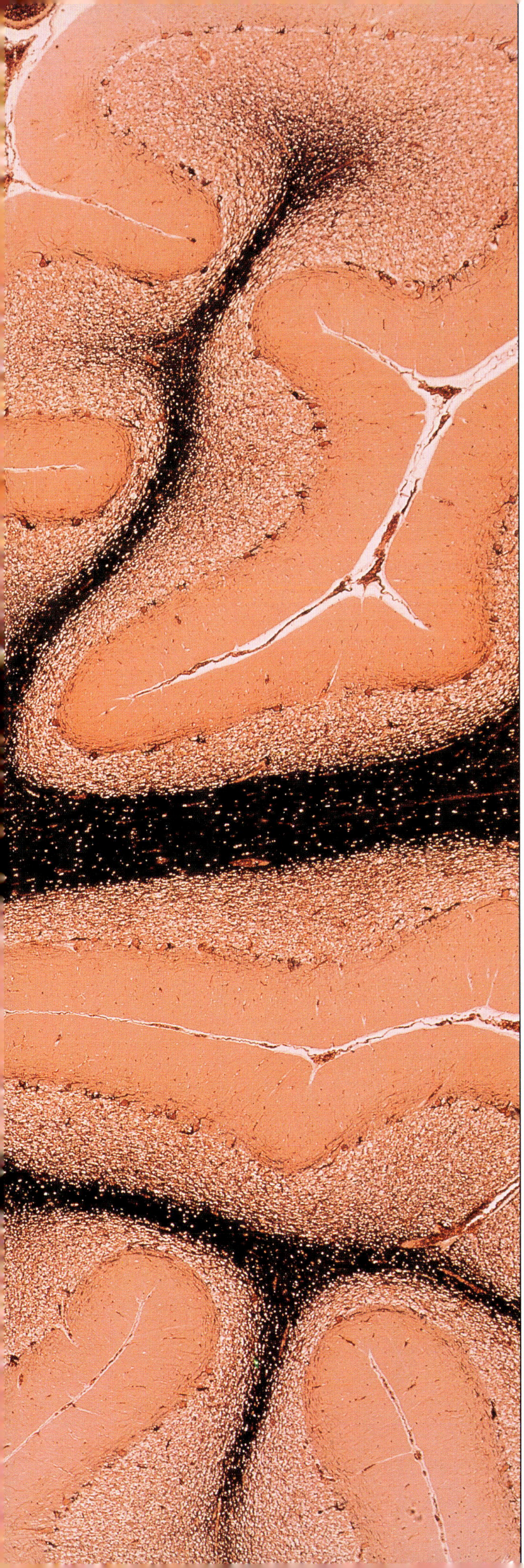

The CONTROL NETWORK

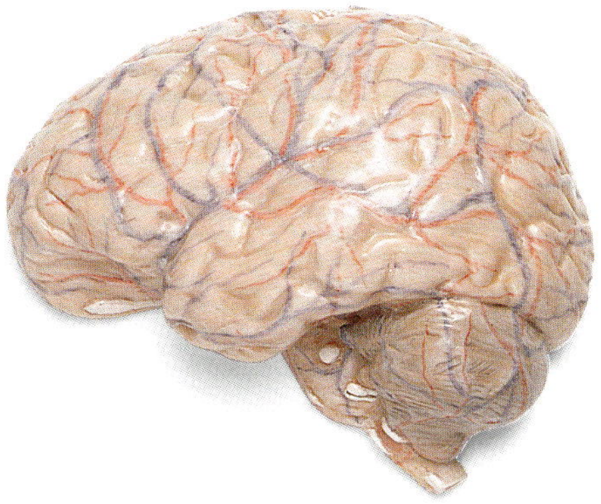

The ultimate bio-computer
Gray and wrinkled, and the same weight as a large grapefruit, the human brain (above) is the control center for all body functions. The smaller, darker part on the lower left is the cerebellum (its interior is shown close up at left). It coordinates nerve signals for complicated body movements.

THE VAST, COMPLEX MAZE of nerves that makes up the human brain controls all body processes—both conscious and autonomic (automatic). The brain receives information from the sense organs and other body parts in the form of tiny electrical nerve signals. And it sends out information in the same form. The outgoing information controls muscle movements and body functions. The brain is responsible for your intelligence, creativity, memories, perceptions, reactions, and emotions.

THE BRAIN AND NERVES

SCIENTISTS HAVE LEARNED AN ENORMOUS AMOUNT about the workings of the human body. But many mysteries remain about the part that allows us to gather this knowledge, the powerful brain. The brain has a huge number of jobs. Its automatic functions include the control of heartbeat, digestion, and dozens of other body processes that happen every minute. Its conscious functions (those you are aware of) are as varied as catching a ball, recalling a memory, and creating a work of art.

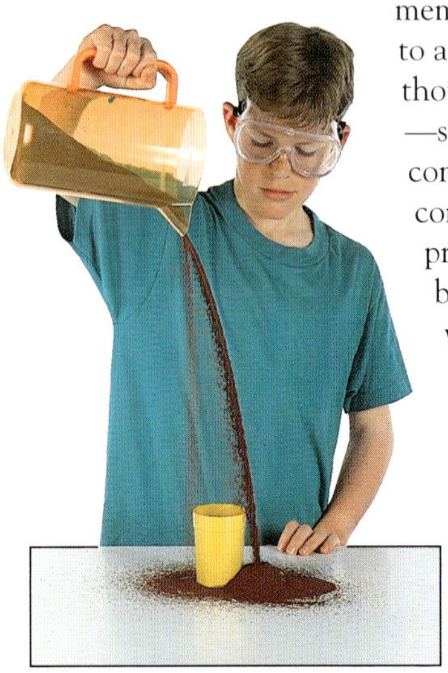

You may have forgotten how you learned simple actions such as pouring from a pitcher. "Relive" the experience of learning by trying to pour a different substance from a different height (p.133).

The brain is the center of all mental processes, from a fleeting memory of a face or smell, to a task that requires great thought and concentration —such as working out a complex puzzle. You are conscious (aware) of these processes. However, your brain does much more, without your realizing it. It controls your body functions such as the heartbeat, breathing, and digestion. It monitors the concentrations of substances such as glucose and carbon dioxide in blood, adjusts water and nutrient levels, and brings on feelings of hunger and thirst when supplies of food or fluids run low. Your brain also screens the gigantic amounts of information that are gathered continuously by your senses and filters out all but the most important features. If the brain did not do this, your attention would be overwhelmed.

Our knowledge of the brain is less complete than our knowledge of most other organs. This is partly due to the astonishingly complicated microstructure of this organ. At the microscopic level the brain is incredibly active. It weighs only one-fiftieth of the weight of the body, yet it is so chemically active that it uses up to one-fifth of the body's glucose-sugar energy supply.

Ancient views

In ancient times, many people thought the heart was the center of all the emotions. The brain was not considered important. When the ancient Egyptians preserved a body as a mummy, the heart and certain other organs were carefully put in their own containers. But the brain was pulled out in pieces through the nose and thrown away.

The Greek philosopher Alcmaeon of Croton (born c.500 B.C.) held that the brain, not the heart, was the seat of the senses and the center of intellect. The great philosopher Plato (428–347 B.C.) agreed. But Plato's pupil Aristotle (384–322 B.C.) returned to the view of the heart as the home of thoughts and emotions.

Galen's ideas

Galen (p.13) of ancient Rome believed that the spinal cord, protected by the vertebrae (back bones), was an extension of the brain. He proposed that, through the spinal cord and its branching network of nerves, the brain was "plumbed in" to all parts of the body, especially to the muscles and the sense organs.

Galen suggested that a mysterious fluid substance, "animal spirit," formed in chambers known as ventricles inside the brain, and that it flowed along the nerves to muscles, making the muscles contract (p.57). This theory of brain and nerve function was incorrect, although it was not challenged for more than 1,500 years. It is true that the brain has

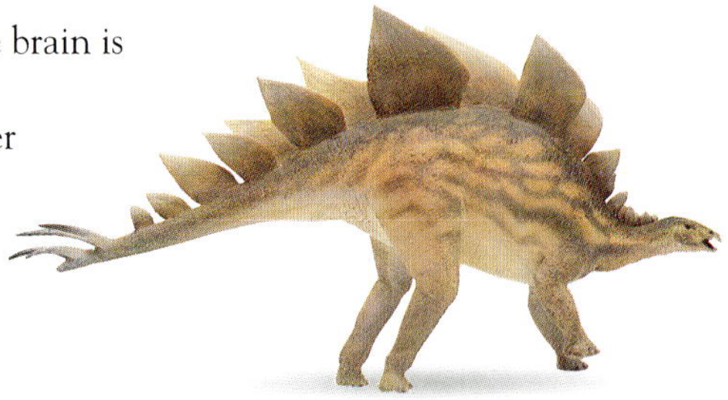

The dinosaur* Stegosaurus *had a tiny brain. But *this was sufficient for its lifestyle of roaming wooded plains. The species survived for millions of years.*

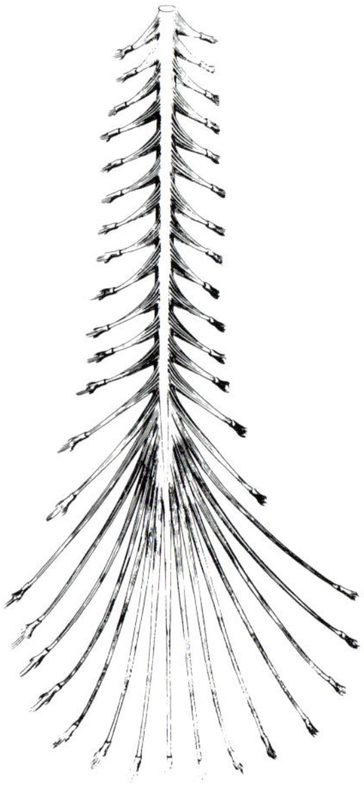

The spinal cord (p.119) inside the *vertebrae (back bones) is the body's main nerve. Its branches extend throughout the trunk (torso) and limbs.*

ventricles, and that the ventricles contain a fluid, called cerebrospinal fluid. But the main role of this fluid is to carry nourishment to the nerve tissues and to collect their wastes.

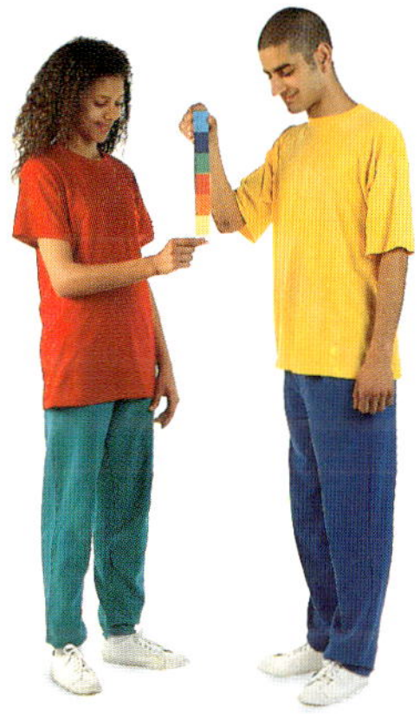

Test your reactions by *making a "react-o-ruler." When you react, nerve signals pass from the senses to the brain and then to the muscles (p.122).*

Nerve cells

With the invention of the microscope in the early 1600's, the brain and nerves were found to be packed with huge numbers of nerve cells, also called neurons (p.119).

By chance, research into nerve cells led to the invention of the electrical battery by the Italian professor Alessandro Volta (1745–1827). Volta's work was inspired by an argument with another Italian scientist, Luigi Galvani (1737–98), about the nature of electricity. Galvani believed that animals produced electricity, whereas Volta was convinced that electricity came from contact between metals and other chemicals. In an experiment, Galvani made a frog's leg twitch by touching it with a metal knife. However, he misinterpreted the result. The leg had not twitched by "animal electricity" generated by the frog. It did so because the contact between the metal and the chemicals in the cells of the nerves and muscles had made a simple battery.

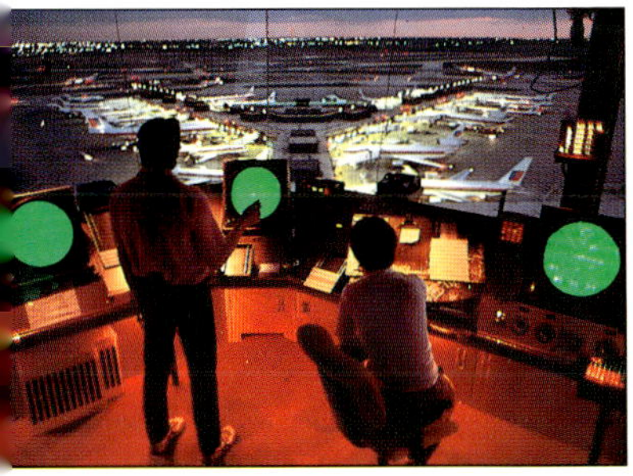

The term "nerve center" refers to the *control center of a complex communications system, such as this air traffic control room in an airport. There are also different nerve centers in the brain that receive messages from each of the senses.*

Volta did further experiments with metals and chemicals, and by 1800 he had produced the first intentional battery. Yet Galvani's theory was correct in a sense – the body does produce electricity in the form of signals to and from the brain along nerve cells, and as electrical "ripples" in heart muscle and other muscles.

Brain parts

The brain has three main structural parts (pp.126–127). These are the cerebellum, the cerebrum, and the brain stem.

The cerebellum mainly coordinates complex muscle movements, from pouring a drink to flying a helicopter.

The cerebrum is responsible for complex thoughts. In humans it is very highly developed. The cerebrum has two wrinkled halves, the cerebral hemispheres. Each of these is divided into five lobes, mostly named from the curved bones of the skull around them. The prefrontal lobes are positioned over the eyes, the frontal lobes below the top of the forehead, the parietal lobes on the top, the temporal lobes on the sides, and the occipital lobes at the lower rear.

The thin surface layer of the hemispheres is known as the cortex. It looks much the same all over, but different areas are specialized for different functions. A wide strip of cortex, running from ear to ear over the top of the brain, receives signals from the skin about touch, pressure, and pain. This strip is called the somatosensory cortex and is the brain's "touch center." Similarly, there are nerve centers for sight, hearing, smell, and taste, and for body movements. These centers are not always related to any particular lobe or any combination of lobes.

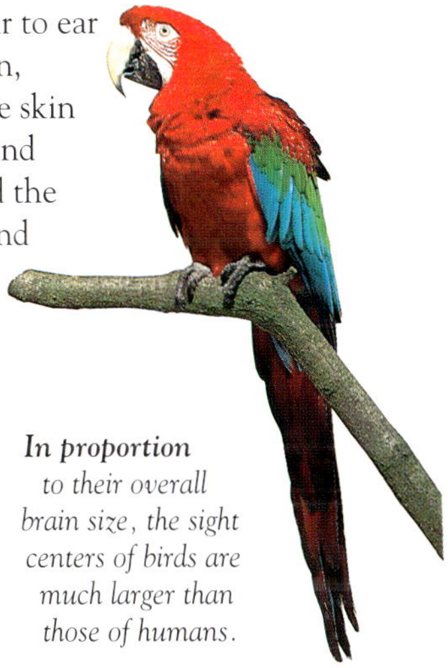

In proportion *to their overall brain size, the sight centers of birds are much larger than those of humans.*

Some parts of the cortex are called nonspecific areas. Scientists have not yet worked out what their purpose is. For instance, the aspects of behavior that we call "personality" seem to be based in the prefrontal and frontal lobes, but they do not seem to have any identifiable center.

The third main structural part of the brain, the brain stem, is concerned mainly with the vital life processes that take place automatically in the body. The brain stem consists of several parts. The hypothalamus, which sits deep in the center of the brain, is a center for homeostasis (p.104). The heartbeat, breathing, and blood pressure are centered in the medulla, the lowest part of the brain stem, which merges into the spinal cord. The point where nerve fibers from the body come together to cross into the upper parts of the brain is the pons.

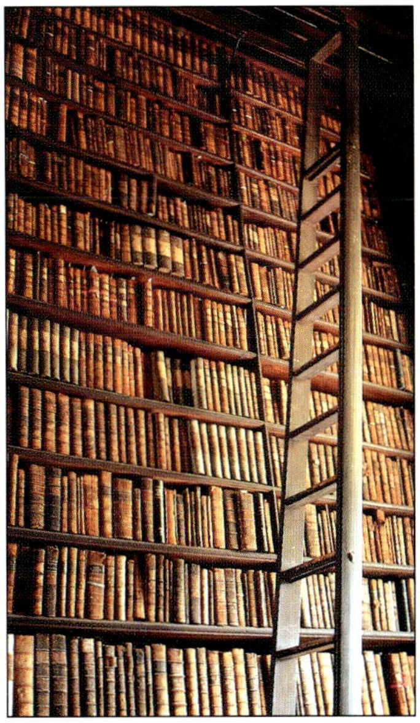

The brain's information store *is as great as that of a library. Scientist believe that in the brain information is organized into various types of memory (p.128).*

The nervous system

LIKE THE circulatory system, the nervous system has branches all over the body. Its nerves divide many times. The thickest nerves look like pieces of cream-colored rope, and the thinnest are narrower than a hair. Nerves are made of bundles of nerve cells (opposite). These cells are specially designed to carry tiny electrical messages. Some nerve cells are called sensory cells. They carry signals from the sense organs, such as the eyes and ears, to the brain, where they are analyzed. Other nerve cells are called motor cells. They carry nerve signals from the brain and spinal cord to the muscles, telling them when to contract and when to relax. Many nerves contain both sensory and motor nerve cells.

■ DISCOVERY ■

René Descartes

The French scientist René Descartes (1596–1650) was a brilliant mathematician and an important philosopher. He believed that there was a connection between the body and the soul (the human spirit) and proposed that a small part of the brain, the pineal gland, linked the two. This idea was incorrect, but another idea Descartes had—that reflex actions (p.120) happen automatically and that they are controlled by nerves—was accurate. He understood that a reflex is caused by signals from a sensory nerve, which travel to the spinal cord and then to a motor nerve, often without entering the brain.

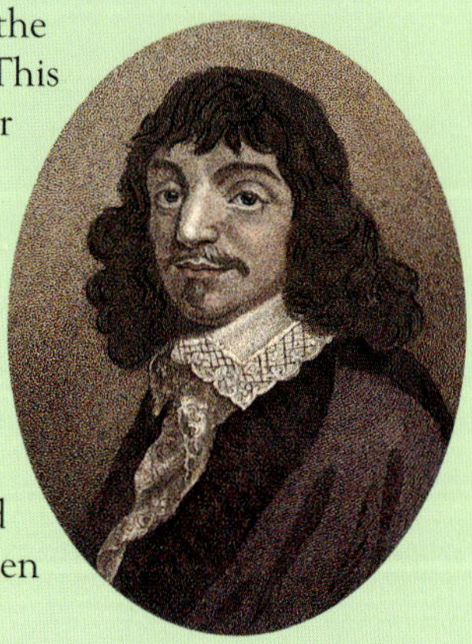

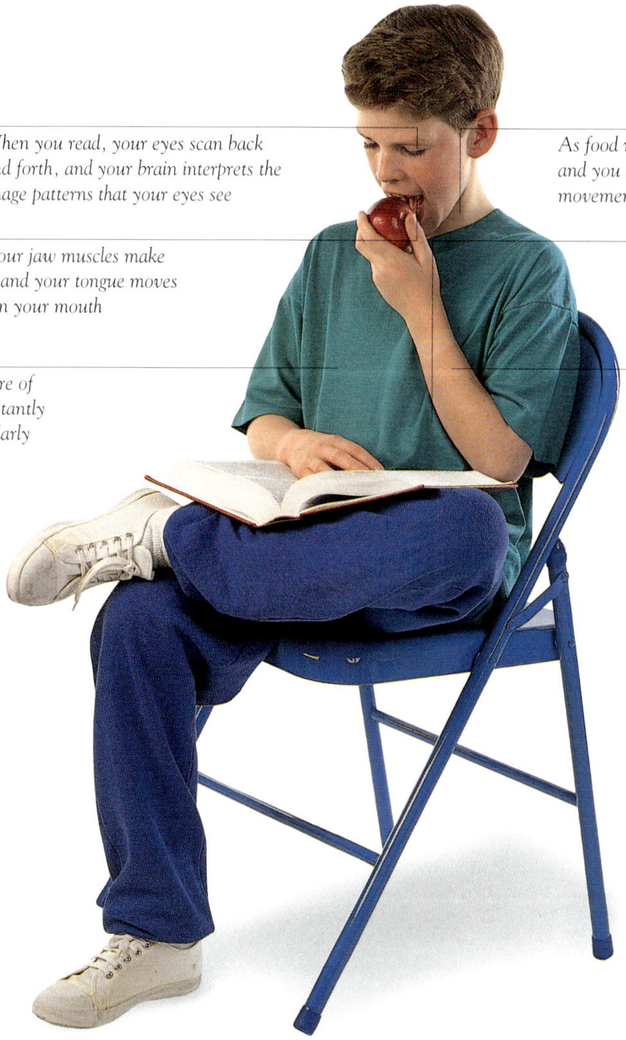

Voluntary actions

When you read, your eyes scan back and forth, and your brain interprets the image patterns that your eyes see

When you eat, your jaw muscles make your teeth chew, and your tongue moves the food around in your mouth

As you sit, you may not be aware of your body posture, but you constantly keep your balance and you regularly change position to rest muscles

Part of the nervous system is voluntary. In other words, the movements and actions that these nerves are responsible for—such as reading, walking, chewing, or sitting upright in a chair—are under your conscious control. You are aware of them, and you can stop or start them at will. Most voluntary actions originate in the cortex (p.127). These actions are controlled by nerves that send signals to the body's skeletal muscles (p.59).

Autonomic actions

As food reaches the back of your throat and you swallow, automatic muscle movements take over

When you digest, your stomach mashes the food you have eaten and muscles in your intestinal walls push it along

Muscles in the walls of the arteries make them wider or narrower to direct blood where it is needed

Part of the nervous system is autonomic, which means that it controls itself. Muscles in body parts such as the arteries, stomach, and intestines work without you thinking about them. You are usually unaware that they are working, and you cannot stop or start them at will. These muscles are under the control of parts of the brain stem (p.126). Autonomic actions are controlled by nerves that send signals to the body's smooth muscles (p.59).

Brain and main nerves

The main nerves of the body branch out and reach every nook and cranny. This system has two main sections. The brain and the spinal cord are together known as the central nervous system. The rest of the nerves, which spread out through the body, are called the peripheral nervous system. The peripheral nerves communicate with the brain via the spinal cord. There are also 12 pairs of nerves, called cranial nerves, that join the brain directly to important parts of the head. These include the cochlear nerves from the ears (p.152) and optic nerves from the eyes (p.139).

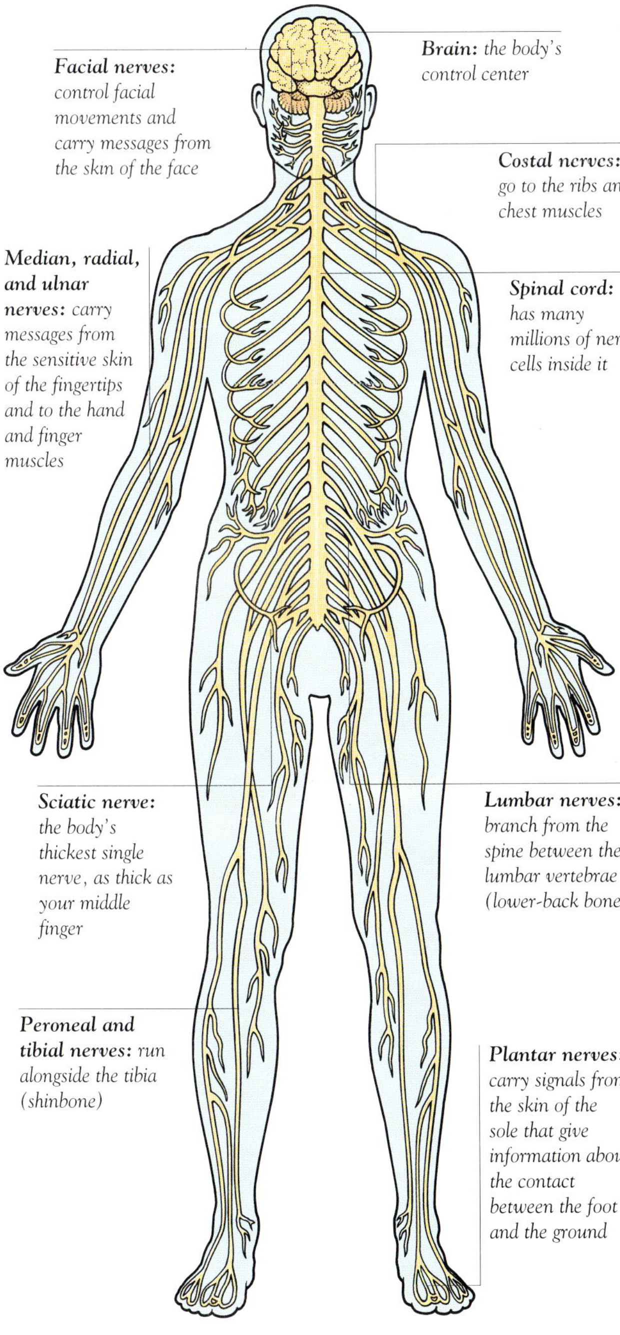

Nerve cells

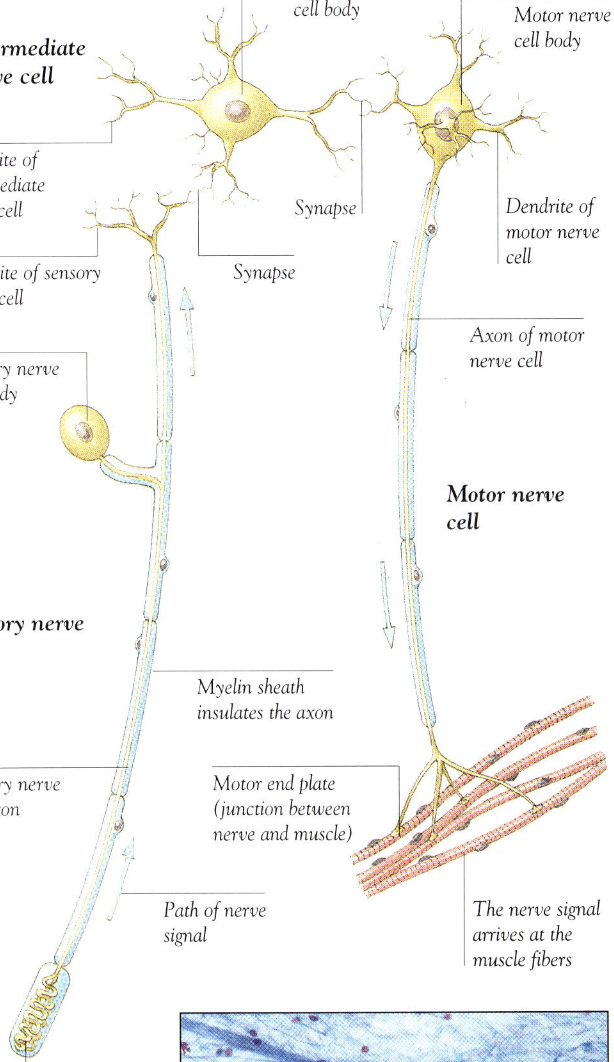

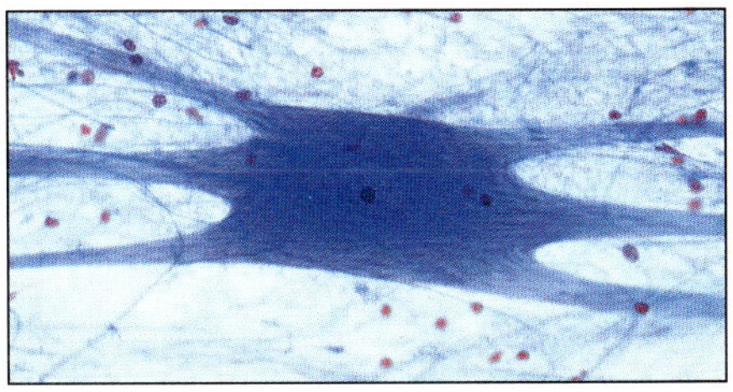

One nerve cell
This is a single nerve cell, seen through a light microscope. The dark blue patch in the middle is the cell body. Three thin dendrites stretch out from either side of the cell body.

The nervous system consists of billions of linked nerve cells (neurons). Each nerve cell has a body (main part), fingerlike dendrites, and a long, wirelike axon. These three elements can be arranged in various ways. Dendrite tips almost touch other dendrites at junctions called synapses. Dendrites pick up nerve signals and send them along the axon to the next nerve cells. In this illustration a nerve signal from a touch sensor in the skin travels along a sensory nerve cell to an intermediate nerve cell, then to a motor nerve cell, which passes it to a muscle.

Reflexes

HAVE YOU EVER been startled by a loud noise that made you jump before you could stop yourself? This is an example of a reflex—an automatic reaction that happens incredibly fast, before you even have time to think about it. A reflex occurs by itself, even if your attention is elsewhere. This is because a reflex is programmed and predictable—you do not have to use your brain to decide what action to take. In a reflex, nerve signals (p.118) are produced by a sense organ, such as the eye or ear, that detects the stimulus (something that provokes action). They go to the spinal cord or the brain, then to the muscles around the body that move in response. Most reflexes are quick responses to possible danger or harm to the body, such as jerking your finger away if it touches something hot.

A bundle of reflexes

Babies cannot control many of their movements, and they cannot feed or clean themselves. But they are far from helpless, as they do many things automatically. A baby is a "bundle of reflexes," several of which are important for basic survival. As you grow, you learn to control or override some of these reflexes. Other types of reflex fade away.

The Moro reflex happens if the baby suddenly falls back or is startled. The baby throws out his or her arms and legs, as if to catch hold of something

Bowel and bladder reflexes expel the contents of these organs automatically when they are full. A child eventually learns to control these actions

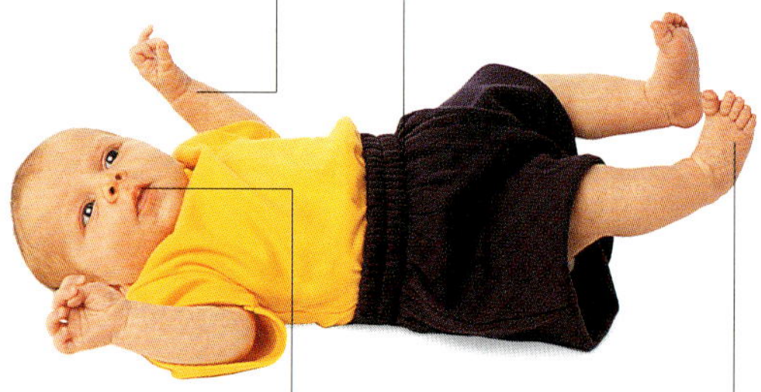

The rooting reflex helps feeding. If touched on the cheek, the baby turns to that side and moves his or her mouth to find the mother's breast or bottle

The stepping reflex happens only in the first few days. If the baby's feet touch a firm surface, he or she makes stepping movements

On the alert

In the animal world there are many possible dangers, such as being attacked by a predator. An animal's senses are tuned to the slightest sound, scent, or movement. Even while feeding or resting, the senses monitor the surroundings. If anything startles the animal, its reflexes are called into action and it is ready to respond at once.

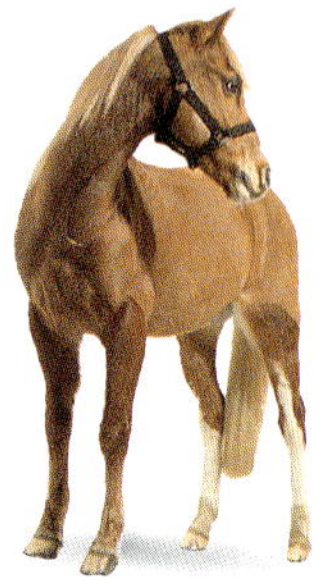

What's that noise?
Even tamed animals such as horses are wary. Hearing a strange sound behind, the horse automatically looks around.

EXPERIMENT

Blinking reflex

See how a sudden loud noise near the face causes the eyelids to close automatically to protect the eyes.

Loud claps
Clap your hands loudly 6 in (15 cm) in front of a friend's face. (No closer, to prevent accidents!) See how your friend blinks immediately. Can your friend override this reflex with practice?

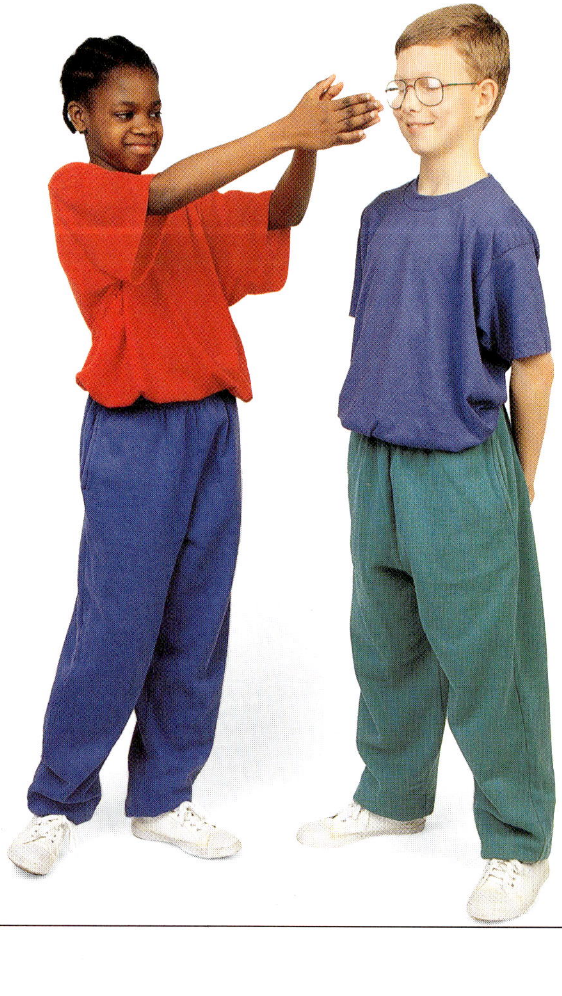

EXPERIMENT

The knee-jerk reflex

Testing the body's reflexes can give a physician useful information about how nerves and muscles work. One simple test is the knee-jerk reflex (below). When your knee is tapped, nerve signals travel from stretch sensors in the knee to the spinal cord and then back to the leg muscles. Meanwhile, other signals travel up the spinal cord to the touch centers of the brain (p.117). As a result, you become aware of your leg's response, but usually too late to stop it from happening.

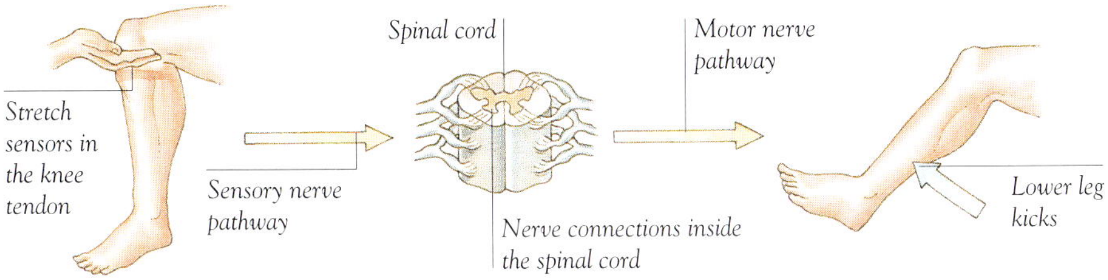

Stimulus
A tap just below your kneecap stretches the tendon (p.185) there. Stretch sensors in the tendon send out nerve signals.

In and out
The signals pass along sensory nerves to your spinal cord. This sends signals back at once along motor nerves.

Response
The signals travel to the muscles in the front of your thigh. These contract and jerk the lower leg upward.

1 SIT IN A CHAIR. Cross your legs so the lower knee fits snugly into the hollow at the rear of the upper knee. Ask a friend to tap your upper knee firmly—on the soft part just below the kneecap—with the edge of his or her open hand.

2 WHAT HAPPENS? Does your lower leg twitch? You may need practice to find the right site. Can you use willpower to stop your knee from jerking?

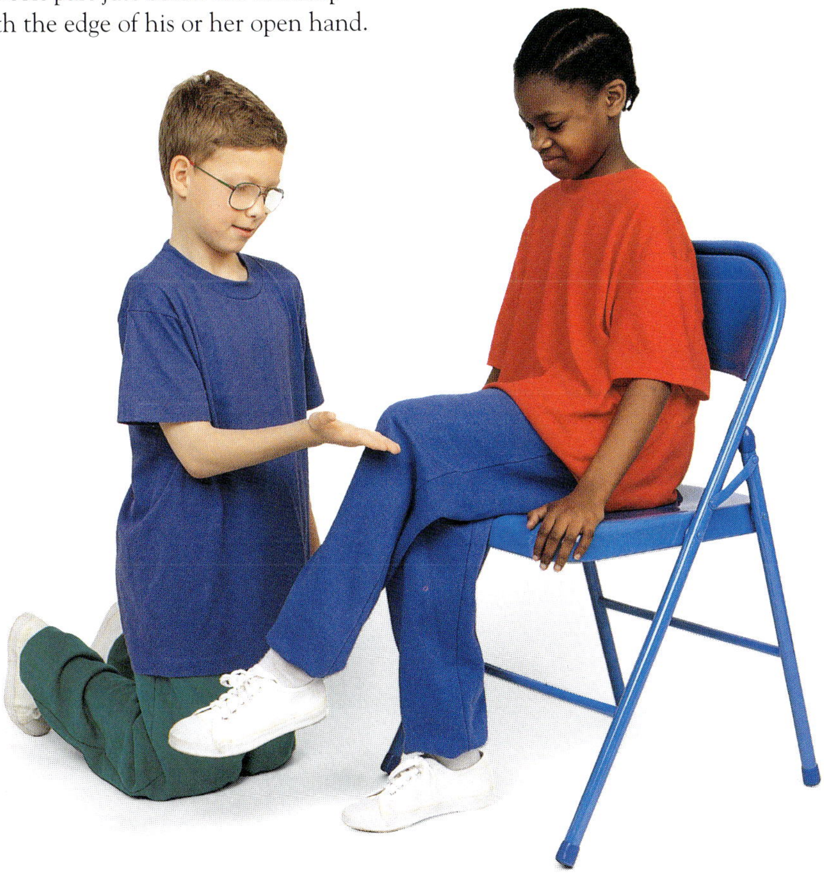

Protecting eyes and face

If an object comes toward your head, you may respond with a sequence of actions, almost without thinking. These actions protect your eyes and other parts of your face in the event of possible danger. The pupils of the eyes also have reflexes that respond to the varying brightness of light (p.141).

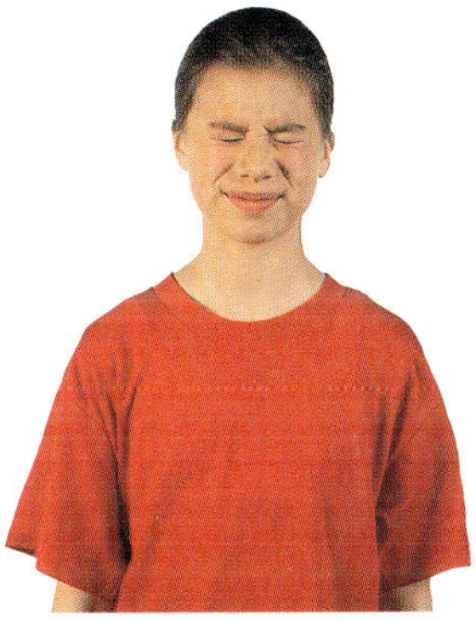

Eyes close
Your eyelids come together and facial muscles contract to tense and toughen your skin.

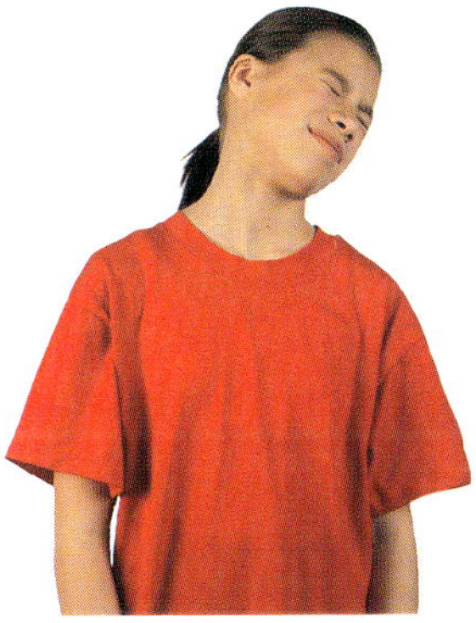

Head jerks
Your neck muscles twist the head back and to the side, so that your face is out of direct line.

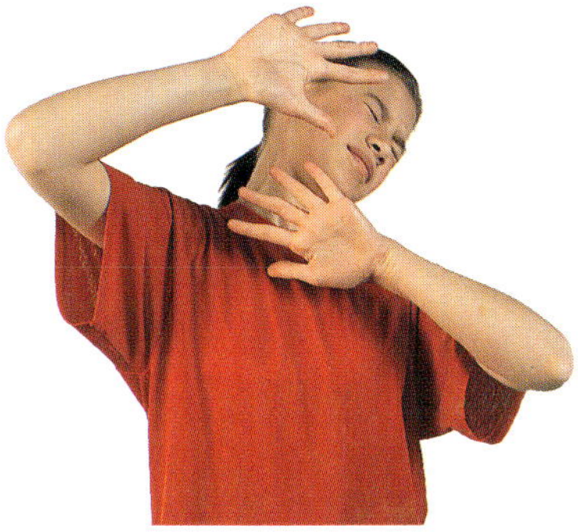

Arms rise
Your shoulder and arm muscles lift your arms and hands in front of your face as a shield.

Reactions

HUNDREDS OF TIMES a day we react to the world around us. When asked a difficult question, we may have plenty of time to think about the answer. At other times, fast reactions are vital, especially in dangerous situations such as driving. At 55 mph (90 kph) on the highway, if an obstruction appears 165 ft (50 m) ahead, a driver has less than 2 seconds to see it, assess the situation, plan what to do, and take action. Each reaction in the body follows the same basic process. A sensory part, such as the eyes, ears, or skin, detects a stimulus. It flashes nerve signals along sensory nerves (pp.118–119) to your brain, at speeds of up to 330 ft (100 m) per second. Your brain becomes aware of the situation, makes a decision, and then sends signals out along motor nerves to your muscles, telling them how to respond.

EXPERIMENT

Reaction time

In this experiment you find out the amount of time it takes to react to a stimulus. Here, the stimulus is feeling your right hand being squeezed. The reaction you must make is to squeeze the hand of a friend on your left. The time between these two actions is your reaction time. Six to ten of your friends must stand in a circle, hands linked. One is the starter. Another has the stopwatch and is the timer.

YOU WILL NEED

- *stopwatch*

Split-second timing

Many sports depend on quick reactions. When a top-ranked tennis player hits a mighty serve, the ball travels at more than 100 mph (160 kph). The opponent has less than a third of a second to note the speed and direction of the ball, move into position, watch for the bounce and ball spin, and swing the racket for the return shot. The more someone practices such fast responses, the more quickly and smoothly the brain, nerves, and muscles can carry them out.

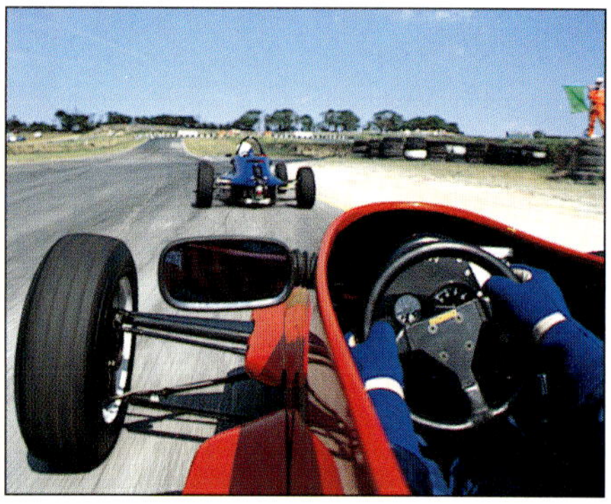

Life or death
Sports such as tennis are rarely a matter of life or death. But automobile racing is. At 200 mph (320 kph), a racing car travels almost 330 ft (100 m) per second. The driver's safety depends on reactions measured in hundredths of a second.

EXPERIMENT

The "react-o-ruler"

Adult help is advised for this experiment

An individual's reaction time is often too fast to measure without complicated equipment. But you and your friends can compare your reaction speeds using this ruler with a colored scale. The idea is to catch the ruler as soon as possible after it starts to fall between your fingers. Record the results. Do you get quicker at first, but then reach a time (color) that you cannot improve?

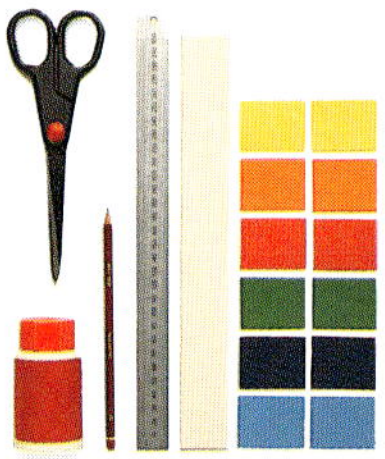

YOU WILL NEED

- *scissors* • *glue* • *pencil* • *ruler* • *12 in x 1 in (30 cm x 2.5 cm) poster board* • *6 pairs of pieces of colored paper 2 in x 1 in (5 cm x 2.5 cm)*

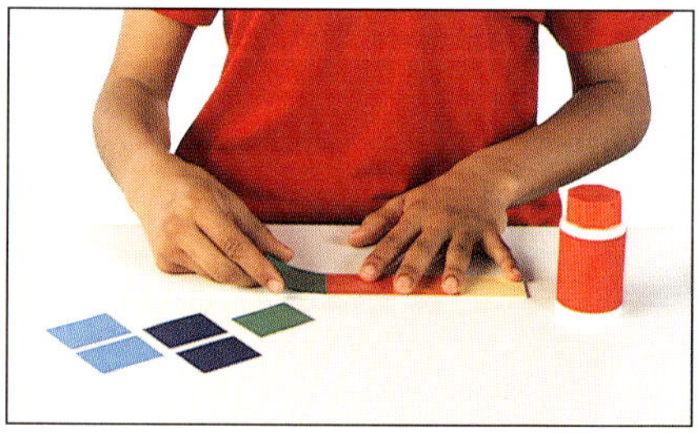

1 STICK SIX of the same-size pieces of colored paper along one side of the poster board. Repeat on the other side, keeping the same color sequence. This is the "react-o-ruler."

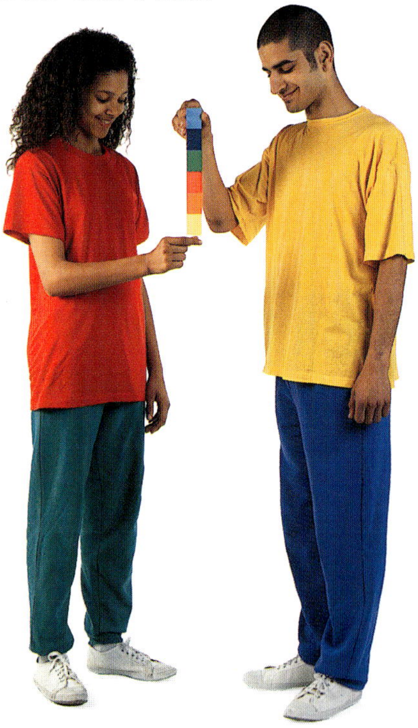

2 GET A FRIEND to hold the react-o-ruler by the upper tip. Place your thumb and forefinger 1 in (2.5 cm) below the ruler, so that it will fall between them. With no warning, your friend lets go of the ruler. You try to catch it by closing your thumb and forefinger as fast as you can. Where are you holding it? The nearer the bottom of the ruler, the quicker your reaction.

Squeezing hands

The starter shouts "Go" and at exactly the same time squeezes the hand on his or her left. As soon as this friend feels the squeeze, he or she squeezes the next person's hand, and so on around the circle. When the starter feels his or her right hand being squeezed, he or she shouts "Stop." Meanwhile the timer starts the watch on "Go" and stops it on "Stop" to get the combined time for all the reactions. To find out the average reaction time of your friends, divide this combined time by the number of friends in the circle. Do your reaction times get faster if you go around the circle twice, or five times? (Do not forget to divide the final time by the total number of hand squeezes.) How much can you improve the times with practice?

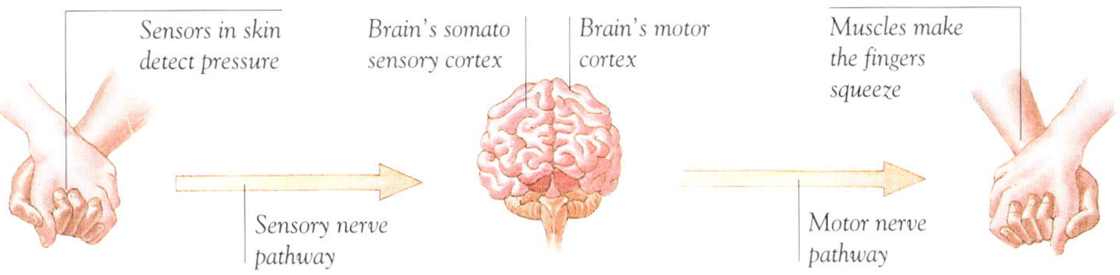

Stimulus

When your right hand is squeezed by the person on your right, your skin sensors detect the increase in pressure. They send signals along sensory nerves, through your wrist, and up your arm and shoulder.

In and out

The sensory nerve signals pass into your spinal cord, then travel up to the somato sensory cortex (p.127) of your brain. It is at this point that you realize that your hand has been squeezed, and you decide to respond.

Response

Signals pass from your brain's motor cortex (p.127), down through your spinal cord, and along motor nerves to the muscles in your hand. The muscles contract and squeeze the hand of the next person in the circle.

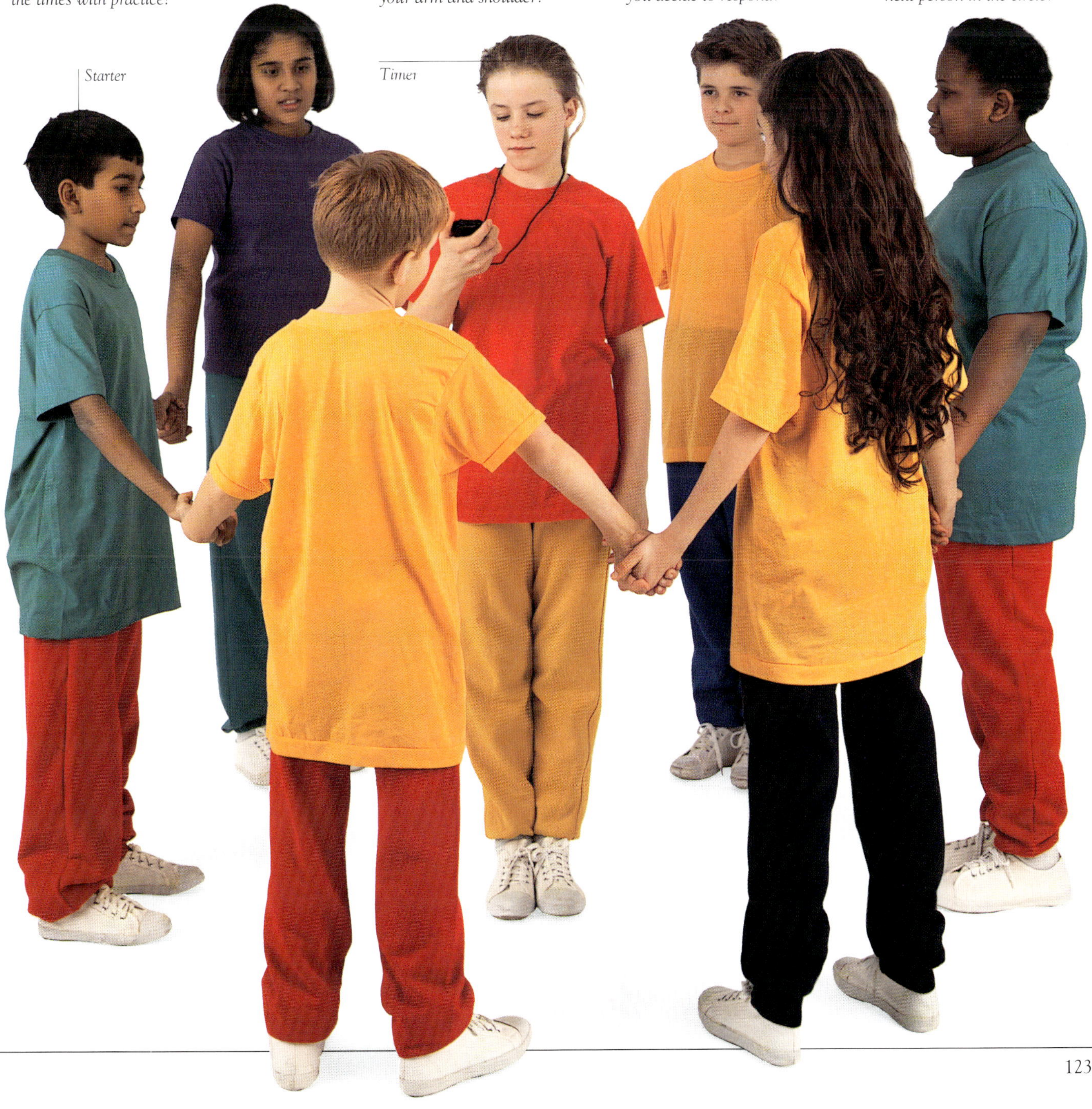

Reactions and decisions

IN A SIMPLE reaction situation, like the "Reaction time" experiment (p.122), only one response is required. But what if you have to decide between two or more responses? Your brain needs a split second to think about them and make a choice before you act. The more complex the choices, the longer the decision time. As with most reaction situations, you get faster with practice.

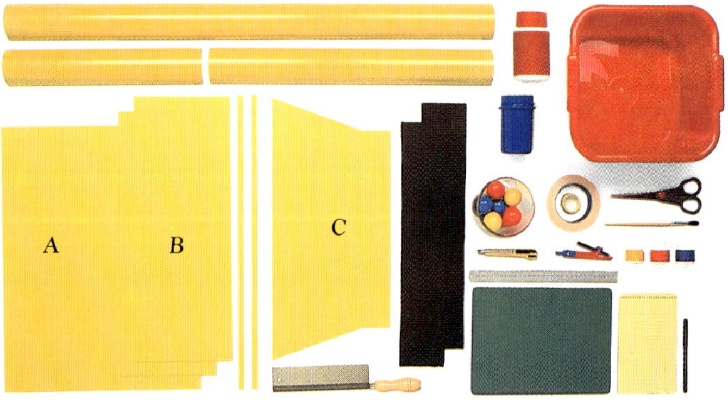

YOU WILL NEED

• for the chute, 3 lengths of plastic gutter (wider than a table-tennis ball), about 40, 24, and 16 in (100, 60, and 40 cm) long • stiff poster board—for the screen front **(A)**, *sheet 20 in x 16 in (50 cm x 40 cm); for the screen sides* **(B)**, *2 sheets 20 in x 8 in (50 cm x 20 cm); for the screen base, 1 piece about 20 in x 12 in (50 cm x 30 cm), shaped as* **C**; *2 thin strips 22 in (55 cm) long • strips of felt • tenon saw • plastic beaker • large bowl • about 12 table-tennis balls painted at least 3 different colors • plastic tape • notepad • metal ruler • pen • double-sided tape • scissors • paintbrush • nontoxic paints • craft knife • compass • cutting mat*

EXPERIMENT

Making decisions

Adult help is advised for this experiment

The amount of time that it takes you to react depends on how rapidly your brain assesses a situation and how many decisions you have to make. You and your friends can test your reaction times by seeing whether you can catch balls as they roll out of a chute. (The chute is lined with felt, so the balls do not make a warning sound as they roll.) This experiment tests how quickly you can react—first, when you have no decision to make because you can catch any ball, and second, when you do have a decision to make, because you are allowed to catch only balls of a certain color. How much quicker can you get with practice? Do you improve as quickly when trying the second part of the experiment as you do when trying the first?

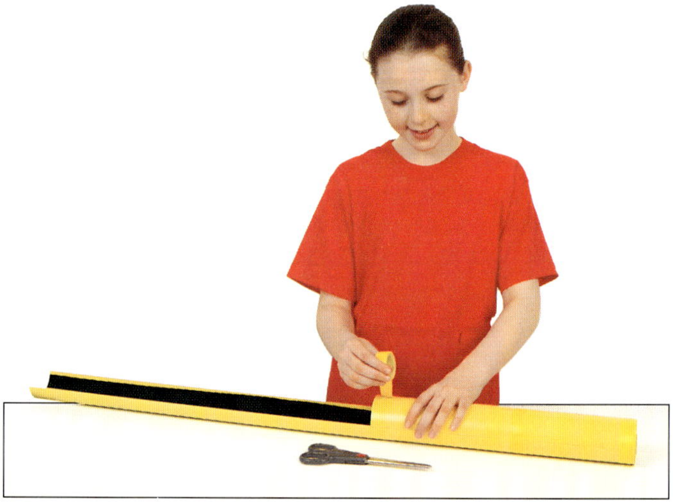

1 LINE THE longest piece of gutter with felt, stuck on with double-sided tape. Place the shortest length of gutter on one end to make a partial tube and attach it with plastic tape.

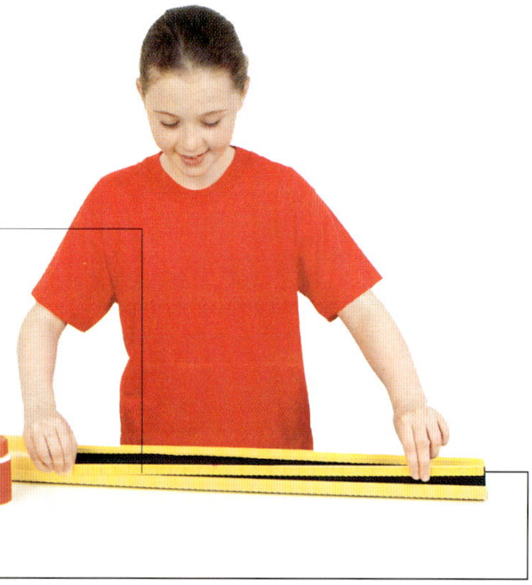

Number the marked intervals on the thin poster-board strips, and position these strips so that the measure starts at the end of the tube

2 DRAW MARKS at intervals of 1 in (2.5 cm) along both thin poster-board strips. Fix them to the outside edges of the exposed portion of the chute with double-sided tape.

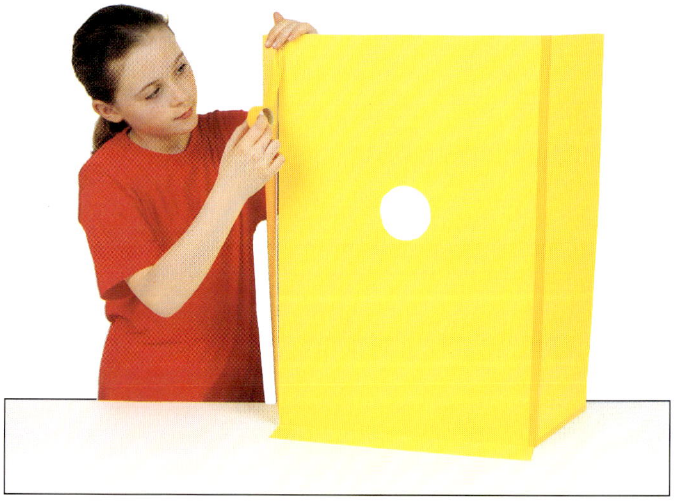

3 CAREFULLY CUT a hole in the screen front, 1 ft (30 cm) from the bottom. Make it slightly larger than the gutter. Tape together the sides, front, and base of the screen.

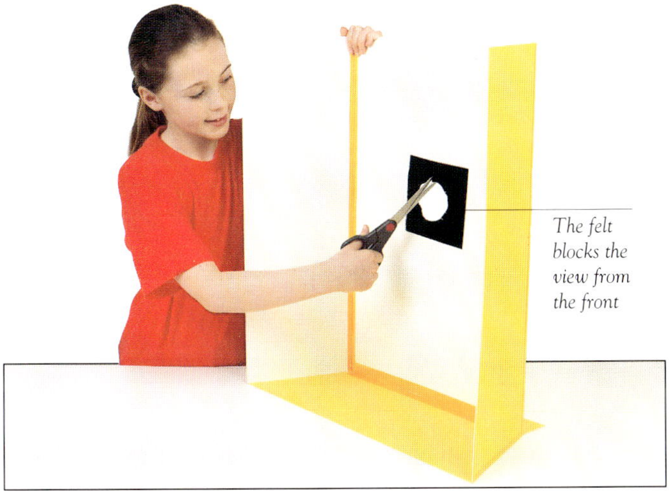

The felt blocks the view from the front

4 CAREFULLY CUT out a square of felt, and tape this behind the screen hole. Trim a hole in the felt, slightly smaller than the gutter. Snip slits into the felt to allow the gutter to be pushed through.

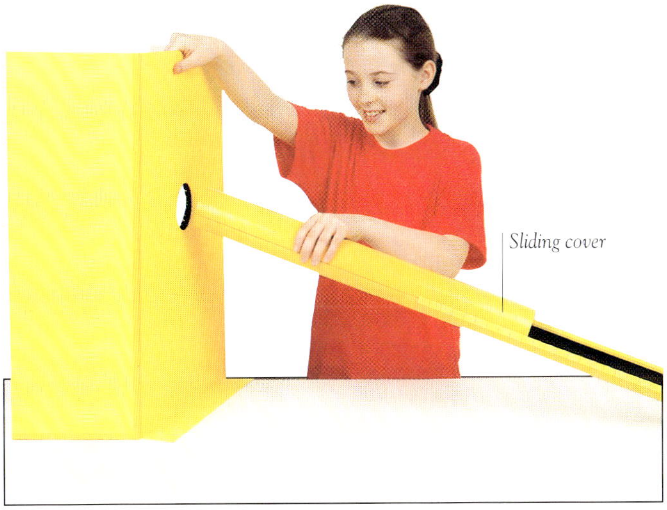

Sliding cover

5 LAY THE THIRD piece of gutter on top of the chute, so that it sits between the measuring strips. This makes a cover that you can slide up and down the chute. Push the chute just through the hole in the screen.

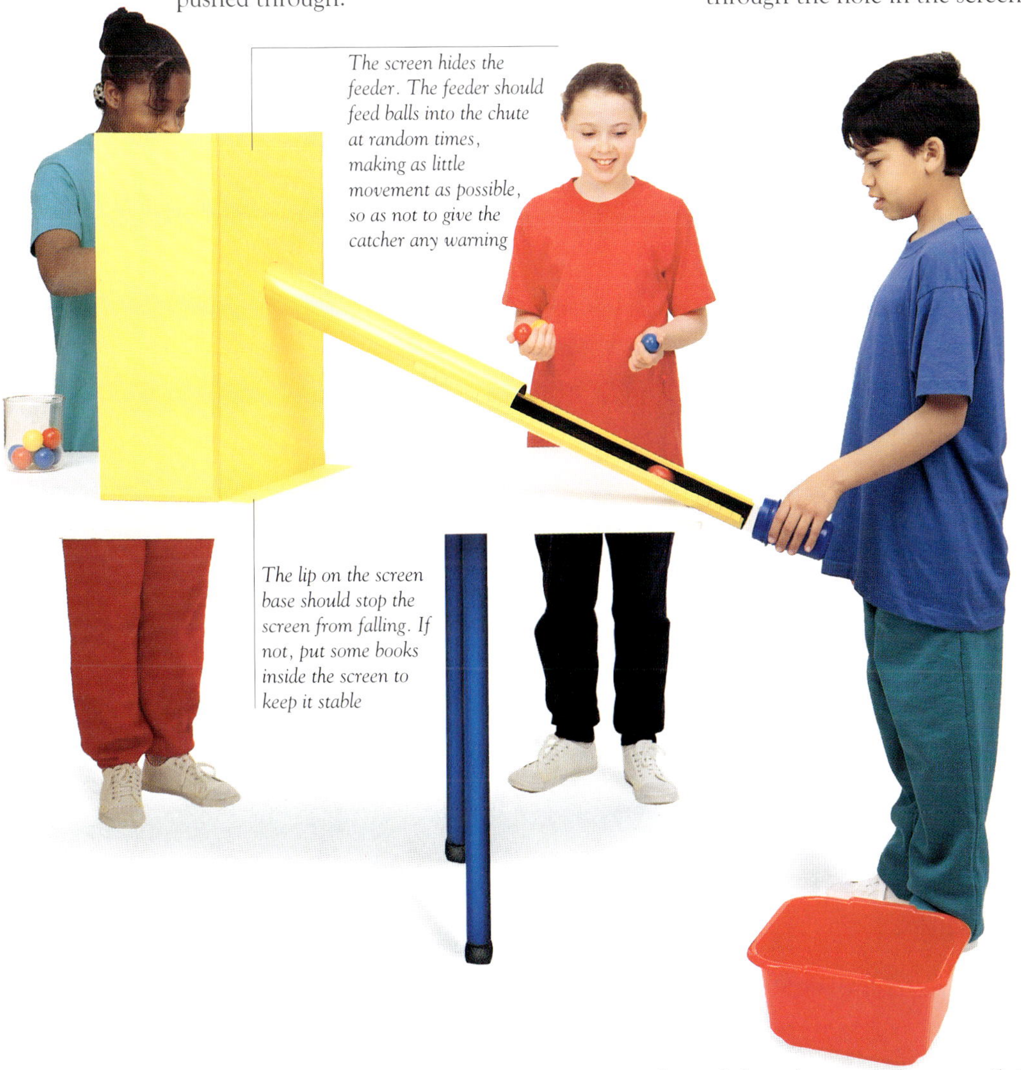

The screen hides the feeder. The feeder should feed balls into the chute at random times, making as little movement as possible, so as not to give the catcher any warning

The lip on the screen base should stop the screen from falling. If not, put some books inside the screen to keep it stable

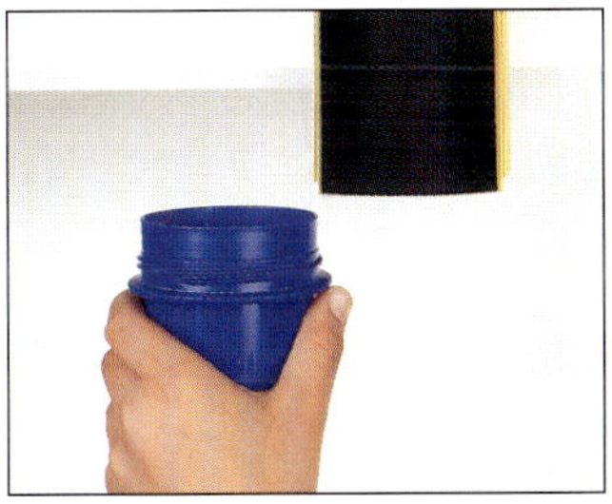

Holding the beaker

For this experiment it is best to place the whole assembly on a tabletop. The lower end of the chute should hang slightly over the table edge. The catcher holds the beaker just to the side of the chute end. After each attempt at a catch, the catcher should move the beaker back out of the way of the chute end. Use the large bowl to hold balls that the catcher misses.

6 SLIDE THE chute cover to expose the maximum amount of open chute. Get one person to feed balls down the chute and another person to try to catch each one in the beaker. Try several successive sets of 10 balls, scoring one for each ball. Does the catcher's score improve with each set? Move the chute cover down one mark on the scale and try again. Keep sliding the cover down until the catcher misses all 10 balls—the limit of her or his reaction time. In the second part of the experiment, the feeder continues to feed all of the balls, but this time the catcher catches only balls of a certain color. Is the reaction time the same as before? What happens if the catcher is allowed to catch balls of two out of three colors?

The brain

A COMPUTER ROOM full of printers, disk drives, and monitors would be still and silent without the central processor itself. Likewise, the body would be lifeless without the brain. The human brain has three main parts. The top part, making up nine-tenths of the brain's volume, is the wrinkled cerebrum. This is the thinking part of the brain. The back part of the brain is the cerebellum, a "mini brain" that deals mainly with balance, posture, and skilled movements. All of the other areas of the brain (including the pons, thalamus, medulla, and hypothalamus shown below) belong to a part of the brain called the brain stem. This joins with the spinal cord below it and the cerebrum above it.

■ DISCOVERY ■

Phineas Gage

For many years experts suspected that the front parts of the brain were involved in personality and the way we behave. In 1848 a discovery occurred by accident in the United States that supported these suspicions. Phineas Gage, the foreman of a road-building team, was injured when gunpowder went off accidentally. The explosion blew a metal rod up into his cheek, through the front part of his brain, and out the top of his skull. Amazingly, Gage survived for 12 years, but his character changed. Once even-tempered, he became prone to rages. His case showed that the frontal lobes of the brain are involved in personality (p.117).

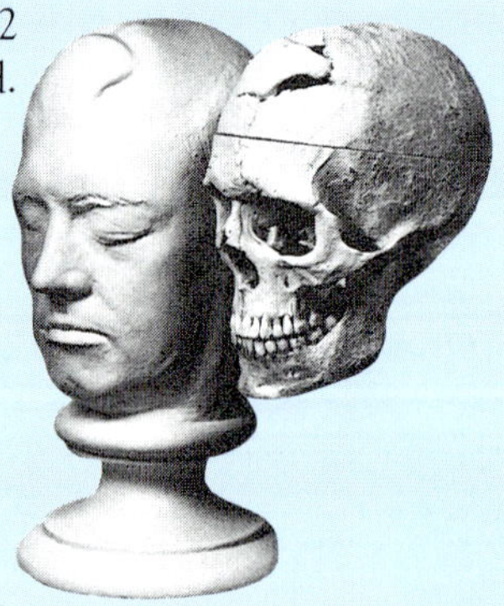

Hole in the head
This is the skull of Gage, beside a plaster cast of his head and face.

Inside the brain

This is a view through the middle of the brain, cut in half from front to back. Each of the two large wrinkled upper parts of the cerebrum is folded downward in the middle of the brain (as can be seen in the brain scan, right). Each of these parts is called a cerebral hemisphere. Some parts of the brain stem form emotions and feelings, some deal with memories (pp.128–129), and others carry out automatic processes or produce basic motivations such as hunger. In the center of the brain is a system of cavities, the ventricles. These are filled with cerebrospinal fluid, which cleans and nourishes brain tissues.

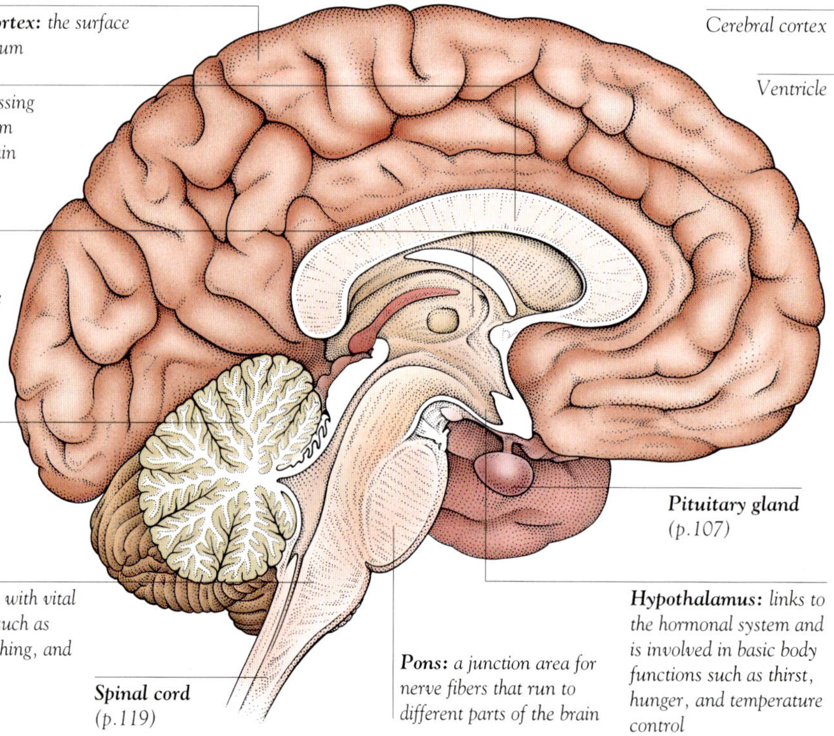

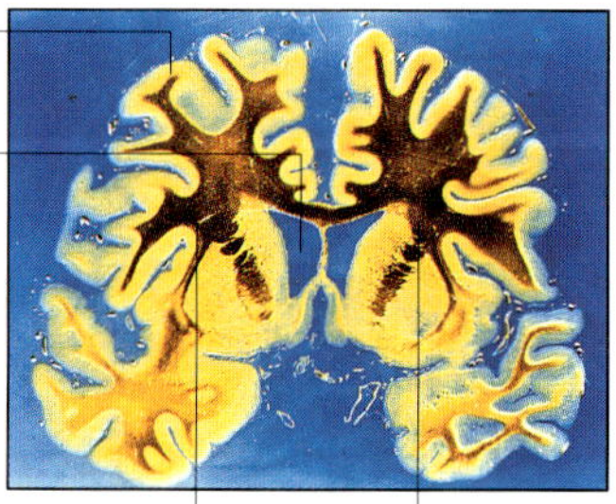

Brain slice
This is a computer-colored photograph of a slice through a brain. The view is from the front. The wrinkled cerebral cortex at the surface of the cerebrum (right), where conscious thought takes place, is shown in yellow. Note how the cerebrum is folded downward in the middle and divided into two cerebral hemispheres.

The cortex

Each cerebral hemisphere has a surface of "gray matter" about ⅛ in (3 mm) thick. This is the cerebral cortex. It is made of billions of nerve cells (p.119), whose axons run to the brain's center and the spinal cord. The cortex is the site of nerve centers for the senses, and of consciousness (awareness), thought, and memory too. Each part of the cortex has a different set of jobs.

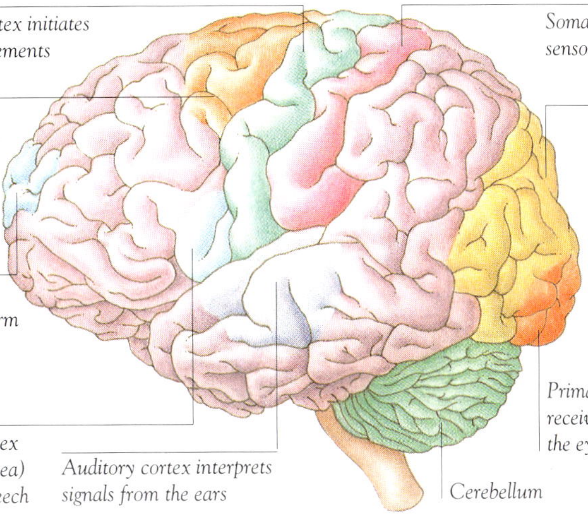

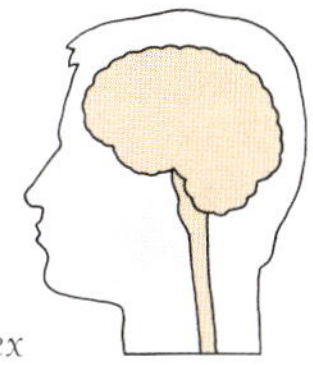

Half the head
The brain takes up the upper half of the head.

Brain size

When compared with the brains of other animals, the remarkable feature of the human brain is not its size—a sperm whale's brain is about six times larger. Instead it is the high proportion of brain size to body size, as well as the way the cerebral hemispheres are folded and wrinkled to give the cortex a large surface area—as big as the top of an office desk. This large surface area means that there is enough space for many highly complex and sophisticated nerve connections.

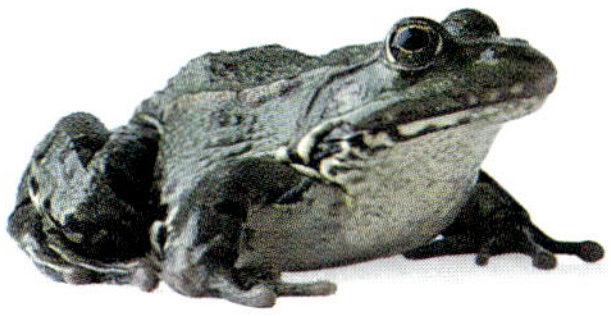

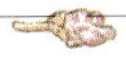

Frog
Most of the frog's small brain deals with basic body processes, coordination, smell, and sight.

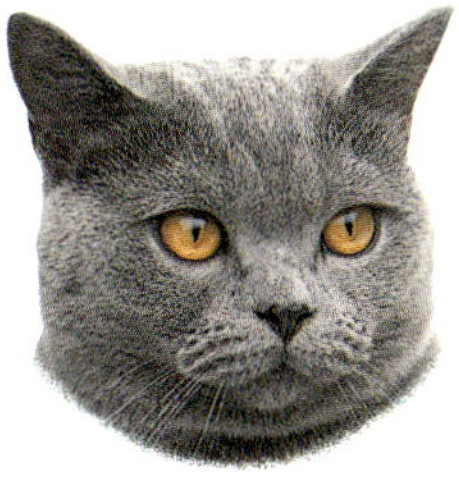

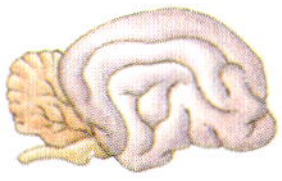

Cat
A cat's brain has a substantial cerebellum, allowing the cat to carry out agile body movements and giving it very good balance.

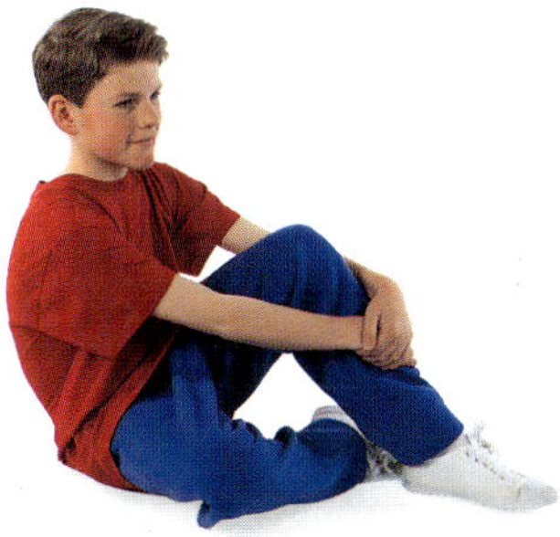

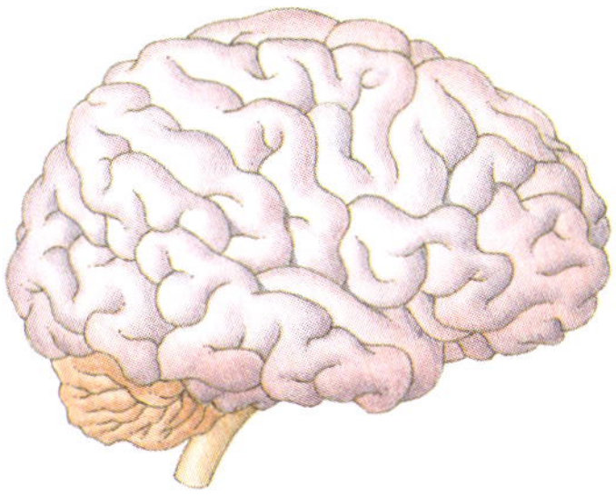

Human
The cerebral hemispheres are so large that they wrap over and cover almost all of the rest of the brain.

EXPERIMENT

Making a mental picture

Adult help is advised for this experiment

The brain's imagination is amazingly versatile. For example, it can construct a mental picture from sound and touch.

You Will Need

- *shallow box with lid* • *cardboard* • *scissors* • *glue* • *marble* • *pad* • *pen*

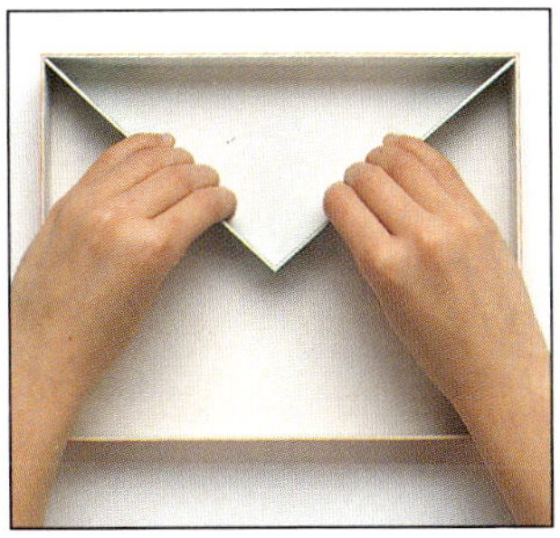

1 Trim the cardboard so that it fits into the box, making a triangular compartment, and glue it in place (left). Put the marble into the compartment, replace the lid, and shake the box to check that the marble stays in the triangle.

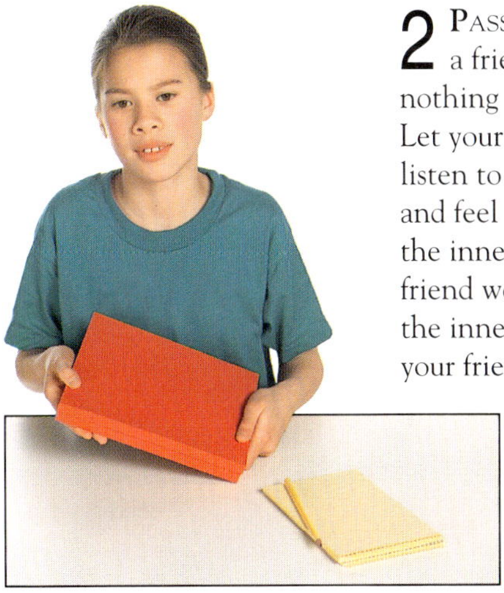

2 Pass the closed box to a friend who knows nothing of the experiment. Let your friend tilt the box, listen to the rolling marble, and feel its impact against the inner surfaces. Can your friend work out the shape of the inner compartment? Ask your friend to draw on the pad the shape that he or she imagines. Now try other shapes of compartment.

Memory

CAN YOU REMEMBER what you had for lunch yesterday? Probably. Can you recall your lunch from 17 days ago? Probably not. The brain has an incredible and very selective ability to remember—and to forget. It is thought that there are several types of memory. Sensory memory (opposite) gives you a constant sense of where you are. Short-term memory (p.130) deals with information you have just received. And long-term memory is a memory for information, sometimes important, sometimes trivial, that you select out over days, weeks, or years.

Long memories

We remember some events for many years. These are often significant times such as exams or birthdays. Memories of them can last for 70 years or more. These memories can be triggered by a chance stimulus of something stored in the memory, or they may be brought back deliberately. Recalling memories now and again helps to refresh them.

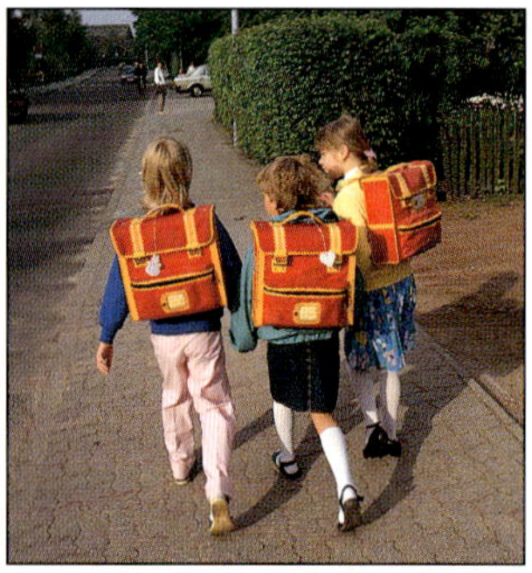

A day to remember
Many people recall their first day at school, but not their second, third, or subsequent days—unless something significant happened.

Memories in the brain

For centuries, scientists could not agree how memory worked in the brain. Recent research has begun to show where different parts of the memory processes take place. However, it does seem that the brain has no single site in which it stores memories. They are spread through several areas, especially around the cortex (p.127). Some of these areas are described here. It may be that different aspects of a particular memory—such as the sights, sounds, smells, and words associated with one event—are stored in different sites.

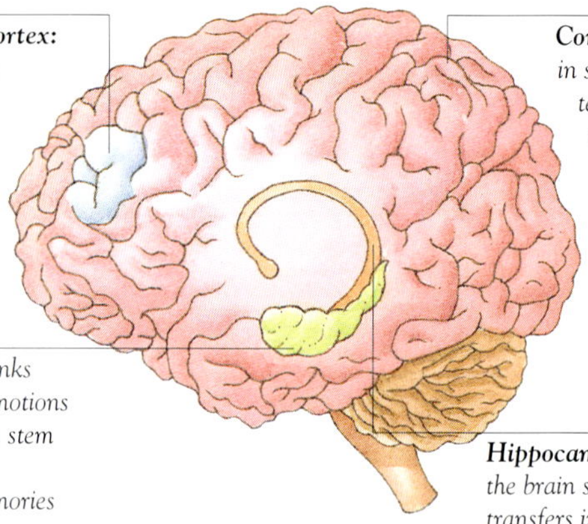

What are memories made of?
This diagram shows some of the brain parts involved in memory processes. It is thought that memories exist as patterns of connections between the nerve cells (neurons) of the brain. The connections occur at synapses (p.119). To store a memory, nerve signals flow along a specific set of routes through certain synapses. This particular memory returns each time nerve signals reactivate and pass again along this set of routes.

EXPERIMENT

Remembering without trying

You often recall things even if you do not consciously try to remember them. In this experiment you can test a friend's memory for faces. The brain seems to have a special facility for remembering human faces, which is very important for identifying people and communicating with them.

YOU WILL NEED

- *20 photographs of faces (or 20 pictures of faces from magazines): the pictures should be of similar size, and all either in color or black-and-white*

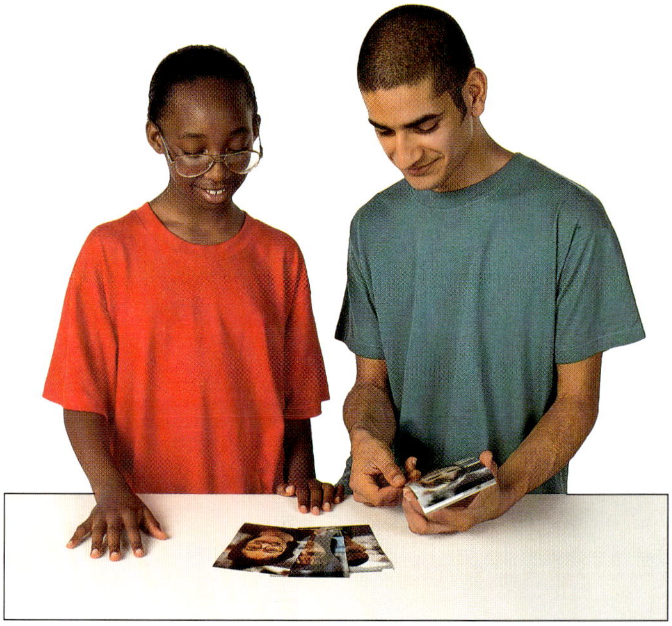

Recognizing faces
Ask a friend to help you, but do not give him or her any details of the experiment. Select 10 of the faces and show them to your friend, one by one, for about half a second each. After a short while, show all 20 faces in any order. Ask your friend to identify the 10 already seen. Even though he or she did not try to memorize the faces, the results should be quite accurate.

Making sense of things

We can remember something much more easily if it makes some kind of sense—that is, if we can see some significance or a recognizable pattern in it. Seeing information as a pattern helps us to remember it from the vast amounts of other information flooding into the brain every second. We cannot remember everything, so we tend to ignore or forget things that have no meaning or that are not important in our lives.

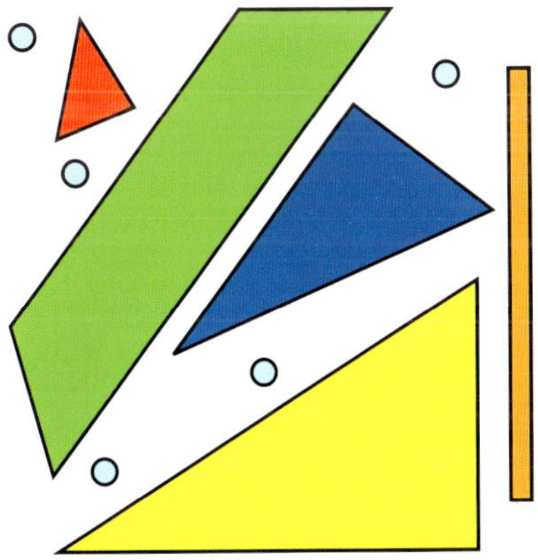

Can you remember this picture?
Study the picture above for 20 seconds, look away, and try to draw it. Can you make a good copy? When the brain sees something, it looks for a pattern or meaning. But this is a meaningless jumble of differently colored shapes. It is difficult to remember.

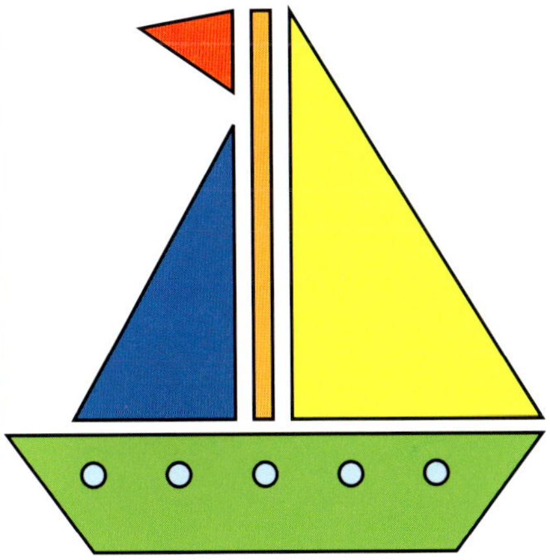

What about this?
You could probably remember and redraw this picture more successfully. It consists of the same shapes as the top drawing. But their arrangement has meaning—a sailboat.

EXPERIMENT

Using sensory memory

Have you ever walked along a street, near a lamppost, when you were distracted and looked away? Did you then turn around and walk on—into the lamppost? This is a rare failure of your sensory memory. This type of memory gives you an awareness of where you are in relation to objects and the space around you, so that you can move around without bumping into things. It lasts only a few seconds and depends mainly on vision. This experiment shows how sensory memory works and how it fades.

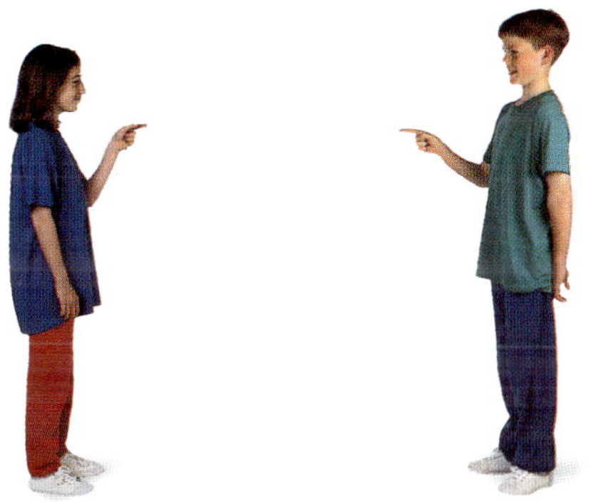

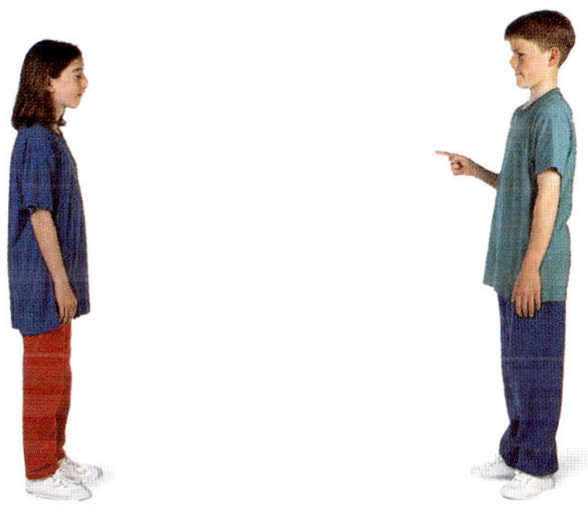

1 STAND FACING a friend, about 7 ft (2 m) away from him or her. Ask your friend to point at you. Now raise your arm and point so that your forefinger is aiming directly at your friend's forefinger.

2 CLOSE YOUR eyes, but try to keep a picture of your friend's position in your mind. Lower your arm. Have your friend "freeze," with his or her eyes open and finger held in the same position.

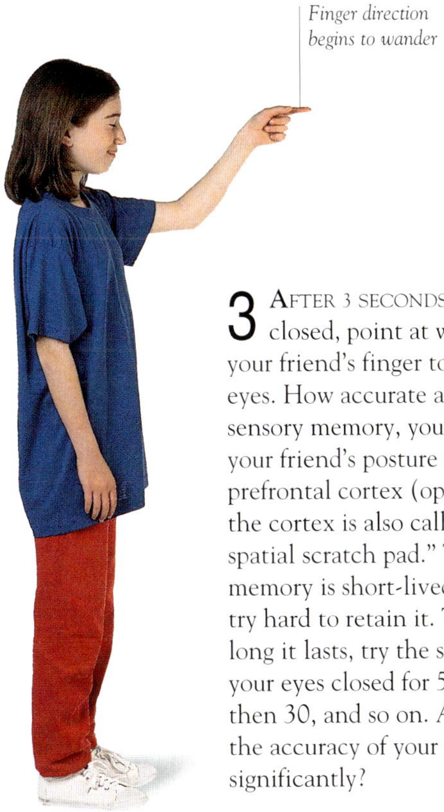

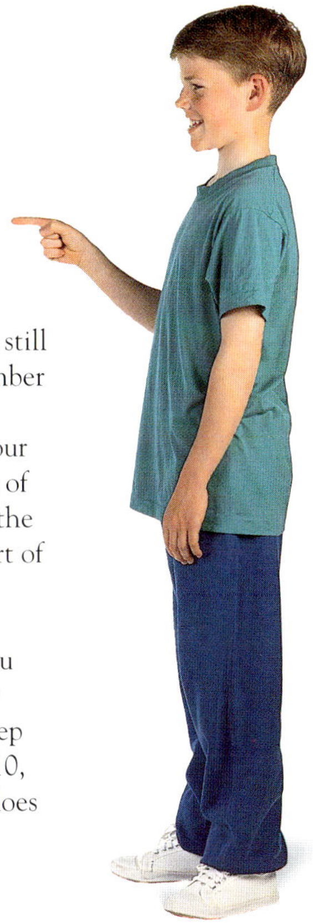

3 AFTER 3 SECONDS, with your eyes still closed, point at where you remember your friend's finger to be. Open your eyes. How accurate are you? Using your sensory memory, you stored a picture of your friend's posture and position in the prefrontal cortex (opposite). This part of the cortex is also called the "visual-spatial scratch pad." The sensory memory is short-lived, even when you try hard to retain it. To find out how long it lasts, try the same test, but keep your eyes closed for 5 seconds, then 10, then 30, and so on. After how long does the accuracy of your pointing fade significantly?

Short-term memory

HOW DO YOU MAKE a telephone call to an unfamiliar number? First you look up the number in the telephone book. Then you repeat the number to yourself as you dial, to help you remember it. You use your short-term memory for this type of task. As its name suggests, short-term memory has a very limited time span. If you look up the telephone number, then wait 5 minutes before dialing, you will probably forget it. But you can keep your short-term memory refreshed by repeating the number to yourself every few seconds. If someone interrupts you during this time, your short-term memory is usually taken over by the new information, and the number vanishes from your brain. The short-term memory has a limited capacity for information, as you can demonstrate with this memory tester.

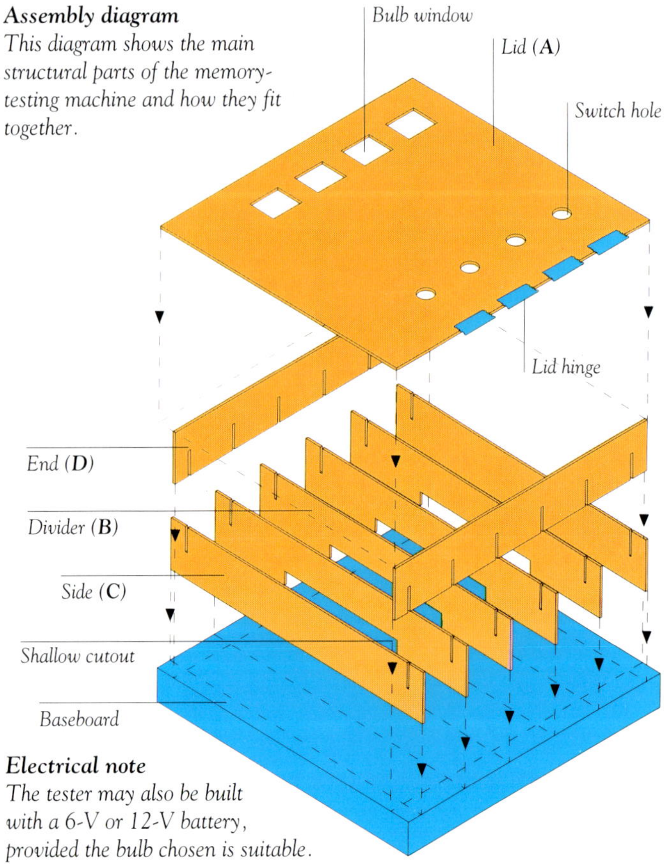

Assembly diagram
This diagram shows the main structural parts of the memory-testing machine and how they fit together.

Electrical note
The tester may also be built with a 6-V or 12-V battery, provided the bulb chosen is suitable.

EXPERIMENT

Make a memory tester

Adult help is advised for this experiment

Make your own memory-testing machine to find out how many items—in this case colored lights in a random sequence—you and your friends can hold in short-term memory. Most people can remember seven or eight items in this way. Can you devise any ways of improving on this?

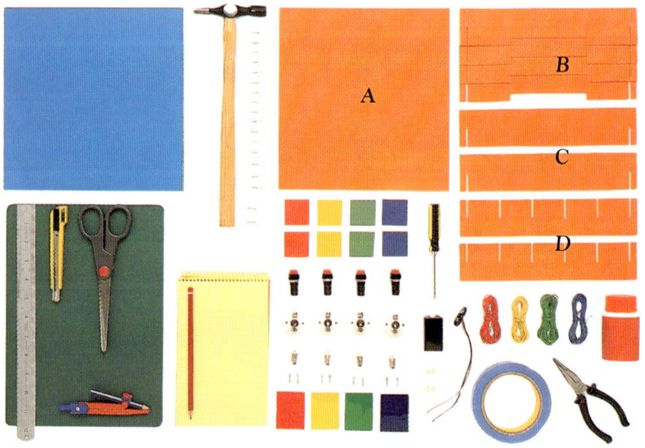

YOU WILL NEED

*• thick softwood baseboard 10 in x 10 in (25 cm x 25 cm) • hammer • 18 U-shaped wire clamps with nails • stiff poster board—for the lid (**A**), 1 piece 10 in x 9½ in (25 cm x 24 cm); for the dividers (**B**), 4 pieces, each 10 in x 2 in (25 cm x 5 cm) with a shallow central cutout and slots 1 in (2.5 cm) long, ½ in (1 cm) from each end; for the sides (**C**), 2 pieces as for **B** but without the central cutouts; for the ends (**D**), 2 pieces as for **C** but with 4 extra slots, equally spaced between the 2 outermost slots • cutting mat • metal ruler • craft knife • scissors • pencil • compass • notepad • 8 squares of paper, sides 1½ in (3.5 cm), in 4 colors (2 of each) • 4 normally open (on-while-pressed) switches • 4 9-V light bulbs and bulb holders • 8 screws for the bulb holders • 4 pieces of cellophane or transparent plastic, 2 in x 1¾ in (5 cm x 4 cm), colored to match the paper squares • screwdriver • 9-V battery • 2 battery-connecting wires with a battery attachment • 2 wire connector blocks • 4 lengths of colored wire • glue • cellophane tape • pliers*

Circuit diagram
Each bulb is connected directly to its own switch by one wire. The other wires from each bulb and its switch go to the battery via the connector block.

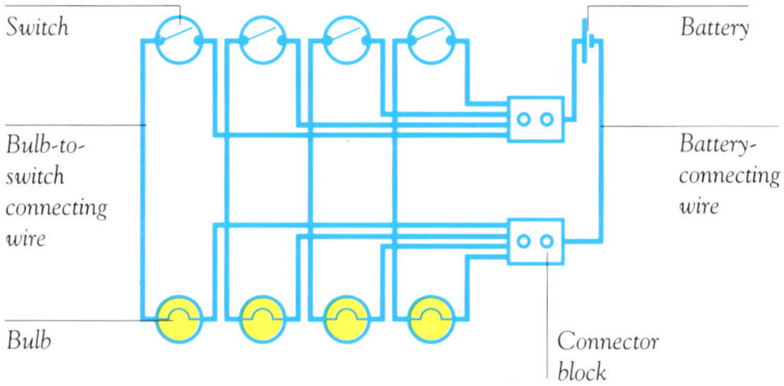

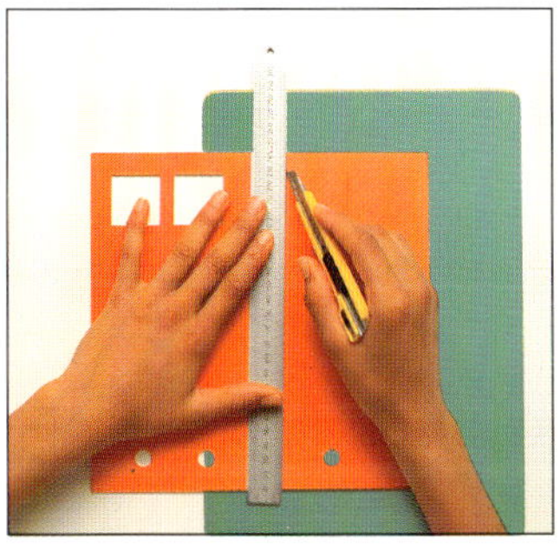

1 ON THE UNDERSIDE of the lid, along one of its longer edges, mark out four 1½-in (3.5-cm) squares. Put one in the top left corner, ¾ in (1.5 cm) from each edge. Draw the next square after a gap of ½ in (1 cm), and repeat for the third and fourth squares. Carefully cut out the squares with the craft knife. The holes that you have made are bulb windows. In line with these windows, carefully cut small holes for the switches, 1 in (2.5 cm) from the opposite edge of the lid.

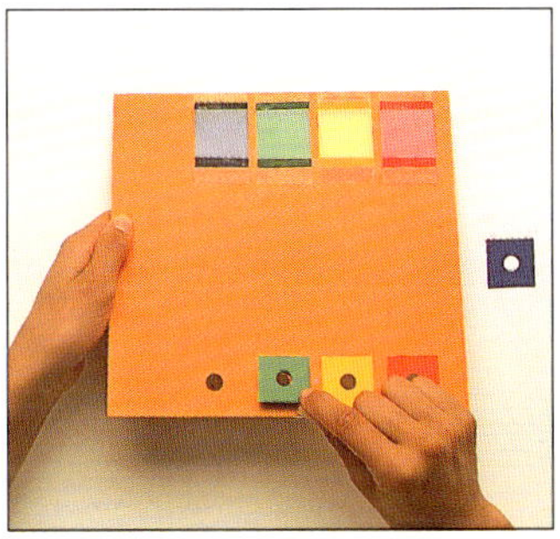

2 ON THE UNDERSIDE of the lid, tape the four pieces of colored cellophane onto the bulb windows. Carefully cut small, round holes in each of the colored paper squares. Glue the squares over the switch holes on both the top and bottom of the lid, to correspond to the positions of the pieces of colored cellophane. The paper square on top of the lid shows the color code for the switch. The paper square on the underside is a color guide for when you connect the wires.

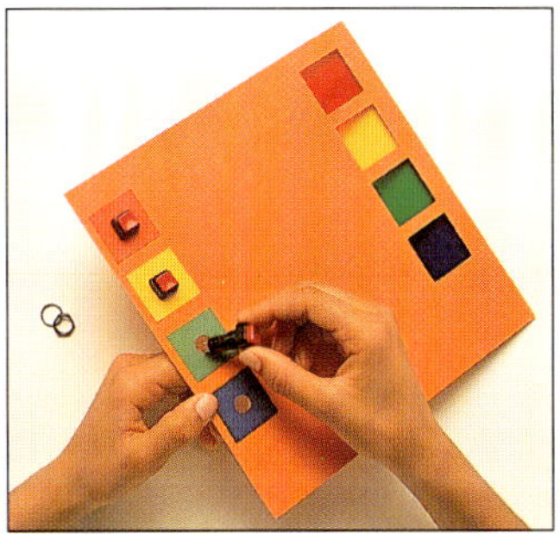

3 INSTALL THE switches. Depending on the way the type of switch is secured, you may need to unscrew a small collar from the stem, and push the switch through from below, before screwing the collar back on again. Or you may need to insert the switch from above, as shown. You can even attach the switch with tape. Whichever method is used, make sure the switch is attached securely enough to cope with the pressure when it is turned on by pressing it down.

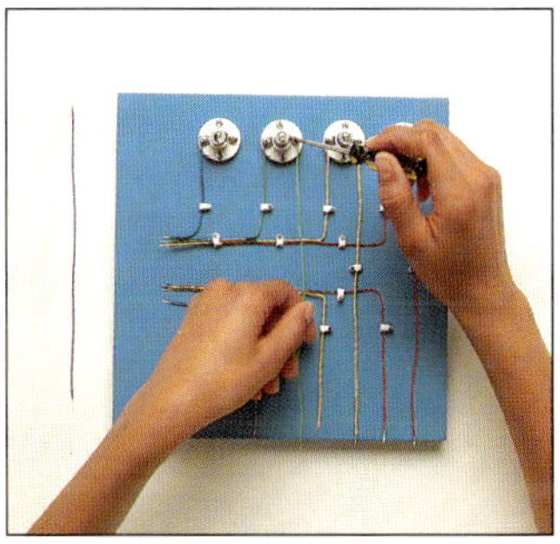

4 SCREW THE bulb holders to the base, so the bulbs will be under their windows. Run wires in L-shapes from the left, where one connector block will be placed, to one contact on each bulb holder. It is helpful if the wire is the same color as the window of the bulb it leads to. Do the same on the other side of the base, leaving the wire ends free to join the switches. Run another wire from the other contact on each bulb holder to its corresponding switch. Secure all wires with clamps.

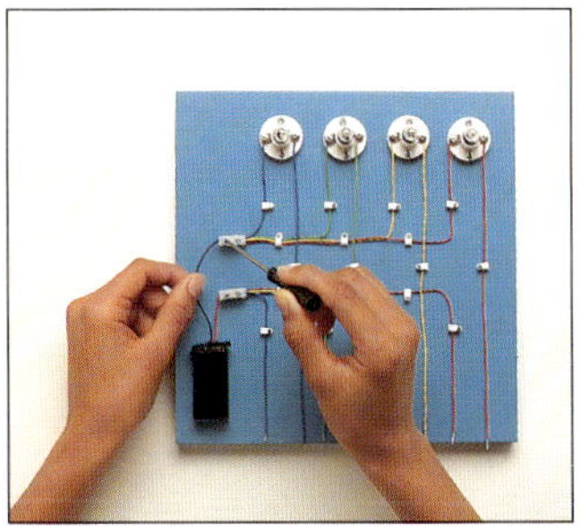

5 TAKE THE ENDS of the four wires from the bulb holders, twist them together, and insert them into one side of one of the connector blocks. Screw the block into the baseboard. Do the same with the four wires that will be connected to switches, using the other connector block. Lie the battery on the lower left of the base. Attach each of the two connecting wires from the battery to a different connector block. Tape the battery in place. Now disconnect one of the battery wires to save power.

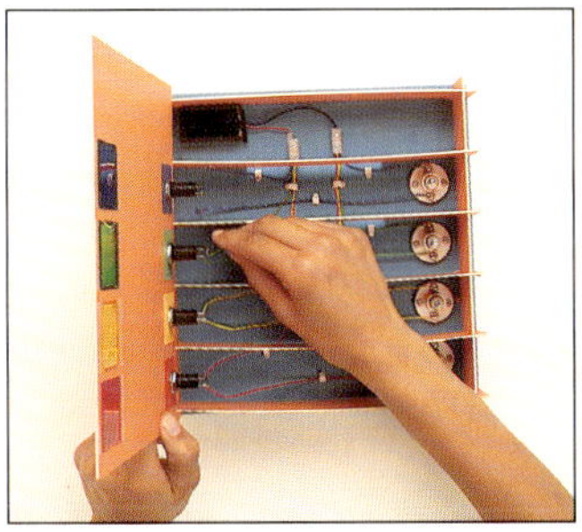

6 SLOT TOGETHER the dividers, sides, and ends as in the assembly diagram (opposite). Glue them together and into position on the base, so that the wires run under the shallow cutouts. Hinge the lid in position with tape, on the edge next to the switches. Connect the free ends of each pair of wires to the corresponding switch. Now reconnect the battery wire, lower the lid, and check that pressing each switch lights the corresponding bulb. The memory tester is now ready to use.

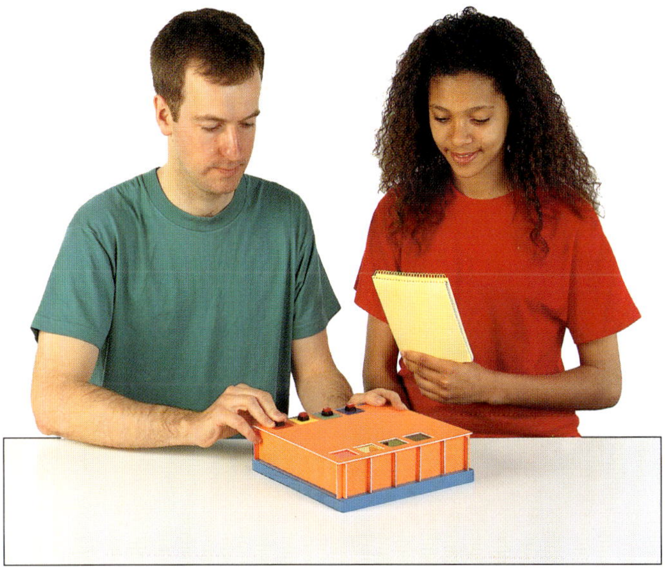

7 WRITE DOWN RANDOM sequences of colors. Begin with two, such as red-blue, and finish with a dozen. Then, as a friend watches, tap out the first of these sequences, so that the lights flash in order. Can your friend repeat the order of lights? Which is the longest sequence your friend can remember correctly? Does your friend improve if you press the switches more slowly? What happens if he or she has to wait before repeating the sequence? Does it help your friend to divide long sequences mentally into several short groups of colors?

Learning

OUR CAPACITY FOR LEARNING depends mainly on the power of our memory. One type of learning involves physical skill, from simple movements such as pouring to complex ones such as writing. These skills are learned through a process of trial and error—we try certain muscle movements, assess the results, and store information on what we have done in memory. Another type of learning involves ideas, inventions, and strategies rather than physical movements. This allows us to plan ahead—to think out, for example, the moves in a chess game. A third type of learning involves transferring facts and figures to the brain's memory, so that they can be recalled later.

Learning to laugh

From the age of only a few weeks, a baby learns to smile and then laugh. The baby learns that these actions produce reactions in those around and give them pleasure. At first the baby's laughter is natural and unaffected. However, as the baby gets older, he or she learns that there are different ways to laugh, from a short chuckle to a loud guffaw, and that these different types of laughter convey different meanings. Learning to laugh is all part of learning to communicate our thoughts, emotions, and intentions to other people.

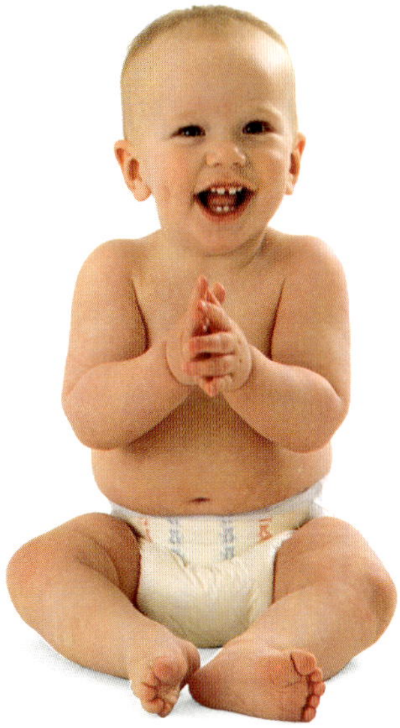

Waiting for a response
A baby may laugh and clap his or her hands to see how other people respond to such actions.

EXPERIMENT

Relearning to write

Writing depends on a series of precise, controlled hand movements. Most of us learn to write with our preferred hand, which we have used since we were very young, for gripping objects and manipulating them. However, the brain can retrain itself and learn to use the other hand—with a certain amount of concentration and effort.

YOU WILL NEED
- *pen*
- *large sheet of paper*

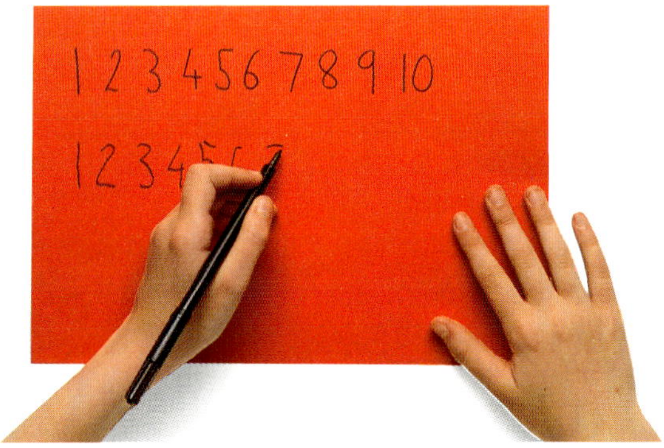

Writing with the wrong hand
With your usual writing hand, neatly write out the numbers 1 to 10, large and clear. Now hold the pen in your other hand. Write the same numbers again below. Are these numbers as neat and tidy as the first set? Keep practicing with this hand, learning to control the pen. Compare your first attempt at writing with this hand to your last. Do the neatness and accuracy of your writing improve?

EXPERIMENT

Learning to draw

Drawing depends partly on physical control and coordination of hand movements. It also depends on the image of the subject that you hold in your mind, especially when you draw from memory. In turn, the accuracy of this image depends on your mental abilities, which usually become more accurate and sophisticated with age, as shown by this simple experiment.

YOU WILL NEED
- *paper*
- *pens*
- *head-to-toe photograph of a person*

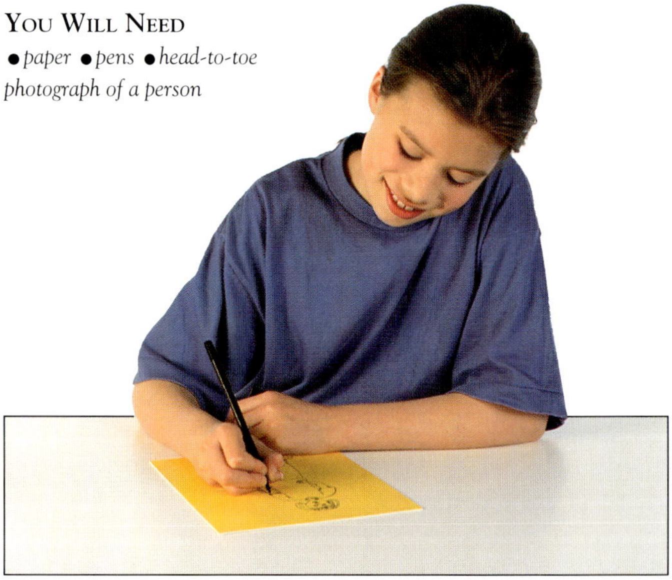

1 ASK FOR THE HELP of friends ranging in age from 3 to 4 years to adulthood. They do not have to be expert artists. Ask them to look at the photograph of a person for a minute, to close their eyes for 30 seconds, and then to draw the main features of the person in the photograph from memory.

Learning to play

As with other games, the basics of chess are relatively simple. Most people can quickly learn the moves for each piece. But learning to play chess well involves memorizing many hundreds of possible moves, as well as possible moves for each of these moves at the next turn, and so on.

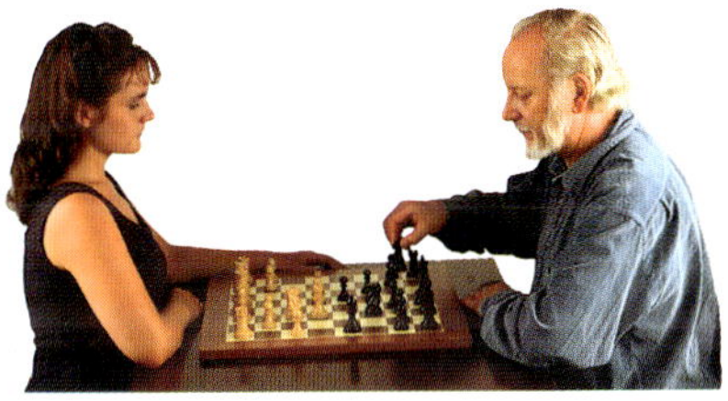

So many combinations
In a chess game, moves must be thought out far in advance. This provides a complex challenge for the brain.

EXPERIMENT

Learning to pour

When you first learned to pour water from a pitcher, you probably spilled most of it. Now you can pour it smoothly. To see the body movements involved in pouring, "relearn" this process by trying to pour from a greater height than usual, and by using sand, which flows in a different way from water. Wear protective goggles to prevent any sand from getting into your eyes. As you tip the pitcher, you must judge where to position it, when the sand will begin to slide out, and how it will fall sideways on its downward journey.

You Will Need

- *large plastic pitcher*
- *plastic beaker*
- *fine sand*
- *protective goggles*

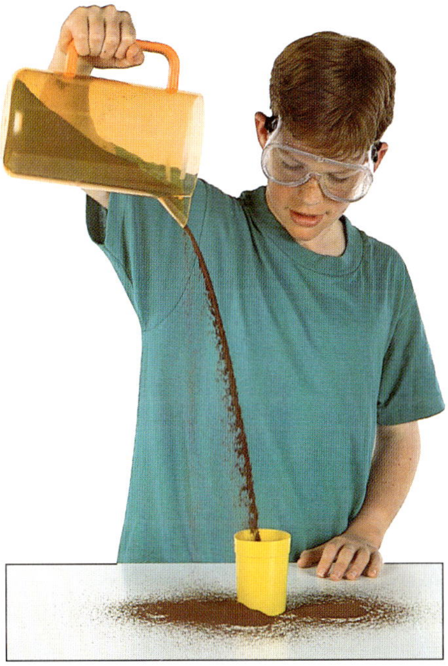

Cascade of sand
Hold the pitcher of sand at head height. Try to pour the sand into a beaker on the table. You must learn to adjust your tipping speed and aim.

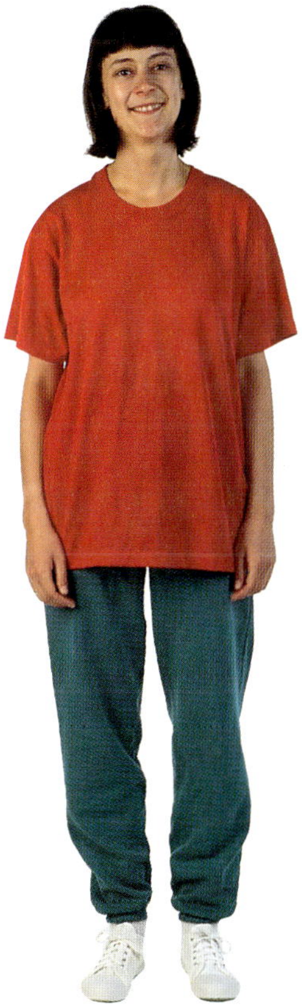

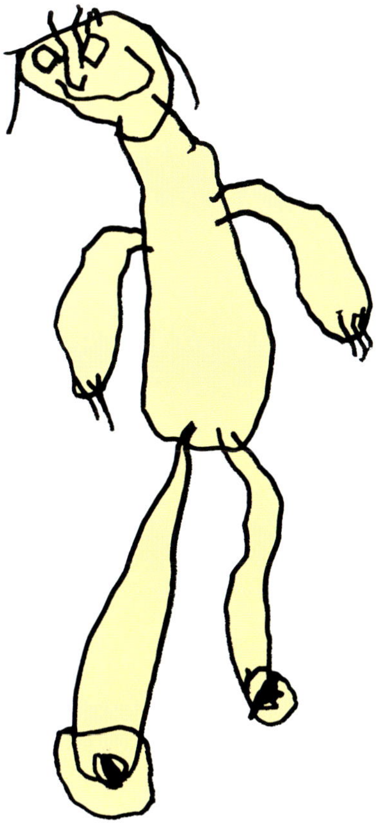

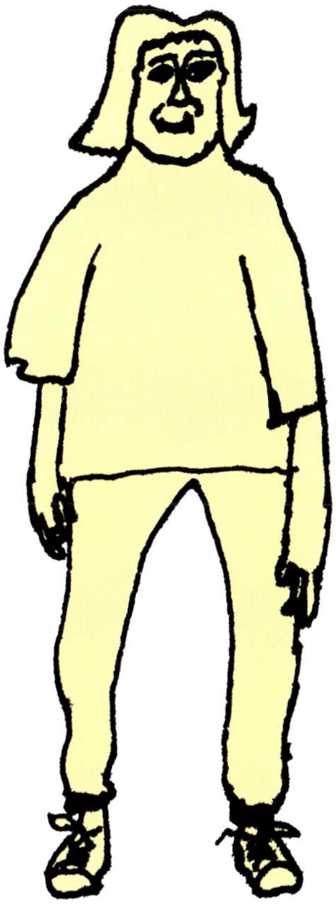

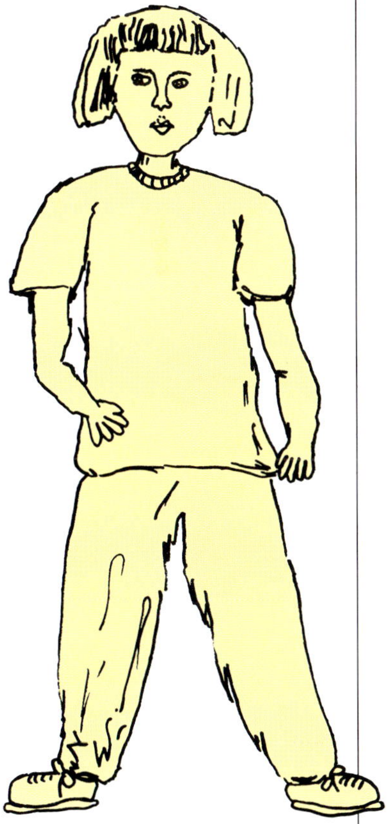

2 Compare the drawings to the original photograph. Which drawing is the most accurate? A sample set of drawings is shown here, based on the photograph above.

By a 4-year-old
This shows a head, body, arms, and legs, but few details, even on the face. Young children may emphasize features that are important in their own lives. The person who drew this was learning to tie shoelaces!

By an 8-year-old
The body and limbs are now more in proportion. The arms and legs connect at the correct places, though one arm is rather long. The face and hair have more detail, and the shoes still figure prominently.

By a 12-year-old
There is greater detail in this picture than in the previous two, and the lines of the drawing are finer. But some features of the photograph have been altered in the memory of this artist. Again, look at the shoes!

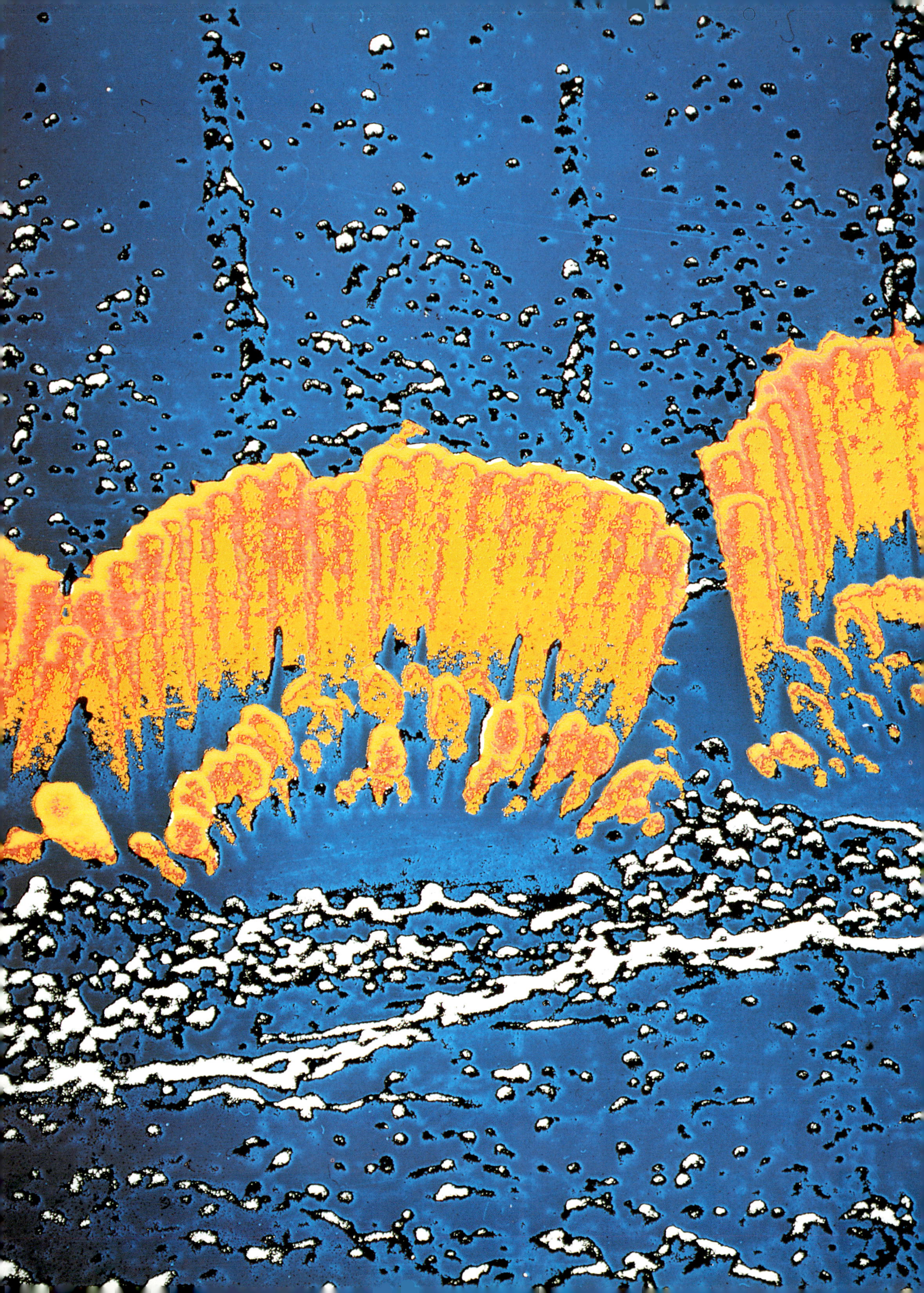

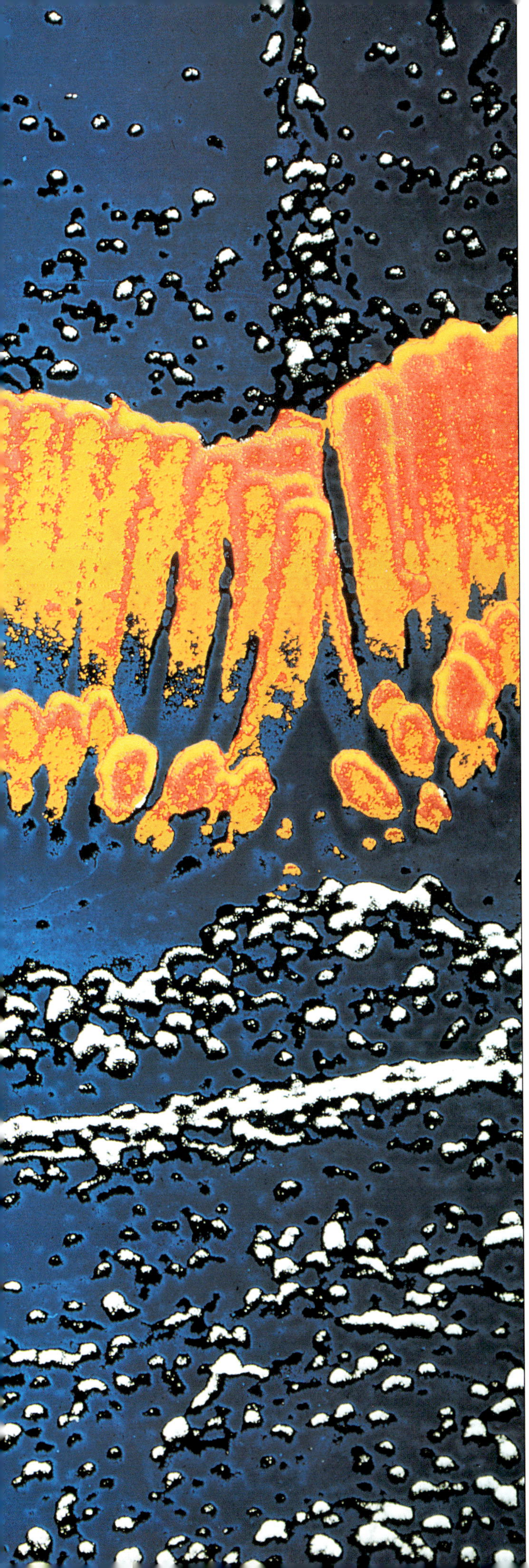

SENSING the SURROUNDINGS

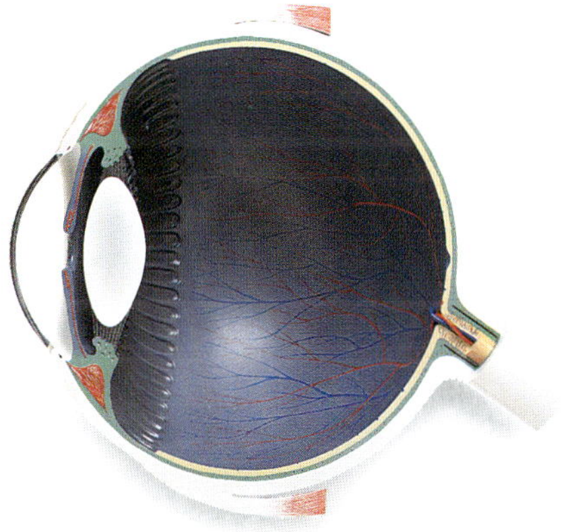

Keeping eyes and ears open

When sound waves enter the ear, many thousands of microscopic hairs deep inside the ear (colored yellow, left) are shaken by a vibrating membrane. The movements of the hairs cause nerve signals to be sent to the brain, which interprets them as sounds. The eye (shown in the cutaway model, above) has more than 130 million light-sensitive cells in its wafer-thin inner layer—the retina.

YOUR SENSES ALLOW YOU TO experience pleasure and pain. They enable you to appreciate art and music, or the smell and taste of a delicious meal. But they are also vital for survival. You can see and hear danger, and feel if you are being harmed. Sense organs transform stimuli such as light rays, sound waves, odors, flavors, or physical contact into a common form of information—electrical nerve signals. These signals are instantly flashed to the brain for interpretation and identification.

THE BODY'S SENSES

ASK SOMEONE TO NAME THE BODY'S SENSES. He or she will probably say sight, hearing, smell, taste, and touch, making a total of five. However, the body has other senses. We are not aware of most of them, since they are part of the automatic control mechanisms that keep internal body conditions stable (pp.104–105). Even the familiar five senses are not as simple as they seem. The sense of touch, for example, provides you with several distinct sensations such as pressure, heat, cold, and pain.

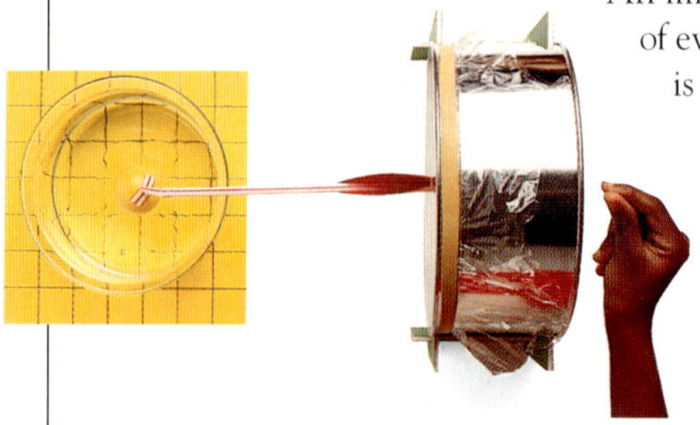

A cake pan and drinking straw show how *sound waves are converted into ripples in the fluid of the inner ear (p.152).*

An important feature of every animal's life is the ability to sense (detect) what is going on in the world around it. Even very simple creatures such as jellyfish and worms can sense light, moisture, vibration, and chemicals. This helps them to avoid possible danger, find food, and seek out suitable surroundings—all actions that are necessary for survival.

Each sense organ—such as the eye, tongue, or skin—converts the information about what it detects into the body's "language" of electrical nerve signals. These travel to the brain along sensory nerves (p.118). In the brain, the signals are sorted and processed, analyzed and interpreted. The signals from each sense organ are dealt with in a specialized center of the brain's cortex (p.127).

The sense organs are chiefly receiver-converters. This means that they receive a sensation and convert it into nerve signals, which go to the brain. Some initial sorting and processing take place, particularly in the eye, ear, and nose, but most interpretation happens later, in the brain. The incoming information is compared with other information already in the brain, in the memory. The brain tries to identify what the senses have detected and decides whether or not it is important.

The vast majority of information that the brain receives is not important, so it is discarded. You only become "aware" of information that does get through this sorting system.

Even when they are working efficiently, our senses detect only a small part of the information available to them. Some animals have senses that are far more acute than ours. For example, a dog can smell many more odors than a human, and at far weaker concentrations. An eagle can see the size and color of a rabbit, when for a human, the rabbit would look like a tiny speck.

Early beliefs

The idea that we have five senses is a traditional one. It goes back at least to the time of the great philosopher Aristotle of ancient Greece (384–322 B.C.), who listed the five over 2,300 years ago. Some early beliefs about certain sense organs seem very strange today. These misconceptions arose partly from a lack of knowledge of the body and partly from a lack of understanding of the nature of light rays, sound waves, odors, and flavors.

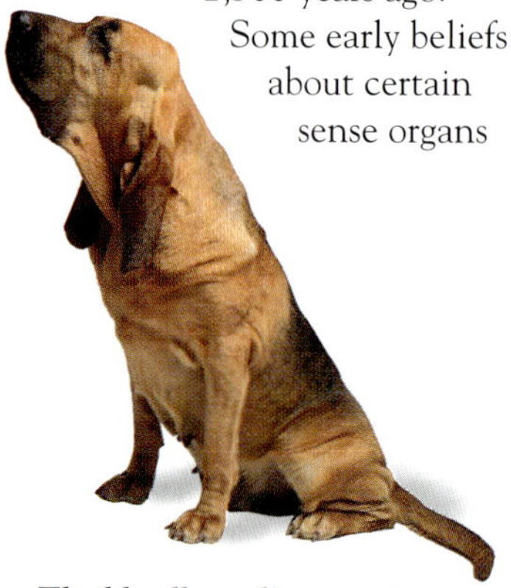

The bloodhound's nose gives a *sense of smell that is hundreds of times more sensitive to certain odors than a human nose.*

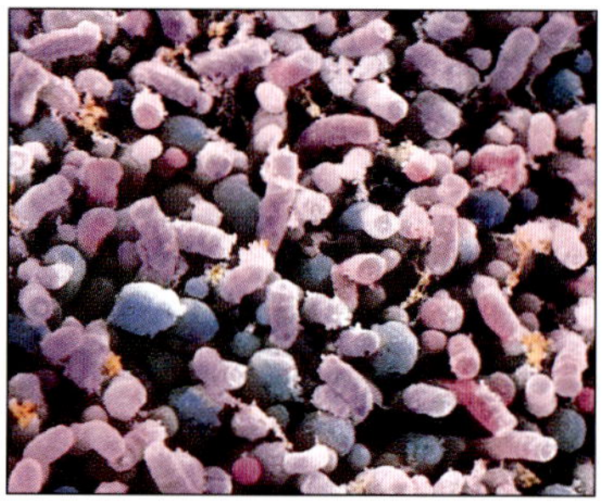

The cells that see, rods and cones, *are packed in the eye's retina (p.139). In this microscope photograph rods have been colored purple and cones blue.*

For example, some ancient Egyptians believed that the body both listened and breathed through the ears. They thought that a substance called "life-breath" entered the right ear, and when the time came, another substance, called "death-breath," entered the left ear.

Many ancient Greeks and Romans thought that we could see because light beamed out of the eye onto the objects that we looked at. In fact, the reverse happens—light rays travel from the object onto light-sensitive cells in the eye.

Renaissance ideas

During the Renaissance there was steady progress in the knowledge that scientists gained about the sense organs.

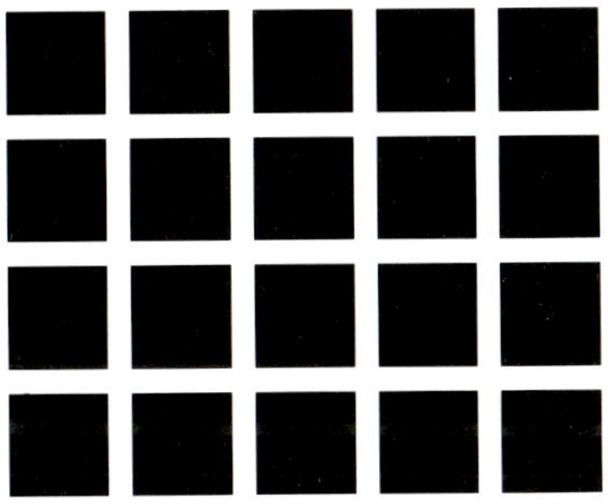

***Look at these squares. Do you see** spots between them? You may, even though there are none. Unusual images like this one can confuse the eye and brain (pp.150–151).*

In 1562 the first thorough book on the ears was written, by the Italian anatomy professor Bartolomeo Eustachio (1520–74). The tube linking the middle ear cavity (p.152) to the throat is called the Eustachian tube in his memory.

Some Renaissance scientists believed that light was detected by the eye's iris (the colored front part) or the transparent lens just behind it. But the Frenchman René Descartes (p.118) showed that in fact the lens focuses an upside-down image onto the

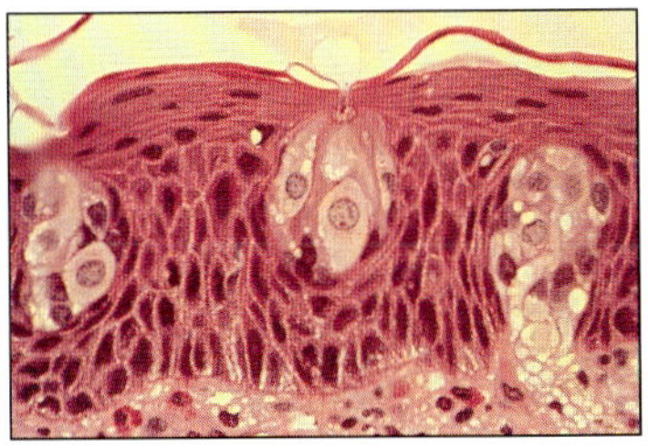

***Onion-shaped taste buds sense the** flavors of food. They are visible in this microscope photograph of a section through the surface of a tongue.*

sensitive retina lining the back of the eye.

Descartes also believed, this time incorrectly, that the optic nerves (p.139) were hollow tubes that carry a mysterious substance called "animal spirit" from the eyes to the brain. In fact each optic nerve, like other nerves, is a bundle of fibers.

Microscopes, invented in the early 1600's, revealed that the eye's retina is crowded with millions of light-sensitive cells of two main kinds—rods and cones (p.142). The Englishman Thomas Young (1773–1829) and the German Hermann von Helmholtz (p.139) believed that there were three types of cones—one type to detect red light, one for green, and one for blue.

However, new research shows that color vision is more complex than Young and Helmholtz suggested. The research shows that what we perceive as a certain color depends also on the colors of surrounding objects.

Chemosenses

Biologists include the senses of smell and taste in a group called chemosenses, because these senses work in a very similar way to each other. Fish and other water creatures rely on chemosenses, because they detect chemicals in the water by smell and taste.

Thousands of microscopic receptors are scattered around the nose and tongue. In the nose they are found on a surface called the olfactory epithelium (p.158). On the tongue they are found on the taste-bud cells (p.160). Each receptor has a pit of a specific shape. Only molecules of a certain chemical are the right shape to fit neatly into the pit. When these molecules slot into the pit, they trigger nerve signals to the brain. This is the "lock-and-key" principle. With many types of receptor pit, shaped to receive a variety of chemicals, your nose and tongue can detect a wide range of substances.

Other senses

Scientists continue to investigate the astonishingly intricate workings of the sense organs. These include not only the main five senses, but other sensors inside the body as well.

Stretch sensors in muscles, tendons, and joints tell the brain about the position and posture of the body. They are part of the proprioceptive sense (p.146). Pressure sensors in certain blood vessels, such as the carotid artery

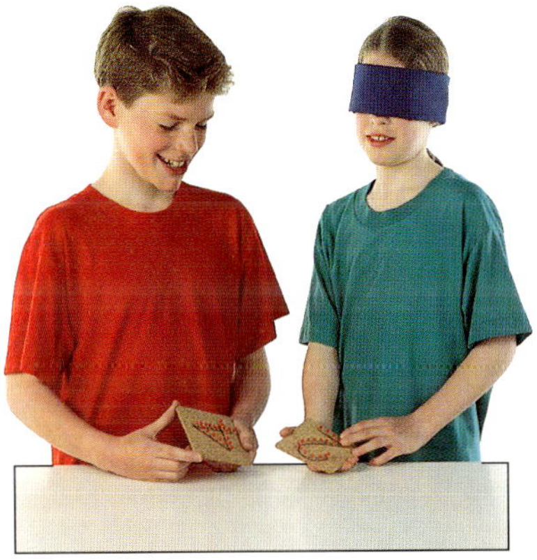

***Skin can help you "see." You can** form a mental picture of an object by touch alone (p.167).*

in the neck, inform the brain about blood pressure. And in the brain, chemosensors monitor concentrations of carbon dioxide, glucose, and other substances in the blood.

Each of these sensing systems is designed to adjust and maintain the environment inside the body automatically. So they leave the parts of the brain that deal with your conscious thoughts free to concentrate on other things.

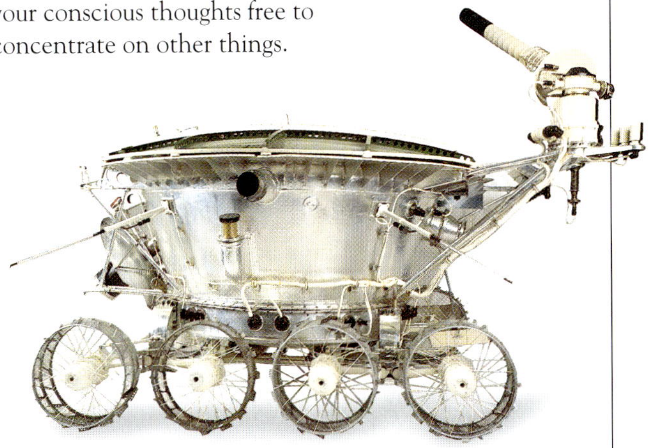

***Many machines can sense things that we cannot, such as** ultraviolet light or magnetic fields. We often make other machines to mimic our own senses. For example, this moon-rover carries cameras and soil samplers to "see" and "feel" the moon's surface.*

The eyes

YOUR TWO EYES provide an incredibly detailed, constantly updated, three-dimensional color view of the world. Light rays enter the eye through the cornea, a domed window at the front. They are detected by the retina, a layer of light-sensitive cells. The retina is not much larger than a postage stamp—and even thinner. From the pattern of light rays, the eye generates patterns of nerve signals and sends them to your brain. The parts of your brain specialized for dealing with sight, the visual centers (p.117), analyze all the information coming in from the eyes. It is your brain that tells you what kinds of shapes and forms, shades and colors, positions and movements you are looking at. The following pages explore the intricate structure and workings of your eyes and brain.

Cleaning the eyes

Tear fluid is made continually in two small, lumpy glands, the lacrimal glands. They are just above the outer side of each eye. The tear fluid oozes from the eyelid each time you blink and washes away dust and germs. The fluid drains into the lacrimal ducts (tear ducts) and then into the nose.

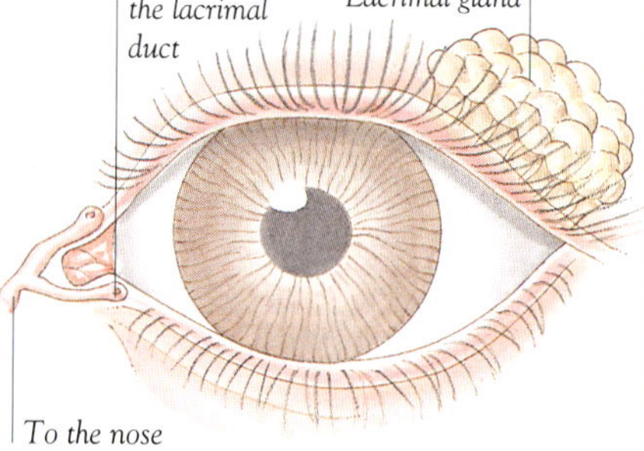

Moving the eyes

As you read these words or glance around, your eyes flick back and forth. Their movements are produced by a team of six long, slim muscles behind each eyeball. The muscles work together to move the eyes in different directions.

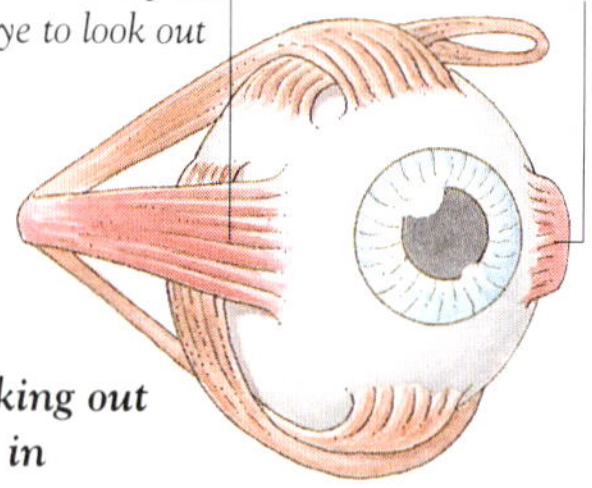

Looking out and in

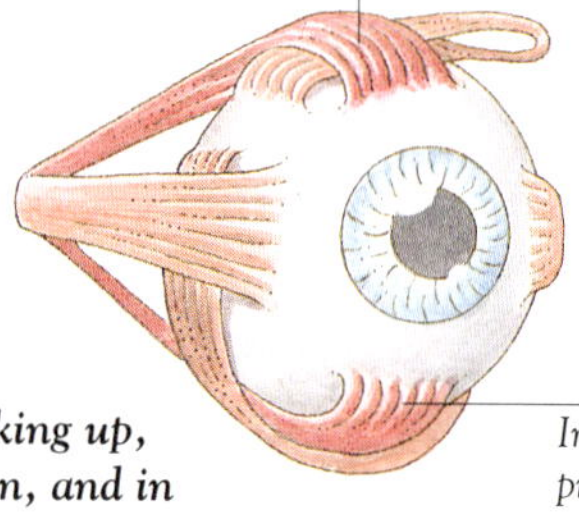

Looking up, down, and in

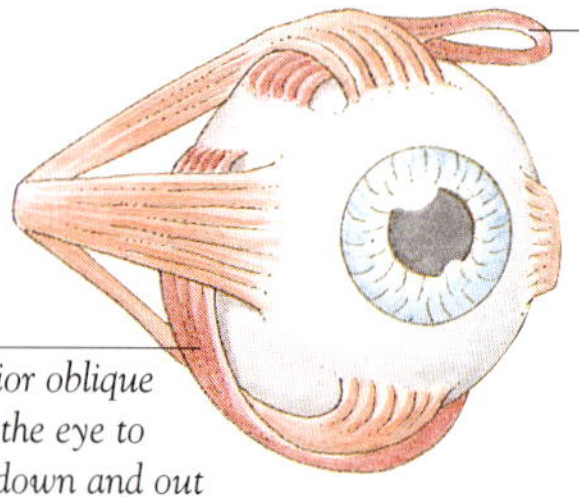

Looking up, down, and out

EXPERIMENT

Looking at your eye

Are your irises both exactly the same color? Can you see the film of tear fluid over the front surface of the eye, the conjunctiva? Can you see into the pupil? Gently pull down your lower eyelid to see the tiny hole into the lacrimal duct.

YOU WILL NEED

- *small plastic-edged mirror*

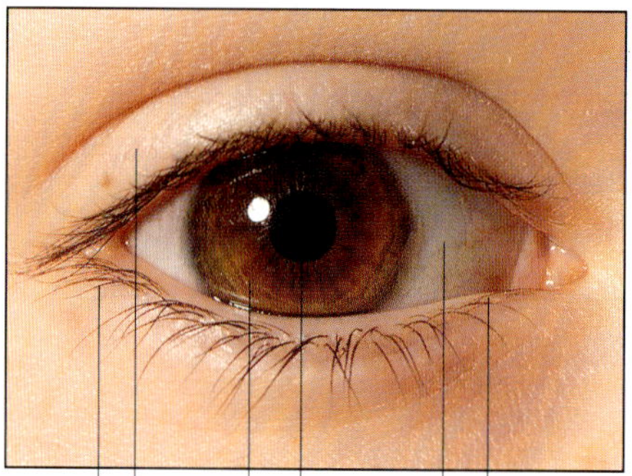

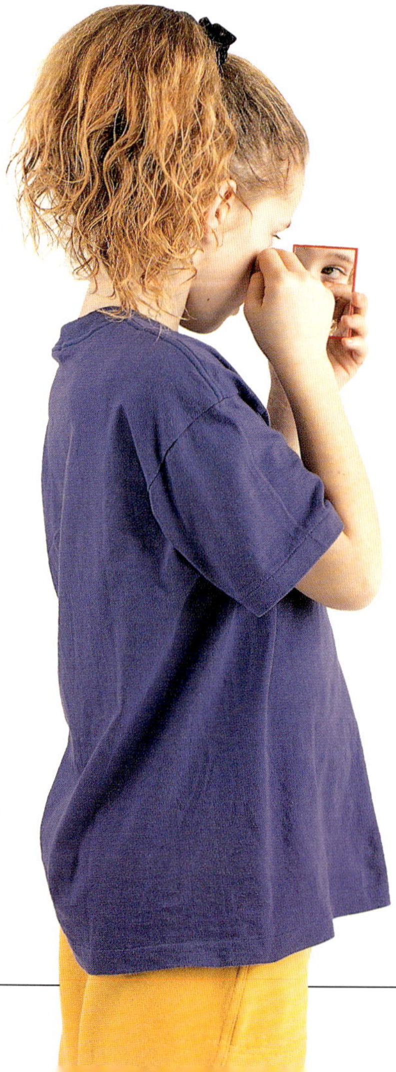

Using the mirror
Stand in good light and look at one eye closely in a mirror. Which parts of the eye can you see?

Inside the eye

This is a cutaway diagram of an eye, seen from above. The eyeball is about 1 in (2.5 cm) wide. Its outermost layer is the sclera, visible from the front as the white of the eye. Within this is the choroid, rich in blood vessels to nourish other eye parts. On the inside of the choroid is the retina. This has light-sensitive cells that detect light rays that have entered the eye through the cornea. The cornea, which partly focuses the rays (p.140), is so transparent that you can hardly see it when looking at your eye in a mirror. Next the light rays pass through a clear fluid, the aqueous humor, and then through the pupil, the central hole in the ring of muscle known as the iris. Then the rays pass through the lens, which focuses them further. They shine through the clear, jellylike vitreous humor that forms the bulk of the eyeball, before reaching the retina.

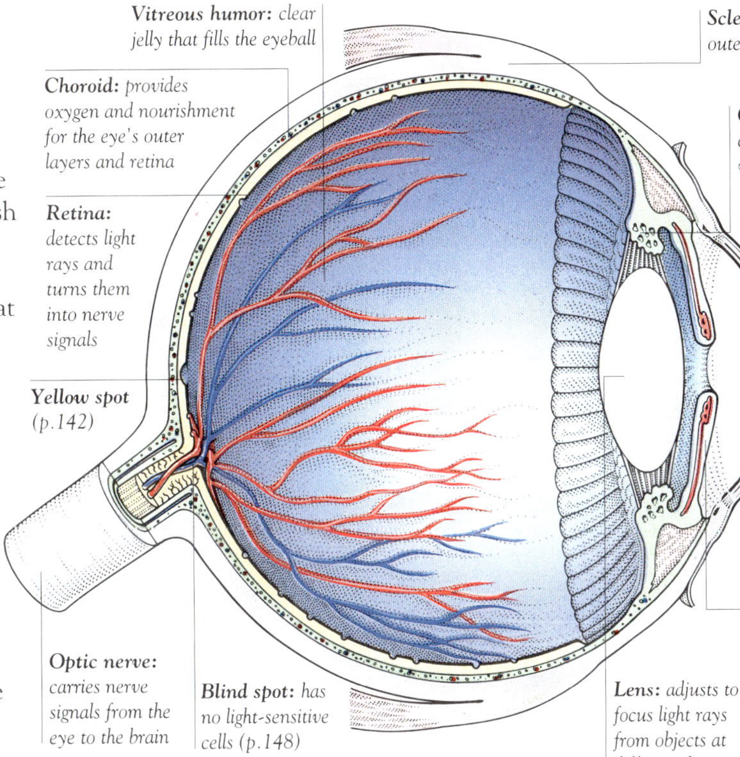

A view into the eye

An ophthalmoscope is a medical instrument for lighting up the inside of the eye and looking into it through the pupil. With it, your doctor can check that the inside of your eye is healthy. The ophthalmoscope also allows blood vessels in the eye to be seen clearly, giving valuable information about the general state of blood vessels in the body.

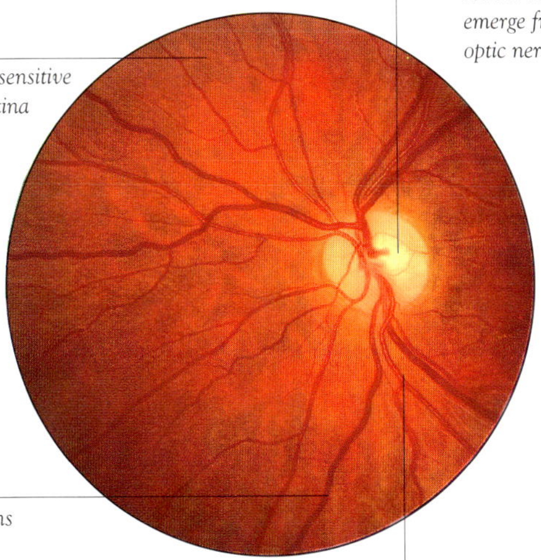

■ DISCOVERY ■

Hermann von Helmholtz

A remarkable German scientist, Hermann von Helmholtz (1821–94), combined work in anatomy and physiology with mathematics, electricity, and optics. In 1850 he measured the speed of tiny electrical nerve signals in living nerves. These, he discovered, travel at about 80 to 130 ft (25 to 40 m) per second, and some go even faster. The next year he developed an early version of an ophthalmoscope (left). Helmholtz also wrote *Handbook of Physiological Optics* (published in several volumes, 1856–66). This book was a landmark in the study of how the eye works. In it he explained how cone cells in the retina contain pigments that are sensitive to one of three different colors of light—red, green, or blue. This is the reason that the eye can see in color.

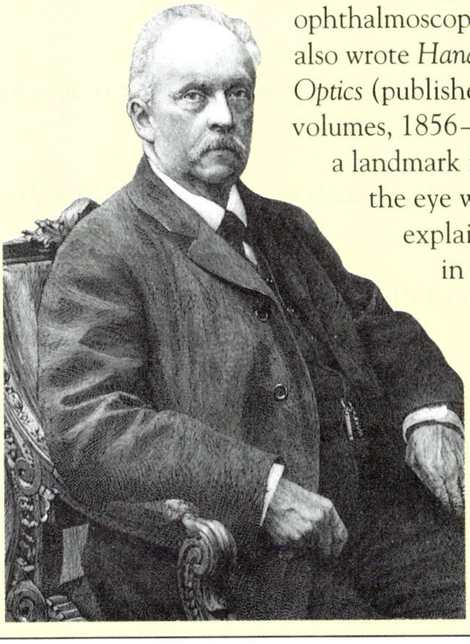

Seeing

WHEN YOU USE binoculars, you adjust them to see things nearby clearly and then readjust them for faraway objects. This is called focusing, and it is done by moving the lenses in the binoculars. The lenses in your eyes also change when they focus on objects at different distances. But the eyes' lenses do not move; they change shape. Ciliary muscles around each lens make the lens fatter (to bend the light rays more) for nearby objects, or thinner (to bend the rays less) for distant objects. The eye also controls how much light enters it. Muscles in the iris shrink the pupil in bright light. This automatic reaction is called a reflex. If the eye did not do this, too much light would enter the lens and damage the delicate retina.

Turning the world upside down

When a newborn baby sees the world for the first time, he or she has no idea of what is up or down, left or right. As the baby reaches out for objects, he or she realizes that when the image of the object falls on a certain part of the eye's retina, then the object is in a certain position. The eye's lens—like any other lens—inverts the image, so that on the retina it is upside down. But the baby never knows anything different. From the very start of our lives we turn images the "right way up" in the brain as an automatic part of seeing.

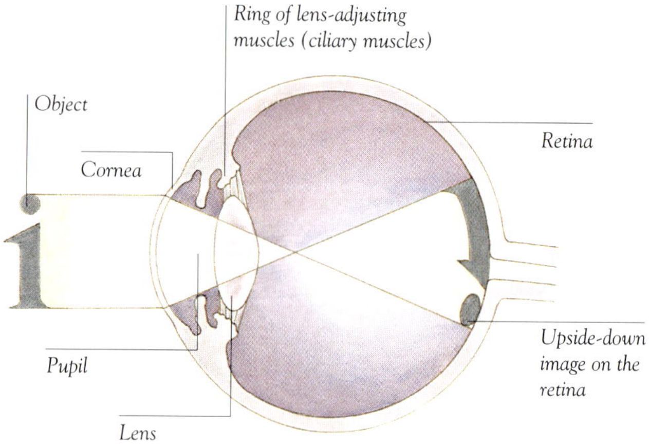

EXPERIMENT

Magnifying-lens eye

Adult help is advised for this experiment

Make an "eye" with a magnifying lens and tracing paper. Move the lens to and fro to focus on objects in the room.

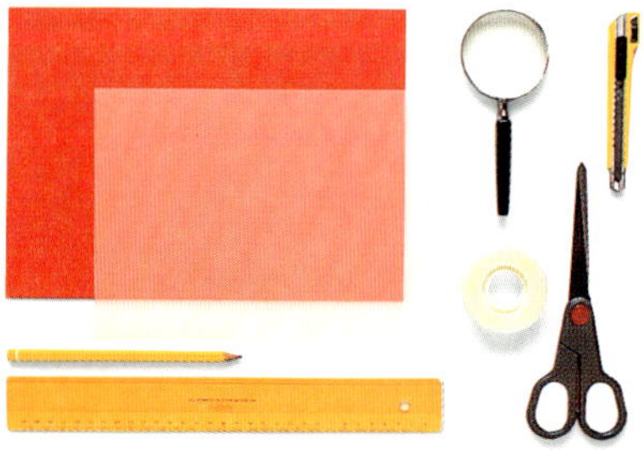

YOU WILL NEED

- *thick poster board*
- *tracing paper*
- *pencil*
- *magnifying lens*
- *craft knife*
- *cellophane tape*
- *ruler*
- *scissors, for cutting tape*

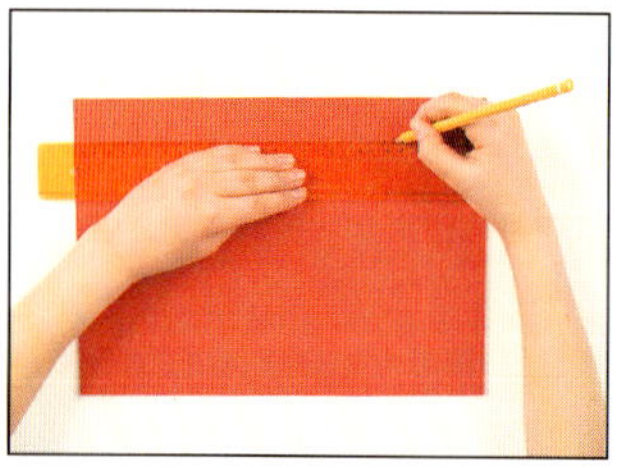

1 USE THE pencil and ruler to draw a window frame around the edges of the sheet of poster board.

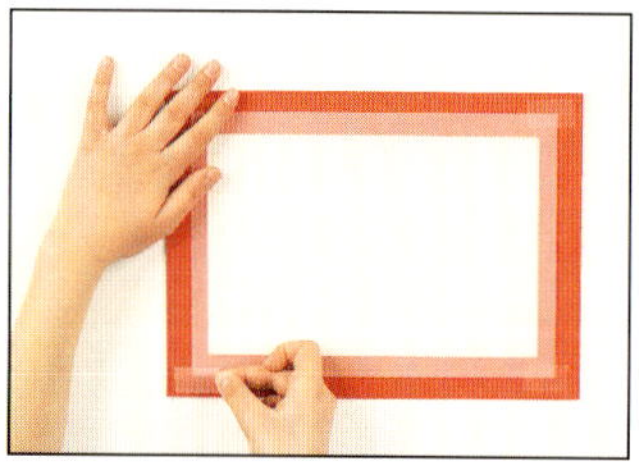

2 CAREFULLY cut out the "window." Tape tracing paper over it. This represents the eye's retina.

3 HOLD UP the frame between your face and the magnifying lens, which represents the eye lens. Look at a bright object, such as a window. Move the lens backward and forward until an image of the object appears on the screen. Is the image upside down? Find another bright object that is nearer. Which way do you need to move the lens to bring this object into focus? Now try an object that is farther away.

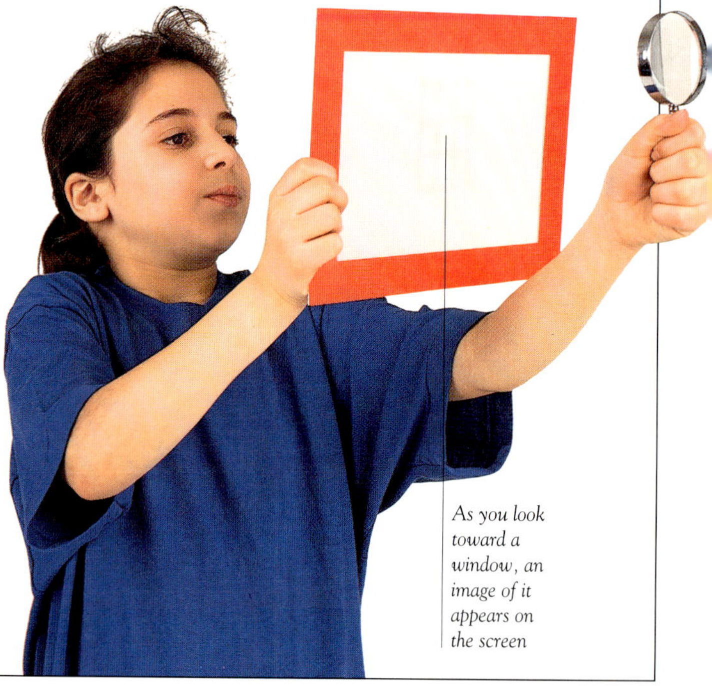

As you look toward a window, an image of it appears on the screen

Seeing sharply

In some eyes the cornea and lens do not focus correctly. In nearsighted eyes, light from distant objects focuses in front of the retina, so images of these objects on the retina itself are blurred. In farsighted eyes, light from nearby objects focuses behind the retina, so these objects seem blurred too. Farsighted or nearsighted people can wear glasses or contact lenses to correct the eye's focus.

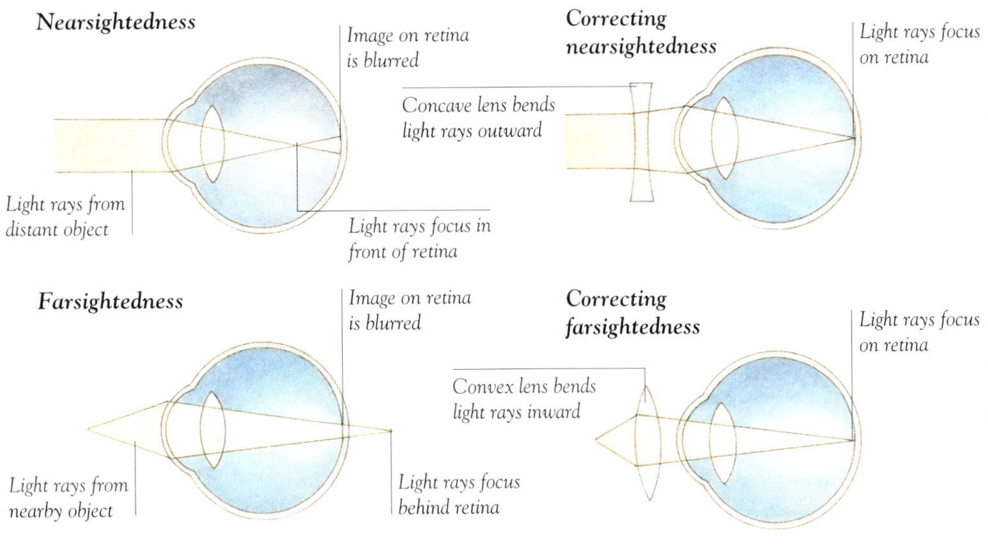

EXPERIMENT

Pupil reflex

Adult help is advised for this experiment

See your own eyes adjust their pupil size to allow in the right amount of light.

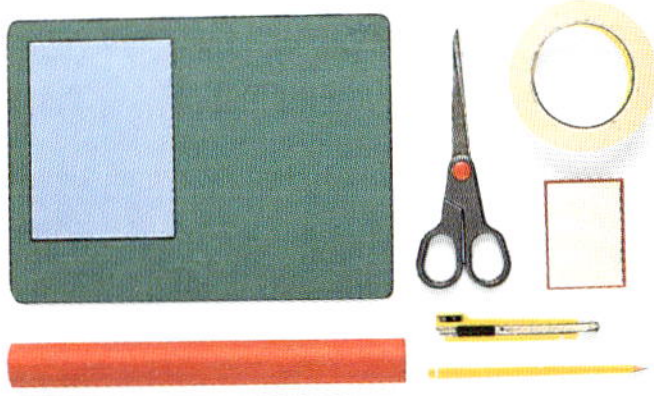

You Will Need

- *cutting mat* • *double-sided tape*
- *rectangular poster-board sheet*
- *small plastic-edged mirror*
- *cardboard tube* • *craft knife*
- *pencil* • *scissors*

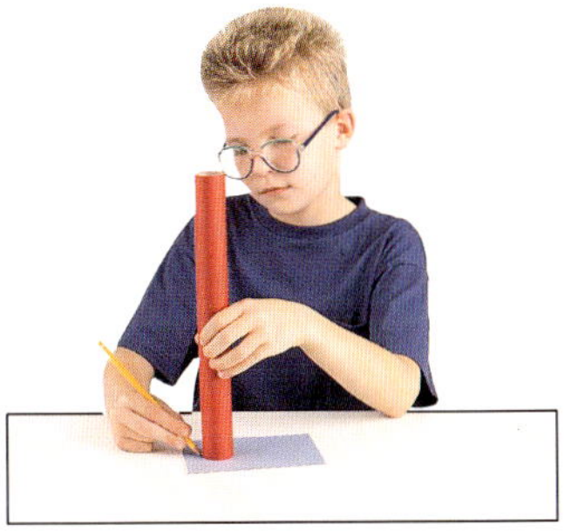

1 Hold the tube near a short edge of the poster board, and draw around it with the pencil.

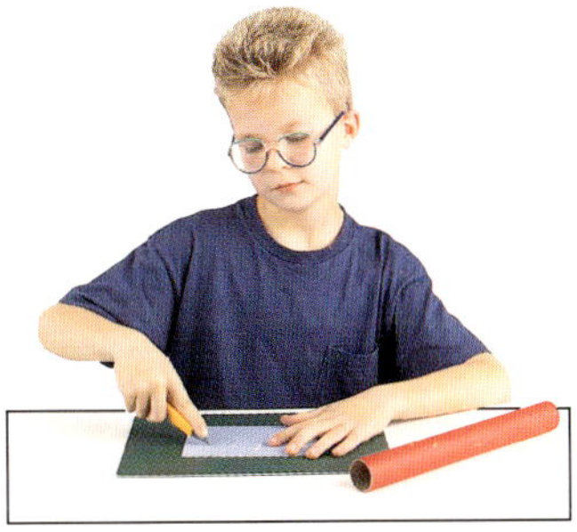

2 With the knife, carefully cut out the circle that you have drawn, so that the tube fits snugly into the hole.

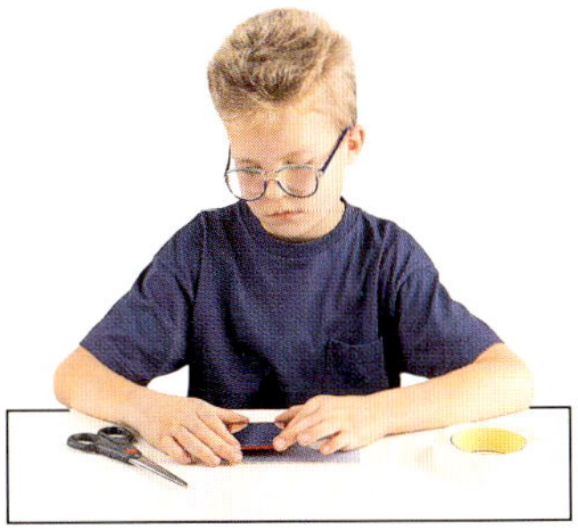

3 Tape the mirror onto the poster board. Its near edge should be about 1 in (2.5 cm) from the tube hole.

4 Push the tube into the hole, and hold it up to one eye, so that you can see your other eye in the mirror. With both eyes open, look at a bright window, then a dark corner. See how your pupil narrows in the light and widens in the dark. What happens if you put your hand over the end of the tube and look toward the window? Because your pupils always widen or narrow together, the pupil that is not covered widens at the same time as the covered one, even though it is looking toward the light.

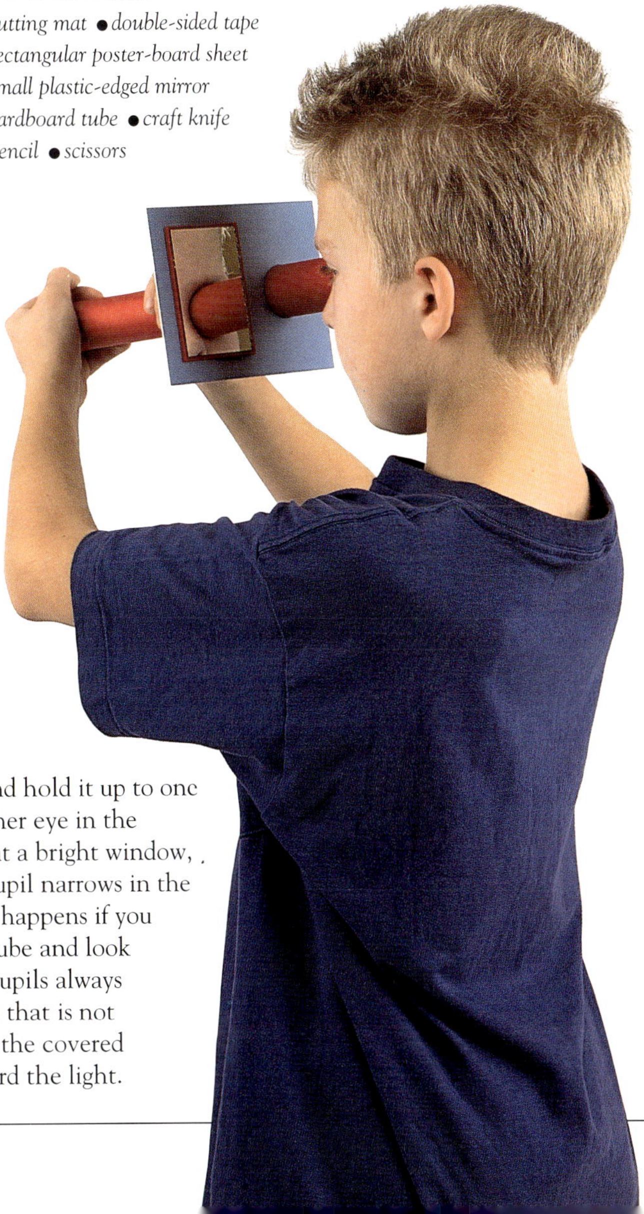

The sensitivity of the eyes

THE AMAZINGLY DETAILED VIEW of the world sensed by each eye is detected by more than 130 million light-sensitive cells in the retina (p.139). When light falls on one of these cells, the cell sends a tiny electrical signal to the brain. There are two types of light-sensitive cell—rod cells and cone cells, so-called because of their shapes. The 125 million rods in each eye are extremely sensitive, even when it is almost dark. But, like black-and-white film, they detect only shades (amounts of light) and not colors. The 6 million cones detect an object's details and colors, but do not work well in dim light.

Retinal rods and cones

Rods and cones are arranged unevenly in the retina. When you look straight at an object, its image falls on an area called the yellow spot, at the back of the retina. This is packed with cones, which see shapes and colors well. At the front of the retina, there are more rods and fewer cones.

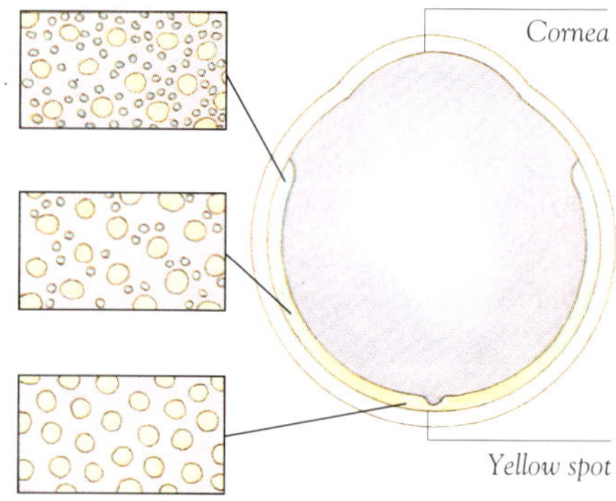

Front of retina
Mostly rod cells, so color vision is poor.

Side of retina
A mixture of rod and cone cells.

Back of retina
Yellow spot is packed with close-set cones.

EXPERIMENT

Fading colors

As light dims in the evening, your vision "grays" and colors seem to fade. This is because the cone cells, which let you see color, do not work in faint light. Instead, you rely on the "black-and-white" rods. Study color fading with this simple test.

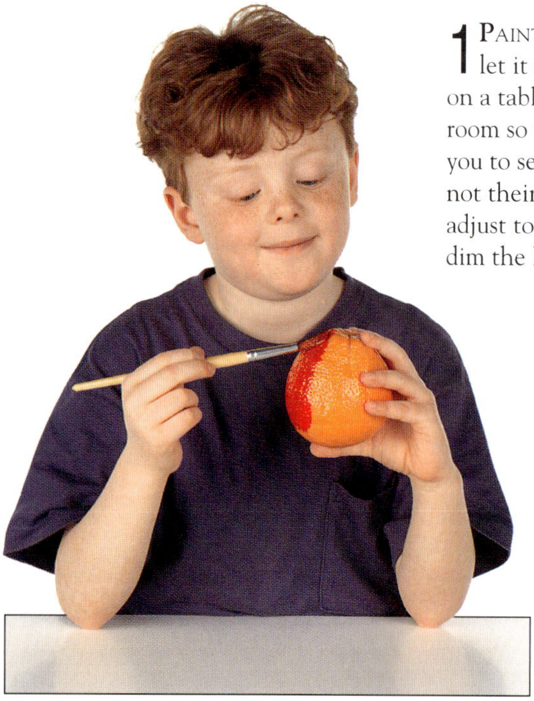

YOU WILL NEED

• *oranges* • *other fruits, such as apples and bananas* • *paintbrush* • *nontoxic red paint*

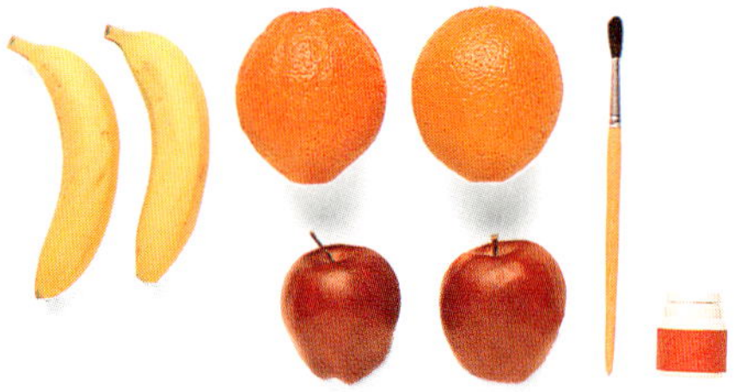

1 PAINT ONE of the oranges red, and let it dry. Put it with the other fruit on a table. Dim the lighting in the room so that it is almost dark, allowing you to see the shapes of the fruits—but not their colors. Give your eyes time to adjust to the new light conditions, then dim the lights further if necessary.

2 ASK A friend who knows nothing of the experiment to enter the room. Wait until his or her eyes adjust to the dim light. Hold up the fruits in a random order, and ask your friend to identify the different fruits and their colors. Now make the room brighter to reveal the color of the painted orange!

EXPERIMENT

The "vision meter"

Adult help is advised for this experiment

The concentration of rods at the sides and cones at the back of the retina means that your eye's sensitivity varies. It changes across its field of vision (the area you see) from side to center. Make a "vision meter" to gauge the point in your field of vision at which you can first see an object—here, a poster-board strip. At what point can you tell the object's color? When can you make out more details?

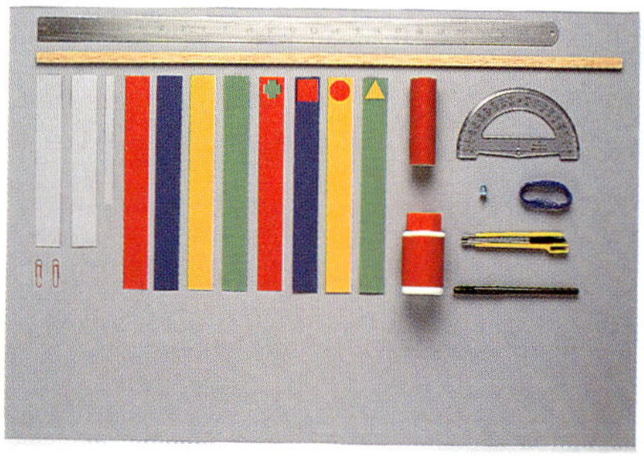

YOU WILL NEED

• *sheet of gray cardboard 30 in x 20 in (75 cm x 50 cm)* • *long ruler* • *28-in (70-cm) wood strip* • *2 strips of gray cardboard 8 in x 1 in (20 cm x 2.5 cm)* • *thin strip of gray cardboard* • *paper clips* • *colored poster-board strips 10 in x 1½ in (25 cm x 4 cm)* • *short wooden rod* • *glue* • *pen* • *protractor* • *map pin* • *thread* • *craft knife*

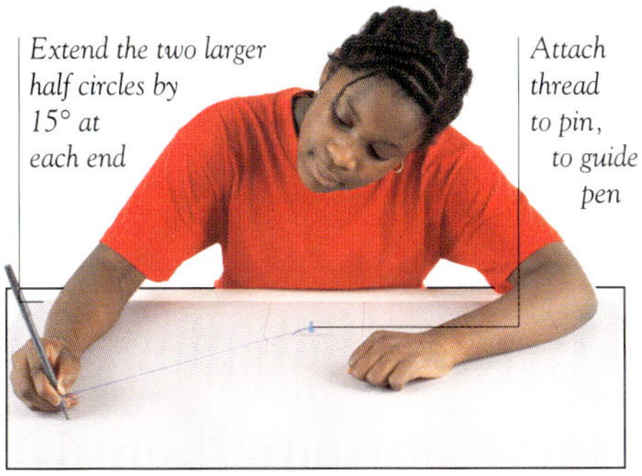

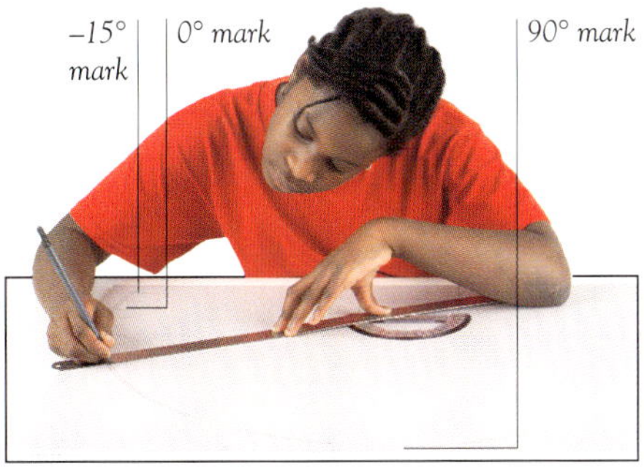

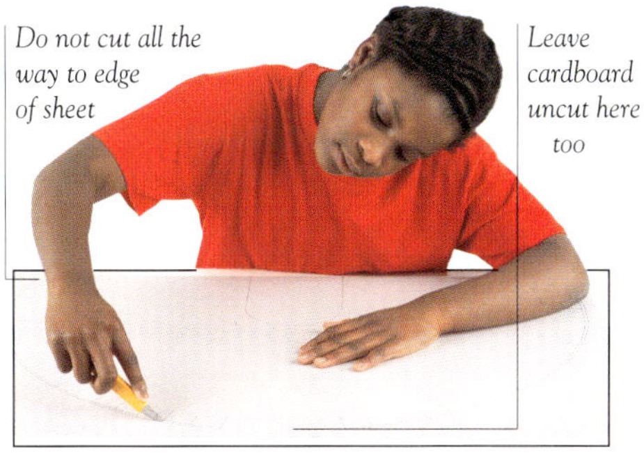

1 MARK A SQUARE with 5-in (12-cm) sides halfway along one of the sheet's long edges. Stick the pin halfway along the square's inner side. Draw three half circles with radii $2\frac{1}{2}$ in (6 cm), $13\frac{3}{4}$ in (34.5 cm), and 14 in (35 cm). Extend the two larger half circles as above.

2 PLACE THE PROTRACTOR with its base parallel to the sheet's long edge and the center of the base where the pin was. Use the ruler, pen, and protractor to mark every 5° around the $13\frac{3}{4}$-in (34.5-cm) half circle and the extra 15° at each end. Label each of the marks.

3 ON A SUITABLE surface, carefully cut out a slot between the two larger half-circles, as well as the extra 15° at each end of the half circles. But do not cut beyond the –15° marks, or for 10° each side of the center line (a line from the pinhole to the 90° mark).

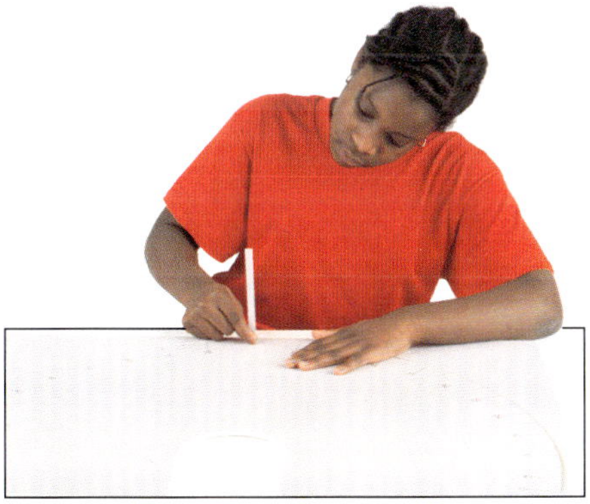

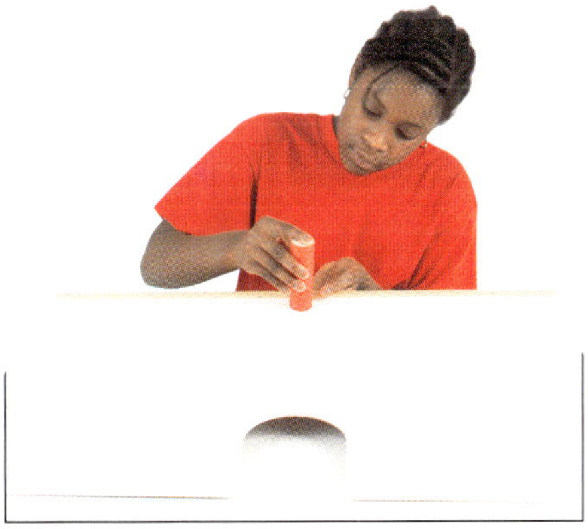

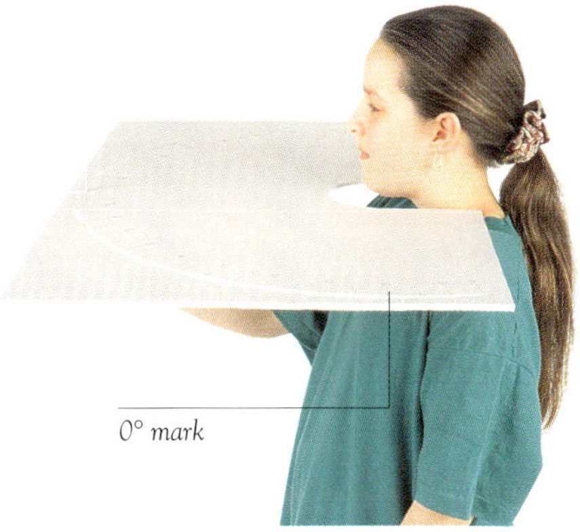

4 CUT OUT the 5-in (12-cm) square and smallest half circle to make a neck hole. Fold a short part of the thin gray strip, and glue it to the sheet at the center line, so that its main part sticks upright. This is the vision meter's sight.

5 TURN OVER the whole sheet. Glue the wooden strip along the long edge opposite the neck hole as a stiffener. Now glue the wooden rod directly under the sight as a handle. The vision meter is ready to use.

6 ASK A FRIEND to wear the vision meter. Make sure that each 0° mark is level with his or her eyes, and that your friend looks directly along the center line at the sight straight ahead.

7 FOLD ONE of the 8-in (20-cm) strips in two, and then fold the tips of each of the two ends outward. This is your test-card holder. Place it in the slit in the vision meter, so that the folded tips stop it from falling through. Now start the experiment. Insert a colored strip into the holder so it sticks upward. This is a test card. Secure it with a paper clip. Your friend must keep staring straight ahead at the sight. Starting from the –15° mark, slide the test card 5° around the slot every few seconds. Note the angle at which the test card first comes into the edge of his or her vision. Can your friend tell you what color the test card is, or do you need to move it farther? Stick shapes on the test cards (like those opposite). At what angles can your friend identify these shapes too?

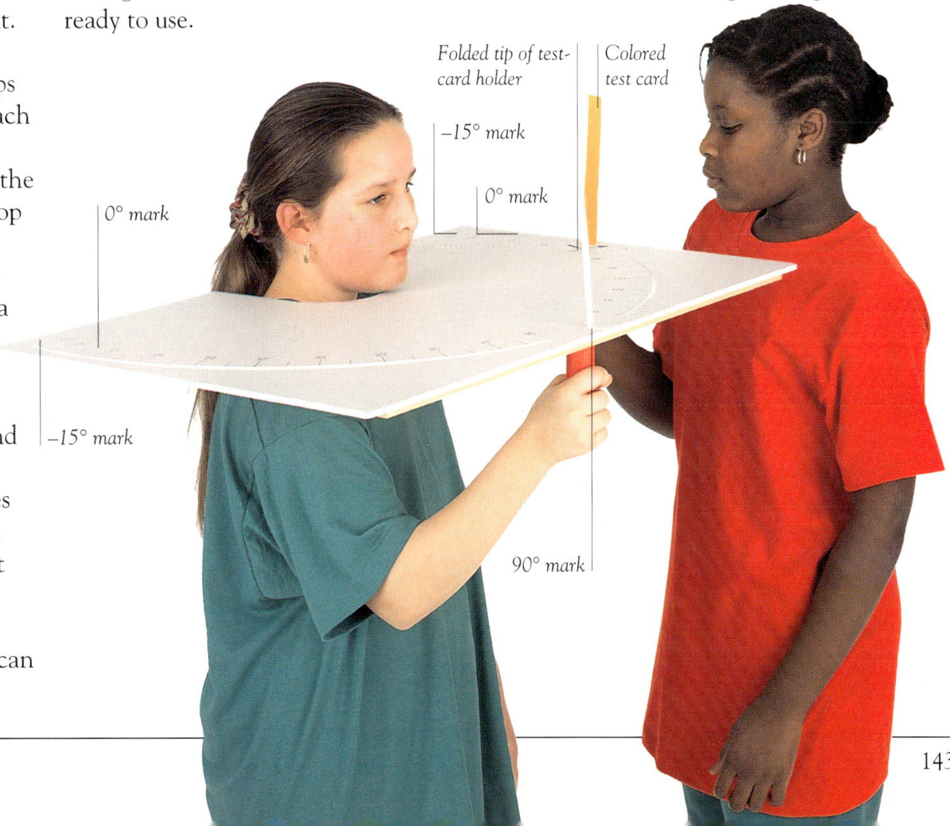

Seeing 3-D images

WHY DO WE HAVE TWO EYES? One reason is that two eyes can judge distances more accurately than one. Each eye's visual field covers a slightly different area, and each eye sees an object from a slightly different angle. The brain receives these two different, overlapping views of an object, but it combines them, so we see only one image. The different angles and surfaces in this combined, 3-D (three-dimensional) image provide clues about how far away the object is. Seeing with two eyes is called binocular or stereoscopic vision.

EXPERIMENT

Two views

Adult help is advised for this experiment

Photographers make "3-D pictures" by printing two slightly different views of the same scene (right), which overlap, but which are in different colors. You can use glasses with colored filters, so that each eye sees only one view. The brain combines the two views into a 3-D scene.

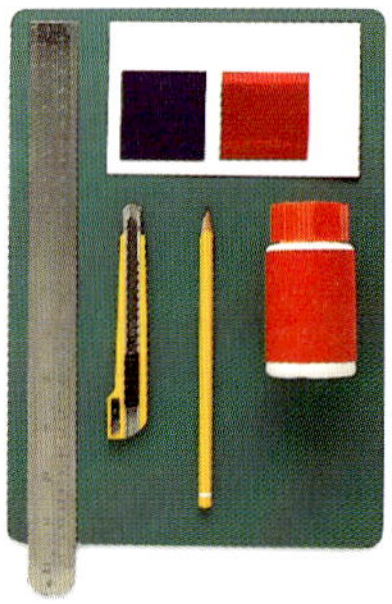

YOU WILL NEED

• cutting mat • metal ruler • poster board 6 in x 3 in (15 cm x 8 cm) • blue and red transparent cellophane from candy wrappers, or the like • craft knife • pencil • glue

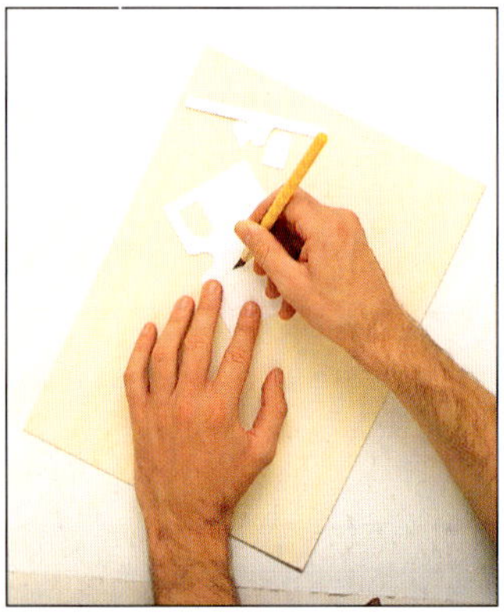

1 DRAW THE SHAPE of some eyeglasses on poster board. Carefully cut them out. Cut out two "lenses" from the cellophane, slightly larger than the lens holes in the glasses. Use blue for the right eye and red for the left. Glue in place on the glasses.

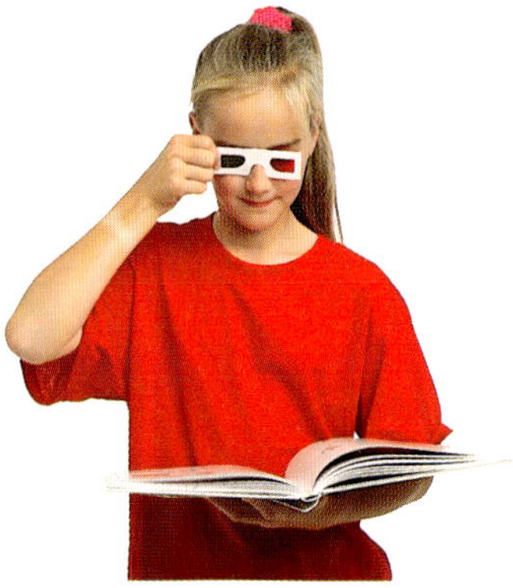

2 LOOK THROUGH your 3-D glasses at the cityscape (right). The blue filter lets only blue light through, so the right eye sees only the blue view. The red filter lets only red light through, so the left eye sees only the red view. Do you see the scene in 3-D?

EXPERIMENT

Holey hand

Normally, the images from your two eyes are very similar. The brain combines them into one view. In this experiment, the images are quite different. One of your eyes looks at your hand. The other eye looks through a tube and sees a small circular part of the scene in front of you. But the brain still combines the two images as usual. So it looks as if you had a see-through hole in your hand.

YOU WILL NEED

• tube about 1 ft (30 cm) long and 1 1/2 in (3 cm) in diameter

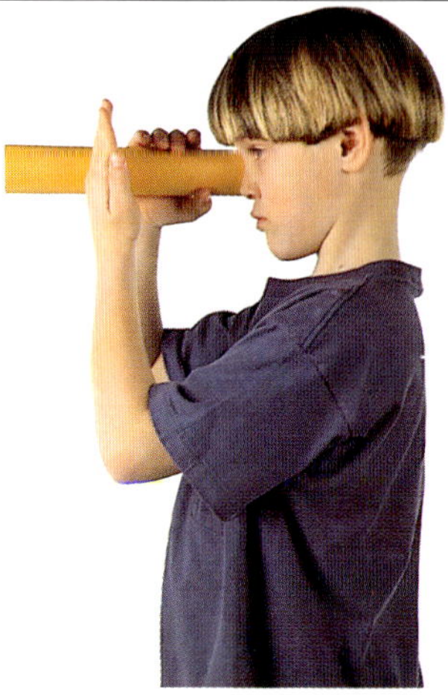

Two views into one

Keep both eyes open. Hold the tube up to one eye. Place your other hand at the side of the end of the tube, with the palm facing you. Slowly bring your palm toward you along the side of the tube. You should see a hole appear in the middle of your hand.

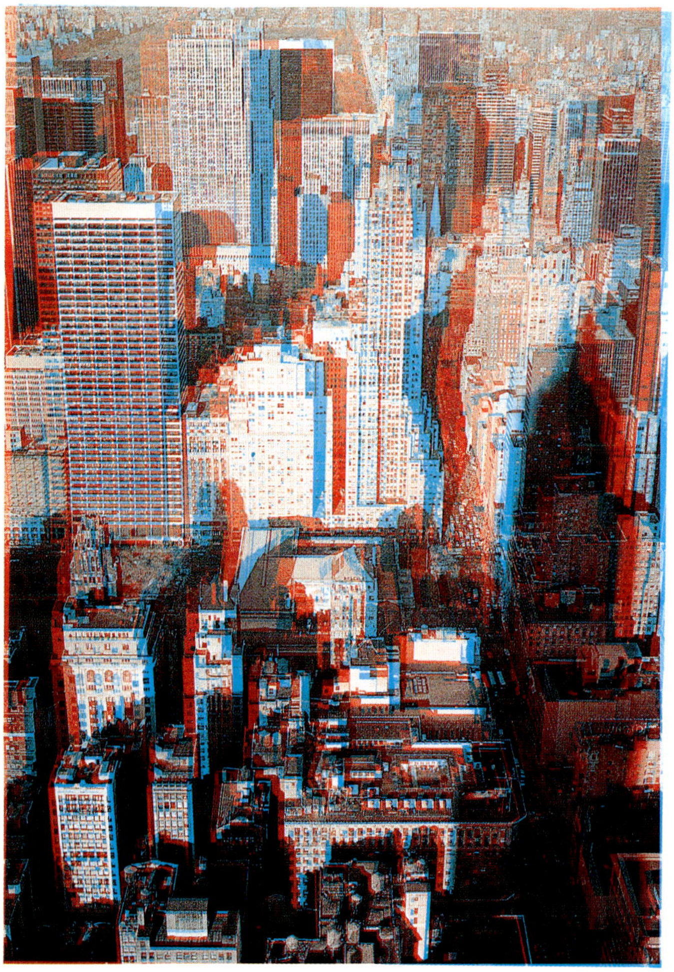

Combining views

Look at an object, such as a die, about 1 ft (30 cm) away. Cover one eye, then the other, as you study it. Each view is different, because each eye looks at the object from a different position. See how the angles of the object's edges and the shapes of its surfaces alter slightly between the two views. Each eye sends different messages to the visual cortex (p.127), which has two sides. The two sets of messages combine in the brain to give binocular vision.

Visual pathways in the brain
Turn this page sideways so that you are looking in the same direction as the person in the diagram. The pictures A, B, and C show the view that you would expect to see with the left eye, the right eye, and both eyes respectively.

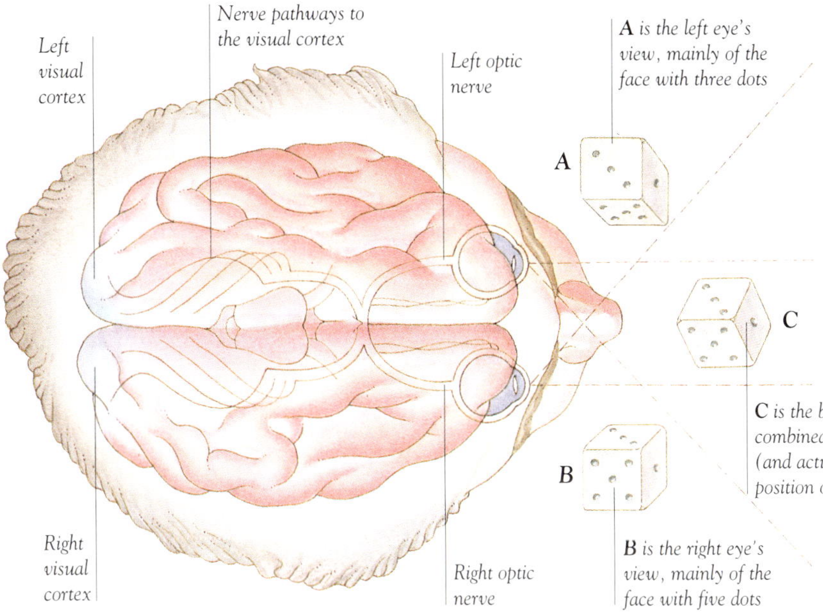

EXPERIMENT

Judging distance

Adult help is advised for this experiment

In this experiment you aim to hit a target with balls of modeling clay. Your binocular vision helps you judge distances accurately, while the same test is difficult with one eye covered.

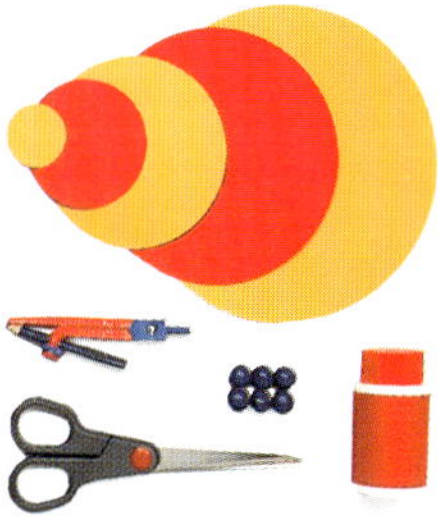

You Will Need

- *colored paper or poster board*
- *compass*
- *pencil*
- *balls of modeling clay*
- *scissors*
- *glue*

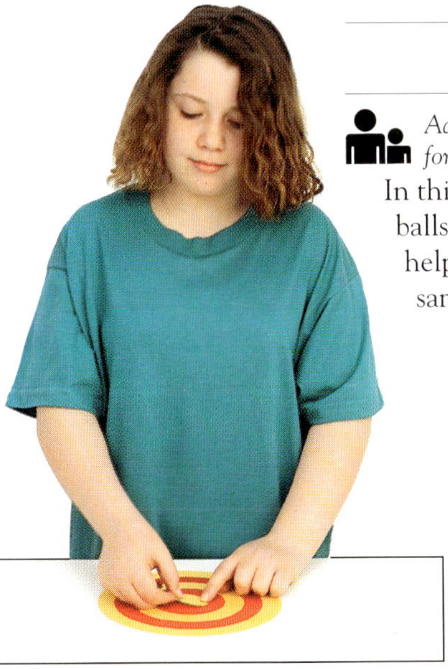

1 Draw and cut out five circles of paper. Make the first 2 in (5 cm) in diameter, the next circle 2 in (5 cm) larger, and so on. Make alternate circles different colors. Glue them together to make a target.

2 Place the target on a table. Stand about 4 ft (1.2 m) away, and cover one eye. A friend holds a ball over the table. Ask the friend to move the ball left or right, forward or backward, so that the ball drops onto the target. Is it easier to hit the bull's-eye with one eye or two?

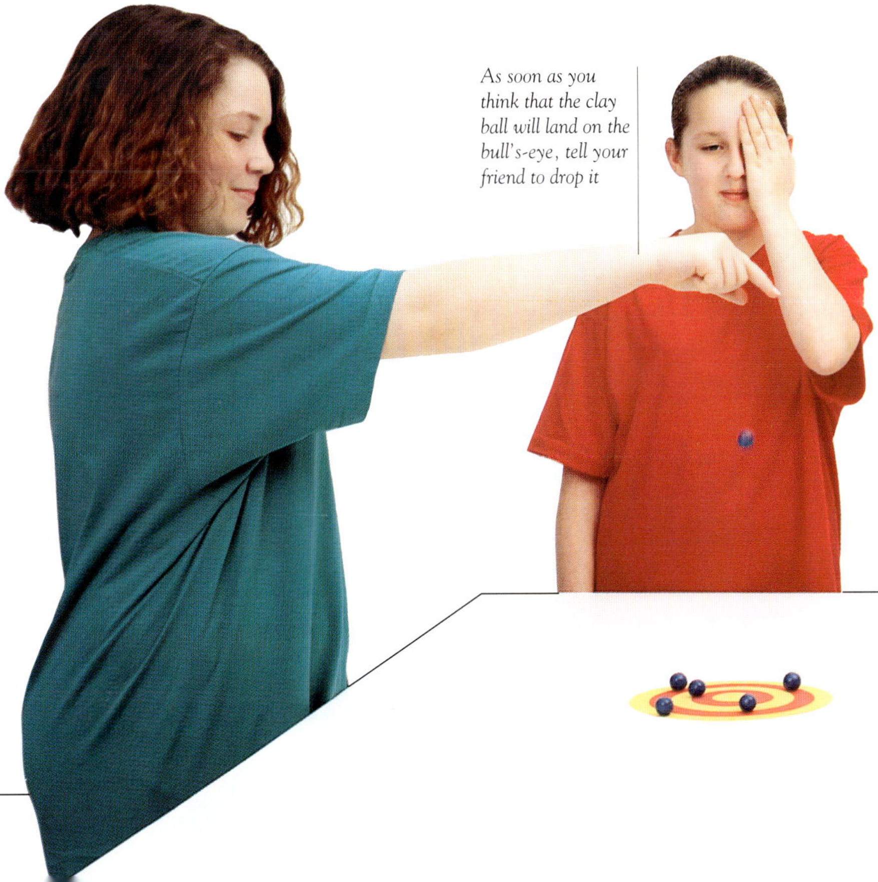

As soon as you think that the clay ball will land on the bull's-eye, tell your friend to drop it

Eyes and coordination

CLOSE YOUR EYES. Without looking, you can sense the positions of your head, neck, torso (trunk), and limbs. This is because millions of microscopic stretch sensors, called proprioceptors, in the muscles and joints are continually sending nerve signals to your brain. These signals tell the brain which muscles are relaxed or contracted, and which joints are bent or straight. However, sometimes this inner awareness of body position (proprioception) is not accurate enough. To get a good sense of the positions of your hands and arms, for example, you regularly look at them. This is especially important when you are making precise movements or carrying out rapid, coordinated actions such as catching a ball (opposite). It is called hand-eye coordination, though in fact the brain is the vital link between hand and eye.

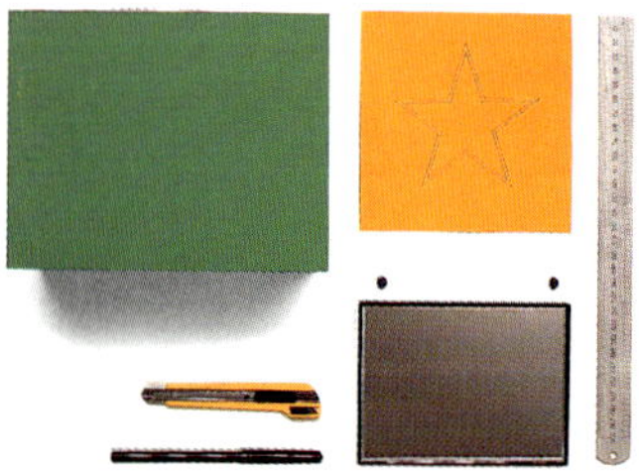

YOU WILL NEED

• cardboard shoe box • several sheets of paper • craft knife • felt-tip pen • modeling clay • plastic-edged mirror to fit inside the shoe box • metal ruler

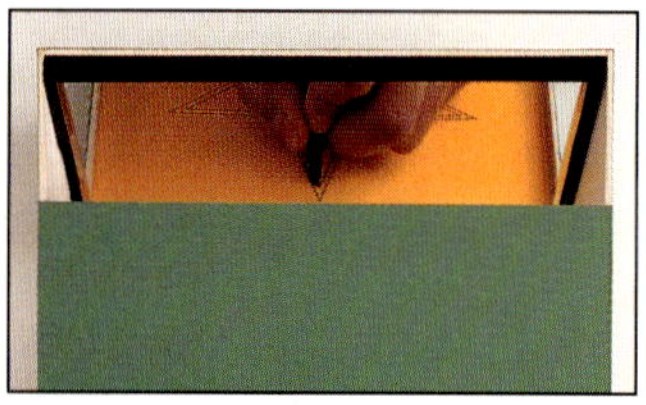

Adjusting the mirror

Before you start to draw, look through the top hole to check that you can see the stars reflected in the mirror. If not, adjust the angle of the mirror by moving the clay blobs.

EXPERIMENT

Mirror drawing

Adult help is advised for this experiment

You use your eyes to monitor the marks you make when you draw or write and to check small adjustments. But in this experiment your eyes are tricked as you draw a star shape, because your hand movements are reversed in a mirror. See how confusing and frustrating this can be.

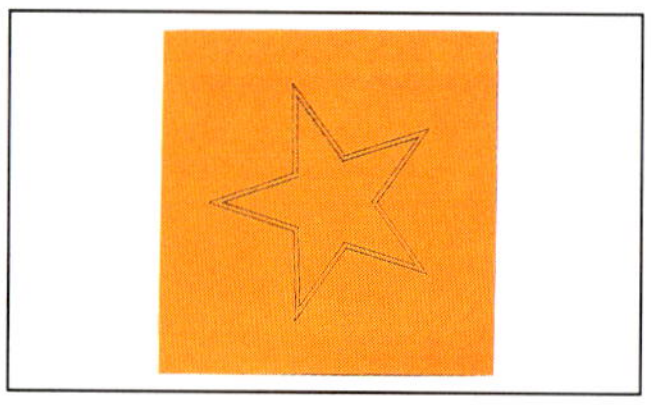

1 USING THE felt-tip pen, draw two neat stars, one slightly inside the other. Do this on several sheets of paper. (The paper should fit inside the shoe box.)

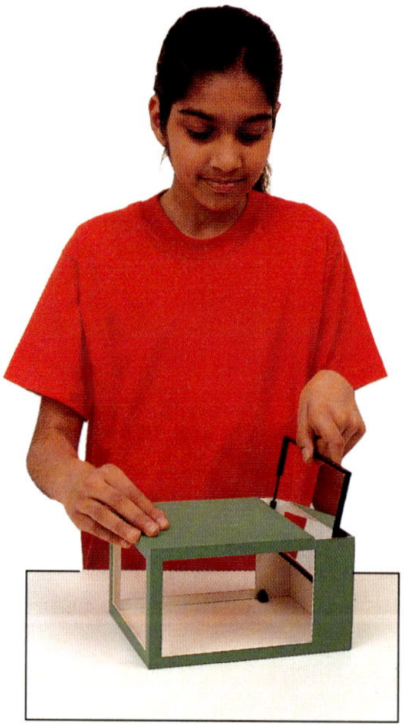

2 VERY CAREFULLY cut four rectangular panels from the shoe box, using the craft knife and ruler. Make sure that you use a suitable cutting surface. Remove the panels shown on the left: most of one of the ends of the box; three-quarters of each side nearest the cut-out end; and one-quarter of the top, farthest from the cut-out end. This is your drawing chamber. Slide the mirror through the top hole, and lean it at an angle against that end of the box. Use blobs of modeling clay to prevent the mirror from sliding down into the box.

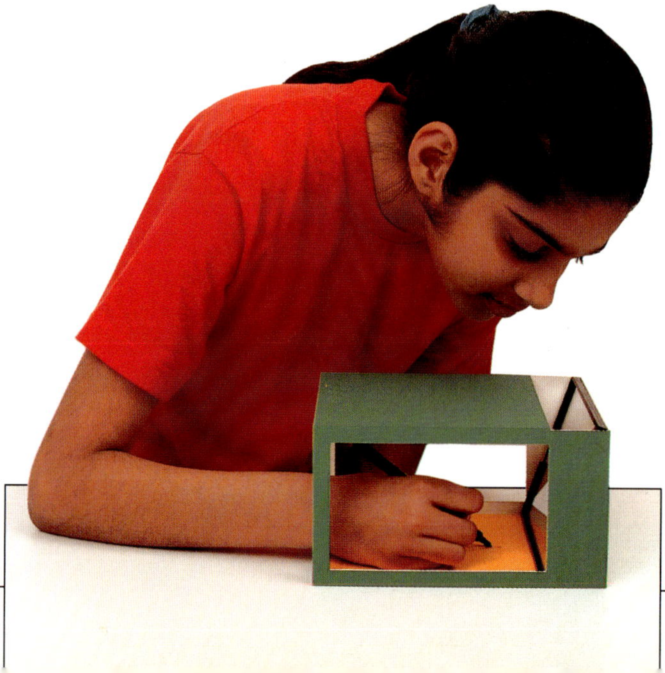

3 PLACE ONE of the star shapes in the drawing chamber. Hold your pen inside the chamber. Now try to draw a new star between the existing two sets of lines, watching your hand in the mirror only. Looking in the mirror, your eye gives your brain information about the hand's position—but it is the reverse of the information sent by your proprioceptors. So you may mean to move your hand one way, yet it goes the other! Does your drawing improve with practice?

EXPERIMENT

Keep your eye on the ball

Watch a friend throw a tennis ball up and catch it. He or she watches the ball on the way up and down. The hands are positioned exactly in the line of the ball's falling path. If your friend looks away while the ball is in the air, a secure catch is much more difficult.

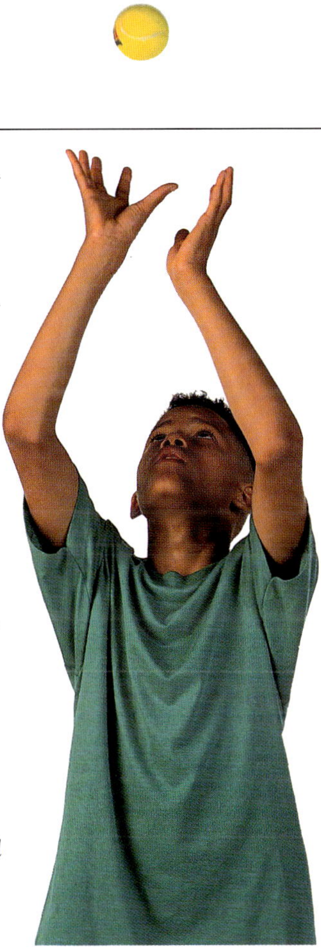

Holding out hands
The eyes watch the ball, while the brain monitors the positions of the arms and hands by the inner proprioceptive sense, and adjusts the arm and hand muscles. At the last moment, the eyes see both ball and hands together. Now try to throw and catch a ball with your eyes closed. Is it possible?

EXPERIMENT

Which finger is which?

Your eyes watch your hands to confirm their positions as monitored by your proprioceptors (stretch sensors, opposite). But if your hands are in an unfamiliar position, the information from proprioception and your eyes may not match—often with confusing results.

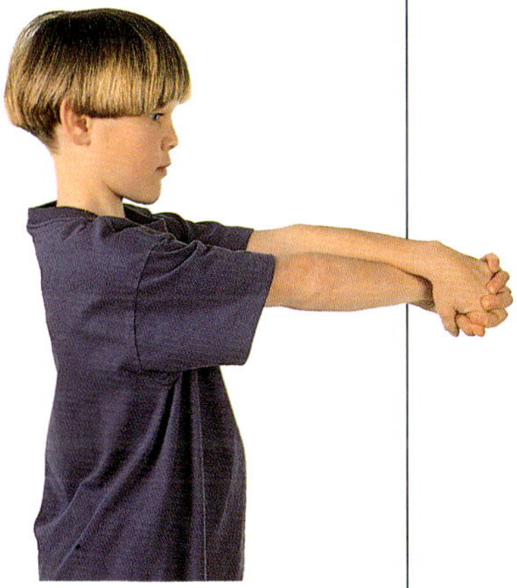

1 HOLD YOUR ARMS out and crossed so that the palms meet. Interlock your fingers.

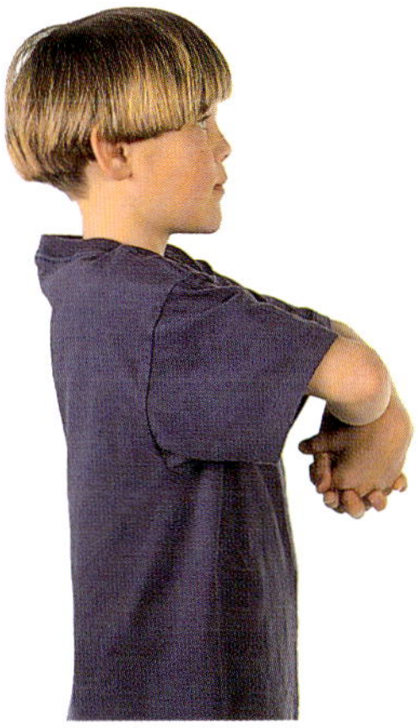

2 BEND YOUR ELBOWS to move your hands down and in toward your body.

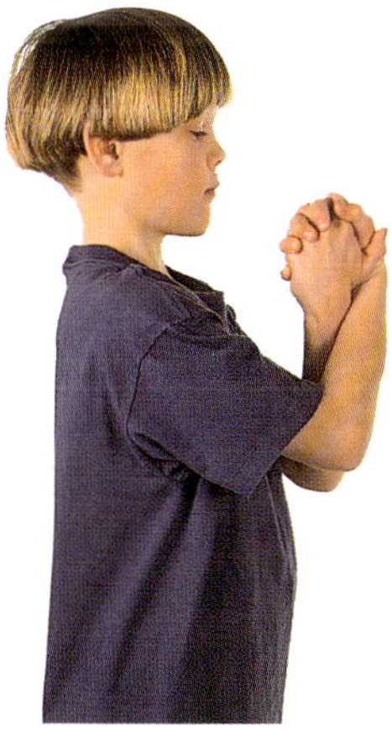

3 KEEP BENDING your elbows and wrists so that your hands come up past your chest.

4 HOLD YOUR fingers in this position. Ask a friend to point to one finger, without touching it. Try to move that finger quickly. Did you move the correct finger? Is it easier if your friend touches it?

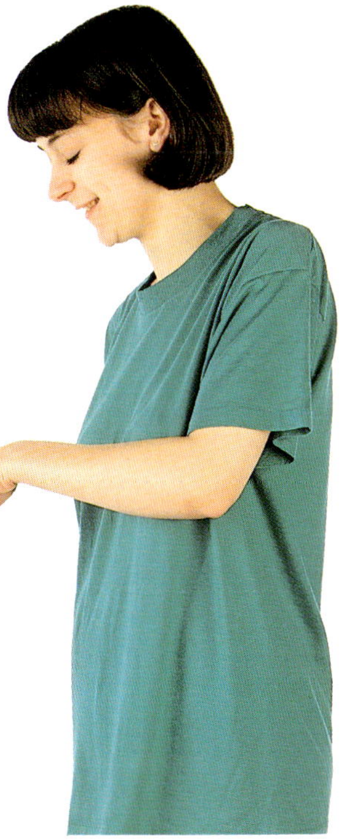

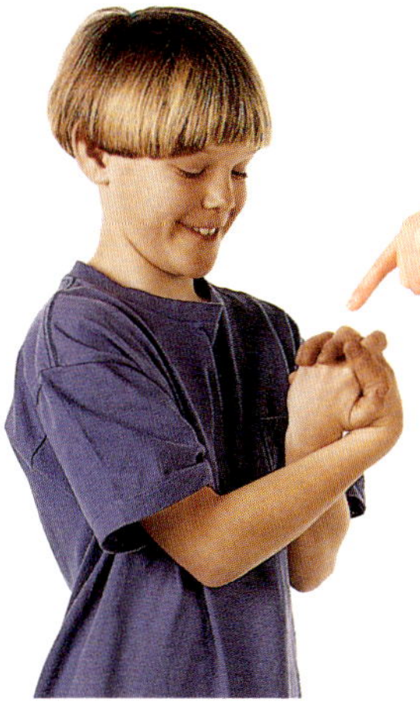

EXPERIMENT

Writing without seeing

As you write, your eyes continually scan the sizes, shapes, and positions of the letters. You make adjustments as you go along. If you close your eyes, you no longer have this visual feedback, so your writing may become messy.

YOU WILL NEED
- *pen*
- *large sheet of paper*

Writing blind
On the paper, neatly write something familiar, such as numbers from 0 to 10. Then write the numbers again, but with your eyes closed. Are the letters as evenly sized, shaped, and spaced as the first version? Muscles and joints can give some feedback about hand movements and positions, but the eyes provide precise detail.

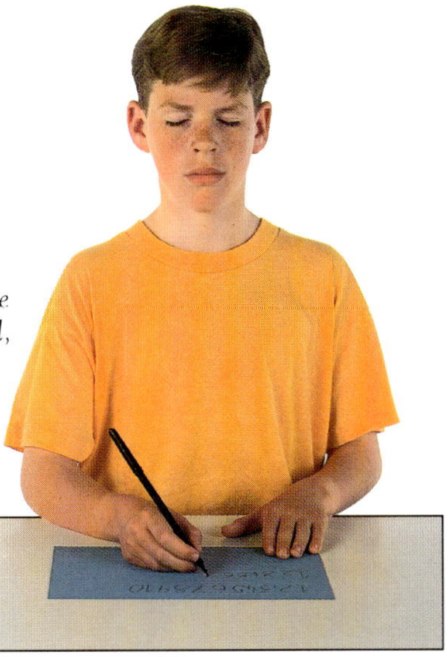

The limits of the eyes

PROFESSIONAL PHOTOGRAPHERS change their cameras and lenses for different tasks, such as achieving a wide field of vision or photographing in dim light. No single lens is suitable for all shots. In the same way our eyes have limitations—many of which are due to their design and structure. For example, objects that are moving very quickly appear blurred to us. Also, there are areas in our field of vision (the area we see) that are blank. If the brain could not "fill in" these areas, we would see patches of shadow.

EXPERIMENT

Seeing what isn't there

Adult help is advised for this experiment

This experiment reveals the hole that the blind spot causes in vision. It also shows how the brain fills in the blank area using information from the colors, shapes, and patterns around it.

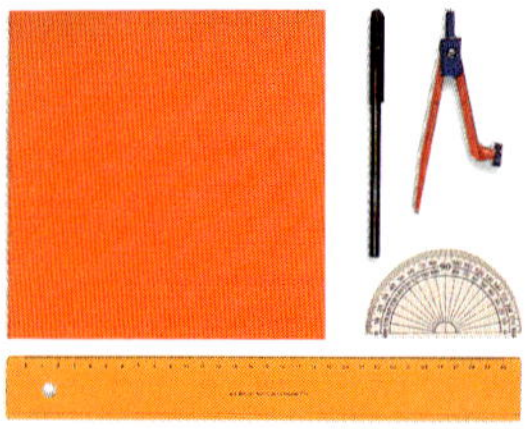

YOU WILL NEED

- *sheet of poster board about 8 in x 8 in (20 cm x 20 cm)*
- *ruler*
- *felt-tip pen*
- *compass*
- *protractor*

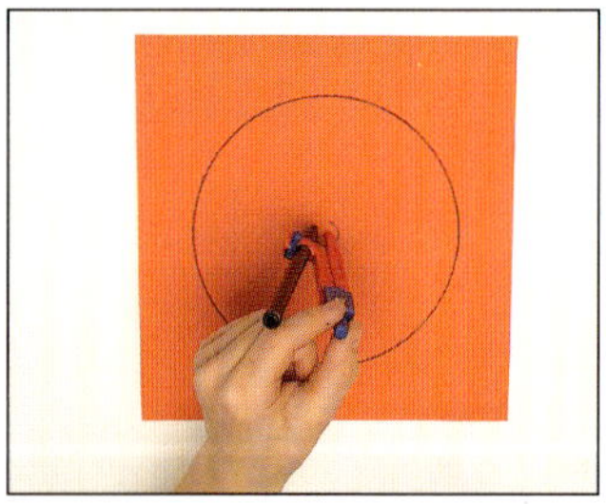

1 WITH THE compass, draw two concentric circles of diameters 6 in (15 cm) and ¾ in (2 cm) on the card.

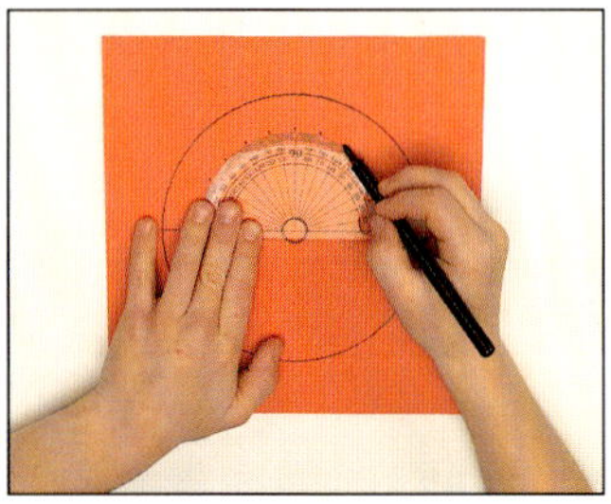

2 PLACE THE center of the protractor on the center of the circles. Draw marks at 15° intervals all around. Do the same with the protractor upside down, so you have 24 marks in a full 360° circle.

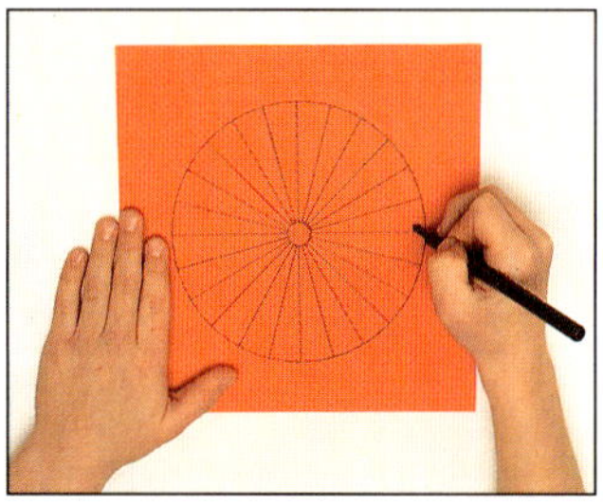

3 DRAW A line from each 15° mark to the compass hole to make a spoked-wheel pattern, leaving the central circle empty. Mark a spot near the end of the right horizontal spoke, as shown.

The blind spot

As you look around, you seem to have an uninterrupted view. But each eye has a blank area in its field of vision. This blank area is due to the blind spot—where the optic nerve and its blood vessels join the retina (p.139). There are no light-sensitive cells on that part of the retina, so images are not detected there. We do not normally notice the blind spot for several reasons. First, an image that falls on the blind spot of one eye is usually seen by the other eye. Second, our eyes are continually darting around, so they rarely look at the same scene long enough for the brain to notice the gap. Third, the brain learns to fill in missing parts of the image (left).

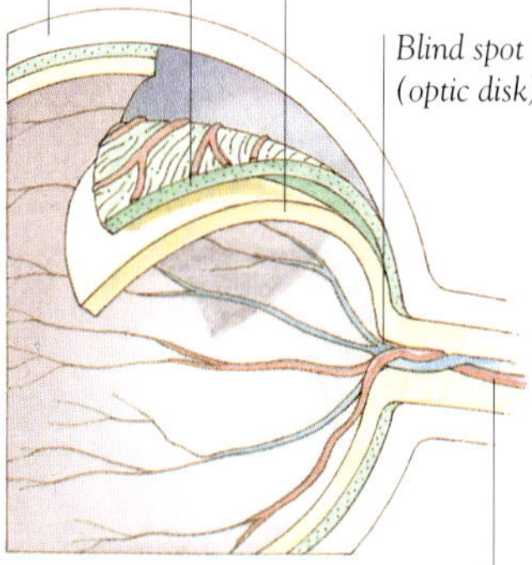

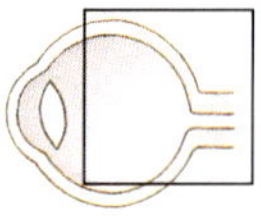

Blind spot position
The illustration above is an enlargement of the rear of an eyeball (right).

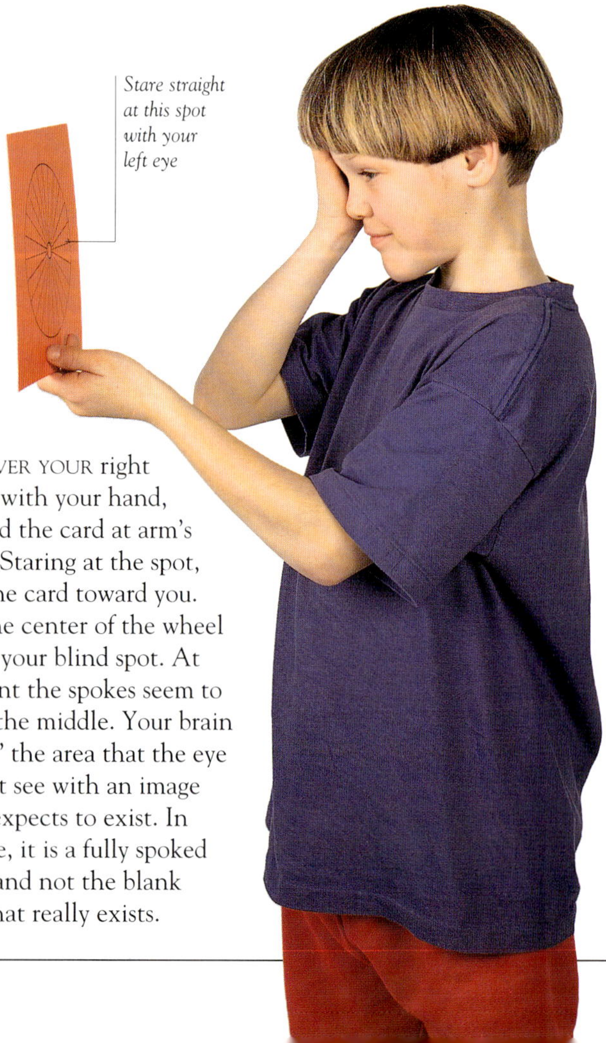

4 COVER YOUR right eye with your hand, and hold the card at arm's length. Staring at the spot, move the card toward you. Soon the center of the wheel falls on your blind spot. At this point the spokes seem to join in the middle. Your brain "fills in" the area that the eye does not see with an image that it expects to exist. In this case, it is a fully spoked wheel, and not the blank circle that really exists.

Complementary colors

The retina has three types of cone cell (p.142). Each type mainly detects only one color of light—red, green, or blue. However, our perception of the color of an object is affected by other factors, such as how long we look at it. Cones may stop working after they have been exposed to their color for a long period of time. The other cones then take over, and if we look away from the object, we often see a "ghost" color that is different from the original. This is called a complementary color. Which complementary colors do you see after you stare at the picture below?

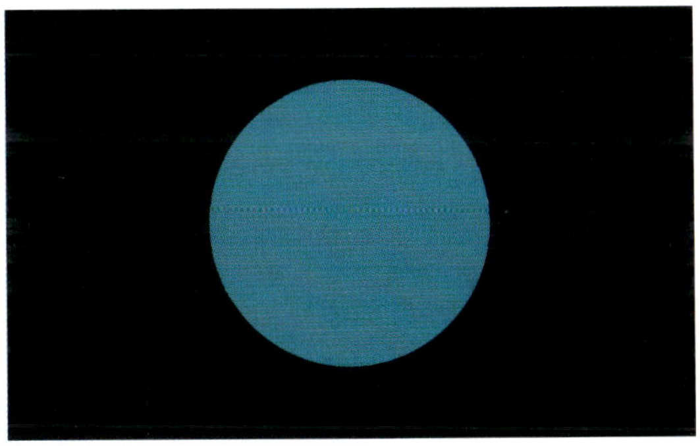

Find the Japanese flag
In bright light stare at this picture for 20 seconds, then look at a blank white surface. Can you see an after-image in complementary colors?

EXPERIMENT

Seeing your own retina

This experiment should not be attempted by children alone. Ask an adult to hold the candle for you

The retina has blood vessels that cast shadows on the light-sensitive cells beneath. However, we usually concentrate on images formed by light shining through the central area of the lens. This light always casts shadows in the same places on the retina, so the brain learns to fill in the gaps in vision made by them. But a light source that comes from the side and jumps about, such as a candle flame, can reveal these shadows.

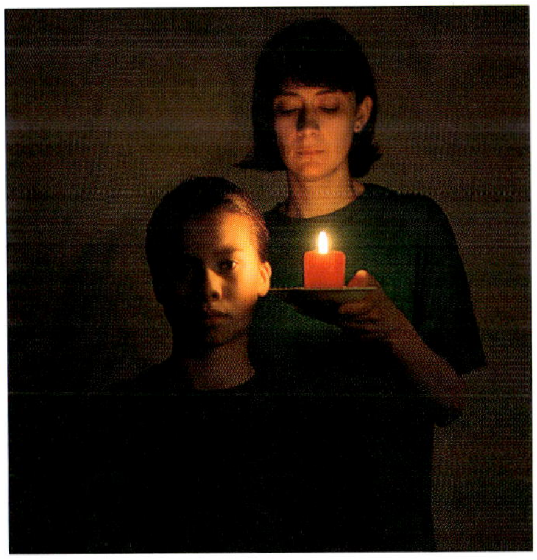

Retinal shadows
In a dark room an adult helper holds a candle 6 in (15 cm) from the side of your head (but no closer), level with your eyes. Look straight ahead. You may see shadows of retinal blood vessels. The brain is unused to the flickering light coming from the side, so it is unable to fill in the gaps made by these shadows.

EXPERIMENT

Seeing a blur

Adult help is advised for this experiment

The eye's rod and cone cells respond to light by sending nerve signals to the brain. The nerve signals are caused by a chemical reaction set off by the energy in light. Each rod or cone cell needs a recovery period to re-form its chemicals before it can make another signal. This recovery takes no more than a few thousandths of a second. Even so, the scene that you see can change in a much shorter time. As you look at something, some cells are responding while others are recovering. So fast-changing images seem to blur together into a continuous sequence. Study this blurring effect with a spinning disk.

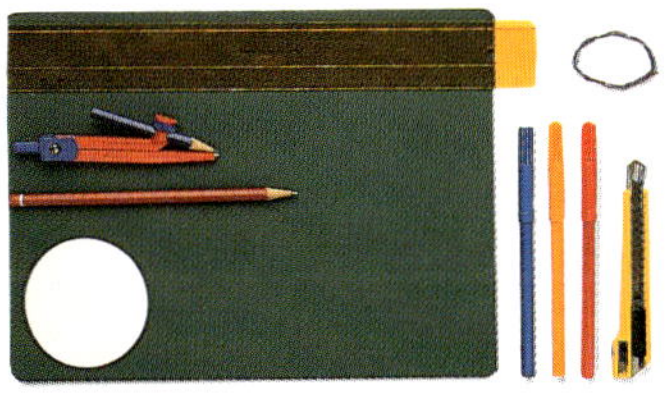

YOU WILL NEED
- *cutting mat* • *compass* • *pencil*
- *white poster board* • *string or thread* • *ruler* • *craft knife*
- *colored felt-tip pens*

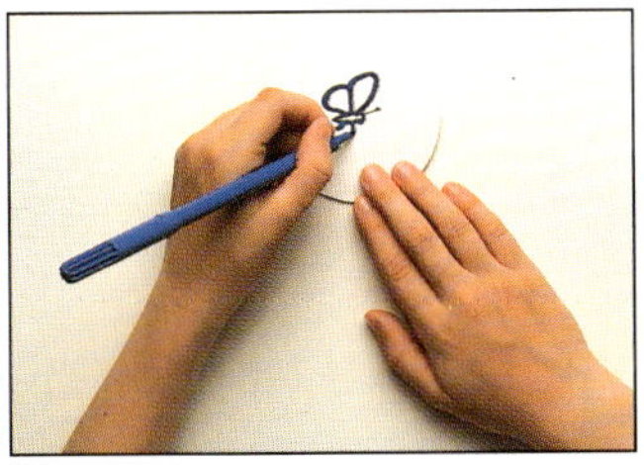

1 USE THE compass to draw a circle about 3 in (8 cm) in diameter on the poster board. Cut out the circle to make a disk. Draw a butterfly on one side and a flower, in a different color, on the other.

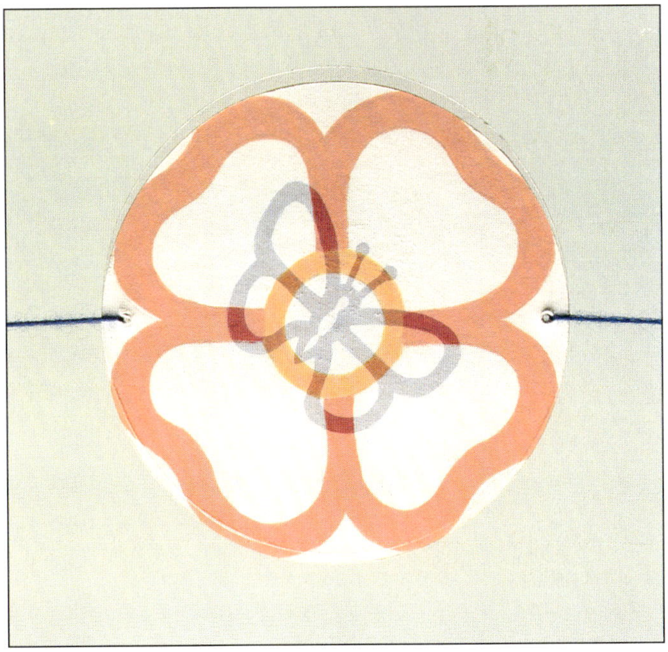

2 MAKE TWO HOLES, at opposite edges of the disk. Feed equal lengths of string through each hole, and tie the ends of each length to form a loop. Hold the loops in your hands, and whirl the disk to twist the strings. Now pull on both strings. As they untwist, the disk spins so fast that the two sides blur into one image. See how the butterfly seems to sit on the flower.

Tricking the eyes and brain

FROM BIRTH, WE LEARN to look and make sense of what we see. The brain devises various ways and methods of interpreting and making sense of the images detected by the eyes. When the eyes see an unusual or novel series of images, the brain may not be able to interpret them in the usual way. The results can be very confusing, as shown by the "visual tricks" on these pages.

EXPERIMENT

Expanding disk

Adult help is advised for this experiment

If a spiral on a disk is spinning one way, your brain gets the impression that the disk is expanding. If the spiral turns the other way, it seems to contract. In a short time, your brain gets used to this movement. If you quickly look at something else, then it too may seem to expand or contract for a moment.

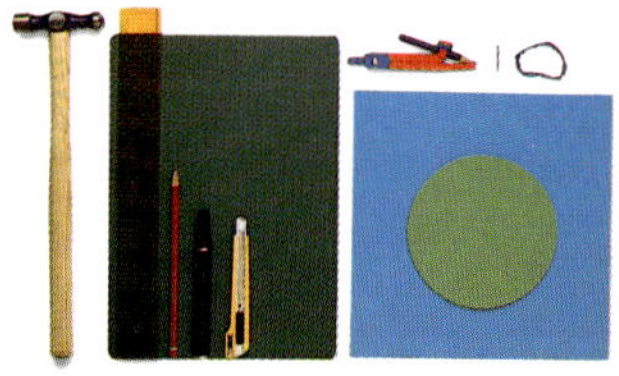

YOU WILL NEED

• hammer • cutting mat • ruler • sharpened pencil • thick marker • craft knife • compass with pencil • nail • thread • wooden board • thick poster-board square with sides of 6 in (15 cm)

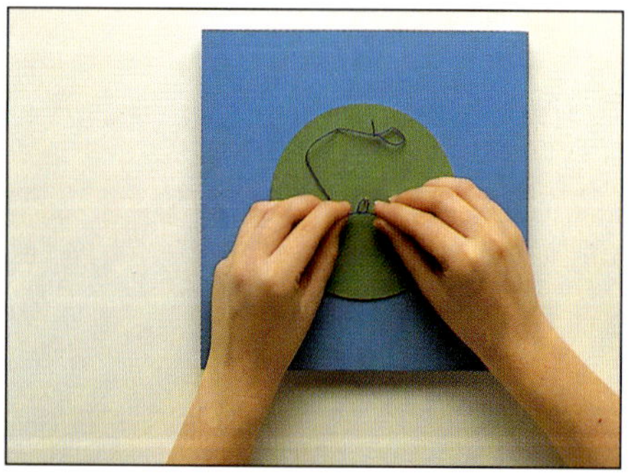

1 DRAW A CIRCLE on the poster board with the compass, and cut out a disk. Hammer the nail through the disk center a short way into the wood board. Tie a loop in one end of the thread to fit the marker barrel. Tie the other end to the nail. Put the marker barrel in the loop.

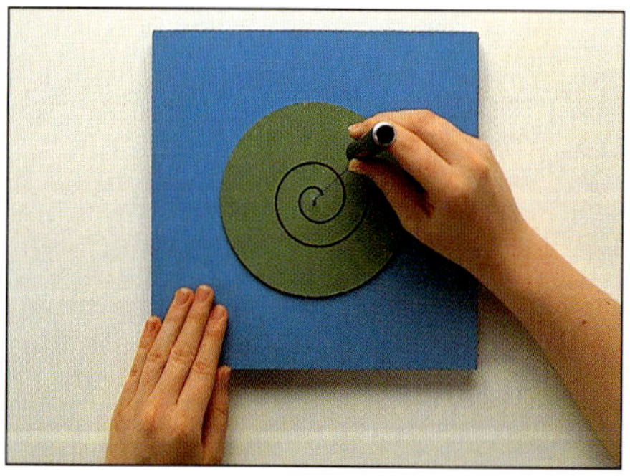

2 TWIST THE marker so that the thread winds neatly around the barrel, pulling the marker toward the nail, but without marking the disk. Then make a spiral with the marker, by drawing in a circular motion as the string unwinds. Keep the string taut as it unravels.

3 REMOVE THE nail and push the sharpened pencil through the center of the disk, so that about 1 in (2.5 cm) sticks out below. With your fingers, twist the pencil steadily on its point to spin the disk. Does the disk seem to expand or shrink? Twist the disk the other way. Is the effect reversed? Watch the disk as it "expands" for 20 seconds, then quickly look at a stationary object nearby. Does the object seem to expand or shrink?

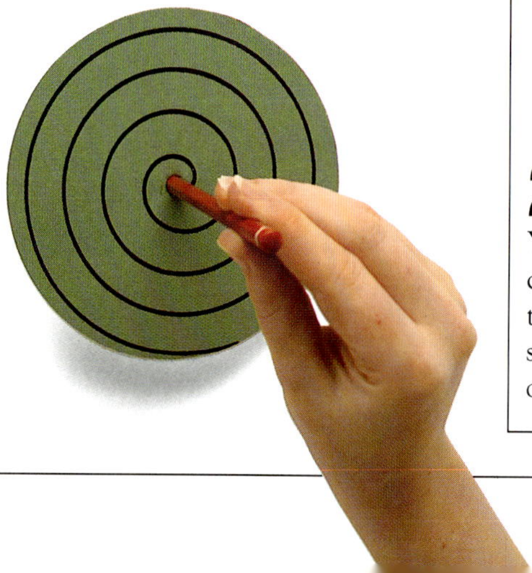

EXPERIMENT

Moving circles

Adult help is advised for this experiment

When you look at close-set circles, their lines become confused and your brain may imagine spinning motions that do not exist.

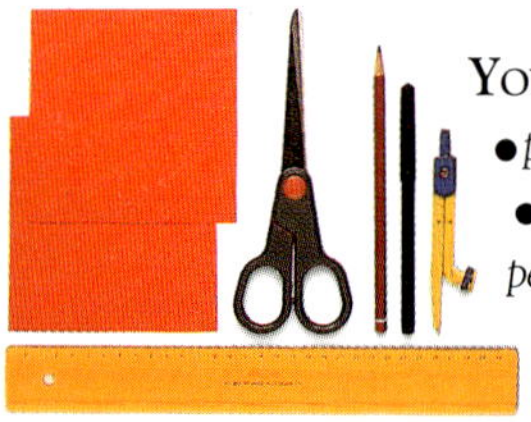

YOU WILL NEED

• poster board • scissors • felt-tip pen • ruler • compass • pencil

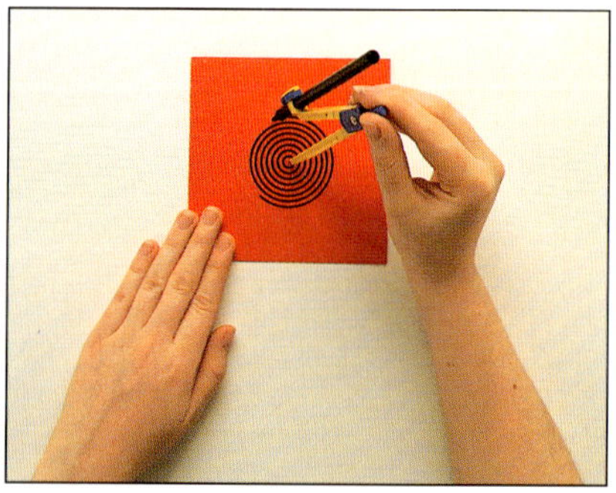

1 WITH A COMPASS and pen, draw 12 concentric dark circles on a poster-board square at intervals of ⅛ in (5 mm). Begin with one 1 in (2.5 cm) wide. Repeat on another square.

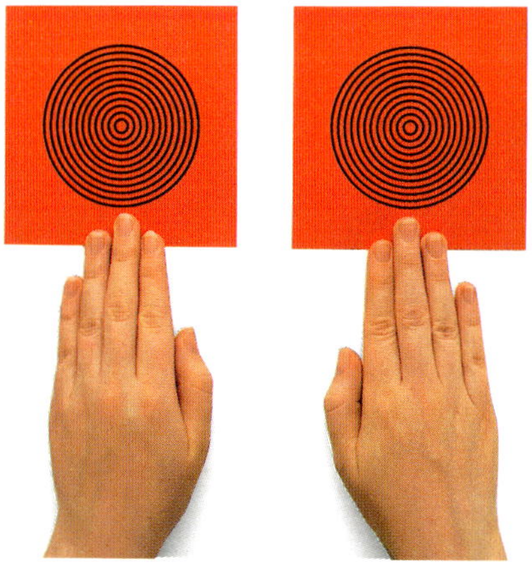

2 ON A SMOOTH surface, move one of the squares in small circles. Your brain cannot follow the fast-changing positions of the lines, and the circles appear to rotate. Hold the squares next to each other and move one. Is there any effect on the other?

EXPERIMENT

Colors from black and white

Adult help is advised for this experiment

When microscopes were first invented, lens makers had some problems. For example, a glass lens bends some colors in the light spectrum more than others. This produces colored edges around objects seen through the lens. A solution is to combine two or more lenses to correct the difference.

The eye's own lens can produce similar effects, and sometimes we see colors that don't really exist.

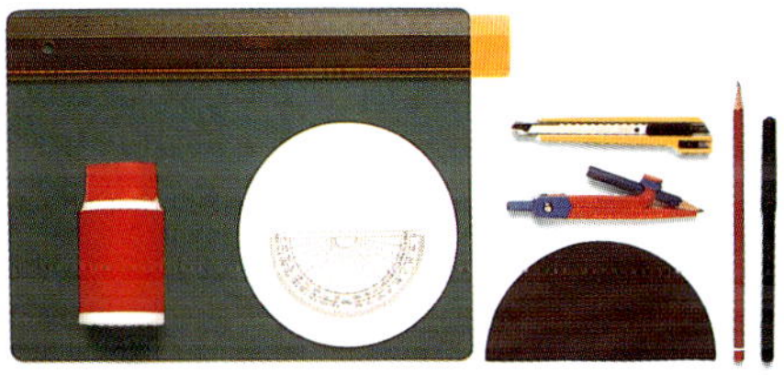

YOU WILL NEED

• *cutting mat* • *ruler* • *glue* • *white poster-board disk 6 in (15 cm) in diameter* • *protractor* • *craft knife* • *compass with pencil* • *black poster-board semicircle to match white disk* • *sharpened pencil* • *thick, black felt-tip pen* • *eraser*

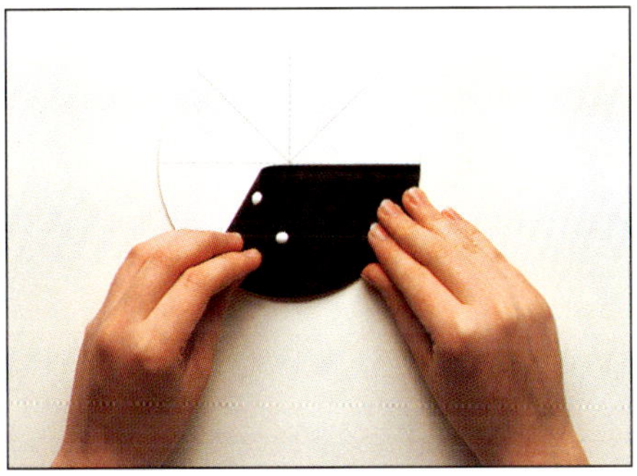

1 DRAW A LINE through the center of the white disk. With protractor and pencil, divide half of the disk into four 45° segments. Dab some glue onto the black semicircle, and stick it to the other half of the white disk.

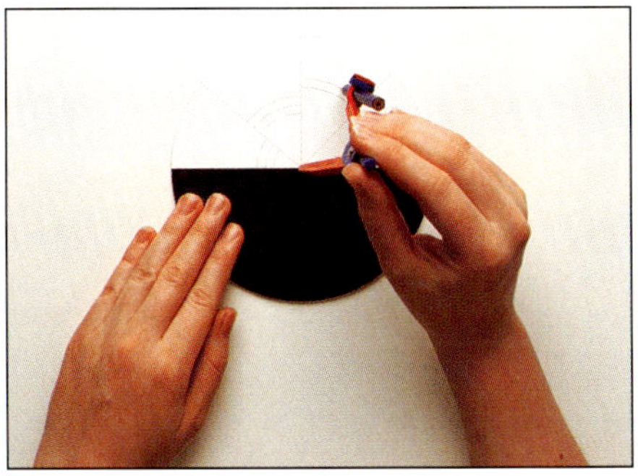

2 DRAW THREE arcs in one segment, 3⁄16 in (5 mm) apart. Begin ½ in (1.5 cm) from the center. Draw three more in the next segment—the same distance apart. Begin 3⁄16 in (5 mm) farther out.

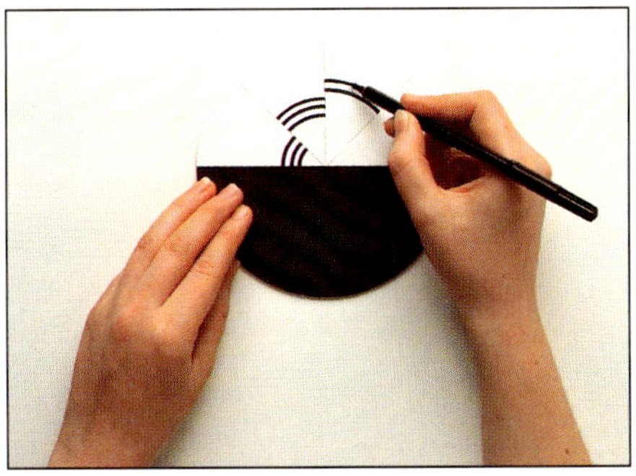

3 REPEAT TO make four sets of three arcs in pencil. Carefully draw over each one of the pencil arcs with the felt-tip pen, as shown. Now erase the pencil marks from the disk.

4 PUSH THE pencil through the disk, so that about 1 in (2.5 cm) sticks out below. Spin the pencil. What do you see? The black arcs are all different lengths, so each one spends slightly more or less time in your vision than its neighbor. With each revolution the arcs are replaced by the black semicircle. The combined effect is that colored edges appear as the arcs pass by the eye's lens, although the disk is only black and white. What happens if you spin the pencil at different speeds?

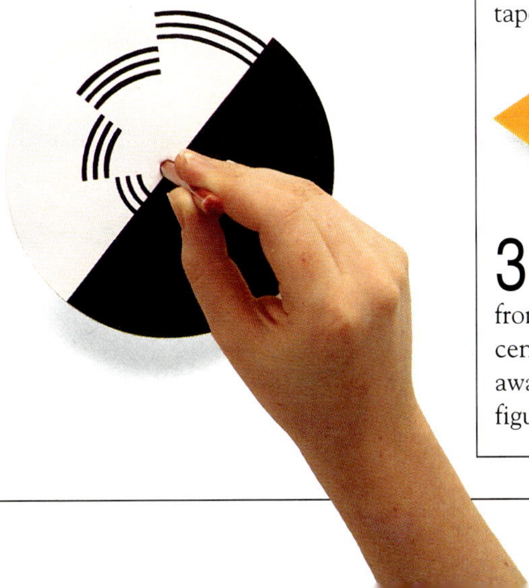

EXPERIMENT

Thiéry's figure

Adult help is advised for this experiment

To understand an object's shape we use clues such as surface shadows. If there are no shadows, a structure can seem ambiguous—that is, you can interpret it in different ways. One such structure is called a Thiéry's figure. You can make one yourself.

YOU WILL NEED

• *poster board* • *scissors* • *tape* • *protractor*

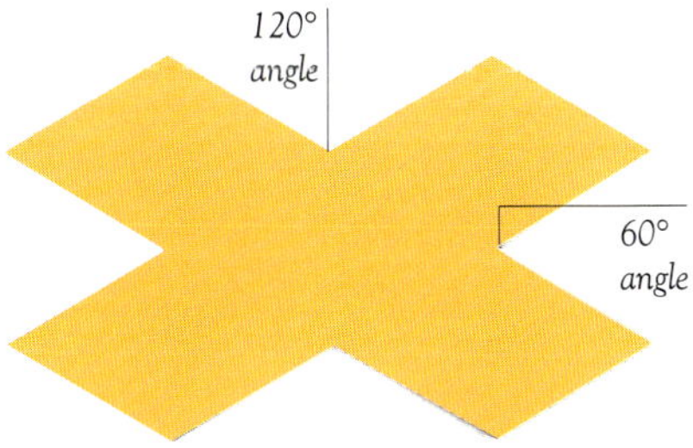

1 CUT OUT a cross of poster board, as above. The cross is made of five diamonds, each with 60° and 120° angles, and 2 in (5 cm) sides.

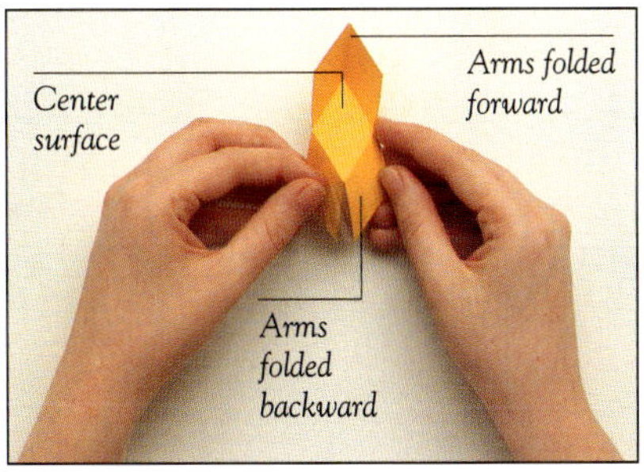

2 FOLD TWO arms forward, and tape together. Fold the other two arms backward, and tape these too. (Stick tape to one side of the figure only.)

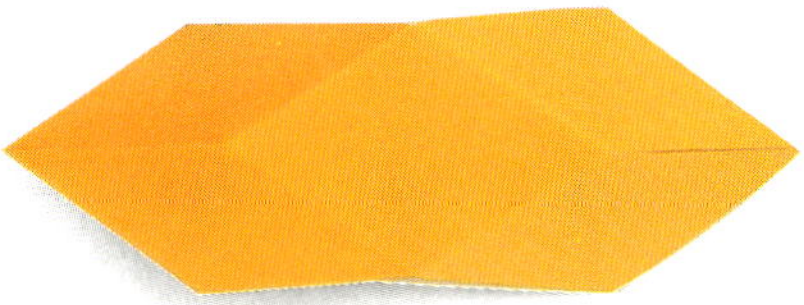

3 POSITION THE figure, untaped side forward, in dim light that comes from several directions. Does the center surface seem to slope toward or away from you? Can you turn the figure inside out in your mind?

The ears and hearing

HAVE YOU EVER been in a truly silent place? Even in the quietest countryside, there are still sounds, such as wind, singing birds, and buzzing insects. Sound travels as invisible waves through the air. Your ears are specially designed to detect sound waves, turn them into nerve signals, and send these nerve signals to the brain, which analyzes them and identifies the sound.

The ear flaps (pinnae) on the sides of your head are the most obvious, but least intricate, parts of your hearing system. Each ear flap funnels sounds along a small tube, the ear canal, to the hidden parts of the ear inside your head. These delicate inner parts—the eardrum, tiny ear bones called ossicles, and the cochlea—are contained in an area about the size of your thumb's tip, just behind each eye.

Some animal ears are more sensitive than ours to certain sounds. For example, we cannot hear the deep, low-pitched rumbles that an elephant detects or the high-pitched squeaks that dogs and bats can hear.

EXPERIMENT

Make a model ear

Adult help is advised for this experiment

Sound waves consist of vibrations of the gas molecules in the air. You cannot see them because the gas molecules are too small. But you can "see" sound waves by converting the invisible vibrations of molecules in the air into visible vibrations in the form of ripples in a fluid. This is exactly what happens in the ear (below). In this model ear the large, flexible plastic-wrap surface acts as the eardrum. When you make sound waves, it vibrates and makes the straw rock to and fro very fast. The straw works like the ossicles (ear bones). Attached to a table-tennis ball, it makes ripples in the water in the bowl, which represents the fluid in the cochlea. Try sounds of different pitch (highness or lowness), like a high squeak or a low growl. Do the the ripples change in size or number?

Inside the ear

Sound waves pass along the ear canal to the eardrum, a piece of thin skin about the size of your little finger's nail. The waves make the eardrum vibrate. The vibrations pass along a chain of three tiny bones, the ear ossicles, which bridge a small air space called the middle ear cavity. The ossicles then transfer the vibrations into the fluid that fills the coiled, snail-shaped cochlea. As the vibrations ripple through fluid in the three chambers inside the cochlea, they shake a delicate membrane that runs along its whole length. Attached to the membrane are microscopic hairs, embedded in hair cells. When the membrane shakes, it pulls the hairs and causes the hair cells to make nerve signals, which pass to the hearing centers of the brain (p.117). The part of the cochlea containing the hairs and hair cells is called the organ of Corti.

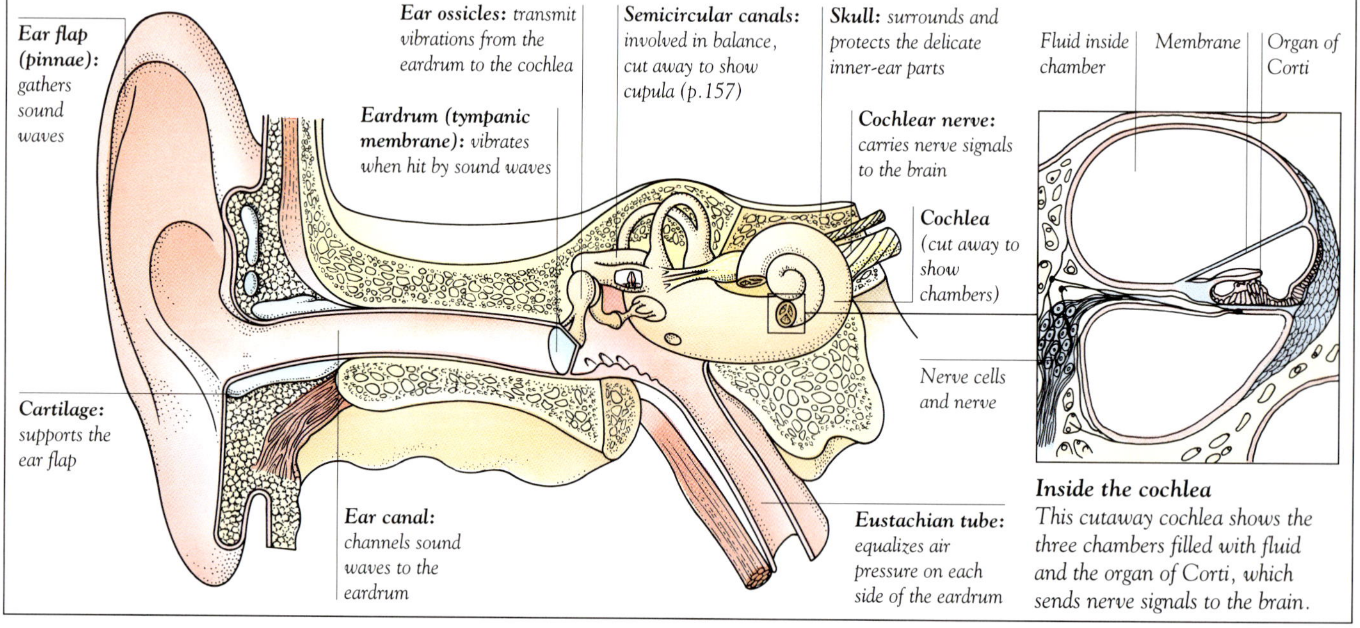

Inside the cochlea
This cutaway cochlea shows the three chambers filled with fluid and the organ of Corti, which sends nerve signals to the brain.

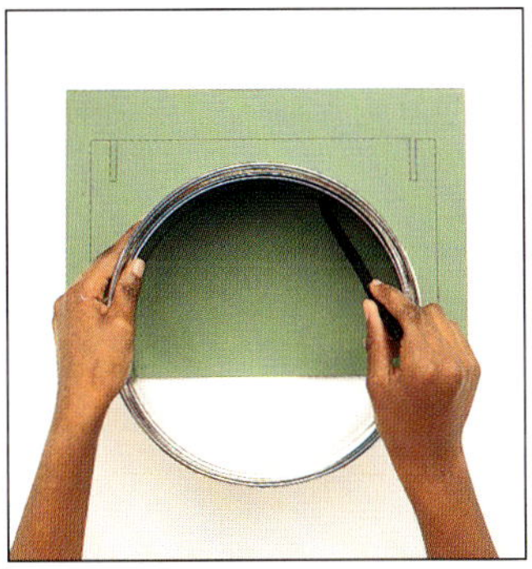

1 DRAW A RECTANGLE with two slits on thick poster board. Then draw around half of the cake pan, as shown. Carefully cut out the drawn shape. Now do this again.

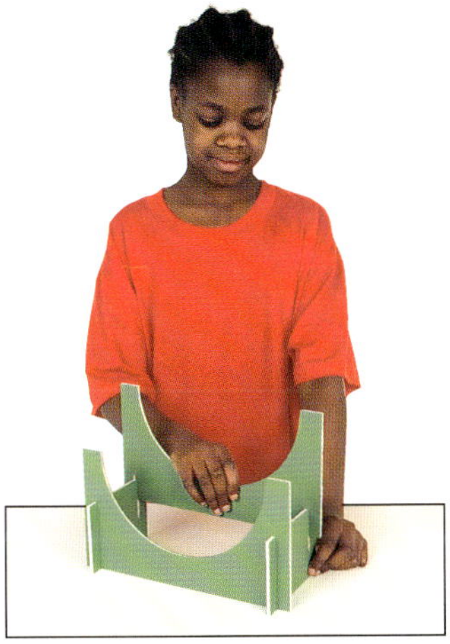

2 CUT TWO rectangles out of poster board, each with two slits at either end of the top edges. Join all the poster-board pieces at the slits. This is the stand for the "ear."

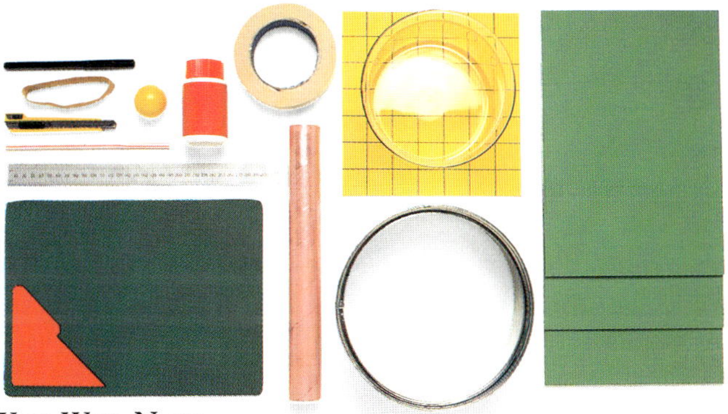

YOU WILL NEED

- *pen* • *rubber band* • *craft knife* • *double-sided tape* • *glue* • *water* • *table-tennis ball* • *bendable drinking straw* • *metal ruler* • *cutting mat* • *thin poster board* • *plastic wrap* • *glass bowl* • *detachable cake pan sides* • *thick poster board* • *poster board with a grid of squares drawn on it*

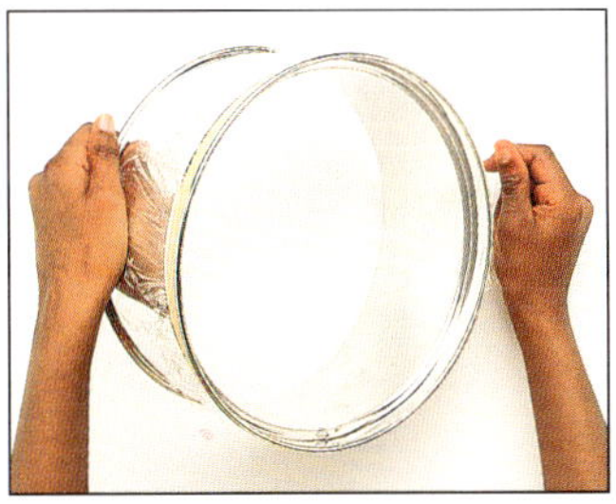

3 PUT A LARGE piece of plastic wrap over one end of the pan. Hold it in place with the rubber band, and make sure it is stretched tight.

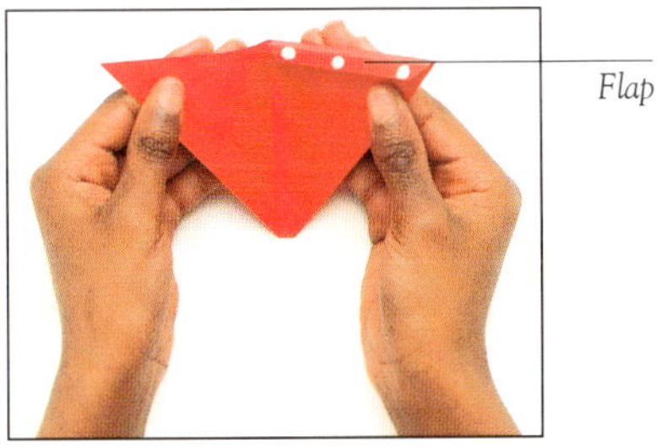

4 CUT A LARGE triangle of thin poster board, with a flap along half of the long edge. Fold the triangle in two. Dab glue on the flap.

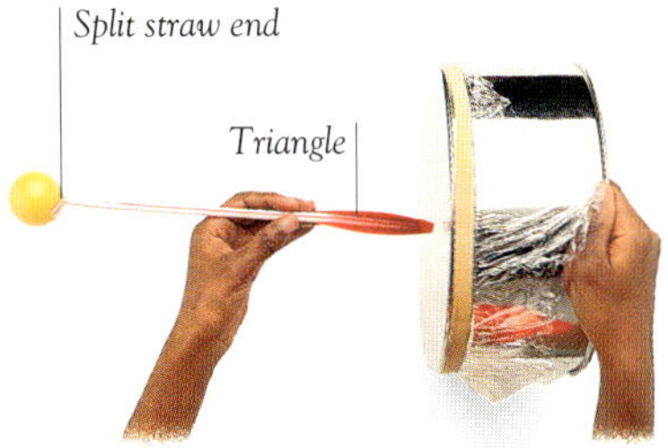

5 GLUE ONE END of the straw to the inside of the triangle. Split the other end of the straw. Use double-sided tape to attach this split end to the ball and also to attach the triangle to the plastic wrap. Make sure the end of the straw is at the center of the circle.

6 PLACE THE PAN on its stand, so that the ball just dips into water in the bowl. Put the poster-board grid below the bowl to make it easier to see ripples. Make lots of different sounds behind the drum, and watch the water's surface. Do different sounds make different ripples?

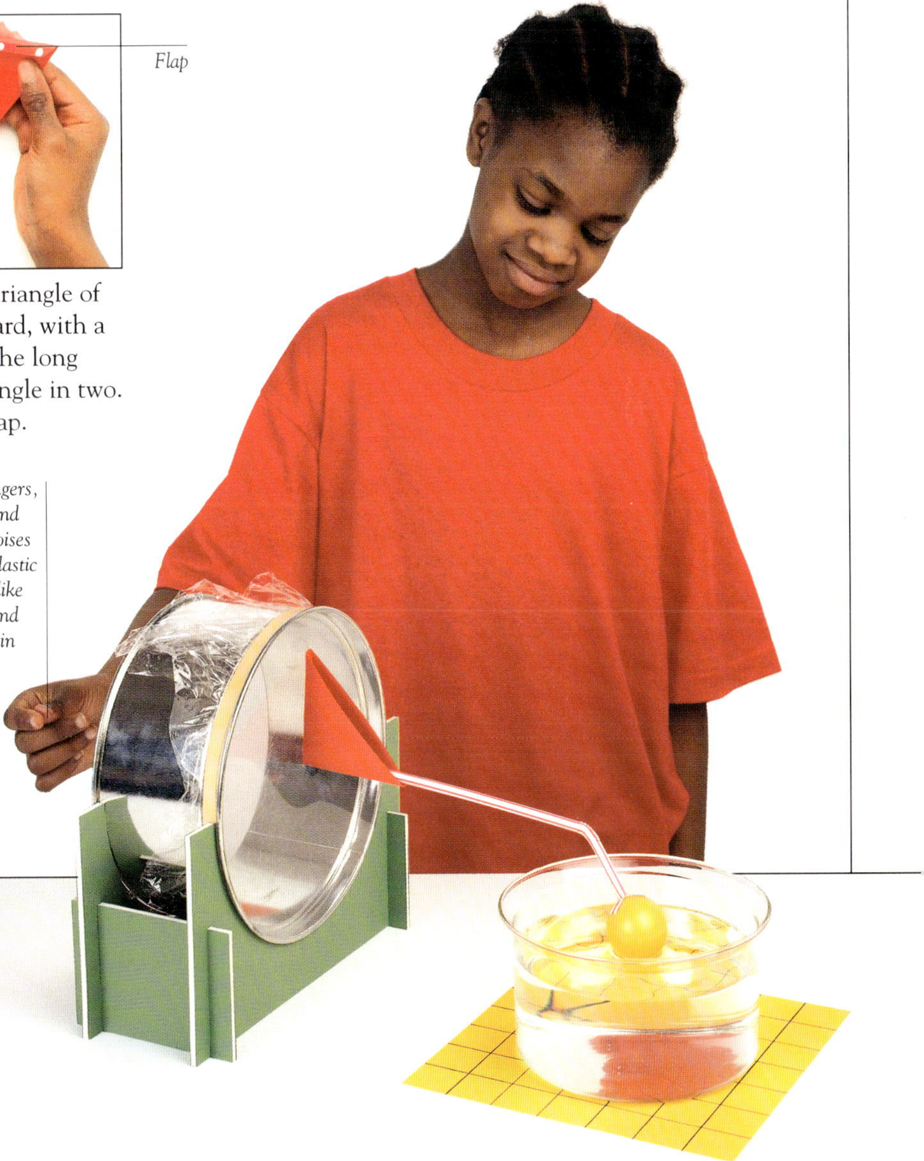

Click your fingers, clap, shout, and make other noises to make the plastic wrap vibrate like an eardrum and create ripples in the water

Judging sounds

EVEN UNDER WATER you can hear certain sounds—noises from above and sounds from within the water. This is because sounds travel not only through air but also as vibrations through liquids and solids. In fact this happens in the bones and fluid inside your own ears (p.152). When you speak, sound vibrations from your larynx (p.71) travel to your ears both through the air and through bones and body fluids in your neck and head. This alters the quality of the sound, which is why your voice seems different when you hear it on a tape recording compared with when you speak. Sound waves also take time to travel. The split-second difference between a sound reaching one ear and then the other helps you to judge where it comes from.

An unfamiliar voice

Make a recording of your own voice and listen to it carefully. You may find that your voice sounds unfamiliar, because you detect the recording's vibrations only through the air, not through your neck and head too, as when you hear your own speech.

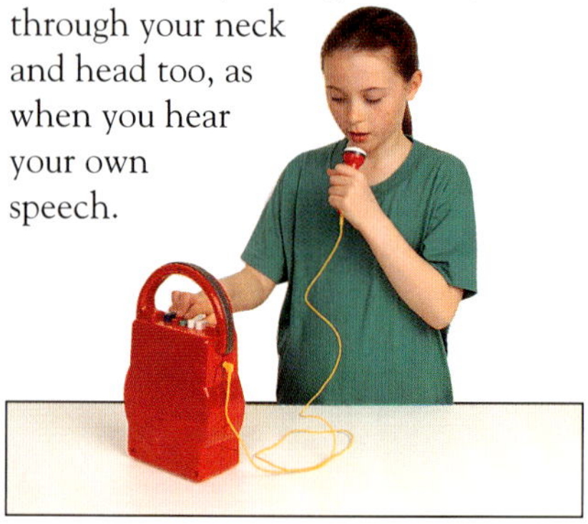

EXPERIMENT

Hearing through solids

Adult help is advised for this experiment

The medium (substance) through which sounds pass can have startling effects on what they sound like to you. Sounds travel at 1,125 ft (343 m) per second through the air, but they travel over 4 times faster through water, and almost 15 times faster through steel! Although sounds travel fast through liquids and solids, many liquids and solids do not convey the full range of a sound's high and low notes, compared to air. This is why sounds coming through water or solids sometimes seem muffled. In this experiment you can investigate how sound waves carried by different materials are different from one another.

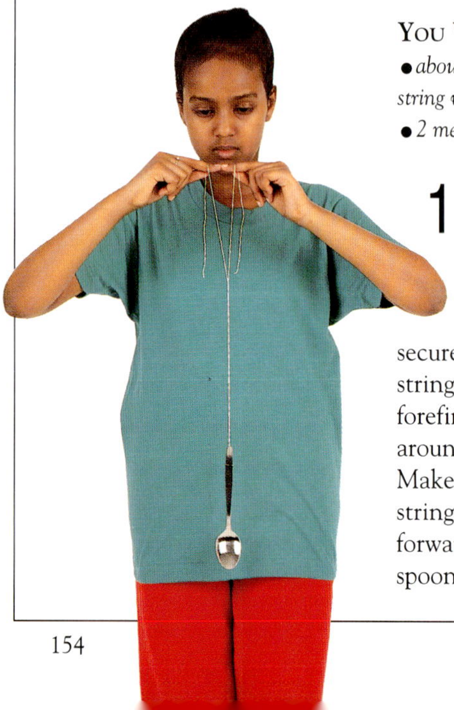

YOU WILL NEED

- *about 3 ft (1 m) of string (kite string works well)*
- *modeling clay*
- *2 metal spoons*

1 TIE ONE spoon handle to the string, halfway along the string's length. Press a blob of clay onto the string on the spoon to secure it. Wind one end of the string around one of your forefingers, then the other end around the other forefinger. Make sure the two lengths of string are equal. Now lean forward, so that string and spoon hang freely.

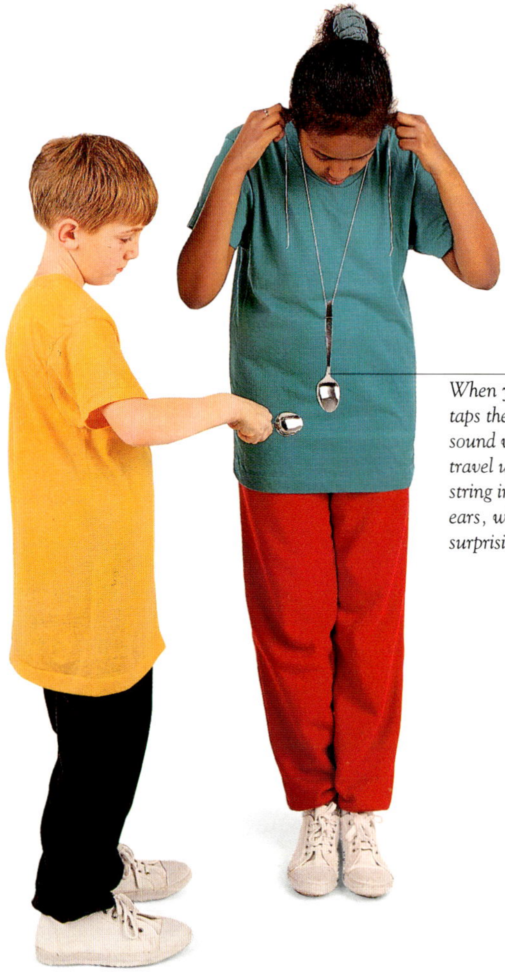

When your friend taps the spoon, sound waves travel up the string into your ears, with surprising results!

2 PLACE YOUR FOREFINGERS lightly on the entrance to each ear. Ask a friend to tap one spoon gently with the other. What kind of sound do you hear? What happens when you use yarn, wire, or rubber bands instead of string?

EXPERIMENT
Judging the direction of sound

When sound waves arrive at one side of your head, they reach one of your ears slightly before the other. Your ears and brain detect this time difference, so you know the sound's direction.

You Will Need
- *blindfold*
- *chair*

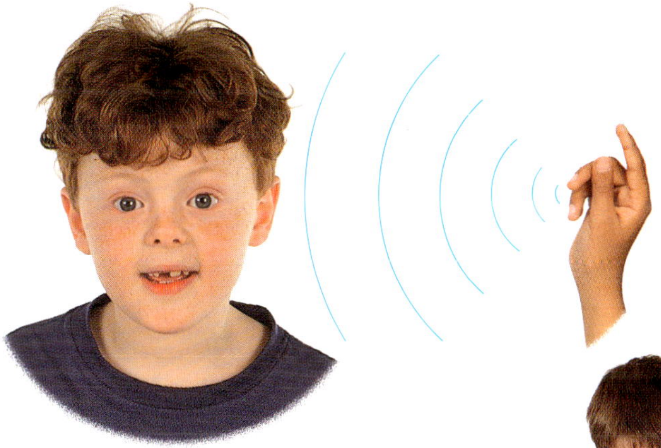

Split-second timing
The time gap between sound waves reaching one ear, then the other, is less than one-thousandth of a second. But the ears and brain still detect it.

EXPERIMENT
Sound mix-up

If a sound comes from directly in front, above, or behind you, it is difficult to work out its direction. This is because the sound waves reach both of your ears at the same time.

Clicking fingers
Sit blindfolded. Ask a friend to click his or her fingers above, behind, or in front of you, but always in line with the center of your body. Can you point to the sound source each time?

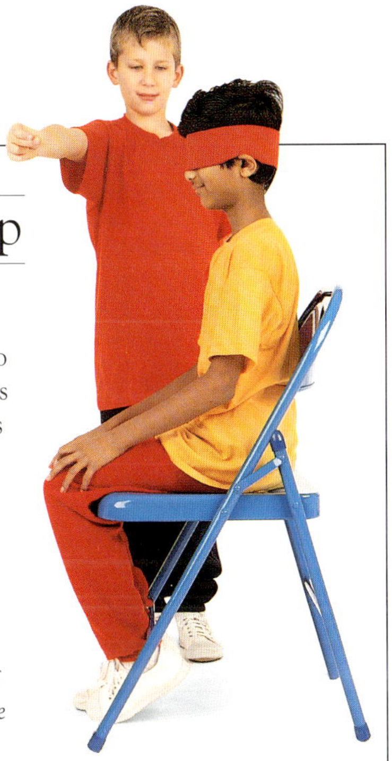

Pointing out the sound source
Get your friends to sit in a circle around someone who is blindfolded, so that he or she cannot see the sound source. In a random order, each person should click his or her fingers. The blindfolded person points to where he or she thinks the sound comes from. In which parts of the circle are the guesses most accurate?

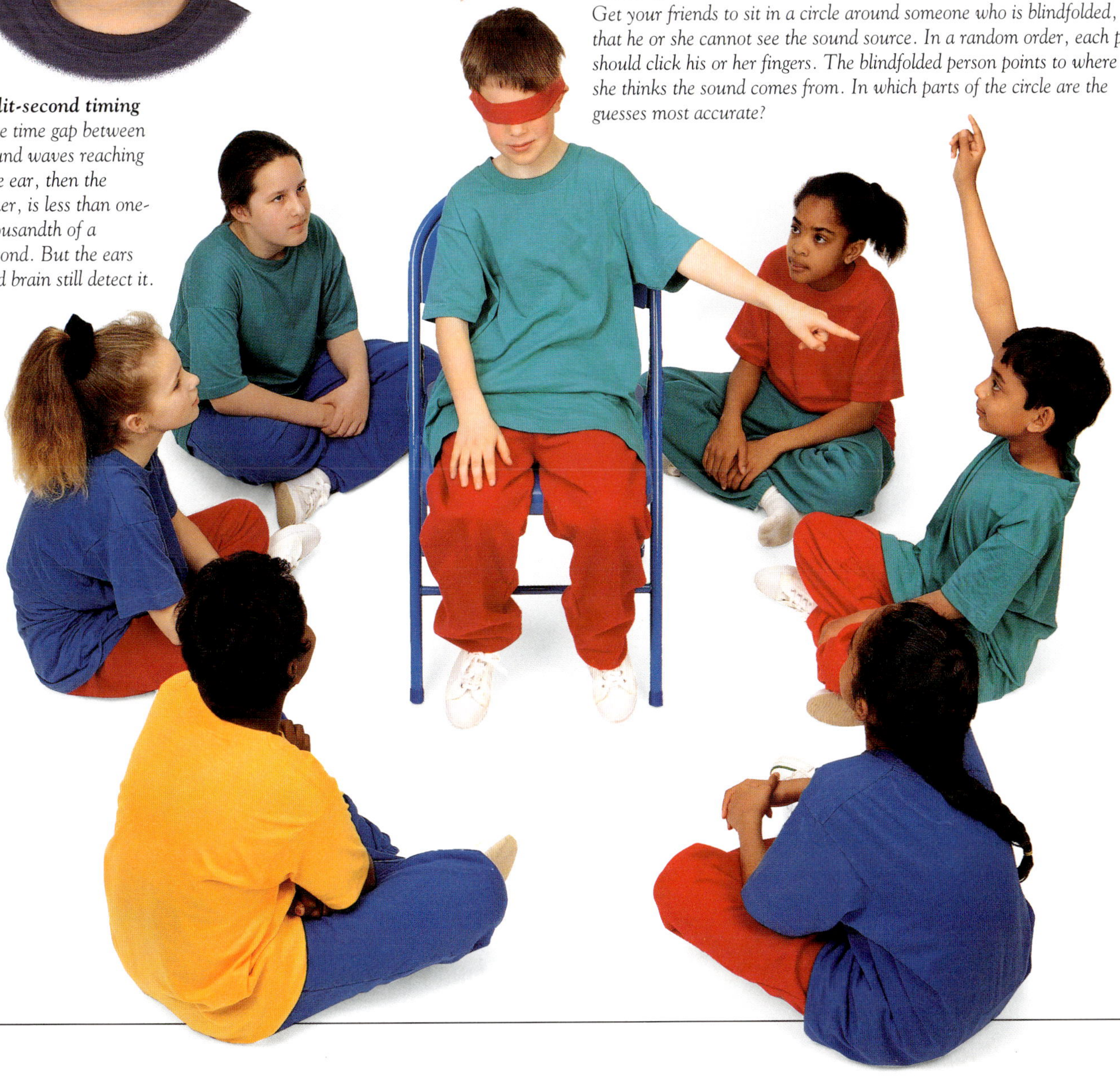

Balance

IF ANIMALS SUCH AS DOGS OR CATS try to walk on their back legs, their unsteady movements show how difficult this is for them. Yet you walk on two legs almost without thinking. Your ability to balance is not a single sense, like eyesight. It is a continuous process, by which your brain receives information from sensory parts all over your body. These parts, described on other pages, include the semicircular canals and other parts of your inner ears, stretch detectors in your muscles and tendons, pressure sensors in your skin, and your eyes, which provide important visual information. Your brain builds up a picture of your body's position and posture in relation to the downward force of gravity. It constantly sends signals to your muscles to adjust the positions of your head, torso (trunk), and limbs.

Any way is up

High in space, the force of the Earth's gravity fades to almost nothing. Astronauts and anything in a spaceship that is not fixed down float about, weightless. There is no up or down. Conflicting signals coming from the inner ears, eyes, skin, muscles, joints, and other body parts confuse the body's balance process. Some astronauts feel dizzy and even nauseated for a time, a problem known as space sickness. This is similar to the motion sickness that you may feel in a car or boat.

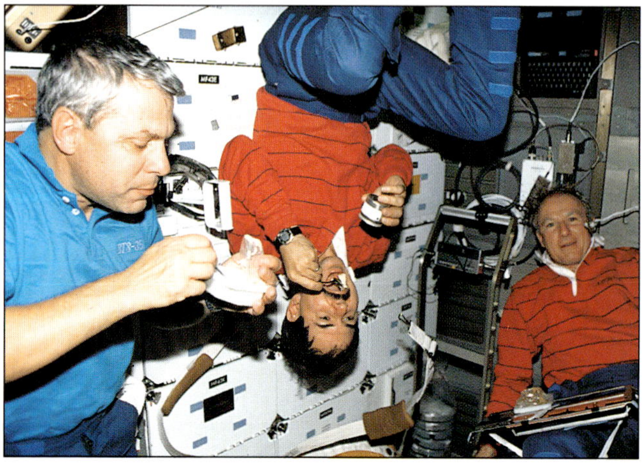

Keeping upright

Stand on one leg and tie your shoelace. Do you find it difficult? It will be at first, although you can probably do it with practice. Take note of how your body continually sways almost off balance. The different parts of the balance mechanism (below) send a constant stream of signals to your brain. Your brain assesses your body's position every split-second and tells your muscles to pull your weight back into a steady position. After standing on one leg for a time, the muscles in that calf and foot may begin to ache, because they each have to work harder than when you stand on two legs.

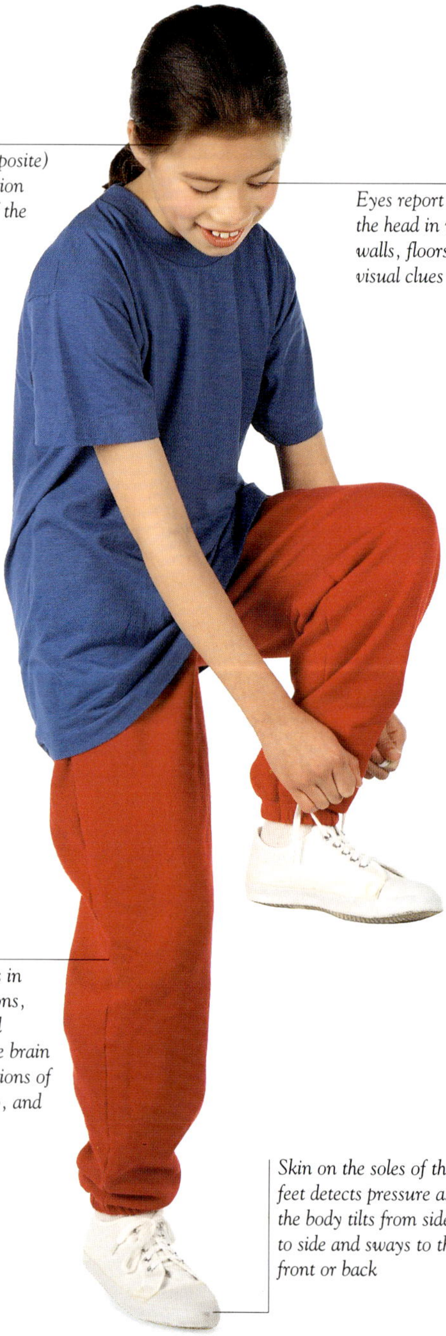

Ampullae (opposite) sense the position and motion of the head

Eyes report the position of the head in relation to walls, floors, and other visual clues

Stretch sensors in muscles, tendons, and joints send messages to the brain about the positions of the neck, torso, and limbs

Skin on the soles of the feet detects pressure as the body tilts from side to side and sways to the front or back

Motion detectors

Deep inside each ear (p.152) are three liquid-filled, C-shaped tubes called semicircular canals. As you move your head, the liquid lags behind the wall of each canal, in the same way that, when you turn a cup of water, the water moves more slowly than the side of the cup. The liquid bends a jellylike blob, called the cupula, in the bulge known as the ampulla, at one end of the canal. This bending moves hairs embedded in the cupula. These are rooted in nerve cells, which send signals to the brain as the hairs move. All of the canals respond to most head movements, but each of them is also especially suited to one particular type of movement.

Inside semicircular canals and ampullae

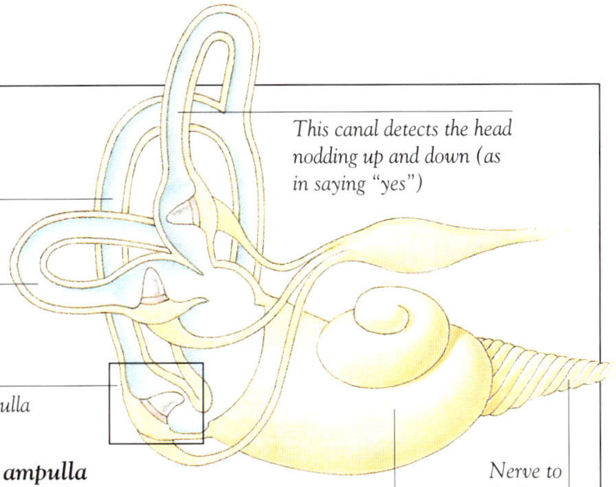

Inside an ampulla

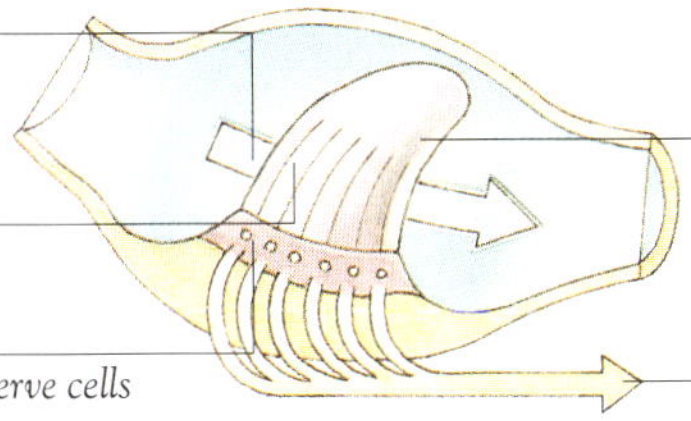

EXPERIMENT

Losing balance

Adult help is required for this experiment

If you take away one part of the balance system, then another, and another, it becomes more and more difficult to carry out even simple tasks, such as standing up straight! In your bare feet, try the four steps shown here. Be sure an adult stands nearby, ready to catch you if you fall.

YOU WILL NEED

- *a safe place with no obstructions and a soft floor, such as a thick carpet, soft grass, or sand*
- *cushion*
- *blindfold*

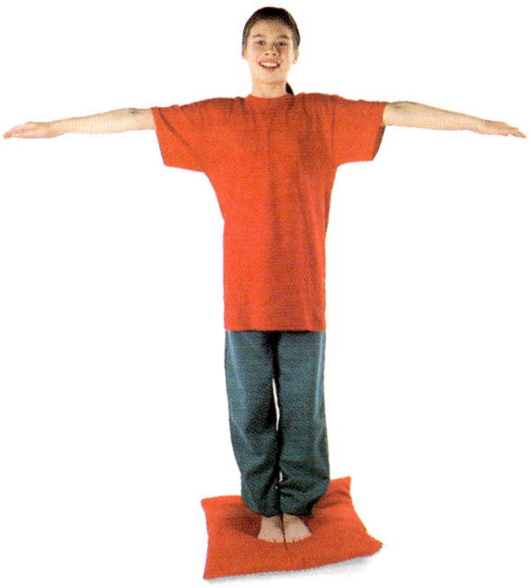

1 STAND ON the cushion. This "blurs" information from the pressure sensors in the skin of the soles of your feet.

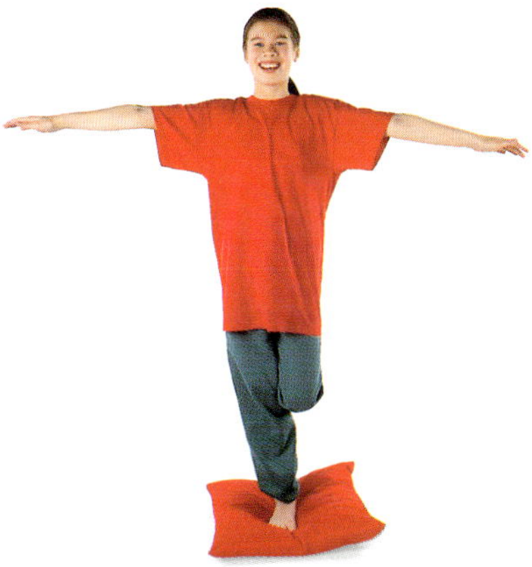

2 STAND ON one foot. Now you have only half of the pressure information from the skin sensors in your feet.

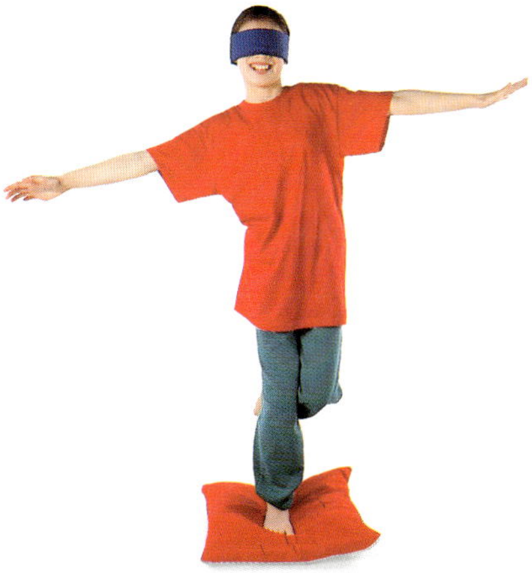

3 ASK AN adult to blindfold you. Now you can no longer see objects and use them to judge if you are upright.

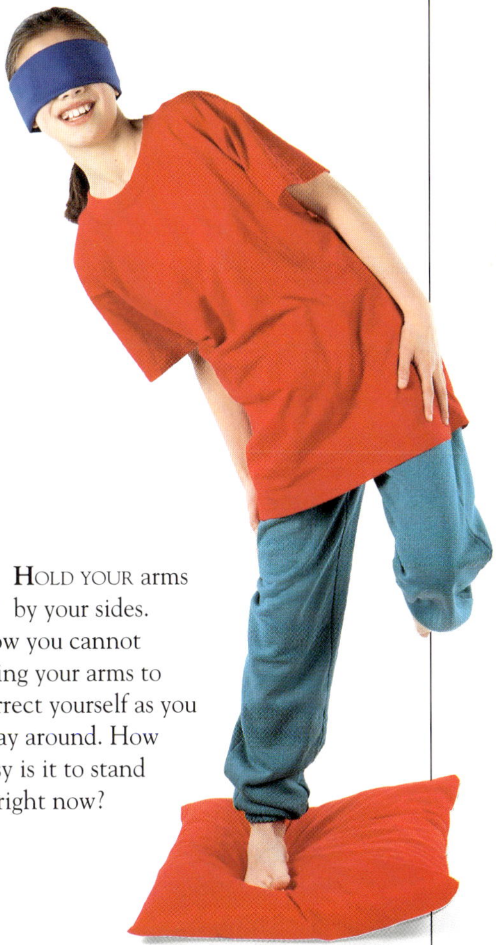

4 HOLD YOUR arms by your sides. Now you cannot swing your arms to correct yourself as you sway around. How easy is it to stand upright now?

The nose and smell

YOUR NOSE IS THE MAIN AIRWAY for your respiratory system (pp.72–73). It is also an important sense organ. For example, it enables you to identify smells, such as smoke, that indicate danger. Inside your nose (p.183) is the olfactory epithelium—a postage-stamp-size patch of nerve cells that have hairy projections. The projections are covered with receptors sensitive to odor molecules in the air. There are probably at least 10 million receptors in your nose—of at least 20 different types. Each type senses a different range of smell molecules. When the receptors detect an odor, they send nerve signals along the olfactory (smell) nerve to the smell center in the brain (p.117). This analyzes the signal pattern and identifies the smell.

EXPERIMENT

Telling by smell

Adult help is advised for this experiment

Your sense of smell works closely with your sense of taste (p.160) to give you information about the foods and drinks you consume. You also identify foods by sight. When you look at something to eat, you often get a good idea of how it will taste. This experiment shows how difficult it can be to identify foods and other smelly substances by smell alone—without the help of taste or sight. Other smells, however, will be very familiar to you. Which smells are easy to identify?

Smell alone

Carefully cut the substances—the cut surfaces will give off fresh odors. Put them on saucers, and cover them with the glasses, so that the odors do not form a confusing mixture in the air. For each substance, remove the glass and hold the saucer while a blindfolded friend (who has not seen the substance) tries to tell by smell what it is. Are foods easier to identify than nonfoods?

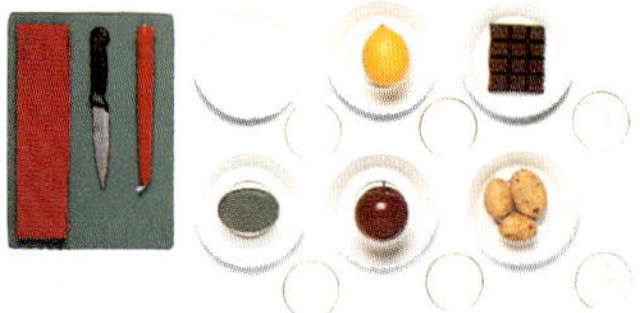

YOU WILL NEED

- *cutting board* • *blindfold*
- *kitchen knife* • *6 saucers*
- *everyday substances with odors, such as wax candle, lemon, chocolate, soap, apple, and potato*
- *6 glasses*

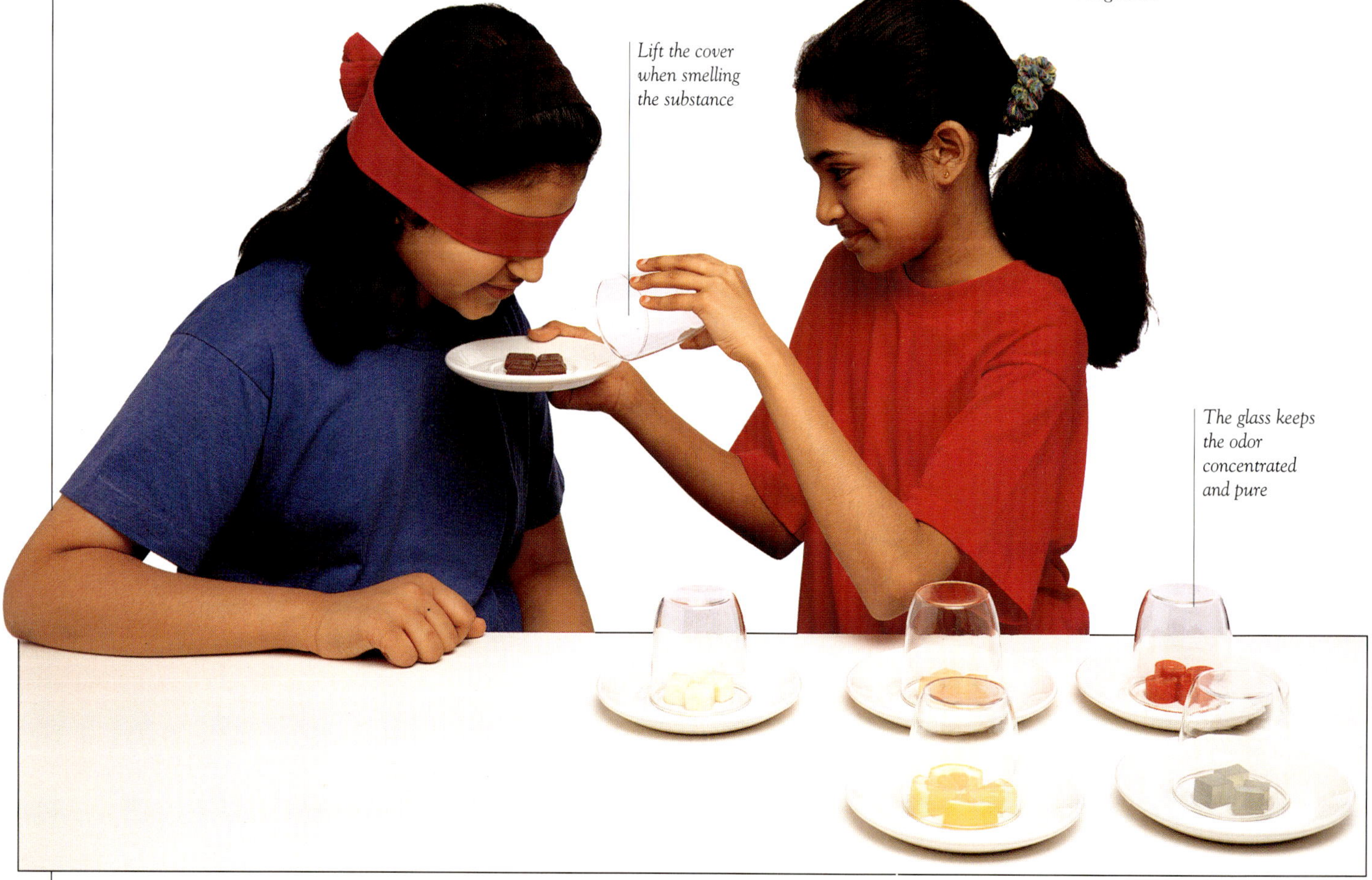

Lift the cover when smelling the substance

The glass keeps the odor concentrated and pure

EXPERIMENT
The smell threshold

There are smells in the air all around us. But most are too weak for the human nose to detect. There must be more than a certain number of odor molecules in a specific volume of air before you can sense an odor. This number is called the smell threshold concentration. You can test a friend to find out what the smell threshold is for vanilla extract and other familiar substances. At each stage of the experiment, air the room.

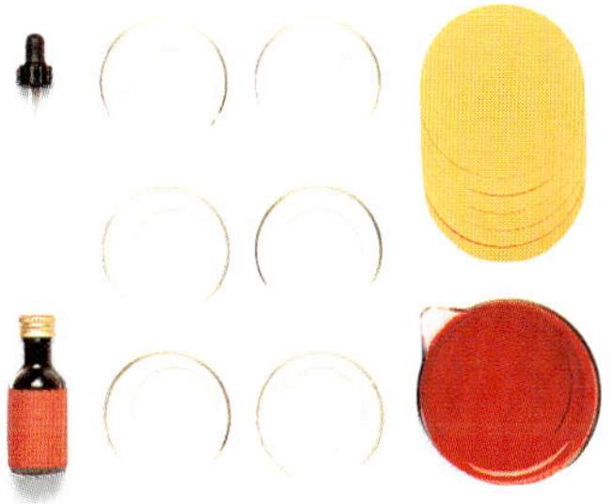

You Will Need
●dropper ●substance with a characteristic odor, such as vanilla extract (you can try others, too, such as banana or strawberry flavoring) ●6 glasses ●poster-board circles to cover the tops of the glasses ●large pitcher of water

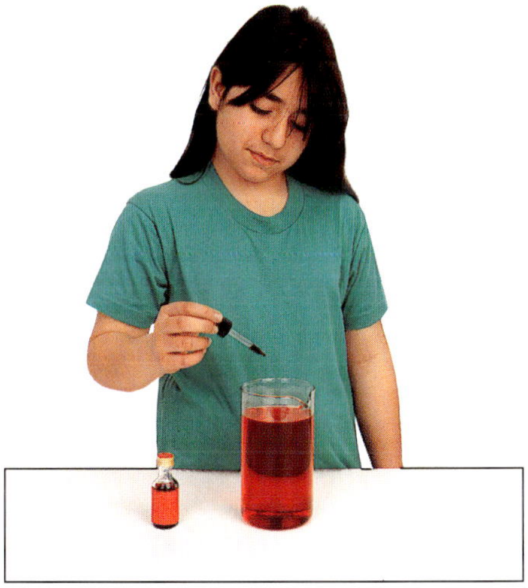

1 Put 10 drops of vanilla extract into the pitcher of water. (The water in these photographs has been colored, so you can see the concentrations.)

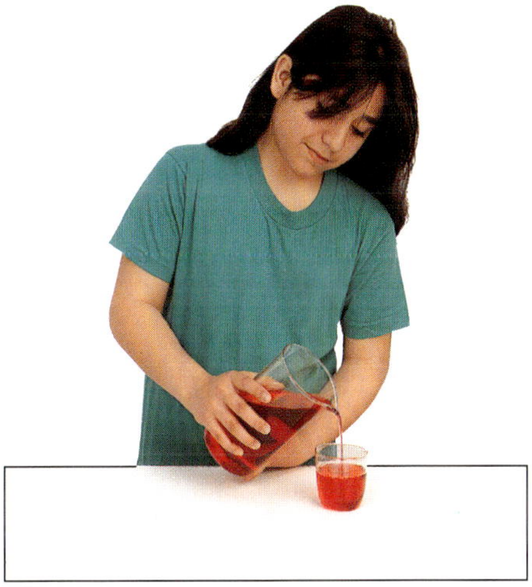

2 Fill a glass with the solution. This is the strongest concentration. Cover it with a poster-board circle. Half empty the pitcher, and fill it up with water.

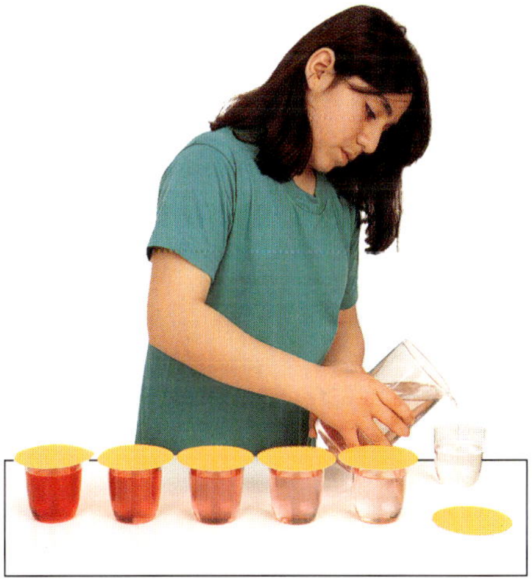

3 The pitcher now has half-strength vanilla. Pour this into another glass. Repeat Step 2 until you have 6 glasses, with lower and lower concentrations.

A trained nose

A person with a "trained ear" can pick out instruments in an orchestra. In the same way, learning to identify certain odors is called having a "trained nose." In fact, when you identify something by smell, it is not your nose you have trained, but your brain's ability to remember smells.

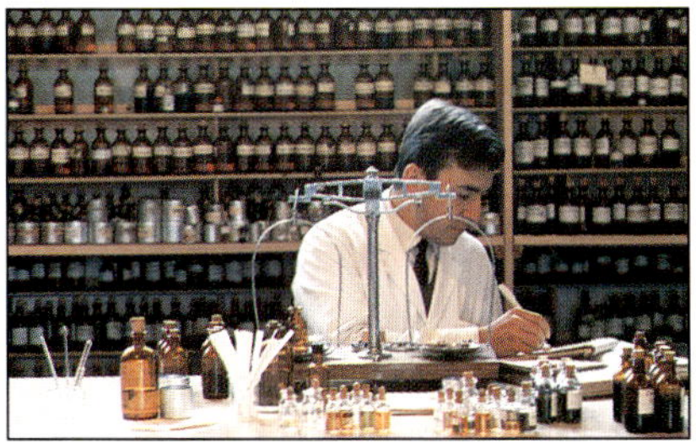

Blending smells
This perfume expert blends scents to make a new product. Wine makers, chefs, and many others need similar smelling skills.

4 Ask a friend to smell the weakest solution. Can he or she identify it? The friend should try the next strongest, and so on, until the odor is identified—then take a breath of fresh air. Next, ask the friend to smell the solutions from strongest to weakest. Is the threshold at which the odor disappears the same as the one at which it appeared when smelling from weak to strong?

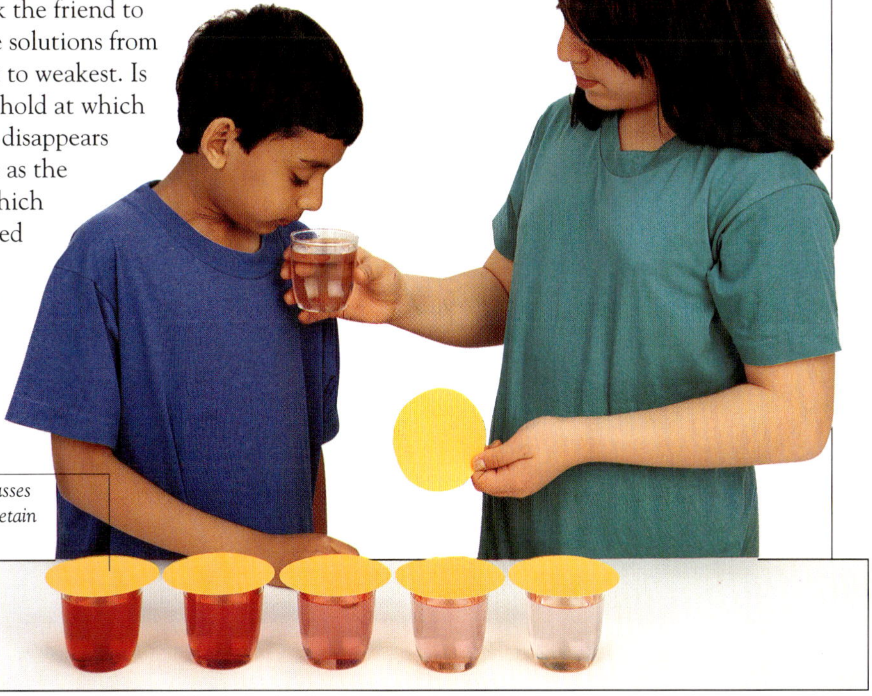

Keep the glasses covered to retain the odors

The tongue and taste

YOUR SENSE OF TASTE is governed by several thousand microscopic onion-shaped clusters of cells called taste buds, scattered mainly over the surface of your tongue. The taste buds detect four basic flavors, using flavor sensors on the surfaces of their cells, similar to the odor receptors in the nose (p.158). The four flavors are sweet, sour, salty, and bitter. The substances in food that carry flavors must be dissolved in saliva before they can seep down into the taste buds. This is why you can taste dry foods, such as crackers, only after chewing them. The taste buds send nerve signals to your brain's gustatory (taste) center, part of the touch center (p.117). This analyzes the signal pattern, so you can identify the taste.

Taste alone

Peel and cut the foods into cubes of equal size, to remove identifying clues such as their shape or skin texture. Ask a friend to be the taster and to wear the blindfold and nose clip, so that he or she cannot see or smell the food. Using the toothpick, rub a food cube on the taster's tongue for 5 seconds. Can the taster identify the food? Ask the taster to rinse his or her mouth out with water. Then try the other foods. When you have finished testing with each food, repeat the process, but without the taster wearing the nose clip. Is it easier to identify the foods?

EXPERIMENT

Telling by taste

Adult help is advised for this experiment

Much of what we think of as taste is a combination of the taste sense and other senses, such as temperature and texture sensations in the mouth, smell, and even sight (p.162). Find out which foods you can identify using your taste buds alone.

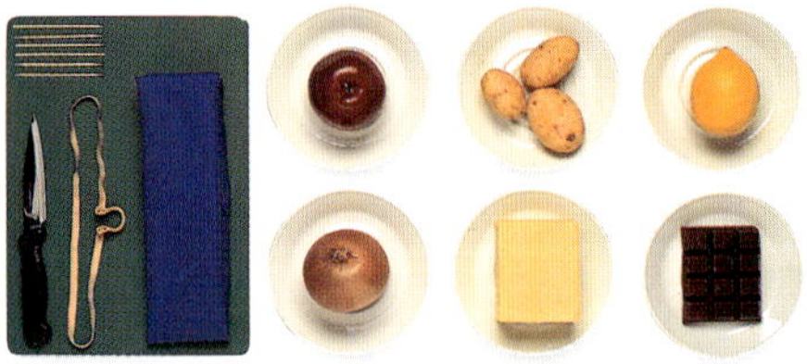

YOU WILL NEED

- *cutting mat* • *toothpicks* • *kitchen knife* • *water* • *nose clip* • *blindfold* • *saucers of foods such as apple, potato, lemon, onion, cheese, chocolate*

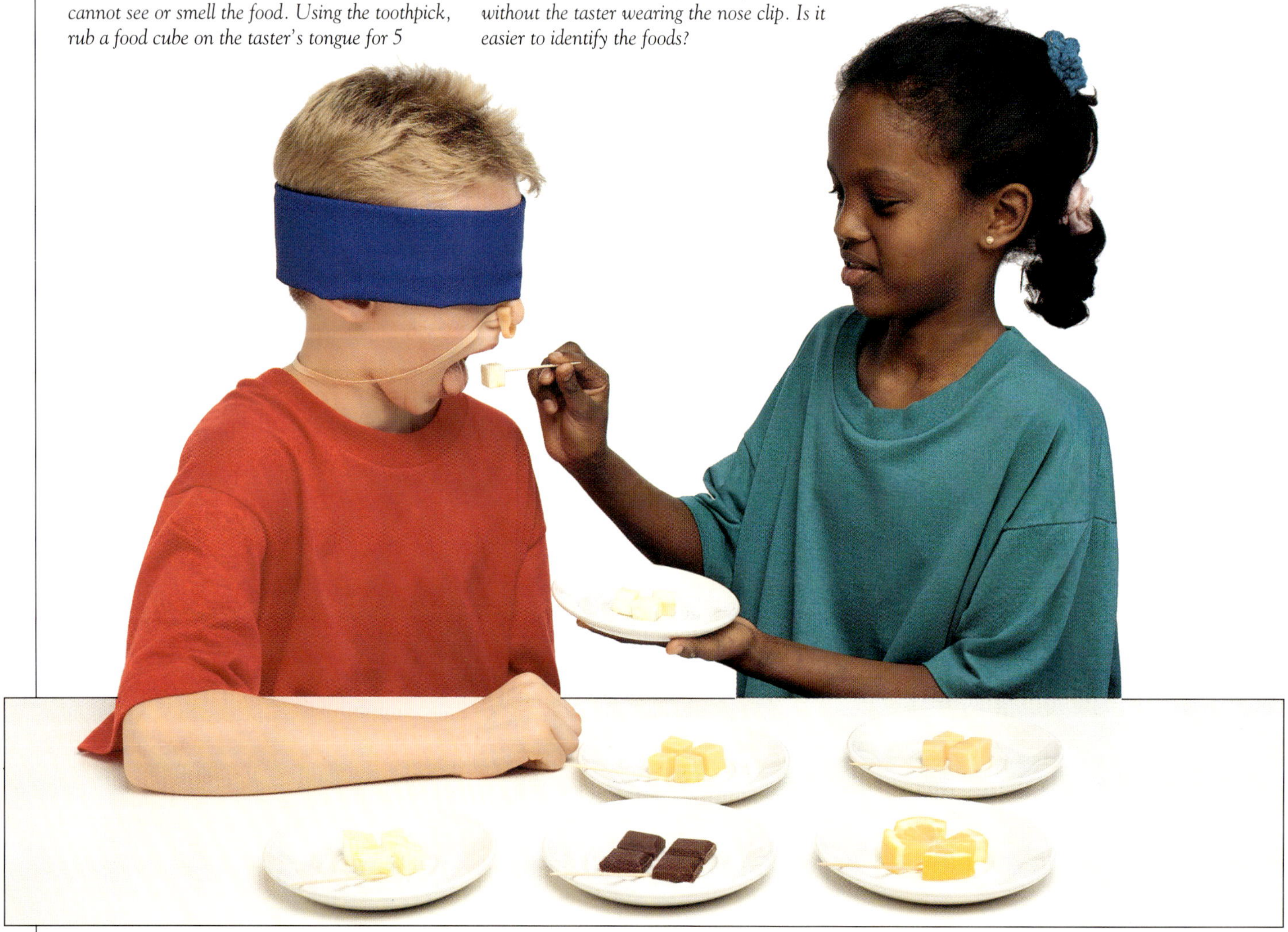

Tongue, papillae, and taste buds

Look at your tongue in a mirror. Most of its upper surface is roughened by projections of various shapes, called papillae. These help to grip food and move it as you chew. At the front of the tongue you can see two types of papillae. The larger ones are fungiform papillae and the tiny hairlike ones are filiform papillae. At the back of the tongue are 8 to 12 large, rounded papillae called vallate papillae. Most of our taste buds are sited in tiny pores between and on the papillae.

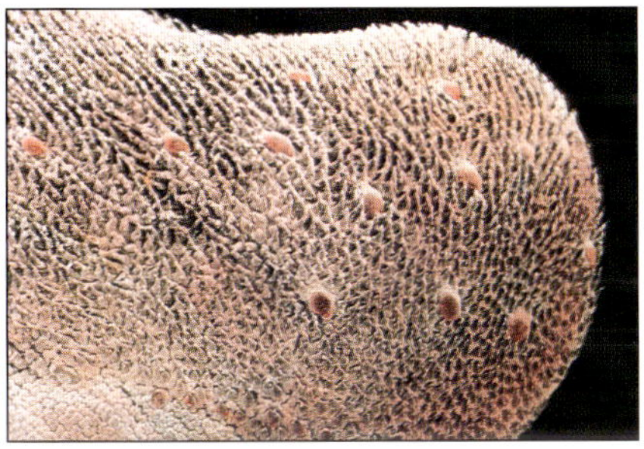

The tongue surface
The electron microscope shows frilly filiform papillae and larger fungiform papillae.

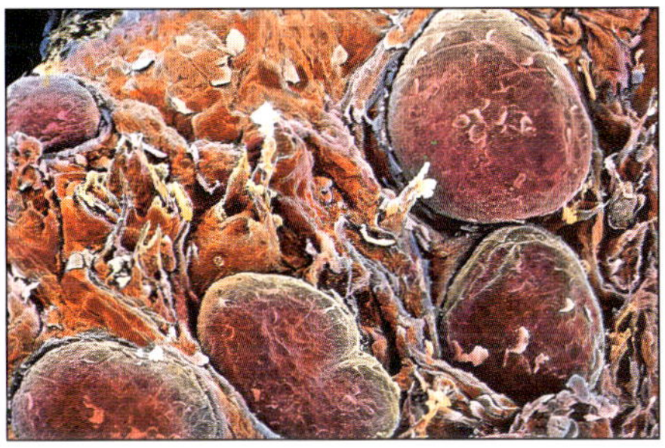

Close-up of papillae
Greater magnification reveals thin, cone-shaped filiform papillae among rounded fungiform ones.

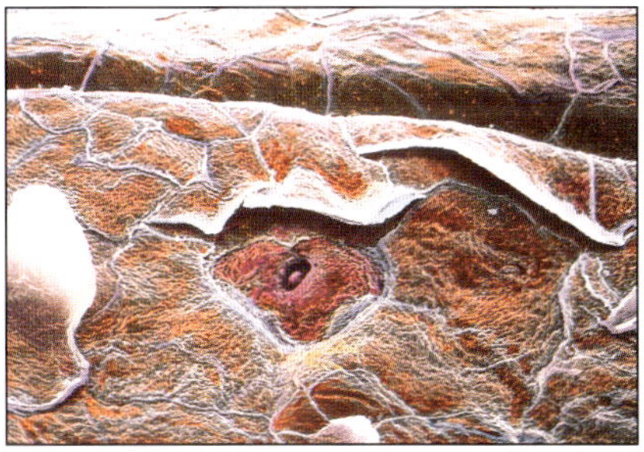

Taste bud
An even closer view shows the opening to a taste bud, set into the surface of a papilla.

Super-mobile muscles

The underside of the tongue is rooted at the back to the bones and muscles of the throat. But the main body of the tongue is extremely mobile and flexible. It consists mainly of eight interwoven muscles within the tongue itself and another eight muscles that join the tongue to the surrounding parts. These muscles can contract in various combinations to give the tongue a huge variety of shapes. Tongue flexibility is important for eating and essential for speech.

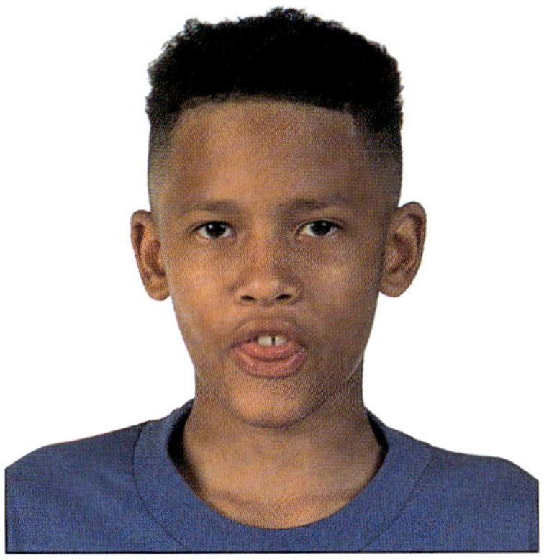

The "th" sound
Watch your tongue in the mirror and feel the different shapes it makes as you speak. For example, to make a "th" sound (above) it comes forward between the teeth.

EXPERIMENT

How one taste masks another

Some flavors are so strong that even when they are present in small amounts, they mask or block out other flavors. However, the other, weaker flavors do not disappear completely. This experiment shows how salt masks out an equally strong second flavor, sugar. But, as you taste solutions of sugar that become increasingly strong, you may be able to detect that another flavor is present.

You Will Need
- *saucer of table salt*
- *saucer of sugar*
- *4 glasses of fresh water*
- *2 teaspoons*

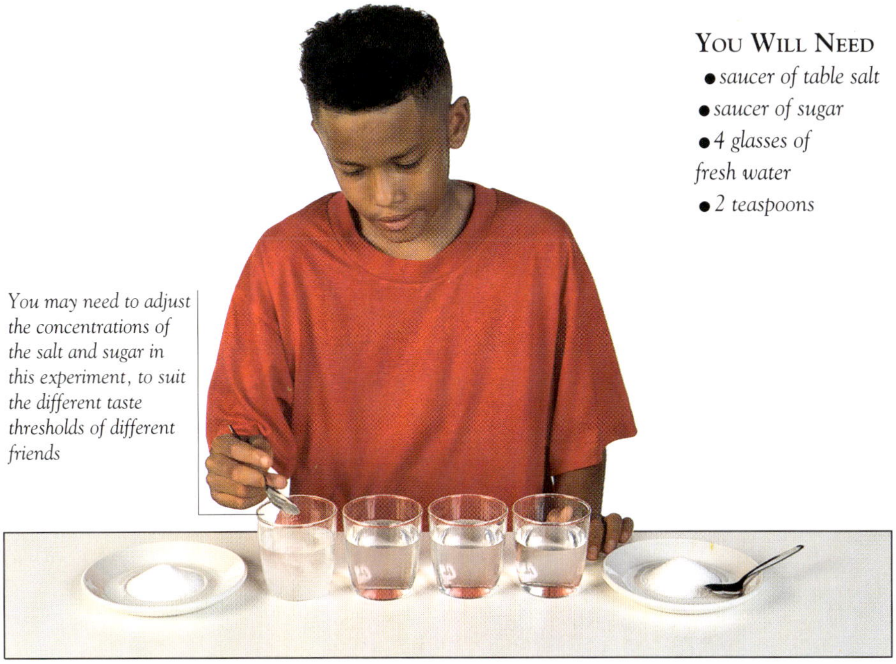

You may need to adjust the concentrations of the salt and sugar in this experiment, to suit the different taste thresholds of different friends

1 Stir half a teaspoon of salt into each glass of water. Stir sugar into all four glasses, putting half a teaspoon in the first, one in the second, one and a half in the third, and two in the fourth.

2 Ask a friend to sip the solutions, beginning with the weakest. In which one can he or she taste a second flavor behind the salt? In which one can he or she identify it as sugar?

Taste expectations

THE TASTE BUDS ON THE TONGUE and the taste centers of the brain (p.117) work together to tell you the flavors of the foods you eat. You also use sensors in the mouth and gums, similar to those involved in the sense of touch (p.164), to detect the hardness, temperature, and consistency of food as you chew. However, what you think you taste when you put food in your mouth also depends a lot on your own likes and dislikes. You are born with some of your taste preferences (opposite), but many other preferences can be accumulated over years of experience and memory. For instance, you may enjoy certain foods because you associate them with happy events from the past. The color and texture of a food and its strength of flavor also influence whether you like its taste.

EXPERIMENT

Fading flavors

When you first taste a flavor, it may seem very strong. But after continually tasting the same flavor over a few minutes, it seems to become weaker and you notice it less. This is known as habituation, and it also occurs with other senses such as smell and touch. You can demonstrate habituation of taste with solutions of sugar of two different strengths.

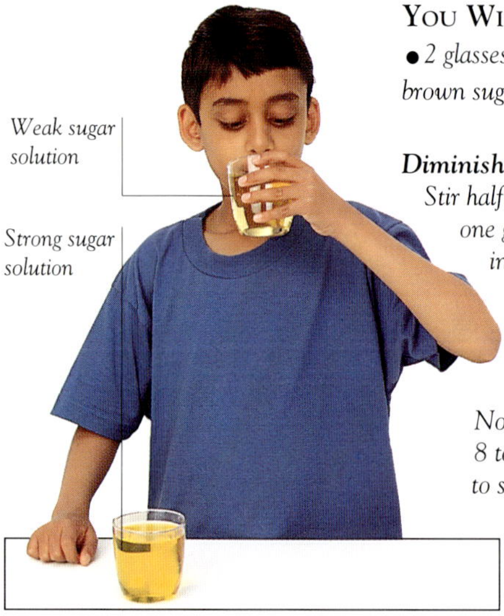

YOU WILL NEED
- *2 glasses of water*
- *white or brown sugar*
- *teaspoon*

Diminishing flavor
Stir half a teaspoon of sugar into one glass and three teaspoons into the other. (The water has been colored here for clarity.) Sip the weaker solution, and note how strong the flavor seems. Now sip the stronger solution 8 to 10 times, then go back to sip the weaker one again. Does it taste as strong as it did the first time you tasted it?

An appetizing sight?

Usually, we look at something before we taste it. This is important because we can check with our eyes that the food is edible and has not gone bad. The sight of food also has a strong effect on what we expect it to taste like. Children often do not want to eat certain foods because of the way they look—perhaps they look slimy or are strange shapes or colors. This attitude may have evolved in prehistoric times, as a way of self-protection, when humans had to hunt and forage for food. It would have made them suspicious of unfamiliar foods, until they were sure these were safe to eat. However, in the modern world, most foods are specially grown and prepared. There is no excuse for not eating your vegetables!

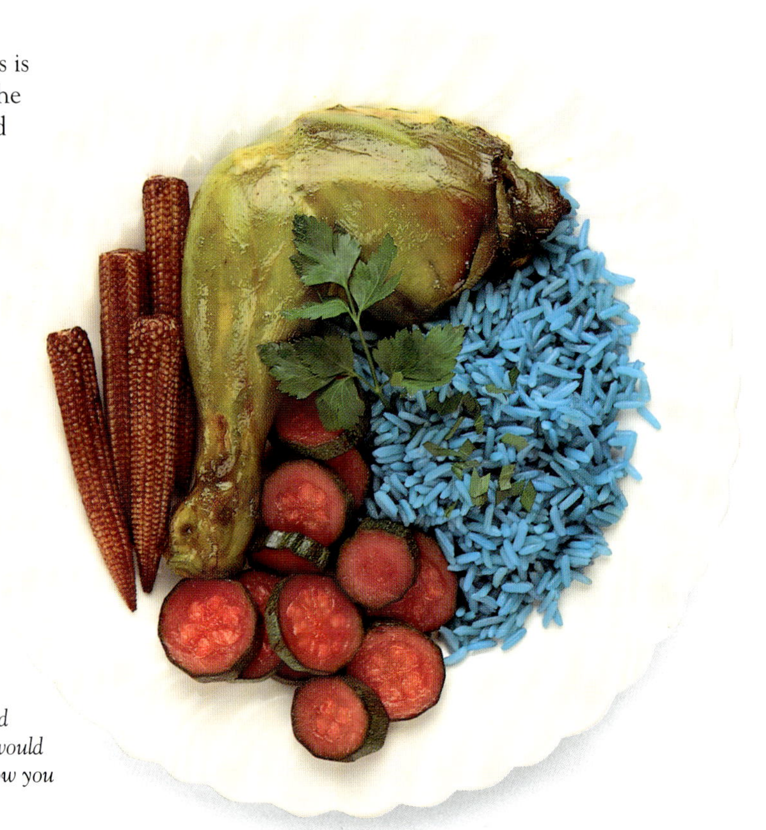

Color confusion
There is something very strange about this meal of chicken, baby sweet corn, zucchini, and rice! Each food is the wrong color. The chicken is green, the baby sweet corn is brown, the zucchini is red, and the rice is blue. In fact, the foods are colored with safe flavor-free food dyes and taste perfectly normal. But would you eat them? What food looks like has a strong influence on how you think it will taste.

Likes and dislikes

What we eat depends on many factors, such as cultural tradition, food prices, and what we need for a balanced diet. But sometimes people—particularly young children—do not think about these factors. They eat what they want to. Generally, children prefer sweet flavors. Which of the foods below are your favorites? How about your friends? Do you think that you have chosen the most nutritional ones?

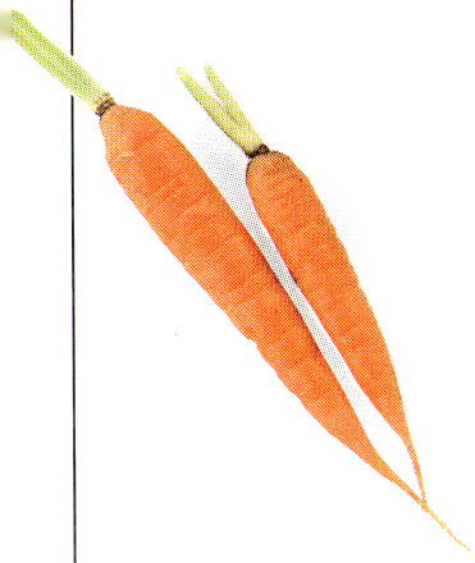

Carrots

Cheese

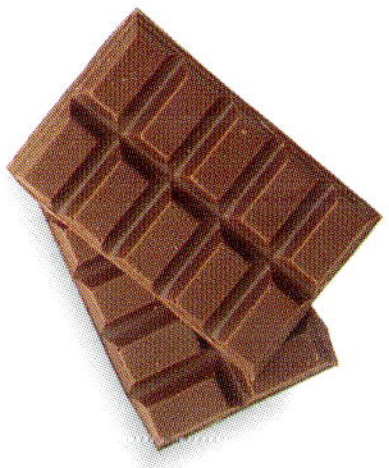

Chocolate

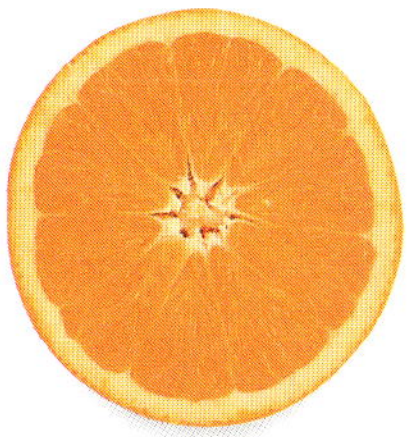

Orange

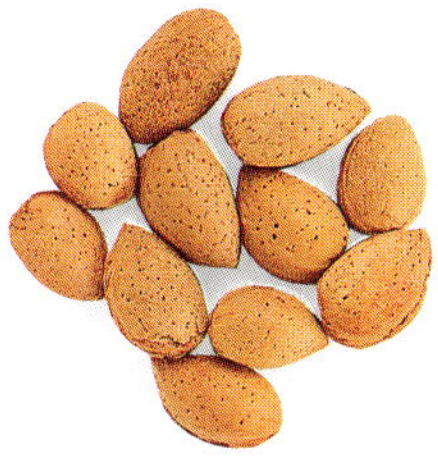

Almonds

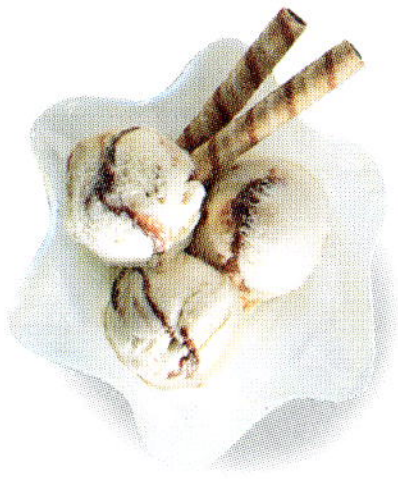

Ice cream

EXPERIMENT

A lemon-flavored potato

Adult help is advised for this experiment

In the food we eat, there are many clues to tell us what the food is. But you can confuse the brain by combining the flavor of one food with the texture of another.

YOU WILL NEED

- *small cube of potato*
- *lemon juice* • *toothpick*

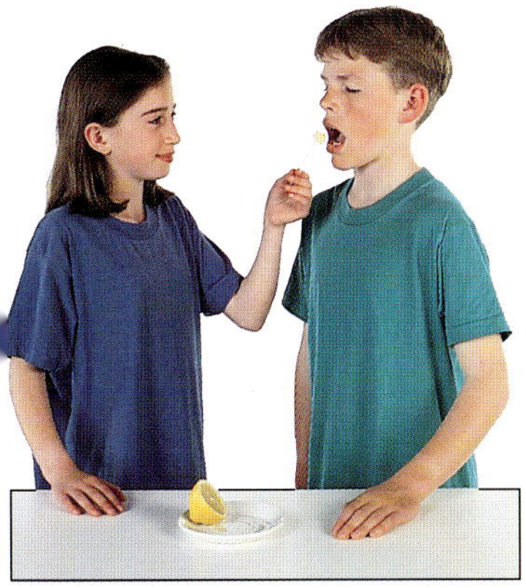

Taste confusion

Soak the potato in lemon juice for 10 minutes. Put it on a toothpick, and give it to a friend to eat. Make sure your friend's eyes are closed, so that he or she cannot see the food. Does your friend identify the food as potato or lemon? The brain receives conflicting information from different sensors, making it difficult to identify the food.

EXPERIMENT

Flavors and concentrations

Each of us has our own favorite flavors. But the strength or concentration of a flavor also has an effect on how much we like it. Some flavors are pleasant if they are weak, but become less so as they get stronger, while other flavors tend to taste better when they are stronger. You can study how the strength of a flavor affects how much you like it, by using the contrasting flavors of salt and sugar. When you do the experiment, make sure you do not take more than a small sip of each solution. (Do not drink all of the solution or you will feel sick.) Ask friends to try the experiment too. Do you find that most people have similar preferences? Do older and younger people have different preferences?

YOU WILL NEED

• *4 glasses of water* • *sugar* • *table salt* • *teaspoons*

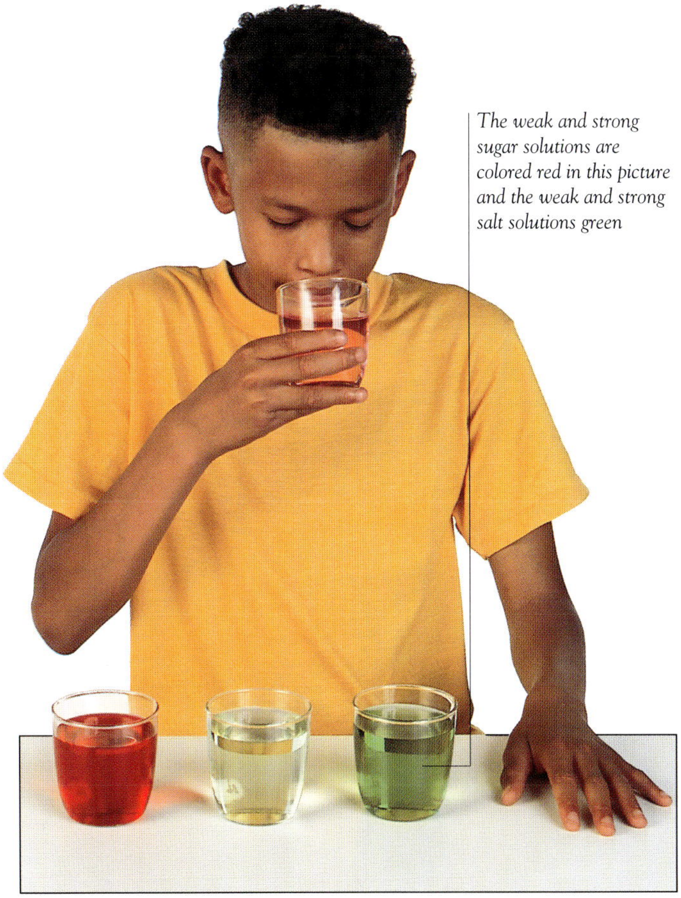

The weak and strong sugar solutions are colored red in this picture and the weak and strong salt solutions green

Sweet and salty

Stir half a teaspoonful of sugar into one glass and three teaspoonfuls into another. Do the same with the salt, stirring half a teaspoonful into the third glass, and three teaspoonfuls into the fourth. Sip the weaker sugar solution first. Then try the stronger one. Rinse your mouth with fresh water, then taste the salt solutions in the same order. Which do you like most and which least? Most people prefer stronger sweet flavors and weaker salty ones.

Touch

YOUR SENSE OF TOUCH allows you to feel incredibly light sensations, such as a fly on your hand, as well as very heavy ones, such as a weight dropped on your foot. The sensation of touch comes from millions of microscopic touch sensors scattered all over the skin. In some places, such as the fingertips, the sensors are close together, so these parts are very sensitive. In other places, such as the back, the sensors are quite far apart. When the sensors are pressed, vibrated, or stimulated by heat or cold, they generate nerve signals that flash to the brain (p.117).

EXPERIMENT

Fading touch

If you are wearing socks, can you feel how high they are on your legs, without looking? Perhaps not. You did feel the socks when you first put them on, but the feeling soon fades. This fading is called habituation. It also happens with smell (pp.158–159) and taste (pp.160–163). Habituation dulls your senses to a continuing stimulus. You become aware of something only when it changes.

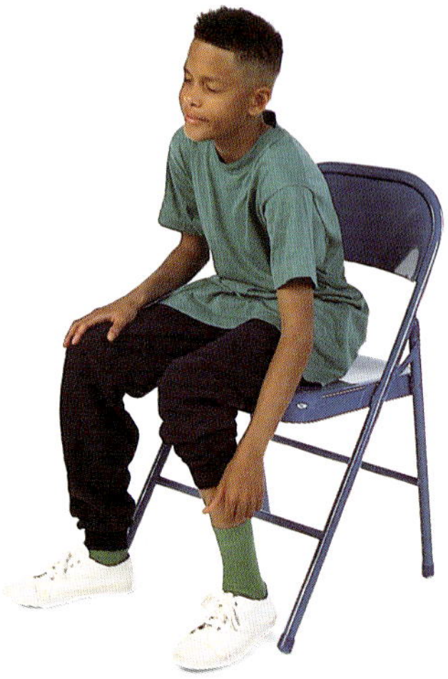

Forgotten feeling
With eyes closed, can you point exactly to the tops of your socks?

Types of touch sensor

The microscopic sensors in the skin are at the ends of nerves. The sensors are specially designed to convert physical sensations into tiny electrical nerve signals. Although we may think of touch as a single sense, there are a number of different types of touch sensor, each of which delivers a different pattern of nerve signals. The different sensors give us a wide variety of information about objects, such as their hardness, wetness, and surface texture.

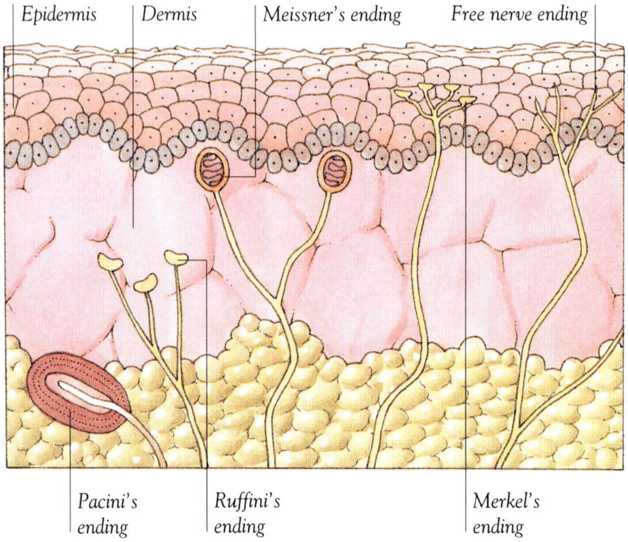

Kinds of stimulation
Each type of touch sensor responds to several kinds of stimulation. But the sensors do have specialized jobs. The deeply set Pacini's endings react mainly to heavy pressure. Merkel's endings respond best to medium pressure. Meissner's endings respond well to light pressure and small, fast vibrations. Ruffini's endings sense changes in temperature and pressure. When free nerve endings are activated, you feel pain.

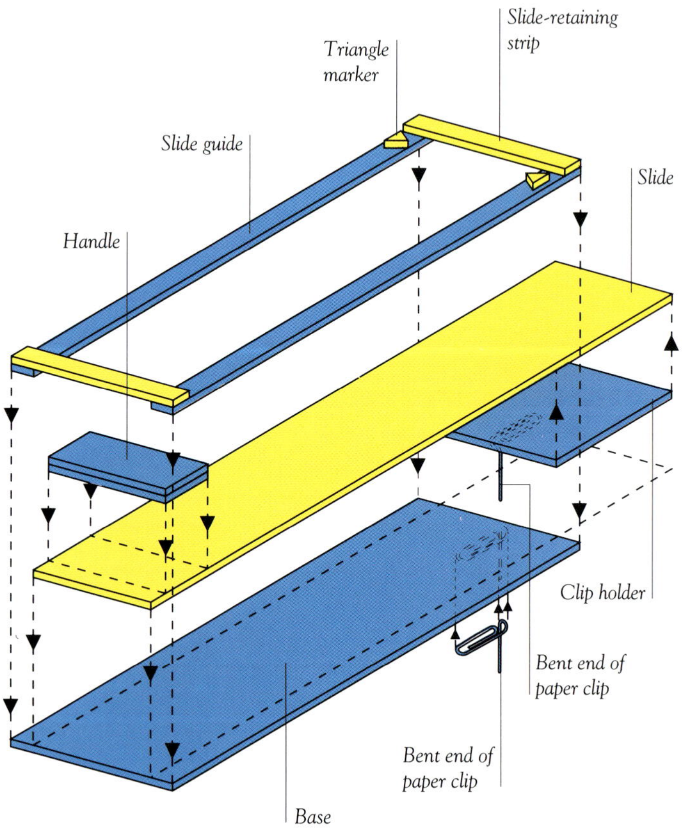

Putting the touch gauge together
Use thick poster board to make the gauge. When you tape or glue the slide guides to the base, make sure that the slide can move backward and forward between them. Tape the two paper clips to the edges of the base and clip holder so that the straightened vertical ends are touching each other.

EXPERIMENT

A touch map

Adult help is advised for this experiment

To feel the surface texture of something, you probably use your fingertips, rather than the back of your hand or your forearm. The fingertips are extremely sensitive to light touch, due to closely packed microscopic skin sensors. Investigate the sensitivity to light touch of different parts of the body by making a touch gauge. Create a touch-sensitivity "map," by sketching a rough outline of a body and marking your results on it.

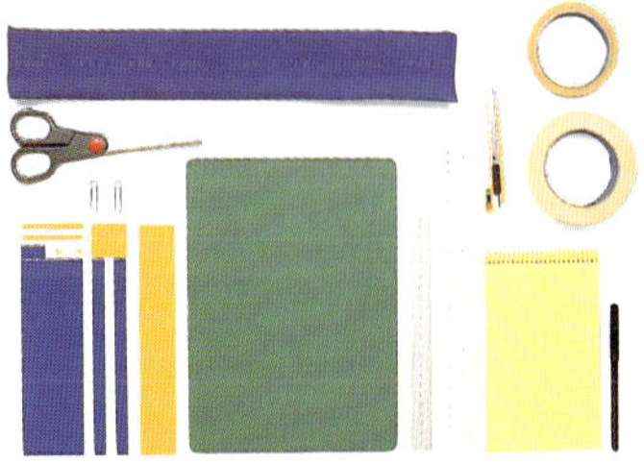

You Will Need

• blindfold • scissors • 2 paper clips • poster board—for the slide-retaining strips, 2 pieces 2½ in x ¼ in (6 cm x 0.5 cm); for the handle, 2 pieces 1½ in x ½ in (4 cm x 1 cm), glued one on top of the other; for the clip holder, 1 piece 1½ in (4 cm) square; for the slide guides, 2 pieces 8 in x ½ in (20 cm x 1 cm); for the slide, 1 piece 9½ in x 1½ in (24 cm x 4 cm); for the base, 1 piece 8 in x 2½ in (20 cm x 6 cm) • 2 poster board triangles about ½ in (1 cm) tall • cutting mat • metal cutting edge • ruler • craft knife • cellophane tape • double-sided tape or glue • notepad • pen

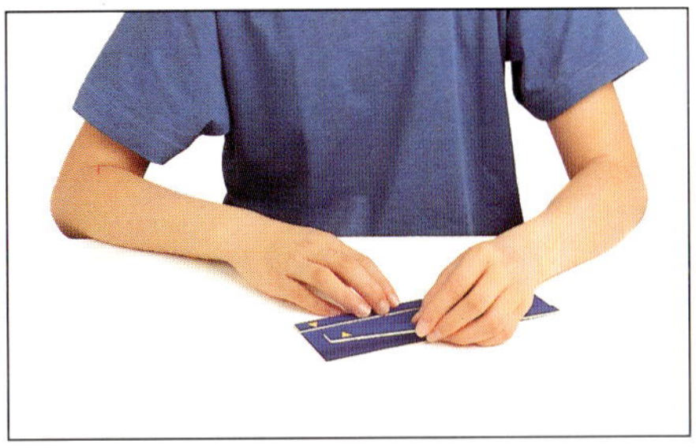

1 STICK THE TWO triangles to the slide guides, ½ in (1 cm) from the end, with double-sided tape or glue. Tape the guides to the base, with enough room to fit the slide between them.

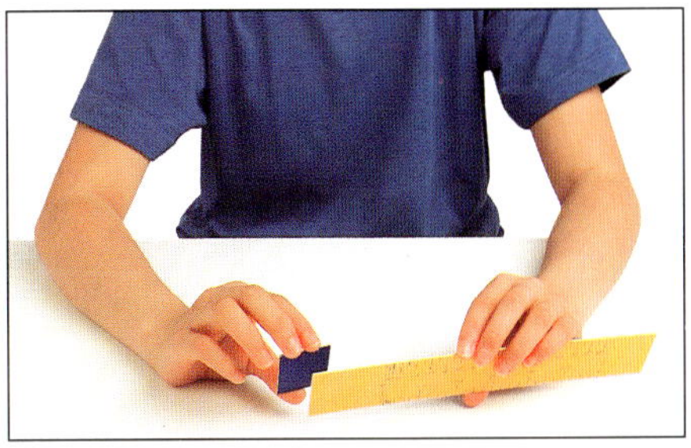

2 DRAW A SCALE 6 in (15 cm) long—with divisions of ¼ in (0.5 cm)—on the slide, starting 2 in (5 cm) from one end. Tape the clip holder to the same end of the slide, on the reverse side.

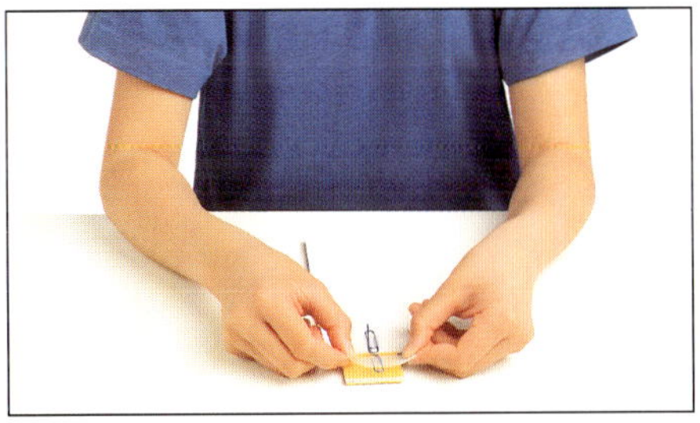

3 PLACE THE SLIDE between its guides, with the scale facing upward, and the paper triangles pointing to zero on the scale you have drawn. Turn over the gauge. Straighten out half of each paper clip, and bend it up at a right angle. Tape one bent paper clip end to the edge of the clip holder and the other to the base, so that the straight ends of the clips stick up vertically, touching each other.

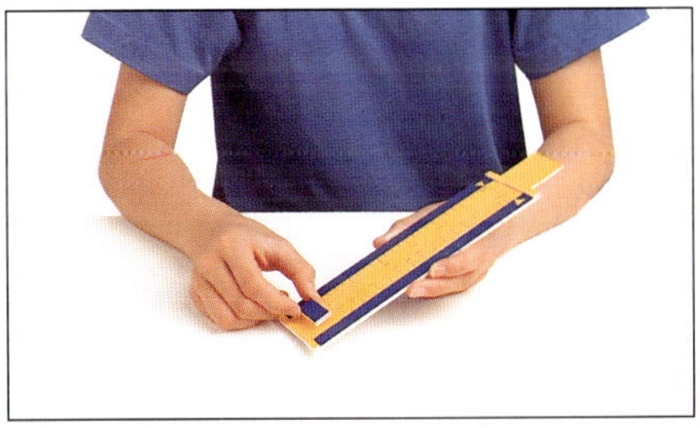

4 TAPE THE slide-retaining strips across each end of the upper side of the gauge, so that they hold the slide to the base, but allow it to move. Then tape the handle to the slide at the opposite end of the scale to zero. Check that the slide moves freely in the guides, and that when zero on the scale aligns with the triangles, the points of the paper clips are exactly together.

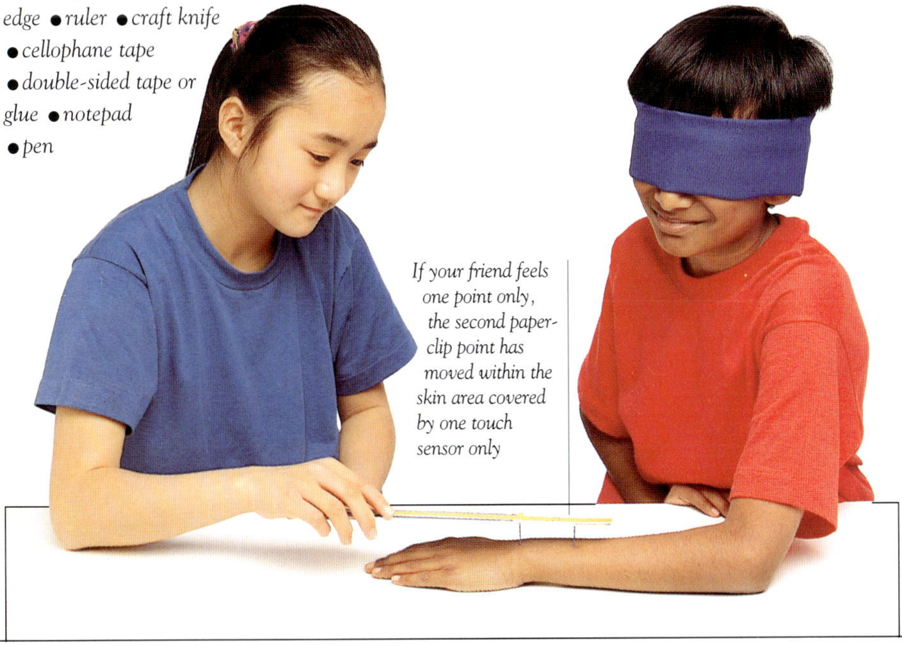

If your friend feels one point only, the second paper-clip point has moved within the skin area covered by one touch sensor only

5 YOU CAN READ the gap between the paper-clip points on the scale of the touch gauge. Ask a friend to wear a blindfold. Begin with the maximum gap between the paper-clip points. Press both points lightly on the outside of the forearm, making sure they touch the skin at exactly the same time. Your friend then tells you whether he or she feels two points or one. If the answer is two, reduce the gap slightly, and try again. Repeat until your friend can feel one point only. When this happens, read the gauge and note the gap between the two points. This gives an indication of the distance between touch sensors at the site. Repeat the whole process for other skin sites, such as the upper arm, wrist, and finger. Which parts of the body are most sensitive, with the greatest concentration of touch sensors?

The touch picture

YOUR SENSE OF TOUCH is a more complicated sense than it might seem. Think of the difference between feeling a warm cat and a cold lump of ice. The different microscopic sensors (p.164) in your skin respond to different stimulations, such as changes in temperature, light touch, or heavy pressure. They send complex patterns of nerve signals to your brain. Your brain assembles an overall "touch picture" from these nerve signal patterns. You describe different aspects of this touch picture with words such as "cold" and "warm," "soft" and "hard," "rough" and "smooth," "dry" and "moist." To learn more about the things that you touch, you use the information from other senses, particularly sight. Imagine how you would hesitate before touching an object that you knew nothing about. You would be sensible to do this—it might be burning hot!

EXPERIMENT

Telling by touch

Adult help is advised for this experiment

Focus on the sense of touch by blocking out other senses that usually accompany it. Use a nose clip and blindfold to block out smell and sight. Then feel various everyday things to find out whether you can identify them by touch alone.

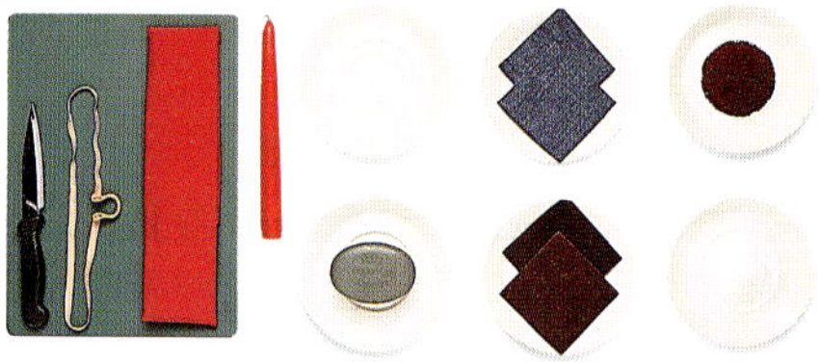

YOU WILL NEED

- *cutting mat* • *small kitchen knife* • *nose clip* • *blindfold* • *saucers* • *samples of everyday substances, such as candle wax, denim, coffee, soap, leather, and sugar*

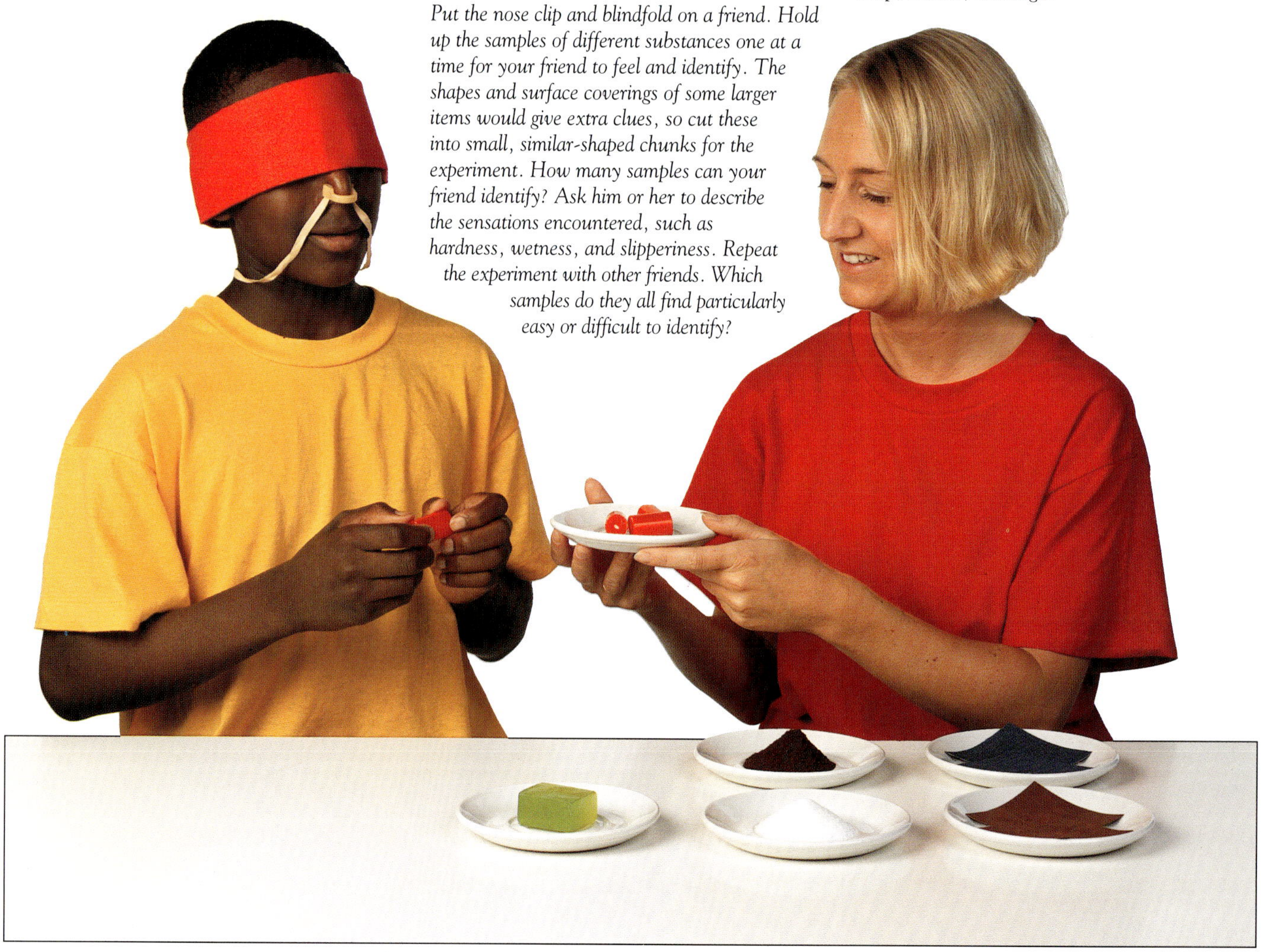

Touch alone

Put the nose clip and blindfold on a friend. Hold up the samples of different substances one at a time for your friend to feel and identify. The shapes and surface coverings of some larger items would give extra clues, so cut these into small, similar-shaped chunks for the experiment. How many samples can your friend identify? Ask him or her to describe the sensations encountered, such as hardness, wetness, and slipperiness. Repeat the experiment with other friends. Which samples do they all find particularly easy or difficult to identify?

EXPERIMENT
Reading by touch

Adult help is advised for this experiment

Fingertips are very sensitive to touch. You can use them to "read" numbers or letters made of map pins stuck into cork tiles.

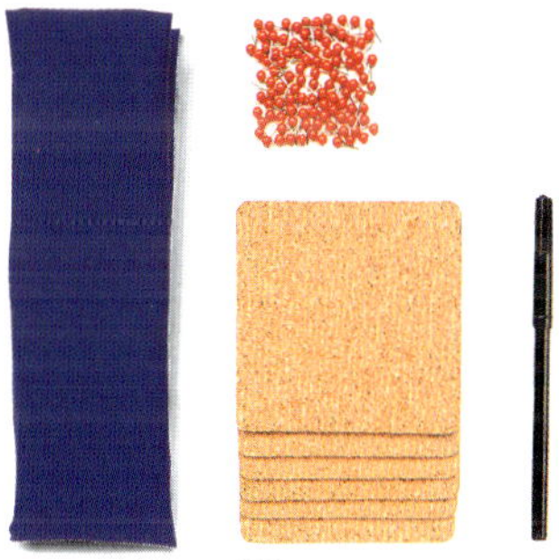

YOU WILL NEED
- *felt-tip pen* • *plastic-headed map pins* • *blindfold* • *cork tiles*

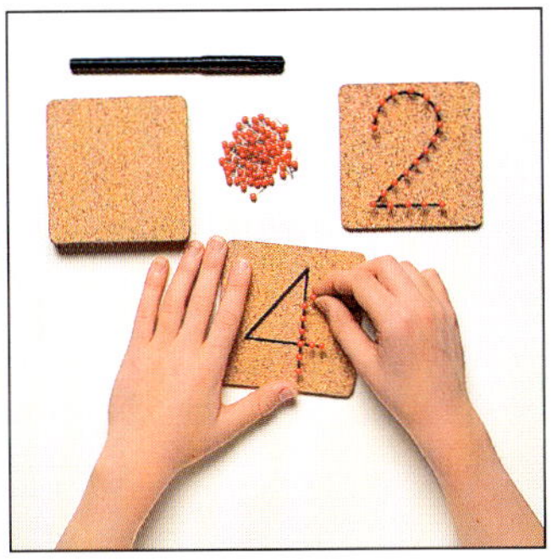

1 USING MAP pins, you can make a system similar to the Braille system (below right) with its patterns of raised dots. Draw a large number or letter on each cork tile. Use simple shapes such as L, O, and 1, and also complex ones such as G, Q, and 4. Make all the figures the same size. Now push the pins into the numbers and letters to make their shapes. Do not push the pin points right through the cork tiles.

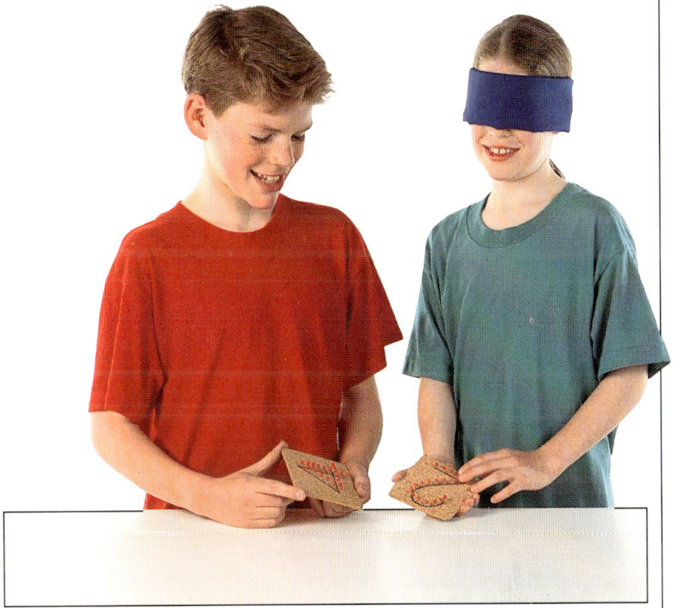

2 BLINDFOLD A FRIEND, and hand him or her the cork squares, one at a time. Ask your friend to feel the pattern of pinheads, and see if he or she can read each letter or number. Which ones are easiest? Does your friend get quicker and more accurate with practice? What happens if you hand over the letter or number upside down?

EXPERIMENT
Blurring the sense of touch

When you look through a window with frost on it, what you see is indistinct. Thick gloves create a similar effect for the sense of touch. Wearing gloves makes it more difficult to feel and identify objects. But there are clues that you can still use, even when blindfolded—such as weight, shape, and hardness.

YOU WILL NEED
- *padded or wool gloves*
- *similar-shaped objects, such as a tomato, walnut, golf ball, potato, and table-tennis ball*

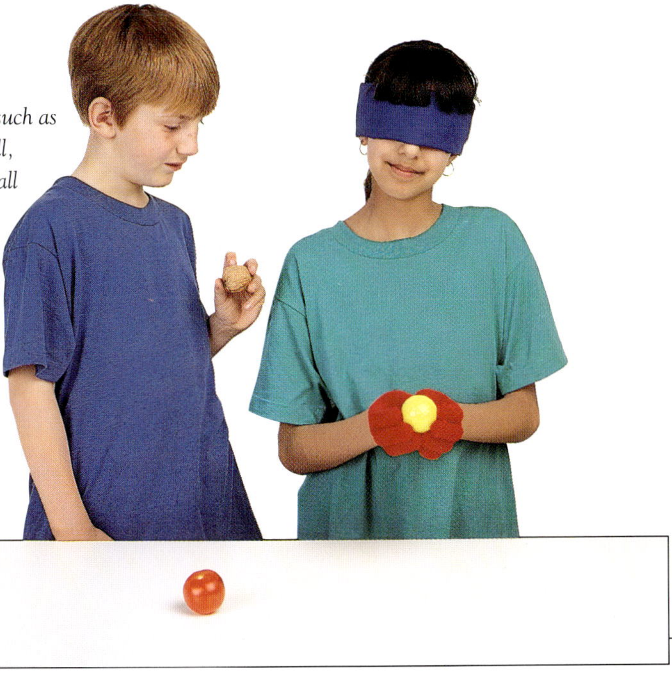

Dulled sensations
Blindfold a friend. Ask him or her to put the gloves on. Pass over a series of objects to feel and identify. Are soft things easier to name than hard ones? Does it help to smell or bounce the objects?

The Braille system

Braille is a reading system for blind people. Patterns of raised dots in groups of up to six (as on a domino) are felt by the fingers. Each pattern represents a number, a letter, or a group of letters. The method is named after its French inventor, Louis Braille (1809–52), who lost his sight when he was 3 years old.

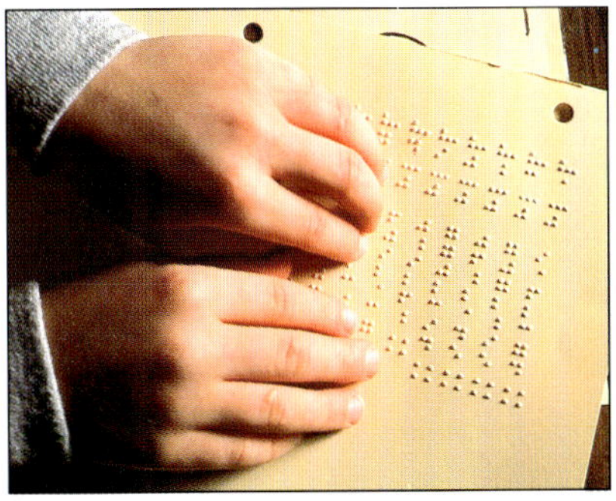

Two-handed reading
Braille is read by the sensitive fingertip skin. Usually, one hand reads the dots while the other hand feels ahead for the next line.

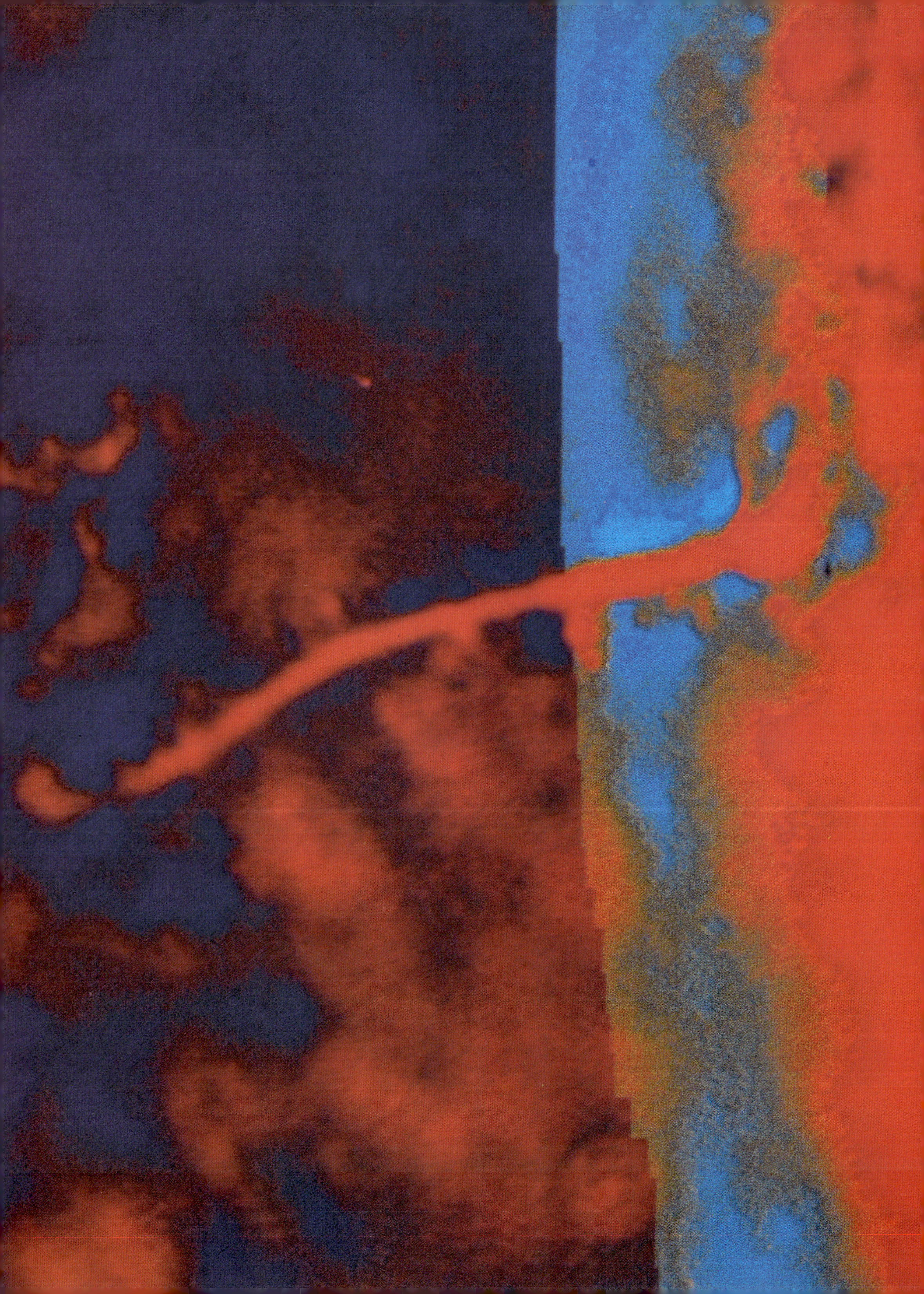

The BODY'S LIFE CYCLE

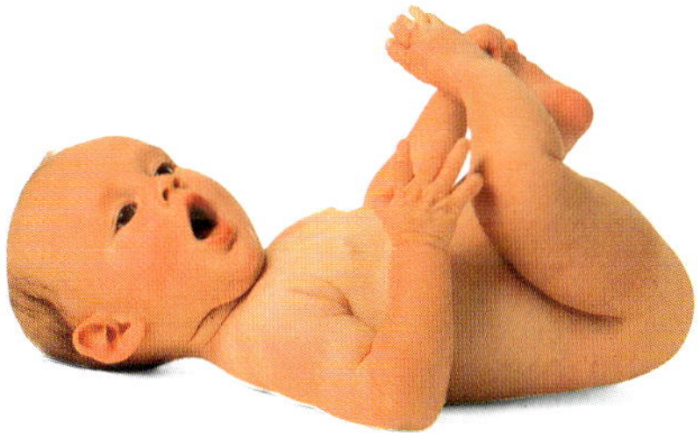

Egg to baby
The human ovum (egg cell) is one of the largest cells in the body—it is just about visible to the naked eye. If a male's sperm cell enters the female's ovum, the egg is fertilized (a sperm is shown at the very point of entry, left), and it develops in the mother's womb. Nine months later, this tiny egg will be a living, breathing, crying new baby (above).

DURING ITS LIFE, THE BODY progresses through well-defined stages. A baby grows from a tiny egg, develops in the mother's womb, and enters the outside world at birth. He or she grows through infancy, childhood, puberty, and adolescence, and matures through the adult years. Finally, the only certain thing about life is that it will end. But the reproductive process brings about new human beings. Parents pass on the blueprint of human life to their babies in the form of genes. And a new cycle of life begins.

NEW LIFE AND GROWTH

THE STAGES OF LIFE for a human body are the same as for any type of mammal. They include the coming together of an egg cell and a sperm cell to create a new individual, formation of the main organs while an embryo in the womb, birth as a baby, rapid growth in infancy, and becoming sexually mature and able to produce offspring. Humans also have important life stages based on culture and tradition, such as the school years, parenthood, and retirement.

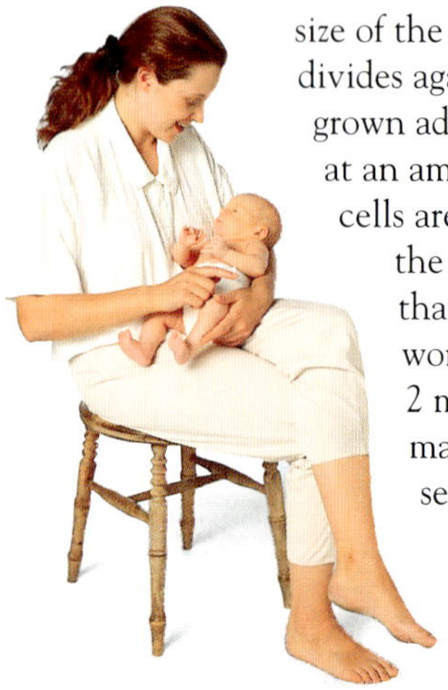

A baby soon learns to smile *at a friendly face, especially that of the mother. Mother and baby recognize each other by smell—from a day or two after birth.*

The cell is the basic unit of life. All living things—plant or animal—are made from cells (pp.24–25). The cell is also the unit of growth. The body grows as its cells divide in two. Each of these new cells enlarges to the size of the original cell and then divides again. Even in a fully grown adult, cell division occurs at an amazingly fast rate. New cells are needed constantly by the body to replace cells that have died or have worn away. For example, 2 million new red cells are made for the blood every second. The cell is also the basic unit of reproduction. Each human body starts out as a single cell, a fertilized egg. These eggs are each smaller than the period at the end of this sentence.

Mother and father

Ancient people realized that after a woman and man had sexual intercourse a baby could be conceived. But their ideas about how this happens were mistaken. For example, Aristotle (384–322 B.C.) of ancient Greece believed that the mother provided only the physical body of the child, which grew from the blood in her womb (uterus). He thought that the role of the father was to provide the "soul" that made the baby alive.

During the Renaissance Leonardo da Vinci (1452–1519) made accurate drawings of how the baby develops in the mother's womb. Unfortunately, his drawings were lost for several centuries, so later researchers did not benefit from them.

Cells from cells

From the 1600's onward, the microscopists turned their lenses to the reproductive process. They discovered egg cells (p.180) and sperm cells (p.185), and saw how a sperm joins with an egg at fertilization (p.172).

Some scientists believed that new cells were made when chemicals gathered together in a body fluid and attracted more chemicals to them, gradually building up a whole cell. However, this theory depended on the false assumption that living organisms can form from chemicals—in other words, from nonliving material. This idea was known as spontaneous generation. The work of scientists such as the Frenchman Louis Pasteur (1822–95) showed that cells do not simply "appear" from nonliving matter.

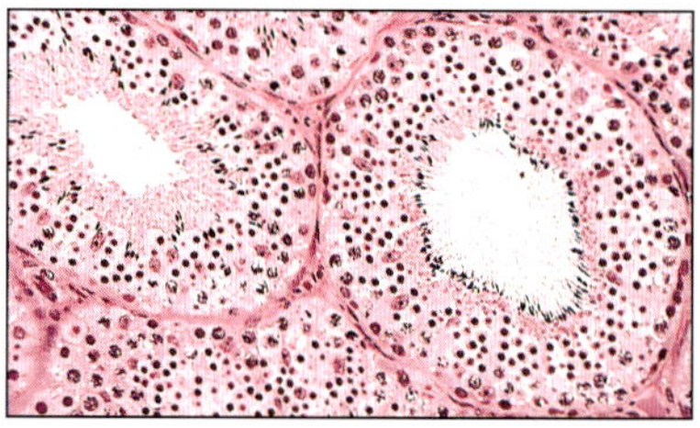

Inside a man's testes there are *coiled tubes (p.23), shown in cross section by this microscope photograph. Millions of sperm cells develop in these tubes, then pass into the centers of the tubes before they are released.*

The German scientist Rudolf Virchow (1821–1902) studied the process of disease at the level of cells and tissues. He supported the idea, now proved correct, that new cells are made by the division of existing cells. He coined the famous phrase: "Every cell from a cell."

Genetics

In 1865 an Austrian monk, Gregor Mendel (1822–84), published his work on the breeding of garden peas. In his writings he explained the basic laws of heredity—how certain traits (features) are inherited by offspring from parents.

Many people believed at the time that the traits of each parent "blend" in their offspring. But Mendel found that, over the generations, certain traits of pea plants do not blend—they either appear or do not. He realized instead that features seem to be inherited as

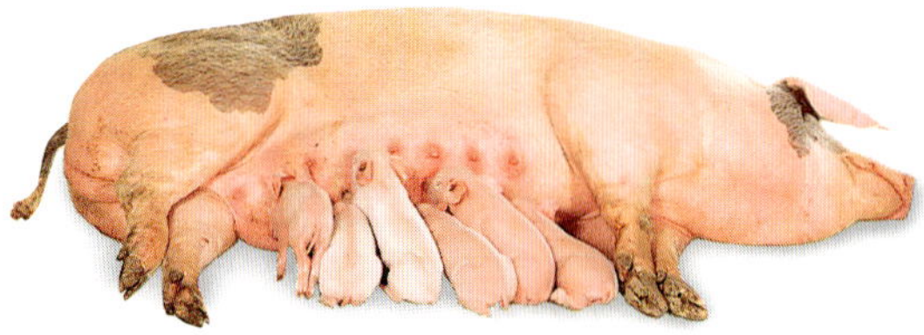

Milk from the mother's mammary glands is the *complete food for baby mammals, such as these piglets. It contains proteins for building up the body, sugars for energy, fats for both, and germ-fighting substances.*

units, which we now call genes (p.176). Sometimes they do not show up in one generation, but reappear in the next. Mendel also realized that some traits are dominant, "overpowering" other traits. However, his theories produced little interest until the 1900's, when Mendel's laws became the basis for the new science of genetics.

We now know that genes are in pairs, and that one member of the pair can be dominant over the other. In a simplified example, each person has a pair of genes that control eye color, one from each parent. If both genes are for brown eyes, the eyes are brown. If both are for blue eyes, the eyes are blue. But if a person has one gene for brown eyes and one for blue, the eyes are not blue-brown. The brown gene is dominant, so the eyes are brown. The ideas of genes and dominance are central to modern genetic research.

By the early 1900's the process of cell division had been studied in great detail. We now know that there are in fact two types.

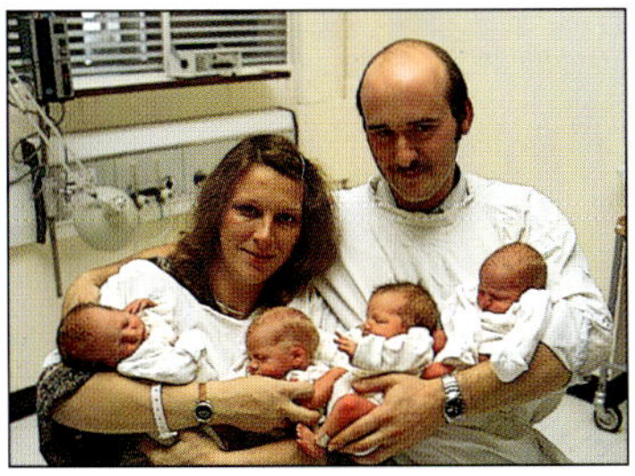

***This set of quadruplets is unusual** because humans generally have only one baby at a time. These babies will have different characteristics, but they will retain a family likeness.*

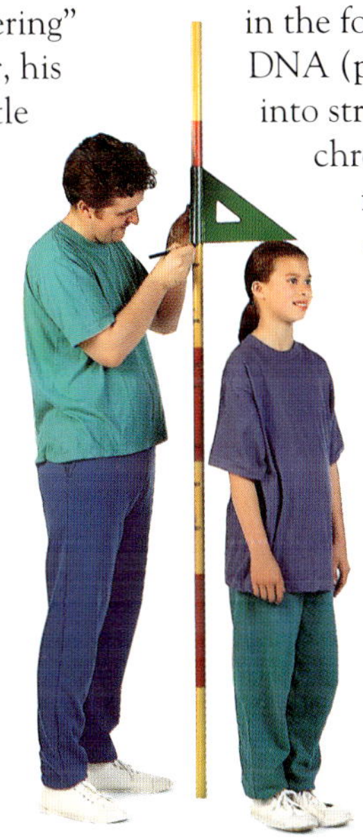

***Do you grow in spurts?** Find out by regularly measuring how tall you are (p.175).*

Mitosis

For growth and maintenance of the body, the cells divide by a process called mitosis. The pairs of genes in each cell, which are in the form of the chemical DNA (p.180), are packaged into structures called chromosomes inside the nucleus. In mitosis, the chromosomes duplicate themselves when the cell is ready to divide, making a second set of gene pairs. The two sets then separate, each moving to one end of the cell. The cell membrane (p.28) grows through the middle of the cell, splitting it in two. So two complete new cells, each with an identical full set of genes, are formed from one parent cell.

Meiosis

The other type of cell division is meiosis. This process has major differences from mitosis. Meiosis produces egg and sperm cells only. There are not two offspring cells; there are four. And each offspring cell contains single genes, not pairs.

Egg cells are made in the woman's sex glands, called ovaries (p.23). Each month, one egg matures, as part of a cycle controlled by hormones (p.106). The mature egg is released from a small bag in the ovary called an ovarian follicle (Graafian follicle) and travels along a tube, the oviduct, toward the womb. If sperm have entered the oviduct as a result of sexual intercourse, fertilization may occur.

Sperm cells are made in the man's sex glands, called testes. These hang in a small sac of skin, the scrotum, below the abdomen. Millions of sperm are made every day. If they are not released they die, break up, and are reabsorbed into the body.

As a result of meiosis, each egg and sperm has a single set of genes. When they join together at fertilization, their sets combine. So each cell in the developing baby has the usual set of gene pairs. We inherit one gene of each pair from our mother and the other from our father. Inherited genes are the reason why we resemble our biological parents.

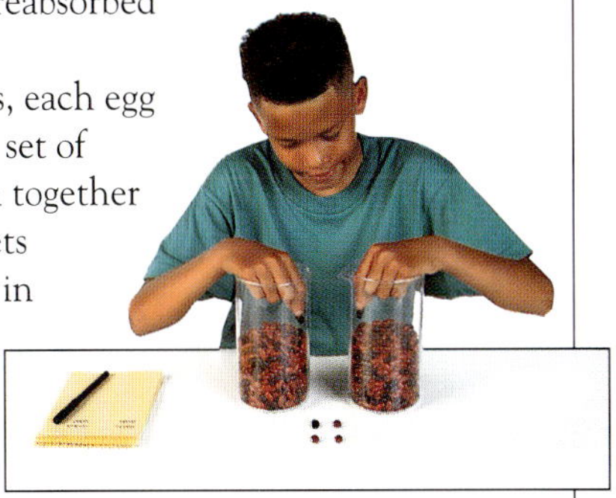

***By choosing pairs of beans from** two jars you can find out the chances of inheriting certain body features, such as a particular eye or hair color (p.177).*

Human growth

During the first 2 months in the womb, all of the baby's major parts and organs are formed (pp.172–173). After 9 months the baby is born. In the processes of birth and early infancy, humans are typical of mammals. For example, the baby feeds on milk made in the mammary glands (after which the mammal group is named) in the mother's breasts. However, the human child soon shows the intelligence that sets us apart from other mammals—by talking, reading, and so on. The next major stage is puberty, which takes place during the teens, when the sexual organs become mature and start to function. After this stage, it is possible to become a parent and begin the cycle of life once again.

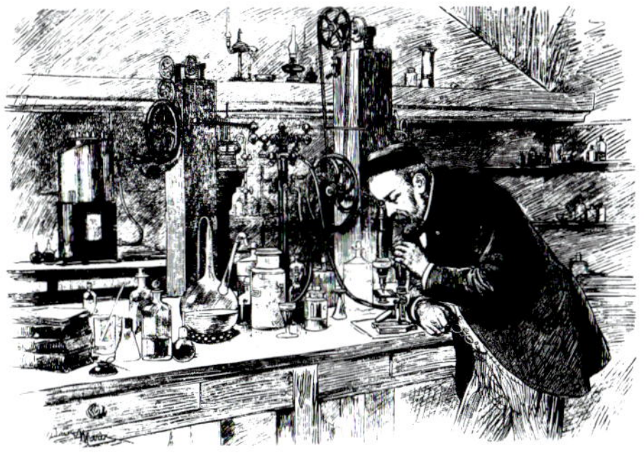

***Louis Pasteur worked in this laboratory.** Scientists such as Pasteur helped to show that life comes from previous life, and that spontaneous generation of new living things from nonliving matter does not occur.*

Reproduction

THE PARTS OF THE BODY concerned with producing babies are together called the reproductive system (p.23). In a mammal such as a cat or horse, a male animal and female animal come together and mate (have sexual intercourse). A sperm cell from the testes of the male fertilizes an egg cell from the ovaries of the female—that is, they join together. After fertilization, the egg grows and develops into a new baby animal in an organ called a womb (uterus), which only female mammals possess. After a period called pregnancy, the baby leaves the womb through the birth canal and is born. Reproduction in humans follows this typical mammal pattern. The human pregnancy period is, on average, 38 weeks from fertilization to birth.

■ DISCOVERY ■

Antony van Leeuwenhoek

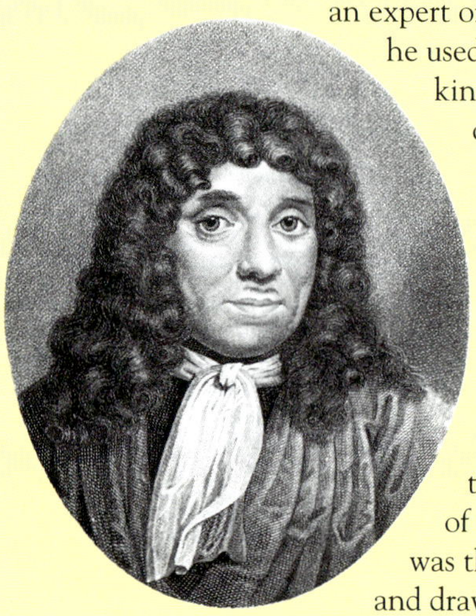

Antony van Leeuwenhoek (1632–1723), the "draper of Delft," was a Dutch textile merchant. He used magnifying lenses, which he made himself, to count the threads in pieces of cloth. His lenses were tiny—many were no bigger than a pea. Van Leeuwenhoek was not an expert on the human body. But he used his lenses to study all kinds of microscopic objects, and the range and accuracy of his observations were astounding. He was one of the first people to see microbes (microscopic organisms) such as bacteria. He studied the movement and size of red blood cells. And he was the first scientist to see and draw sperm cells (below).

Tiny bodies

In the 17th century, some scientists believed that the eggs (ova) of female animals, including humans, contained tiny versions of the parents, waiting to grow into babies. These scientists were called "ovists." After the discovery of male sperm cells, which were originally called spermatic animalcules, other scientists—known as "animalculists"—argued that the tiny beings were not in the eggs, but in the heads of the sperm. Later it was realized that in fact egg and sperm contribute equally to the conception of a baby (right).

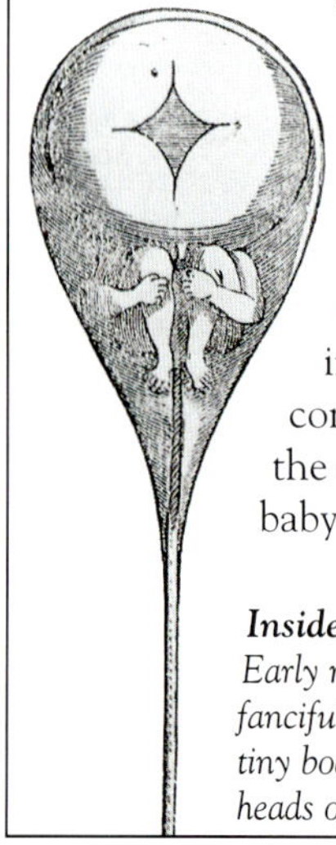

Inside the sperm
Early microscopists made fanciful drawings of imaginary tiny bodies curled up inside the heads of sperm cells.

Fertilization

Sperm cells pass into a woman's body during sexual intercourse. They swim through her womb and into the oviducts (also called Fallopian tubes), which connect the ovaries to the womb. If a mature egg cell is released by one ovary at about this time, the sperm cells are attracted to it. One of the sperm cells penetrates the membrane, called the zona pellucida, that is wrapped around the egg cell. Then the genetic material of egg cell and sperm cell combine (p.171). This event is called fertilization.

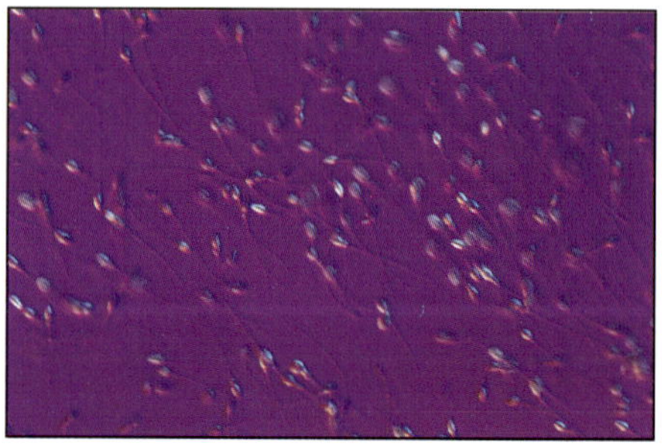

Sperm cells
These tadpole-shaped cells, shown here through a light microscope, are very small (p.26). They swim by lashing their long tails.

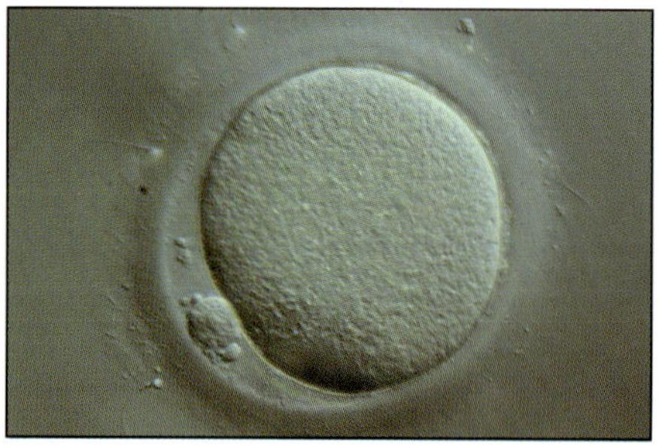

Egg cell
The zona pellucida around an egg cell looks like a halo under a light microscope. After fertilization, the membrane thickens to keep out other sperm.

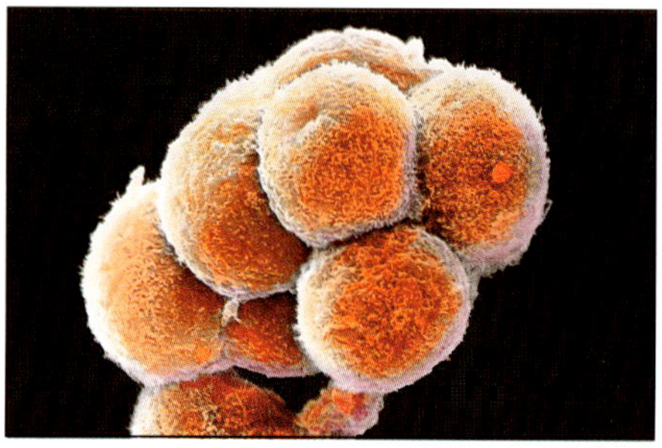

Ball of cells
The fertilized egg cell divides into two cells, then into four, and so on. This electron microscope view shows the ball-like 16-cell stage.

A baby's development

As the fertilized egg continues to divide, each of the cells in the ball becomes slightly smaller. Living on its stored reserves of yolk, the ball floats along the oviduct to the womb. About a week after fertilization, it burrows into the thick, blood-rich womb lining and begins to feed on nourishment provided by the lining. The cells multiply, becoming hundreds in number, then thousands. As they multiply, the cells begin to differentiate—in other words they change into different types, such as nerve cells, muscle cells, and so on. Slowly the baby's body takes shape.

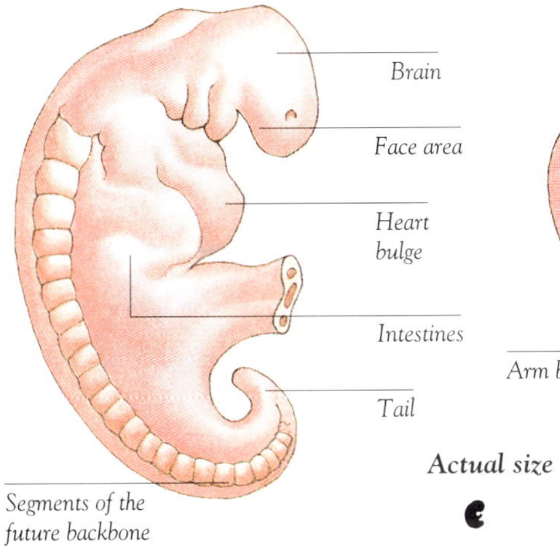

After 4 weeks
The future backbone forms a ridge. The baby has a tiny tail and at this stage is difficult to distinguish from other baby mammals.

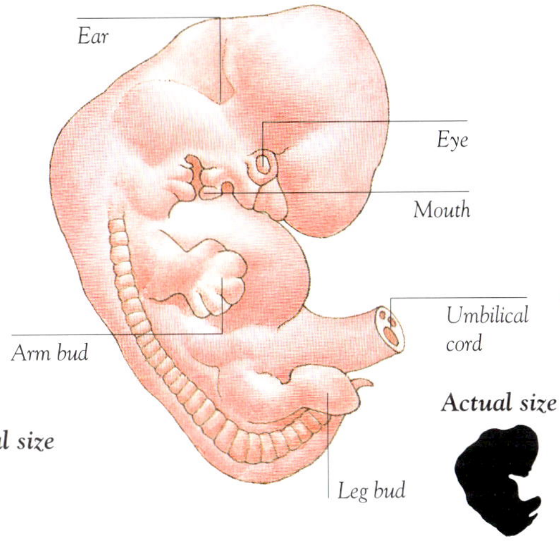

After 5 weeks
The eye is recognizable, but the ear is slitlike. Limbs grow out of the trunk, and the tail shrinks away. At this stage the baby is called an embryo.

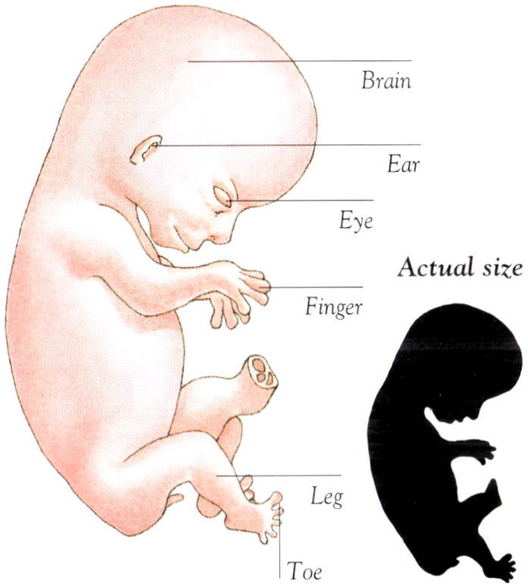

After 8 weeks
From this age, the developing baby is called a fetus. It is only thumb size, yet all its main parts are formed, even fingers and toes.

■ DISCOVERY ■

Reinier de Graaf

The Dutch physician and anatomist Reinier de Graaf (1641–73) studied many body parts, including the pancreas, the gall bladder next to the liver, and the male and female reproductive organs. In 1672 he published a book on the female reproductive system. He believed that he had identified the eggs (ova) as blisterlike swellings on the surface of the ovary. In fact, each of these swellings is a mature follicle (egg container) with the actual egg cell hidden deep within it. The whole structure is called a Graafian follicle in his memory. Each follicle contains fluid that nourishes and cushions the egg and hundreds of other cells that support it. Fertilization occurs when the egg cell is released from the follicle and meets a sperm cell in the oviduct (opposite).

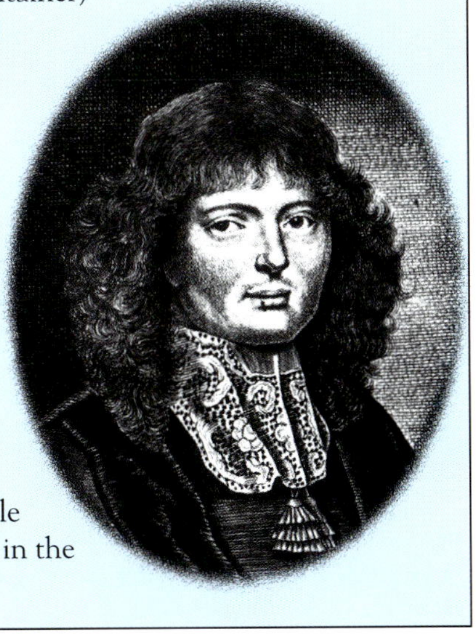

Nourishing the baby

Inside the womb, the baby floats in a pool of amniotic fluid. It cannot breathe air or eat food. Oxygen and nutrients pass to the baby from the mother's blood through the placenta, a disk-shaped organ in the womb wall. Blood flows between the baby and placenta along a flexible tube, the umbilical cord.

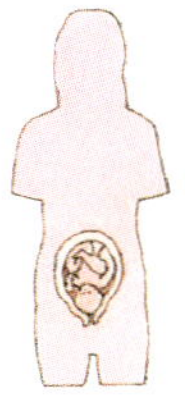

Bulging abdomen
The enlarging womb makes the mother's abdomen bulge.

Ready to be born
This cutaway view shows a baby after 9 months of development.

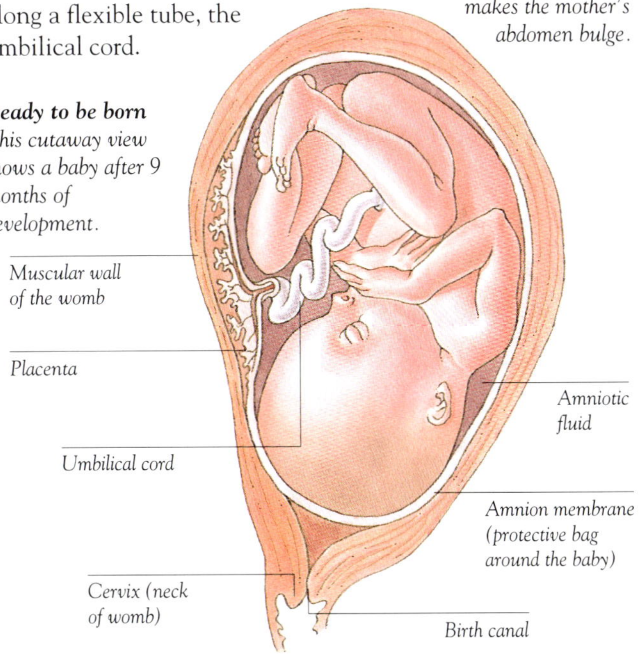

Growth and aging

HAVE YOU WATCHED a young child learning to walk? He or she often topples over. This is partly because the brain, nerves, and muscles have not yet learned how to balance the body. It is also because the young child is "top-heavy." A baby has a very large head in relation to the body compared with an adult. In the womb (p.173), the brain and head develop very early. By the time a child is about 3 years old, the brain and head are more than four-fifths fully grown, yet the body's bones and muscles are only about one-fifth of their adult size. In early childhood the body lengthens rapidly. From about 9 or 10 years, the arms, and then the legs, grow fastest—much more quickly than the torso. There is a rapid growth spurt just before and during puberty (p.171). The average person is physically fully developed by the age of 20 to 25. After 40 to 50 years, the changes of aging become noticeable. The muscles become smaller, there is loss of height, and the skin develops lines and wrinkles.

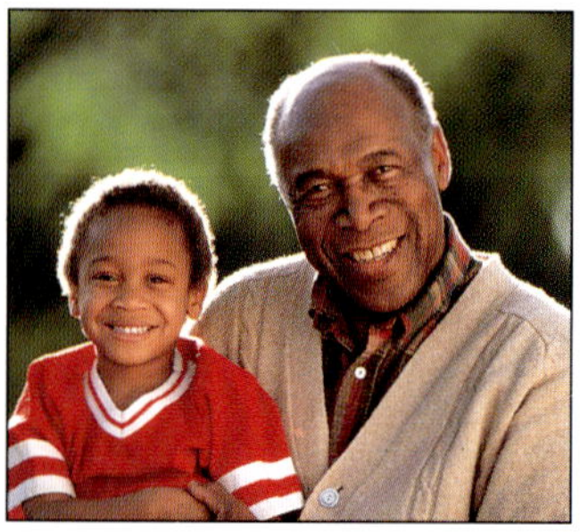

Different but the same
Often, many similarities can be seen in members of a family, even though the people may be at different stages of the aging process.

EXPERIMENT
Growth rate

Adult help is advised for this experiment

See how tall you are and how fast you grow by marking your height with a pen on a measuring pole (made from a length of wood or plastic). Do this at regular times—say every 4 months. Your growth rate is the amount you have grown each year. Does it vary as you get older? Measure the growth rates for your family and friends too. Do people grow faster at certain ages? In particular, try to measure the growth rates of a baby, someone in their early teens, and an older person.

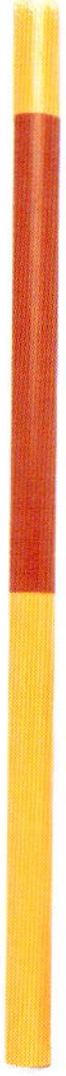

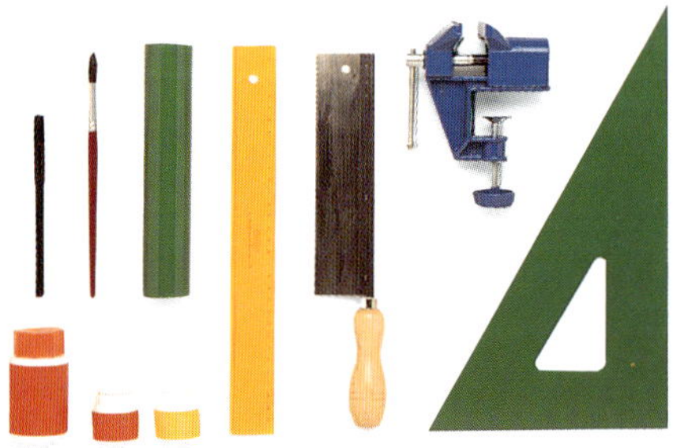

YOU WILL NEED
- *pole $6\frac{1}{2}$ ft (2 m) long* • *pen* • *paintbrush*
- *plastic pipe to slip over the pole* • *strong glue*
- *paints* • *ruler* • *saw* • *vise* • *large set square*

Changing proportions

In this series of photographs, the height of each person—from the new baby to the young adult of 20 years—has been adjusted so that he just fits into the panel. This makes all of the bodies exactly the same height. The photographs allow you to compare the body proportions and to see how they change with age. For example, the baby has a very large head, almost one-quarter of its total height. By adulthood, however, the head is only about one-eighth of the total height. Compare the legs and arms, too. The baby's legs make up roughly one-third of its total height. In a full-grown person they are almost half of the total height. Added to these general changes are many individual variations (pp.16–17). A person may have a relatively long body or long legs throughout his or her life.

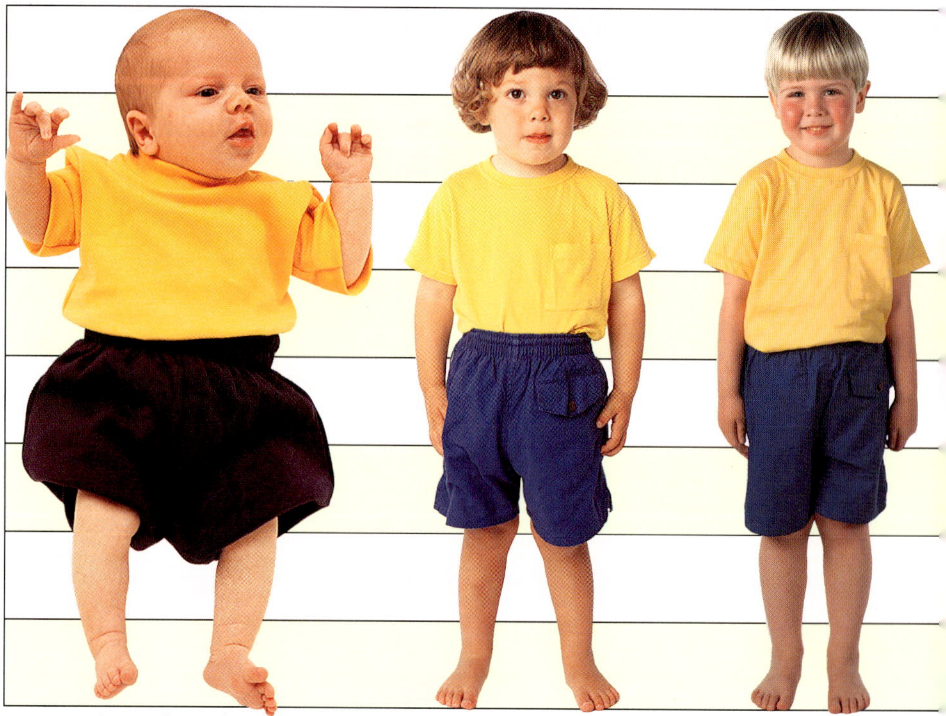

2 months: 1 ft 10 in (55 cm)

2 years: 2 ft 10 in (86 cm)

4 years: 3 ft 8 in (110 cm)

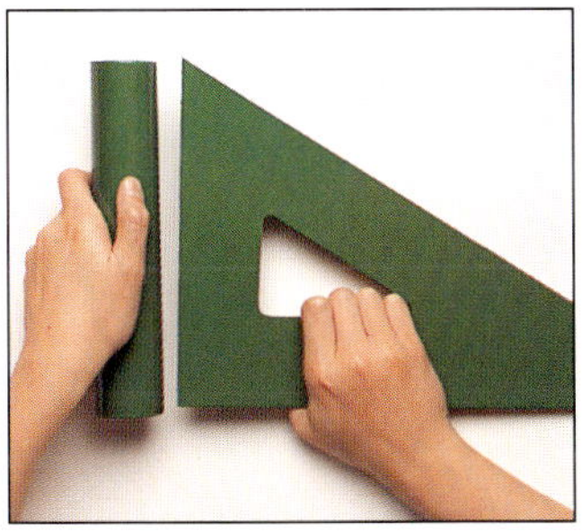

1 ASK AN adult to saw the pipe, held in place by the vise, to the same length as the set square's shortest edge. Glue the pipe to this edge.

2 PAINT THE pole in stripes 1 ft (30 cm) wide, and allow the paint to dry. Slide the pipe onto the pole. Now measure your height. Stand upright next to the pole. Get a friend to slide the pipe down so that the set square rests on your head. The friend marks the pole below the pipe with a line and the date. To check your height, add up the number of whole stripes and measure the extra part of the last stripe with the ruler.

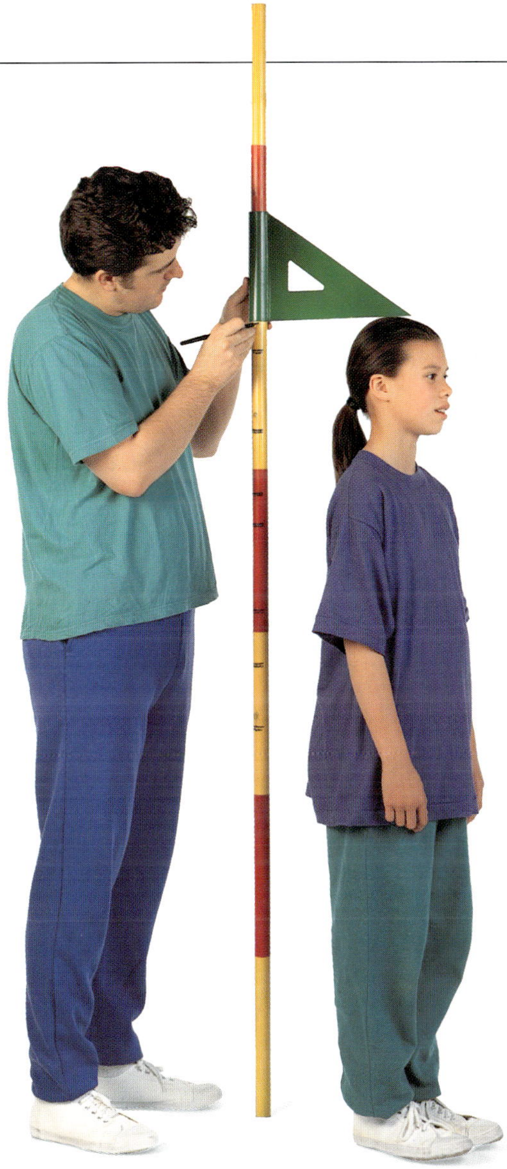

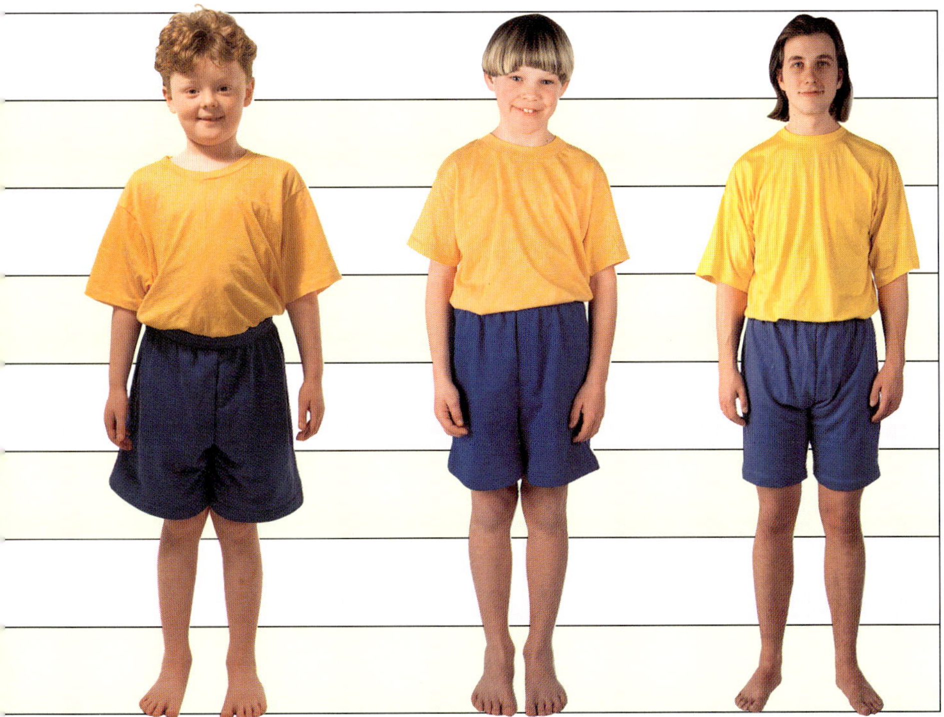

7 years: 4 ft (120 cm)

12 years: 4 ft 10 in (145 cm)

20 years: 5 ft 10 in (175 cm)

Changing faces

These details from self-portraits by the Dutch artist Rembrandt (1606–69) show how he aged over a period of 40 years. Although facial features gradually change during life, we can still recognize the same person after many years from the face's overall shape, proportions, and expressions.

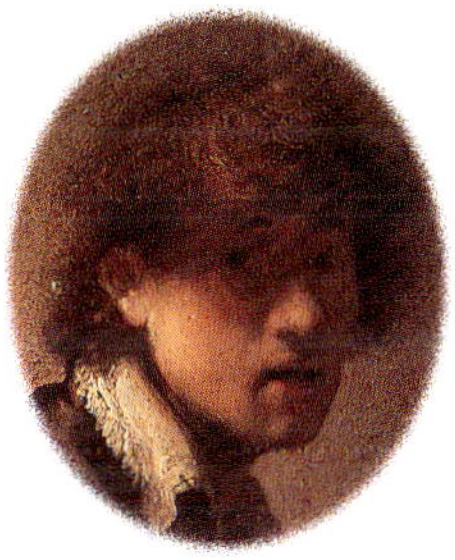

Age 23 (1629)

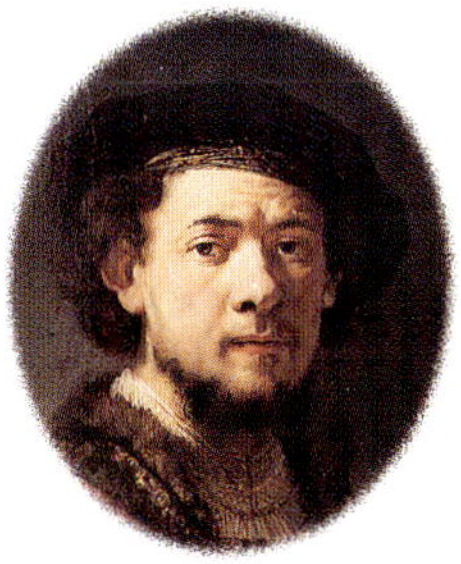

Age 31 (1637)

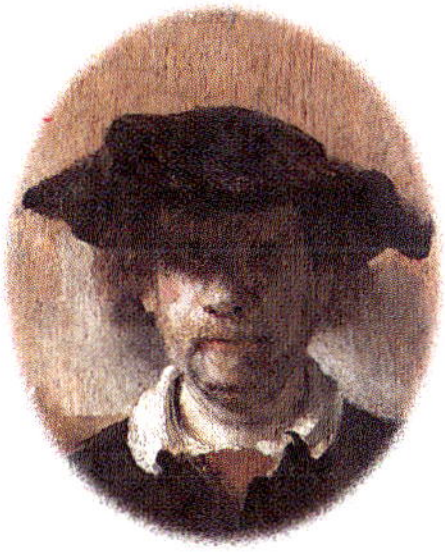

Age 44 (1650)

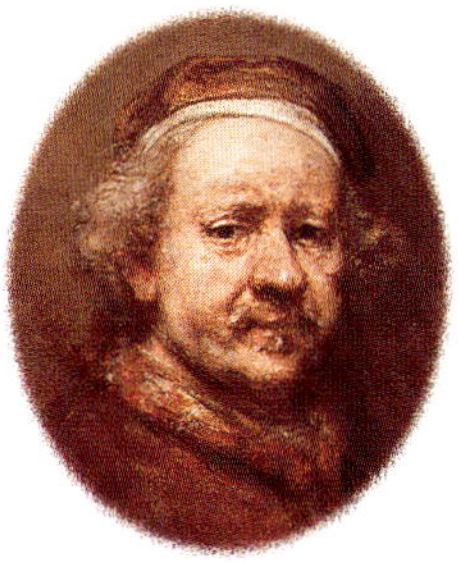

Age 63 (1669)

Genes and inheritance

A COMPLICATED STRUCTURE such as a jet plane or a skyscraper must be built from a set of plans. The body also has "plans," called genes. These contain, in chemical code, all the instructions needed to build and run a body. There are about 100,000 different genes in each body cell. Each gene is a short section of a long molecule called DNA (p.179). DNA is packaged in chromosomes, arranged in pairs in the cell nucleus. However, sperm and egg cells contain not pairs of chromosomes, but single sets. This is due to meiosis (p.182). When a sperm fertilizes an egg, these single sets pair up in a new cell—which multiplies and develops into a baby.

Genes and chromosomes

Each body cell has 46 sets of gene-containing DNA molecules. The DNA molecules are coiled into 23 pairs of X-shaped structures called chromosomes in each cell nucleus.

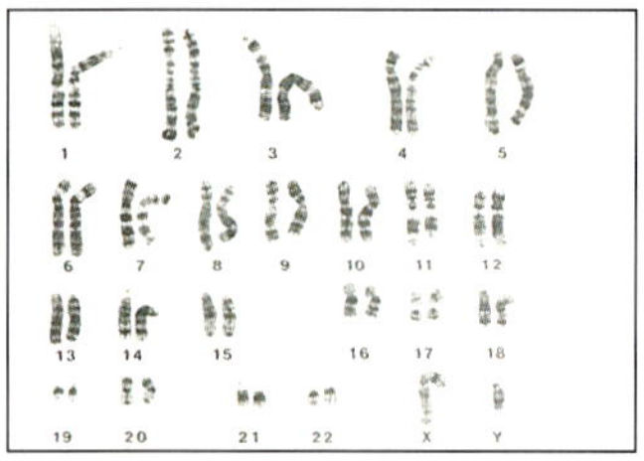

Full set of chromosomes
There are 23 chromosome pairs. One chromosome of each pair comes from the mother, the other chromosome from the father.

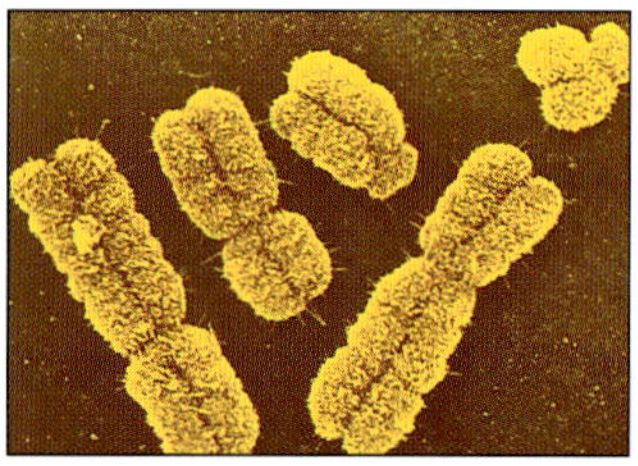

Chromosomes close up
Each chromosome contains a thin DNA molecule, about 2 in (5 cm) long, coiled very tightly and protected by proteins called histones.

Family features

Every human body is unique, from its overall shape to its fingerprints. But most people resemble their biological parents, who are in turn like their parents, and so on. This is because offspring acquire parts of the genetic "body plan" from each parent. This is called inheritance. An example of a feature passed from one generation to the next is the "Hapsburg jaw." Many of the Hapsburgs, a European royal family, had a distinctive lower jaw and chin, as seen in these details from famous paintings.

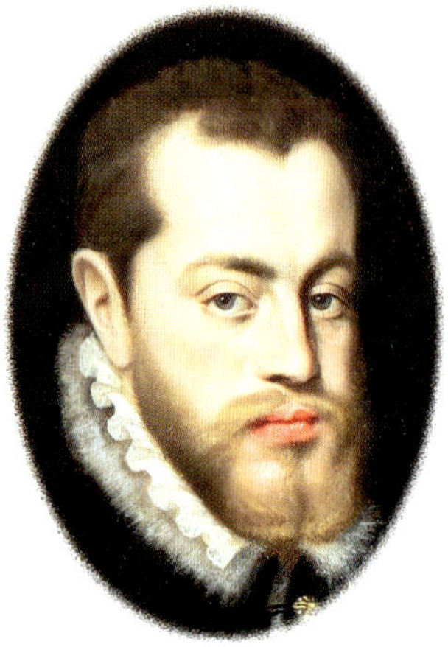

Philip II, King of Spain
Philip II (1527–98), here painted by Antonio Moro, shows the deep chinline that was characteristic of his family line.

Philip IV, King of Spain
Philip IV (1605–65), the grandson of Philip II, here painted by Diego Velázquez, inherited the family jawline and slightly protruding lower lip.

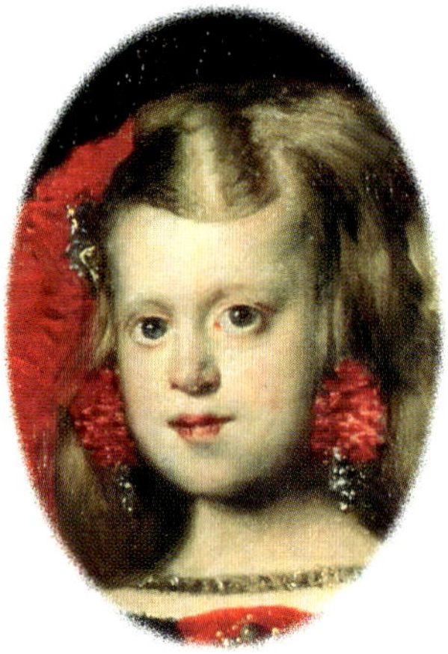

The Infanta Margarita
Daughter of Philip IV, the Infanta Margarita (1651–73), also painted by Velázquez, had very similar facial features to her great-grandfather Philip II.

■ DISCOVERY ■

Francis Crick and James Watson

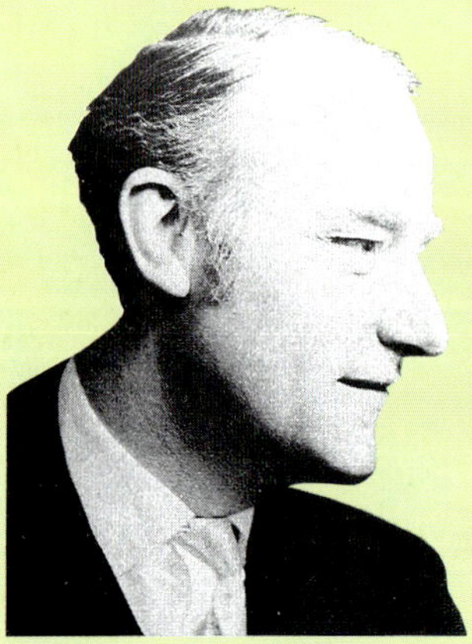

In the 1940's individual genes were discovered to be sections of a chemical called DNA (deoxyribonucleic acid). In 1953 the Englishman Francis Crick (born 1916, left) and the American James Watson (born 1928, right) worked out the structure of a DNA molecule. It is like two corkscrew-shaped staircases, intertwined as a double helix (p.179). Each "staircase" is twisted incredibly tightly. There are 1 million twists in a $\frac{1}{8}$-in (3-mm) length of DNA. When a cell divides, the "staircases" separate, and each makes a mirror image of itself. In this way genes are passed on as cells divide to form new body cells or to produce sperm and egg cells.

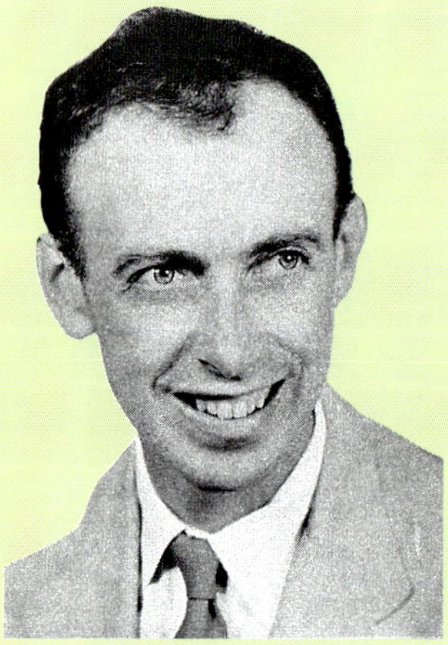

EXPERIMENT

Chances of inheritance

Many of your body features are inherited in a complicated way, following instructions from many interacting genes. However, some features are inherited more simply, involving only one or a few genes. They include eye and hair color and the ability to roll the tongue into a U-shape. This experiment shows how genes from each parent can combine so that their offspring are bound to inherit some genes, but also how the offspring can inherit some genes by chance. In the experiment genes are represented by beans and parents by containers. Any pair of beans in the parent container represents a gene pair. If the offspring has conflicting genes, such as one gene for blue eyes and one for brown—or one black bean and one red here—the body follows instructions in the dominant gene (p.171).

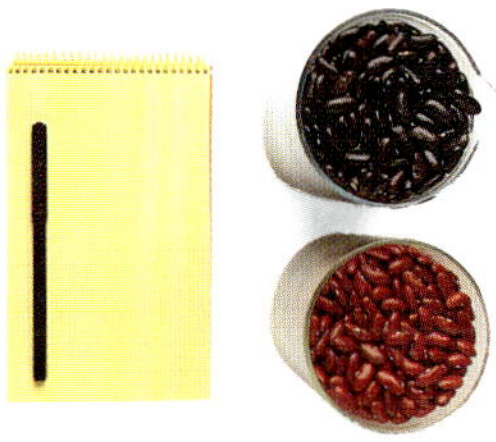

You Will Need

• notepad • pen • 2 large containers • at least 400 small objects of two different colors, such as dried red kidney beans and black beans

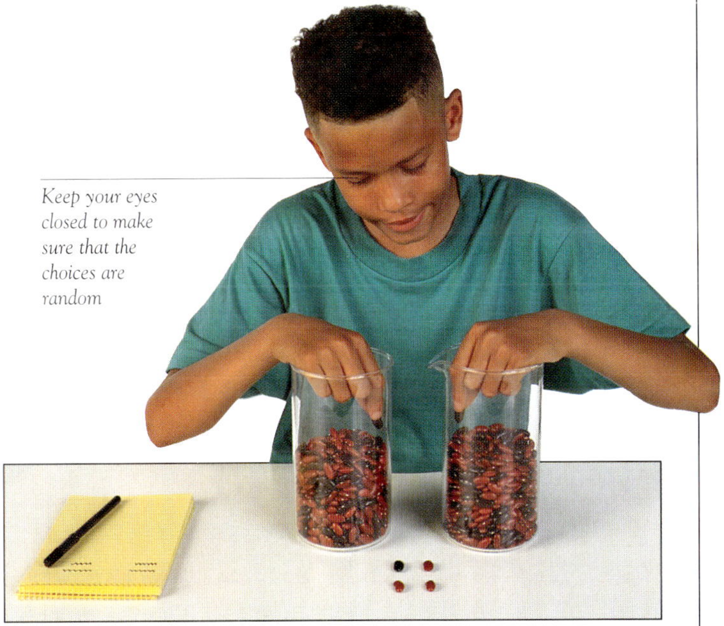

Keep your eyes closed to make sure that the choices are random

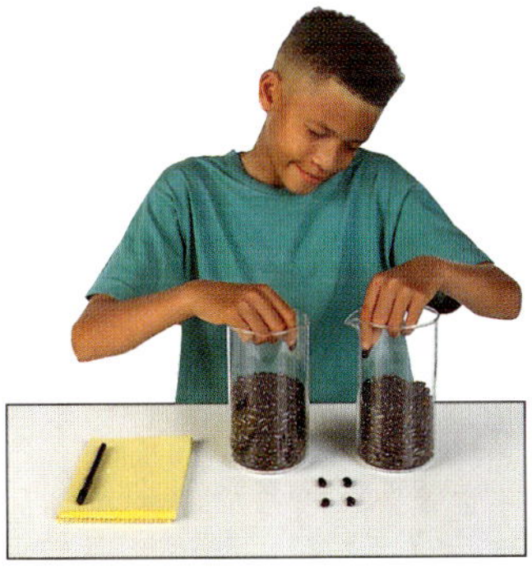

1 PUT BLACK beans in both containers. Take a bean from each to represent the offspring's gene pair. Repeat several times. Note the result.

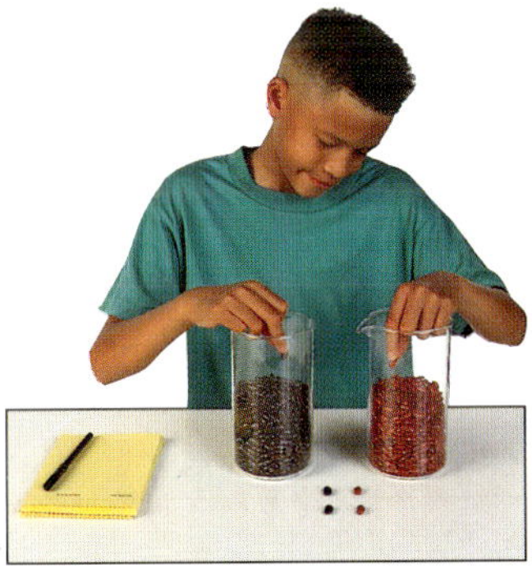

2 PUT RED beans into one container and black ones into the other. Pick several pairs of beans, as in Step 1. Note the result.

3 COUNT EQUAL numbers of red and black beans into each container—say, 100 red and 100 black per container—and mix them well. With eyes closed, take one bean from each container and pair them. Repeat at least 50 times. What are the proportions of black-black, red-red, and black-red pairs?

Both parents have black-black gene pairs

Black genes will be passed to the offspring

All offspring have black-black gene pairs

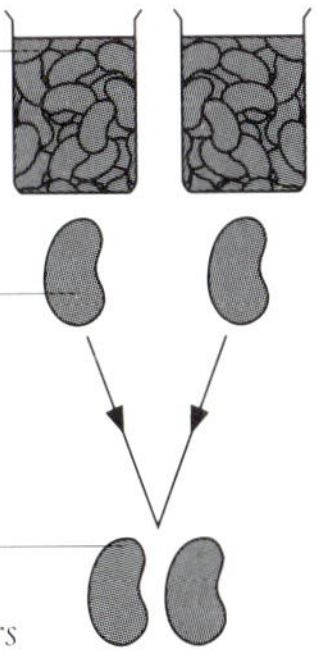

All the same

Genes are in pairs in the body (p.171). In this example, each parent has identical pairs of genes, and both parents are the same. The result is easily predicted. As genes are selected from each pair, from each parent, all the offspring have the same genes as each other and as the parents.

One parent has black-black gene pairs, and one red-red gene pairs

Black and red genes will be passed to the offspring

All offspring have black-red gene pairs

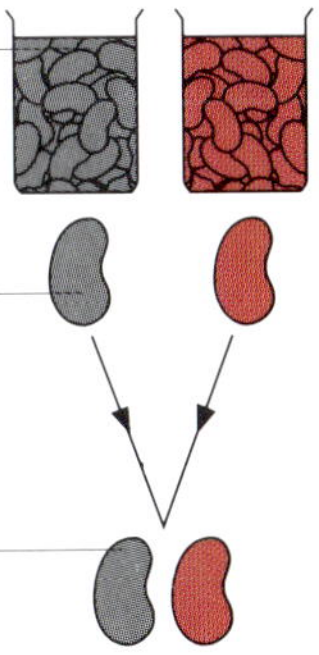

Same again

This time, one parent has identical pairs of genes. So does the other—but the two parents are different from each other. Even so, the results soon become obvious. All the offspring have the same combination of genes, which is black-red. This offspring becomes a parent in Step 3.

Both parents have black-red gene pairs

Each parent can pass on either red or black genes

The offspring have three types of gene pair, in the proportions 1:1:2

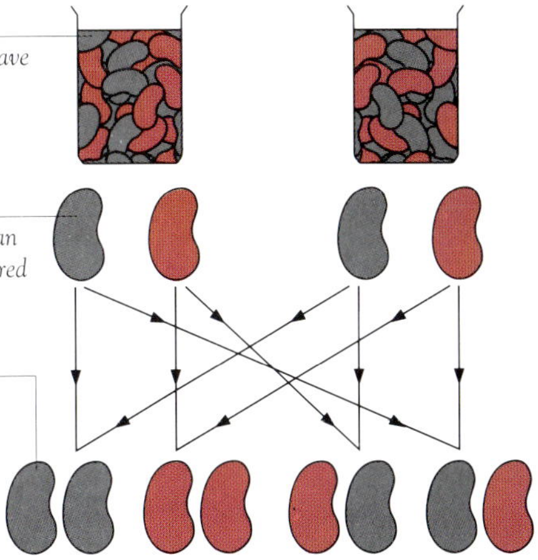

New combinations

In Step 3, both parents are the same—they each have dissimilar pairs of genes, one red and one black. Since the combinations follow the mathematical laws of chance, they produce predictable proportions of each different combination. In the body, for those pairs that are mixed (black-red), the dominant gene will dictate how the body develops.

Using a microscope

THE INVENTION OF THE LIGHT microscope revealed a previously unseen world. Light microscopes are essential scientific tools today in many places, from medical laboratories to school classrooms. A microscope is also useful for several of the experiments in this book. The one shown here can magnify objects by up to 200 times. As you look through a microscope to see tissues, cells, and other tiny objects firsthand, you will better understand your body's structures and the functions of its parts. The basics of microscopy are not difficult to master. Some important guidelines for working with a microscope are described on this page.

The microscope

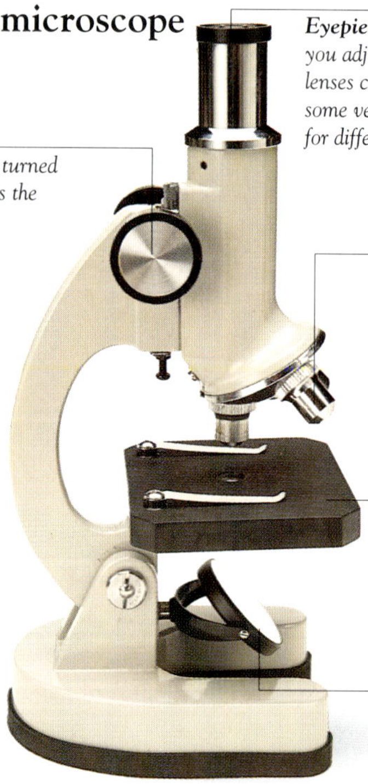

Eyepiece: *moves up and down as you adjust the focus; it contains lenses called the eyepiece lenses (in some versions these can be changed for different magnifications)*

Focus knob: *turned slowly to focus the specimen*

Objective lenses: *on a swiveling turret, with each giving a different magnification, usually from about 50 to 200 times*

Specimen stage: *place the glass slide carrying the specimen here, and secure it with the two clips*

Mirror: *reflects the light source (left)*

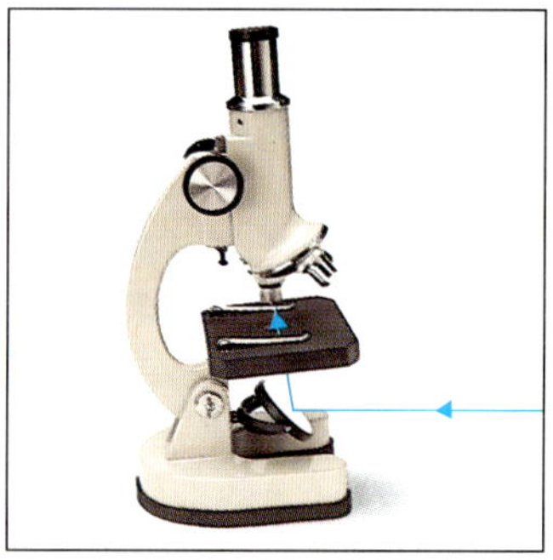

1. Lighting

This type of microscope needs a light source, such as a desk lamp or a powerful flashlight. The mirror reflects the light up through the specimen—as shown by the arrows (left), then through the objective lenses and eyepiece lenses into your eye. Adjust the mirror while looking through the microscope, until you find the most suitable angle for lighting the specimen.

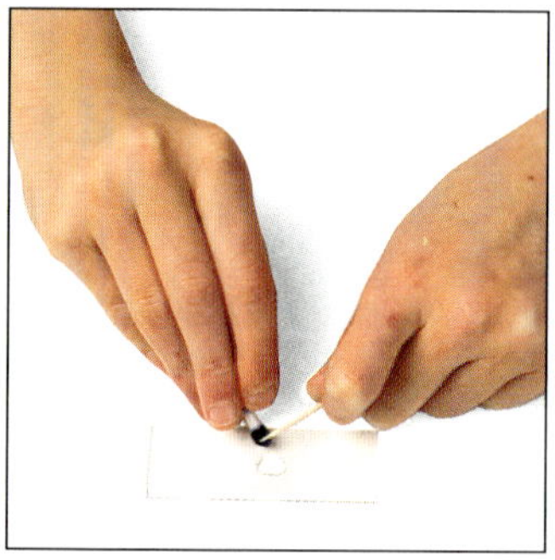

2. Specimen preparation

The specimen should be very thin and not too large. Cut a slice of it, with adult help. It is often useful to add drops of water to the specimen and cover it with a small transparent cover slip. This keeps the specimen from drying out. Rub a drop of water-based ink into the water with a cotton swab, while you lift the cover slip with a toothpick (as left), to stain important features.

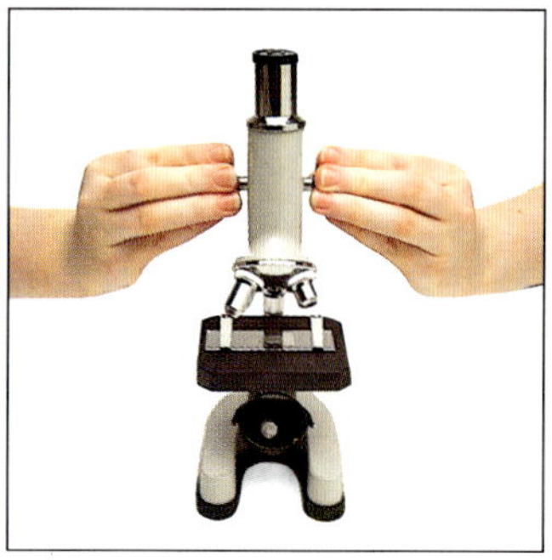

3. Focusing

Put the slide on the stage, with the specimen under the lens. Look through the eyepiece, and turn the focus knob to bring the specimen into focus (sharp view). Higher magnifications give more detail, but they have drawbacks. They need brighter light, the relevant part of the specimen is harder to find, and only a thin layer of the specimen is in focus at one time.

4. Studying

Always check that the objective lens does not move too low as you focus, or it may smash into the specimen and slide. Look away from the microscope every few minutes, to rest your eyes and your neck muscles.

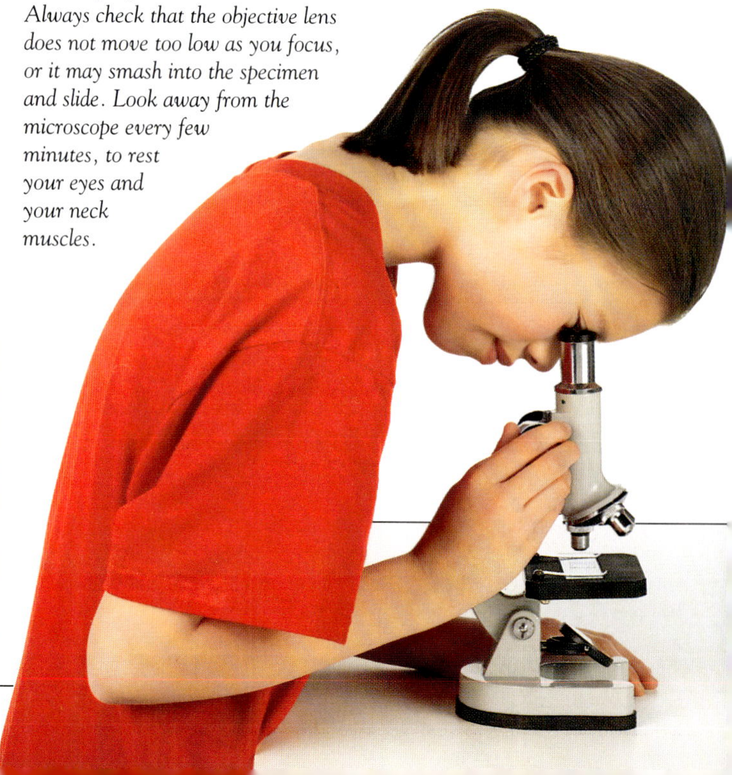

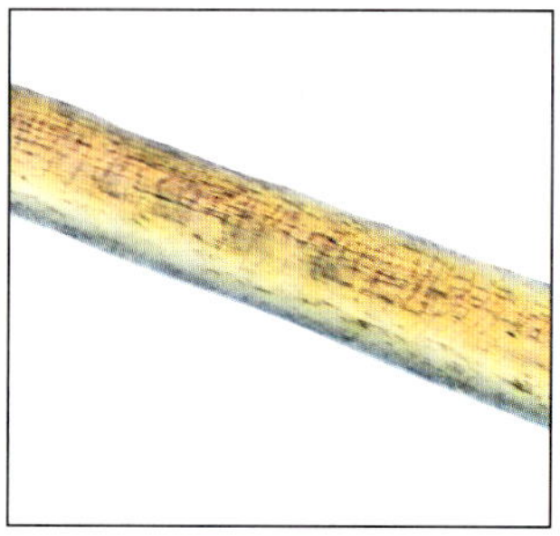

Practice materials

Practice how to use your light microscope by looking at items that you can obtain easily and that are simple to handle, such as this human hair (p.40). Compare your hair to wool, cotton, and artificial fibers. Here you can see that the hair is not smooth, but has tiny scales.

GLOSSARY

The following seven pages explain many of the general terms used in this book. The explanations refer to the human body, although many of the terms also have wider uses—for talking about other animals and in general science. The terms apply mainly to the body as a whole. They do not include, for example, the scientific names of bones or muscles. If you want to find these, turn to the index (pp.186–191). Use the index, too, if you want to find out about a particular body organ, such as the heart, or a body system, such as the digestive system.

ABDOMEN The lower part of the main body (trunk or torso), below the thorax (chest cavity).

ABSORPTION Taking in or soaking up a substance. The intestinal lining absorbs the nutrients from digested food, which are in turn absorbed into the blood and passed to body tissues.

AMINO ACIDS The building blocks of proteins, which are the body's main structural substances and also form enzymes. Different proteins are made from different sequences of amino acids. *See Proteins*.

AMYLASE An enzyme that breaks down the starches in food into their simpler subunits during digestion. *See Enzyme*.

ANATOMIST A person who studies anatomy—the physical makeup and structure of the body (as opposed to physiology—the body's functions and chemistry).

ANTAGONISTIC MUSCLES Muscles that pull in opposite directions, with one member of the pair pulling the bone one way and the other pulling it back.

ARTERY A large, thick-walled blood vessel that carries blood away from the heart. It divides to form capillaries.

ATOM A very tiny particle that cannot easily be split into anything smaller. Everything is made up of atoms. Elements consist of one type of atom only, but most things you see consist of many types of atoms, combined into molecules. *See Element, Molecule*.

BALANCE A mechanism by which the brain receives constant information from many sensory parts around the body, such as the ears, eyes, skin, muscles, and joints. Using this information, the brain adjusts the muscles to keep the body in a stable posture and stop it from falling over.

BILE A body fluid made by the liver and stored in the gall bladder. Bile flows along the bile duct into the small intestine, where it emulsifies the fats in food, so that they can be digested more efficiently. *See Emulsify*.

BLOOD A liquid that is the body's main transport substance. It carries oxygen, nutrients, energy-rich substances, salts, minerals, hormones, vitamins, and various cells, and distributes them to the tissues around the body. It also collects wastes for disposal by organs, such as carbon dioxide for disposal by the lungs and urea for disposal by the kidneys. A pigment called hemoglobin makes blood red.

BLOOD VESSEL A tube that carries blood through the body. The main types of blood vessel are arteries, capillaries, and veins. Each of these is described elsewhere in the glossary.

BONE A strong body part, made chiefly of the protein collagen and various minerals. There are 206 bones in an adult skeleton. Bones are fairly rigid but also slightly flexible. *See Collagen*.

CAPILLARIES Microscopic blood vessels with walls only one cell thick. Oxygen and nutrients pass from the blood in the capillaries to the cells in body tissues. Wastes produced by the cells pass the other way, from tissues into the blood.

CARBOHYDRATES A group of chemicals containing carbon, hydrogen, and oxygen. They include sugars and starches, and are the body's main energy sources.

CARDIO- To do with the heart. The thick muscle that makes up the wall of the heart is called cardiac muscle. A machine that shows the pattern of electrical signals that pass through the heart is called an electrocardiograph.

CARTILAGE A tough, rubbery substance. It lines the ends of bones where they meet in a joint. It also forms structural parts in the nose and the larynx (voice box).

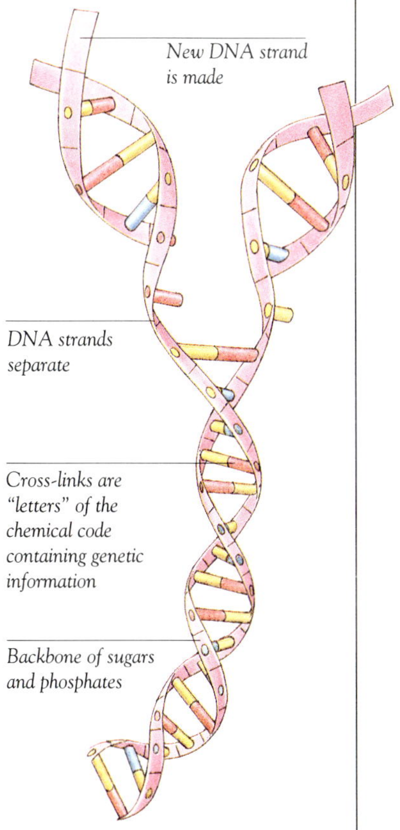

DNA
DNA has a double-helix shape—that is, it is like two intertwined corkscrews. As DNA duplicates itself, each helix separates and makes a mirror image of itself.

Cells The microscopic units, sometimes called building blocks, that make up all living things, including the human body. The body has more than 100 million million cells. A typical cell consists of a cell membrane surrounding a fluid substance called cytoplasm. Each cell contains tiny structures called organelles, such as the nucleus. *See Membrane, Nucleus, Organelle.*

Central nervous system The part of the nervous system that consists of the brain and spinal cord. *See Peripheral nervous system.*

Cervical To do with the neck or a necklike structure. The cervical vertebrae form the backbone in the neck region. The cervix is the neck of the womb (uterus).

Chemical reaction A process in which chemical substances come together, split up, and recombine to produce a new set of chemical substances. Hundreds of chemical reactions happen every second in each cell of the body.

Chromosomes X-shaped structures, containing the substance DNA, found inside cells. DNA carries genes, which have all the information for the structure and growth of the body. *See DNA, Genes.*

Collagen A tough, fibrous protein found in the dermis layer of the skin and in cartilage and bone.

Condensation When gas or vapor changes into a liquid. Usually the molecules or atoms in the gas are very far apart, so the gas is invisible. But in the liquid they are closer together, so the liquid is visible.

Hair
A hair grows from a follicle—a cavity formed by the epidermis folding down into the dermis below.

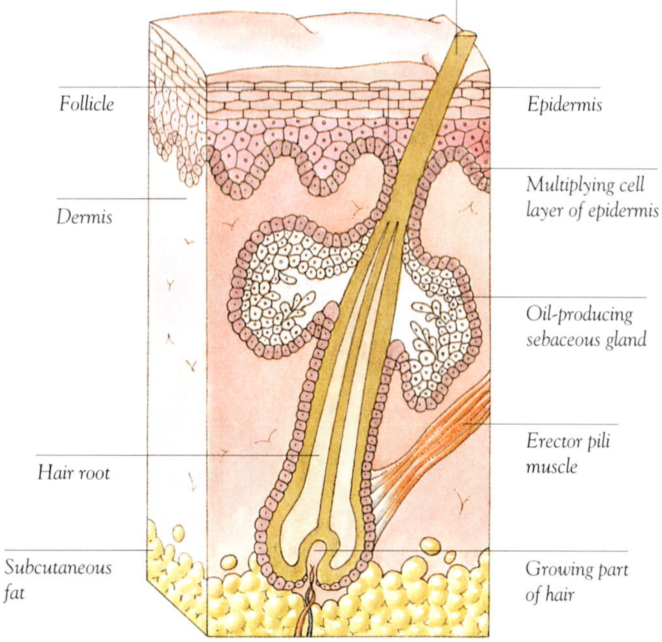

Connective tissue A body tissue that is specialized to connect, support, or fill in between other tissues. Connective tissue is one of the four basic kinds of tissue in the body. It makes up most of bone, cartilage, fat, the lower layer of the skin, and blood. *See Tissue.*

Corpuscle A "small body." This term was used widely by the early microscopists to describe the new objects they saw. Several tiny body parts are still sometimes called corpuscles, such as red blood cells and some of the touch sensors in the skin.

Cortex The outer layer or part of an organ. The cortex of the kidney contains microscopic filtering units called nephrons. The cortex of the brain is a thin gray layer, consisting of billions of nerve cell bodies and nerve connections, where sensations, thoughts, and movements originate.

Dent- To do with teeth. Dentine is the tough, shock-absorbing layer under the enamel covering of a tooth.

Diffusion The spreading out of a substance. The atoms or molecules of the substance move from where they are more concentrated to where they are less concentrated, so that eventually they are spread out evenly.

Digestion The process of breaking down substances into smaller, simpler substances. In the body the digestive system breaks down the large molecules in food into small ones that can be absorbed into the blood.

Digestive tract The long tube that goes through the body from the mouth to the anus. Its main parts are the mouth, pharynx (throat), esophagus, stomach, small intestine, and large intestine.

DNA The abbreviation for deoxyribonucleic acid. This important substance is found in chromosomes inside the nucleus of a cell. It carries all the information, in the form of chemical codes, needed to build a human body and to keep it alive. The information is in units called genes. When any new cells are made (except egg and sperm cells), DNA duplicates itself, so the new cells contain exactly the same genetic information as the originals. *See Chromosomes, Genes.*

Ear The organ of hearing (the auditory sense). The flap on the side of the head is supported by flexible cartilage. Behind is a chamber called the middle ear cavity, set into the skull bones. This contains the tiny ear ossicles, which transfer vibrations from the eardrum. Deeper in the skull are the cochlea, in which the vibrations are converted into nerve signals, and the fluid-filled chambers and canals that contribute to the mechanism of balance. *See Balance.*

Egg cell A female sex cell, made in the ovaries of a woman. Fertilized by a sperm cell from a man, it will develop into a new human being. *See Fertilization.*

Elastin A stretchy, rubbery protein found in the dermis layer of the skin and in other connective tissues.

Joint
A joint is lubricated by an oil called synovial fluid, which is produced by the synovial capsule, a baglike membrane around the joint.

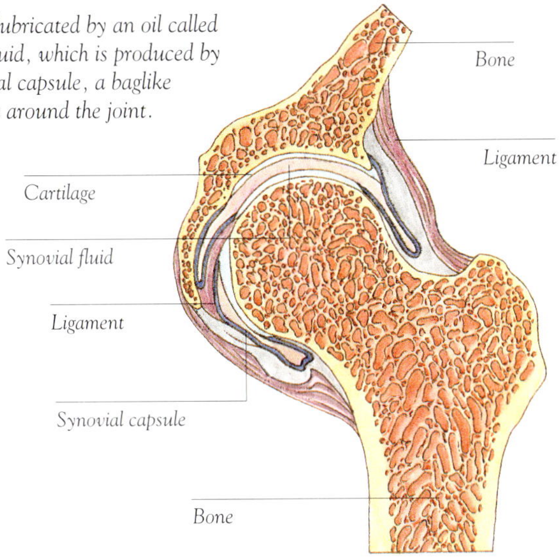

ELEMENT A simple substance that is made up of only one kind of atom, such as carbon, iron, or sodium. *See Atom*.

EMBRYO A baby in the early stages of development in the womb, between about 2 and 8 weeks after fertilization. *See Fetus*.

EMULSIFY To break up a substance such as a fat into droplets, so that chemicals such as enzymes have more surface area to attack.

ENDOPLASMIC RETICULUM An organelle inside a cell. It is the site for making or storing proteins and cell products. Its membrane usually takes the form of a large bag, folded many times. *See Organelle*.

ENERGY The ability to do work, such as moving things or heating them. The body gets its energy from food.

ENZYME A special type of protein that controls a chemical reaction in the body. There are hundreds of types of enzyme to regulate different aspects of the body's chemistry. *See Proteins*.

EPITHELIAL TISSUE Tissue that forms protective coverings or linings for body parts. Epithelial tissue is one of the four basic kinds of tissue in the body. It lines the digestive tract, airways, blood vessels, and other hollow tubes and parts. The skin cells in the epidermis are also epithelial cells. *See Tissue*.

EVAPORATION When a liquid changes into a gas or vapor. Usually, the molecules or atoms in the liquid are very close together, so the liquid is visible, but in the gas they are very far apart, so the gas is invisible.

EYE The organ of sight (the visual sense). The eyeball is a jelly-filled sphere with a lens at the front that focuses light onto the retina, the sensitive layer at the back. *See Retina*.

FATS Types of lipid, one of the body's main groups of chemicals. Fats provide both energy and structural ingredients for cell membranes and many other cell parts. The subcutaneous fat layer just under the skin contains cells that are full of fat. *See Lipids*.

FERTILIZATION When an egg cell from a woman joins with a sperm cell from a man to form a single cell. This cell is a fertilized egg that will develop into a baby.

FETUS A baby during the middle and later stages of development in the womb, between about 8 weeks after fertilization and birth. *See Embryo*.

FIBER A component of food, made mostly of plant material such as cellulose. Fiber cannot be digested to obtain energy or nutrients, but it helps to make digestion work efficiently and keep the intestines healthy.

FOLLICLE A small bag, sac, or cavity. In the skin, a hair follicle is a tiny cavity from which a hair grows. In the ovary, an ovarian follicle (Graafian follicle) is the fluid-filled container for the mature egg cell.

GENES Units of inheritance, passed from parents to their offspring. Genes are the plans for each feature of the body, such as bone shape, intestinal structure, and skin color. Genes are sections of the chemical DNA, packaged into structures called chromosomes, arranged in pairs inside the nucleus of a body cell. Only a selection of the genes in any particular type of cell is active. *See Chromosomes, DNA*.

GENETICS The study of genes: what they are made of, how they work, and how they are inherited. *See Genes*.

GLUCOSE A type of sugar with small, simple molecules. It is obtained from digested food, either directly or through conversion from other types of food nutrients, such as carbohydrates. Glucose is the body's major source of energy and is often called "blood sugar."

GOLGI BODY A tiny organelle, inside a cell, specialized to store cell products and wrap them in membranes, so that they can leave the cell. *See Organelle*.

HABITUATION When the brain learns to ignore repeated signals from a sensor that do not seem to be important. *See Sensor*.

HAIR A long, stiff rodlike structure that grows from a pit in the skin called a hair follicle. Hairs are made mainly of dead cells filled with the tough protein keratin. Hairs protect and insulate the body. Sensitive nerves wrapped around the bases of hairs detect when they are being moved.

HEPATO- To do with the liver—the part of the digestive system that processes and stores nutrients. Hepatocytes are the main types of cell in the liver.

HORMONES The body's "chemical messengers." Made in hormonal glands, they are chemicals that circulate in the blood and stimulate certain body parts—their target organs—into action.

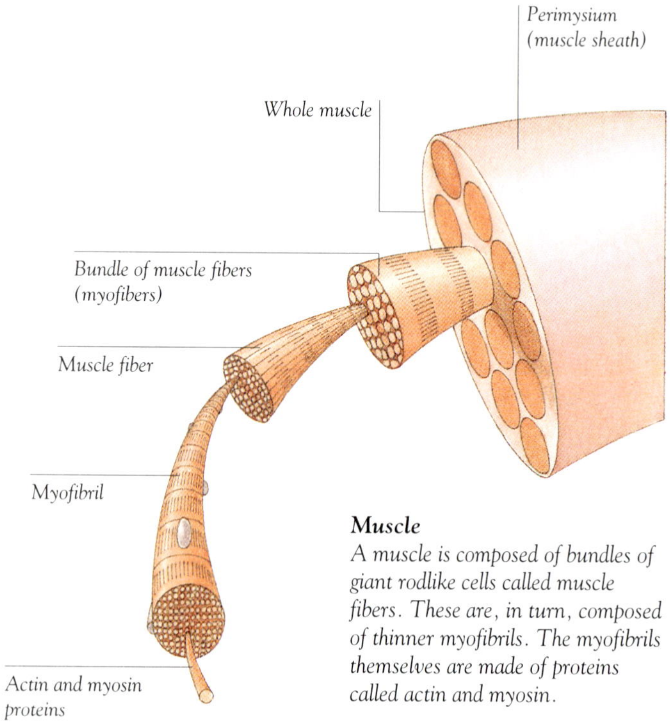

Muscle
A muscle is composed of bundles of giant rodlike cells called muscle fibers. These are, in turn, composed of thinner myofibrils. The myofibrils themselves are made of proteins called actin and myosin.

Joint The part of the body where two bones meet. In some joints the bones are fixed firmly and cannot move, as in the skull. In other joints the bones move smoothly over a limited range. The bones in these types of joint are covered by cartilage and held together by ligaments.

Keratin The tough, hard protein that makes up the body's outer layer of skin, hairs, and also nails.

Lever A simple machine with a rigid bar that pivots (swings) about a point called the fulcrum. A lever makes it easier to move a heavy load. The body's bones work as levers.

Ligaments Tough, elastic straplike parts that attach bones together at a joint, so that they do not come apart.

Lipase An enzyme that breaks down the lipids (fats and oils) in food into their simpler subunits during digestion. *See Enzyme.*

Lipids One of the body's main groups of chemicals. Lipids provide both energy and the structural ingredients for cell membranes and many other cell parts. They are made primarily from carbon, hydrogen, and oxygen. Lipids, which include fats and oils, do not mix with water.

Lobe A distinct rounded segment, section, or part of a structure such as an organ. The liver has two lobes. The cerebrum of the brain has five lobes on each side.

Lumbar To do with the lower back. The lumbar vertebrae form the backbone in the lower part of the back.

Lymph A pale fluid that is like blood, but with certain parts, such as the red cells, removed. It carries nutrients and germ-fighting cells. Lymph is formed from the fluid that collects between cells. It passes through a network of tubes called the lymphatic system and empties into the blood circulation.

Lymph node A kidney-shaped organ connected to the lymphatic system. The largest lymph nodes are up to 1 in (just over 3 cm) long. They store germ-fighting white blood cells and help to clean and filter lymph fluid. Lymph nodes enlarge and harden during some types of illness, when they are called "swollen glands."

Marrow The jellylike substance inside certain bones. It makes new cells for the blood.

Meiosis A type of cell division by which a cell splits into four offspring cells. This type of cell division occurs only to make sperm and egg cells for reproduction. During meiosis, as in mitosis, a duplicate set of the parent cell's gene pairs is produced. However, unlike mitosis, this new set and the original set of gene pairs then both split in two, with the result that each of the four offspring cells has only a set of single genes, not gene pairs. When an egg joins a sperm at fertilization, a complete set of gene pairs is formed. *See Genes.*

Membrane A flexible barrier around or within an object. A cell has a cell membrane enclosing it and membranes inside it too. On a larger scale, most body organs are also covered or lined by membranes, which are themselves composed of layers of cells. For example, there is a membrane around the lungs called the pleura and one around the heart called the pericardium.

Microscope A device that magnifies objects (makes them look bigger). A light microscope uses light rays and can magnify by about 1,000 times. An electron microscope uses beams of subatomic particles called electrons and magnifies by a million times or more.

Microscopist A person whose work involves using microscopes.

Microtubules Scaffolding-like systems of rod-shaped molecules, such as proteins, inside cells. Microtubules give a cell shape and strength, and move parts such as organelles around within the cell.

Mineral A simple chemical, usually an element, that the body needs to stay alive and healthy. Two examples are calcium for strong bones and teeth and iron for healthy blood. *See Element.*

Mitochondrion A tiny organelle, specialized to break down substances from food to provide its cell with energy. *See Organelle.*

Mitosis A type of cell division by which one original cell splits into two offspring cells. It is the normal method of cell multiplication in the body, for growth and to replace cells that die or are lost by wear and tear. During mitosis a duplicate set of the parent cell's gene pairs is produced, so that both of the offspring cells have identical gene pairs. Compare with meiosis. *See Genes.*

Molecule A chemical made from two or more atoms joined together. Some molecules consist of only one type of atom; some have several types. A molecule of oxygen has two atoms of oxygen. A protein molecule has thousands of atoms of various substances, such as carbon, nitrogen, and oxygen. *See Atom.*

Motor nerve A nerve that carries nerve signals from the brain and spinal cord to the body's muscles.

Muscle A body part specialized to contract (get shorter). Muscle tissue is one of the four basic kinds of tissue in the body. It makes up all muscles, from major skeletal muscles to heart muscle and the tiny hair-erecting muscles in the skin. *See Tissue.*

Myo- To do with muscles. A myofiber is a threadlike fiber inside a muscle, and a myofibril is a thinner thread inside the myofiber.

Nerve A long, thin body part that is specialized to carry messages around the body in the form of tiny electrical signals. Nerve tissue is one of the four basic kinds of tissue in the body. It forms the brain, nerves, and parts of the sense organs. *See Motor nerve, Sensory nerve, Tissue.*

Nerve signal A tiny electrical signal that travels along a nerve. Nerve signals move along the membranes of nerve cells (neurons). The strength of a typical nerve signal is between 50 and 100 millivolts—that is, about a 50th of the strength of a flashlight battery. The signal lasts for about 5 milliseconds (a 200th of a second).

Neuro- To do with nerves. A neuron is another name for a single nerve cell.

Nose The organ of smell (the olfactory sense). The protruding part on the face has two nostrils (air holes), a flexible framework of cartilage, and hairs to filter the passing air. Behind is a hole, or chamber, called the nasal cavity, set into the skull bones. This contains the olfactory epithelium, a patch of tiny projections that are linked to nerve cells. Nerve signals are sorted by the olfactory bulb and interpreted by the brain as smells. The nose is the major entrance and exit for air going to and from the lungs.

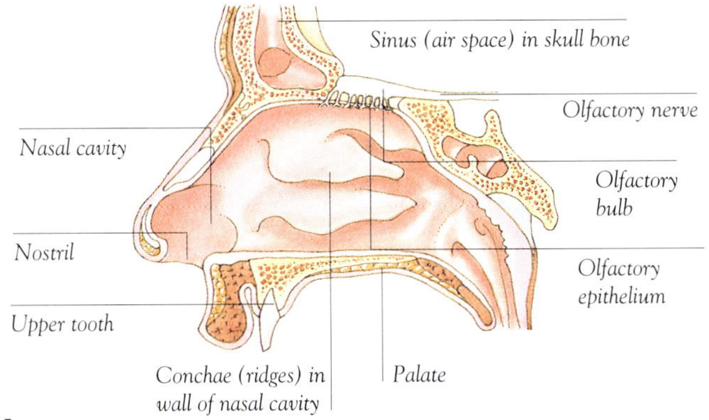

Nose
Behind the outer nose is an air chamber, the nasal cavity, which has the olfactory epithelium in its roof.

Nucleolus A tiny structure inside the nucleus of a cell. The nucleolus transfers genetic instructions from the chromosomes in the nucleus out into the rest of the cell. *See Chromosomes, Nucleus.*

Nucleus A special type of cell organelle, that acts as the cell's "control center." The nucleus contains the cell's genetic information in the form of DNA chemicals packaged into chromosomes. *See DNA, Organelle.*

Nutrients Substances in food that the body can break down during digestion, absorb, and rebuild into its own cells and tissues.

Oils Types of lipid, one of the body's main groups of chemicals. Oils are greasy and do not mix with water. *See Lipids.*

Organ A major structural part of the body that carries out an important role. The heart is an organ that pumps blood. The kidneys are organs that filter wastes from the blood. Most organs are made of collections of tissues. *See System, Tissue.*

Organelle A tiny structure inside a cell that carries out an important role. The nucleus is an organelle that contains genetic information. The mitochondria are organelles that break down substances to provide the cell with energy.

Organic To do with substances containing the element carbon. Carbon atoms are the main atoms of molecules, such as proteins and DNA, that are found in living things. The word "organic" also means substances that are, or were, part of an organism (living thing). *See Element.*

Osmosis The movement of a solvent, such as water, through a semipermeable membrane, through which other substances may not be able to pass. *See Solvent, Semipermeable membrane.*

Osteo- To do with bones. Osteocytes are cells that make the hard material that forms bones.

Pelvic To do with the pelvis, which is the lowest part of the abdomen. The pelvic organs are those in the lower abdomen, such as the bladder and rectum.

Peripheral nervous system The part of the nervous system that consists of the nerves that snake and twist through the body, connecting the brain and spinal cord to the many parts and organs. *See Central nervous system.*

Peristalsis When contents are pushed along a tube by waves of contraction of the muscles in the walls of the tube. Many substances pass through body tubes in this way, such as food through the esophagus and intestines, and urine along the ureter from kidney to bladder.

PHYSICIAN Generally, a medical doctor. The term is sometimes used in contrast to a surgeon, who performs operations.

PHYSIOLOGIST A person who studies physiology—the way the body works and its functions (as opposed to its anatomy, or structure).

PIGMENT A colored substance. Artificial pigments are used in stains, dyes, and paints. The body has its own pigments, such as dark brown melanin, which gives color to skin and hair.

PROPRIOCEPTORS Sensors that respond to body movements and changes in body position and posture. Stretch sensors in muscles, tendons, and ligaments are all types of proprioceptor. *See Sensor.*

PROTEASE An enzyme that breaks down the proteins in food into their simpler subunits during digestion. *See Enzyme.*

PROTEINS The body's main construction substances. They are the structural ingredients of skin, muscles, bones (with minerals), and many other parts. Proteins also form enzymes, which control chemical reactions. Proteins are made from building blocks called amino acids.

PUBERTY The period during which the sexual organs become mature and functional. The male's testes start to make sperm, and the female's ovaries begin to produce mature eggs. Puberty is usually accompanied by a spurt in body growth and various body changes, such as breast development in females and the appearance of facial hair and a deeper voice in males.

PULMONARY To do with the lungs. For example, the pulmonary arteries carry blood to the lungs. The pulmonary circulation is the part of the blood circulation to and from the lungs.

RENAL To do with the kidney. The renal arteries carry blood to the kidneys for filtering and waste removal.

RESPIRATION The process of breathing: inhaling fresh air into the lungs to absorb oxygen and then exhaling stale air. The term "cellular respiration" refers to the sets of chemical reactions inside a cell in which energy-rich substances, such as glucose, are broken down to yield their energy in a form that the cell can use. In cellular respiration the body uses oxygen and produces carbon dioxide as a waste.

RETINA The light-sensitive layer that lines the inside of the rear of the eyeball. Arranged around the surface of the retina are about 130 million special cells, called rods and cones. These change the energy of light rays into tiny electrical nerve signals. These signals are sent along other nerve cells to the optic nerve, which delivers them to the brain.

SCANNER A machine that scans the body, building up an image of its inner parts, line by line. Some scanners beam lines of weak X-rays through the body. Others transmit high-pitched sound, called ultrasound, through the body, or detect how certain body parts react in a strong magnetic field. A computer processes the results and displays them on a visual display unit (TV screen).

SEMIPERMEABLE MEMBRANE A membrane that allows a solvent—in the body, water—to pass through, but prevents other substances from doing so. This selective letting-through process is called osmosis. *See Membrane, Osmosis, Solvent.*

SENSOR A structure that changes some kinds of stimuli into nerve signals. Some sensors are whole organs, such as the ear, which converts sound waves into nerve signals. Some sensors are microscopic bunches of cells, or even single cells, such as the stretch sensors in muscles and tendons, which produce nerve signals when stretched or distorted.

SENSORY NERVE A nerve that carries nerve signals from a sense organ, or another type of sensor, to the brain or spinal cord.

SKELETON The supporting framework of the body. In a developing baby it is composed mainly of cartilage. This changes to bone as the baby grows into an adult.

SKIN The organ of touch and the body's outer covering. The skin's millions of

Retina
The retina is only a few cells thick. Its light-detecting rod and cone cells are linked to the optic nerve by other nerve cells such as the ganglion nerve cell and bipolar nerve cell.

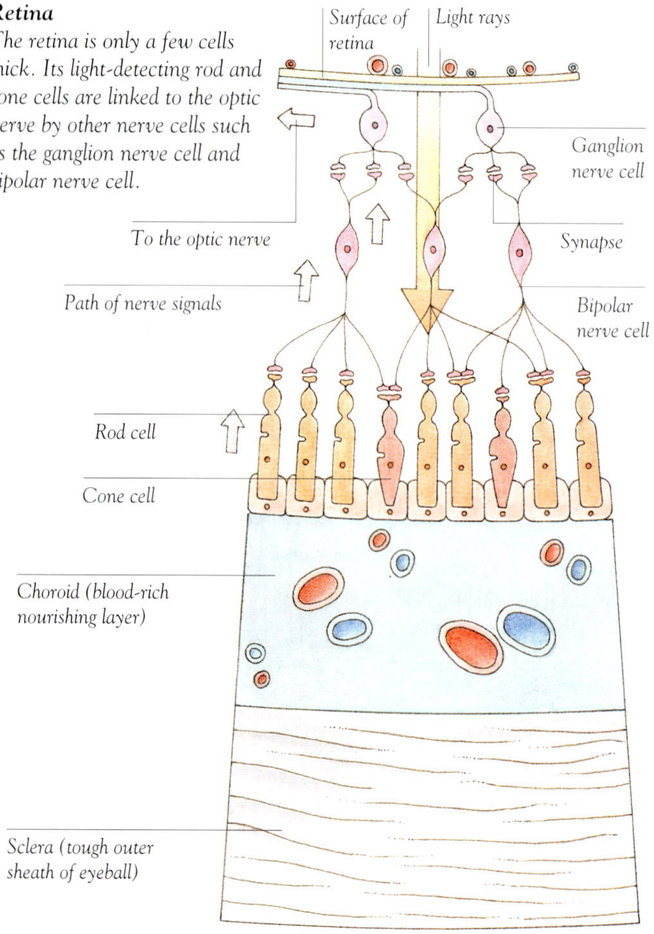

microscopic sensors detect different aspects of touch, such as light touch, heavy pressure, heat or cold, vibrations, and the damage we feel as pain. The skin also protects the body from conditions outside and keeps its fluids in.

Solute A substance, usually a solid, that is dissolved in a solvent. *See Solution.*

Solution The result of a substance (called the solute and usually solid) dissolving in another substance (called the solvent and usually liquid). A common example is sugar (a solute) dissolved in water (a solvent). The atoms or molecules of the solute are freed from each other and can float around, so that the solute frequently seems to disappear in the solvent. An example of a solution in the body is urine, in which urea and other waste products are dissolved in water.

Solvent A substance, usually a liquid, in which other substances are dissolved. *See Solution.*

Species A group of living things whose members can breed with each other, but who cannot breed with any other group. All human beings belong to one species, *Homo sapiens*.

Sperm cells Male sex cells, made in the testes. If an egg cell from a woman is fertilized by a sperm cell, it can then develop into a new human being. *See Fertilization.*

Surface area The amount of surface that an object has. The bigger the surface area of an organ, the more of a substance it can absorb (take in) through this surface. This applies to the insides of the lungs, for absorbing oxygen, and to the insides of the small intestine, for taking in nutrients from food.

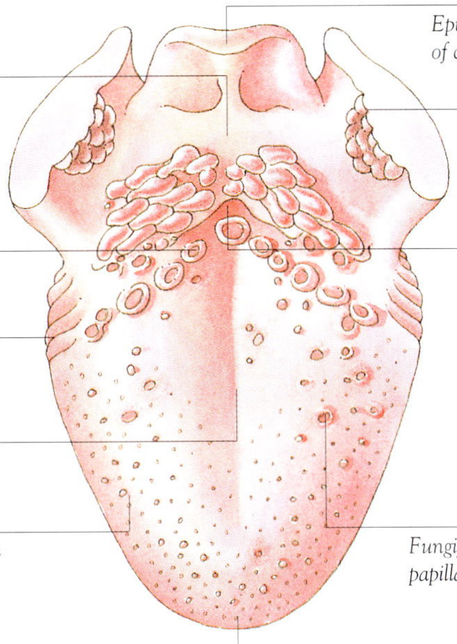

Tongue
The tongue's upper surface is covered by a variety of bumps, called papillae. The tonsils are masses of germ-fighting lymph tissue.

Synapse The tiny gap between two nerve cells (neurons). The two cells do not touch each other. Electrical signals traveling along the nerves change their form at this gap and cross it in the form of chemicals called neurotransmitters. *See Nerve signal.*

System A group of organs or other parts that carries out one major role. For example, the heart, blood vessels, and blood form the circulatory system, which delivers oxygen and nutrients to all body parts and collects their wastes.

Systemic The part of the circulatory system that takes blood to all of the body except the lungs.

Tendon The strong ropelike part of a muscle, where it narrows toward its end and is attached to a bone. Tendons are often called sinews.

Thoracic To do with the thorax (chest). The thoracic vertebrae form the backbone in the chest region.

Thorax The chest—that is, the upper part of the main body (trunk or torso), above the abdomen.

Tissue A collection of similar cells, all of which perform one main function. Strictly, the body has only four basic types of tissue: nerve, epithelial, connective, and muscle; but there are many variations on these types. Each kind of tissue is described elsewhere in the glossary. *See Organ, System.*

Tongue The organ of taste (the gustatory sense). Flavor molecules are detected by thousands of microscopic onion-shaped cell clusters called taste buds. These are scattered on and among the larger bumps and lumps on the tongue, called papillae. Under its surface, the tongue is a mass of flexible interwoven muscles.

Valve A device to control the flow of a substance. A common example is a water tap. In the body, valves in the heart and main veins are one-way valves. They ensure that the blood flows the right way around the circulatory system.

Vein A large, slack-walled blood vessel that carries blood back to the heart.

Vesicle A small, fluid-filled bubblelike structure. In a cell there are numerous vesicles. Made from membranes, they contain items such as fat molecules, or germs that have been engulfed by the cell.

Vitamins Substances that are needed for the smooth running of the body's chemical reactions. Vitamins are not structural or energy containing, but they "oil the wheels" of the body's chemical machinery.

X-rays Invisible waves that can pass through most of the body, except for hard parts such as the bones. A radiograph is an "X-ray photograph" produced when X-rays that have passed through body tissue are exposed on a photographic plate. This leaves bone-shaped shadows where no rays have gotten through.

Index

A

B

C

T

U

V

W

X Y Z

Acknowledgments

STEVE PARKER would like to thank Roger, Bryn, Mukul, Christina, Emily, and the team at Dorling Kindersley for their dedication, hard work, attention to detail, and good humor; Jane for her continuing support; Alan and Martin for being human guinea pigs; and Jim Cameron for his long-lasting inspiration.

DORLING KINDERSLEY would like to thank Tina Brazil, Jeanette Cossar, Fiona Courtenay-Thompson, Neil Lockley, and Des Reid for editorial assistance; Sarah Brigham for design assistance; Richard Walker and Dr. Frances Williams for checking the text; all of the staff and pupils at John Perryn Primary School, East Acton, London; Caroline Brooke and Christine Rista for picture research; Jane Parker for the index; Lyn Rutherford for preparing the meal on page 162.

PICTURE CREDITS
t top; *b* bottom; *l* left; *r* right; *c* center

Allsport 21*cr*. *Mike Hewitt* 54–55
Archiv für Kunst und Geschichte Berlin 175 *cbr*, 175*c*.
Australian Overseas Information Service, London 12*cr*.
Clive Barda, London 107*bl*.
Biophoto Associates 47*tr*, 47*cr*, 47*br*, 103*c*.
Bridgeman: National Gallery, London 175*br*, 176*cr*; *Philip Mould Historical Portraits Ltd* 176*tr*; *Prado, Madrid* 176*crr*.
British Museum 11*tr*.
Bruce Coleman: Fred Bruemmer 113*tc*; *Stephen Krasemann* 113*tl*.
Comstock 10–11.
Mary Evans Picture Library 13*tl*, 22*tr*, 58*tr*, 70*b*, 102*cr*, 110*tr*, 171*br*, 172*tr*, 176*bl*, 176*br*.
Chris Fairclough 128*cl*.
Giraudon Munich Pinothek 175*cra*.
Robert Harding Picture Library 56*r*, 171*bl*.
Hulton Deutsch Collection 17*tl*, 21*c*.
Image Bank: Brett Fromer 25*br*; *John Kelly* 20*cl*.
Mansell Collection 16*bl*, 47*tc*, 91*tr*, 96*t*, 104*r*, 118*tr*, 139*br*.
Ruth Midgley 31.
National Library of Medicine 172*bl*.
National Medical Slide Bank 168–169.
Nature Photographers: Craig Cooper 89*bl*; *Richard Neave* 46*bl*, 46*bcl*, 46*bc*.
Pinsharp 3-d Graphics: Jim Sharp 144*br*.
SPL 87*bl*, 95*tr*, 134–135; *Michael Abbëy* 40*tl*; *Department of Clinical Cytogenetics, Adden Brookes Hospital, Cambridge* 176*cll*; *Biophoto Associates* 176*cl*; *Dr. Goran Bredberg* 134–135; *Dr Jeremy Burgess* 26*tr*, 32*l*, 34*tr*; *CNRI* 45*tl*, 91*cr*, 92–93, 103*cl*, 103*tl*, 114–115, 126*br*; *A.B. Dowsett* 102*br*; *Don Fawsett* 58*tl*; *Fawcett / Hirokawa / Heuser* 85*cl*; *Professor C. Ferland / CNRI* 71*tr*, 71*br*; *Astrid and Hans Friedler Michler* 107*tl*, 119*br*; *Manfred Kage* 42–43, 68–69; *Francis Leroy / Biocosmos* 25*tl*, 94*bl*; *Will and Deni McIntyre* 167*br*; *P. Motta / Department of Anatomy, University of La Sapienza, Rome* 136*tr*, 161*tl*, 161*tc*, 161*tr*; *Professor P.M. Motta and J. Van Blerkom* 172*br*; *NASA* 156*bl*; *NIBSC* 103*cr*; *David Parker* 13*cr*; *David Scharf* 78–79; *Sheila Terry* 30–31; *Gianni Tortoli* 159*bl*; *Jeremy Trew* 24*cr*; *U.S. Department of Energy* 14*tr*
Tony Stone Images: 66*c*, 122*bl*, 174*cl*; *Thomas Brase* 117*br*; *Paul Chesley* 117*bl*; *Keith Wood* 81*br*.
UK Crown / Aspley Ltd (E-Fit photograph) 19*tr*.
Warren Anatomical Medical School Museum, Harvard 126*tr*.
The Wellcome Institute Library, London 28*tr*, 106*tr*, 173*bl*.
Dr. Robert Youngson 139*bl*.
Zefa: H. Sochurek 112*tl*.

ILLUSTRATIONS
Karen Cochran 22*b*, 23.
Mick Gillah 27*t*, 34*b*, 46*r*, 59*t*, 85*t*, 97*c*, 98*b*, 108*b*, 119*l*, 139*t*, 152*b*.
Tony Graham 27*t*, 34*b*, 46*r*, 59*t*, 72*b*, 85*t*, 87*t*, 97*c*, 98*b*, 119*l*, 126*bl*, 139.
Selwyn Hutchinson 22*b*, 23*t*, 23*b*, 72*b*, 106*b*, 126*bl*.
Kevin Jones Associates 108*b*, 152*b*.
John Temperton 14*b*, 15*b*, 16*br*, 18*b*, 26*b*, 39*t*, 34*bl*, 49*r*, 42*bl*, 57*br*, 57*tr*, 58*bl*, 60*b*, 61*tl*, 73*tr*, 84*tr*, 86*b*, 88*br*, 89*c*, 95*bl*, 97*b*, 99*t*, 103*b*, 109*t*, 111*br*, 119*tr*, 121*tl*, 123*tr*, 127*t*, 127*bc*, 128*tr*, 138*bl*, 138*tr*, 140*cr*, 141*tr*, 142*tr*, 145*t*, 148*tr*, 157*tr*, 164*bl*, 173*t*, 173*bl*, 179*br*, 180*bl*, 181*tl*, 182*tl*, 183*bl*, 184*bl*, 185*t*.
Bryn Walls 25*bl*, 27*br*, 28*cr*, 29*br*, 51*b*, 90*br*, 91*br*, 102*b*, 103*t*, 106*b*, 111*t*, 129*l*, 103*bl*, 103*br*, 164*br*, 173*c*, 177*b*.

MODEL MAKERS
David Donkin 2*b*, 6*tr*, 7*cl*, 7*br*, 33*b*, 41, 67, 124, 125, 127*br*, 143, 146.
Christina Betts 2*cr*, 3*b*, 6*bl*, 53, 77*b*, 131, 153, 165.
Bill Gordon Models 115.

MODELS
Roohi Ahmed, Saima Ahmed, Huda Ismail Ali, Charlene Allen, Karen Banton, Jayne Basterfield, Stephen Baverstock, Christina Betts, Nadine Biddulph, Christopher Birch, Jermaine Bowes, Gavin Browning, Rebecca Bunting, Thomas Bunting, Charmaine Dale, Leo Dudley, Lisa Ganpot, Philip Gilderdale, Jassy Gill, Rikki Hassan, Patora Ho, Phillip Hyde, Camay Jones, Chantelle Joseph, Selina Jules, Goran Kanlic, Davina Kirwan, Michelle Kunzi, Joanna Lagou, Jaqui Lamb, Sarah Lillicrap, Majuran Manohasandra, Joanna Mason, Marrion Murray, Bushra Murza, Sophia Nawaz, Megan Norwood, Jennifer Oatway, Aaron O'Connor, Ian O'Herhily, Philip Ormerod, Najad Osman, Richard Palmer, Hetan Patel, Mukul Patel, Priti Patel, David Pluck, Yasmeen Rahim, James Rasmussen, Ashley Rodwell, Kathleen Rooney, Wayne Saunders, Robina Sakhi, Lisa Scanlon, Samantha Schneider, Sobia Shah, Elham Sharoudi, Oliver Stobbart, Nadeem Syed, Jay Tan, Roger Tritton, Aidan Walls, Bryn Walls, Rosie Walls, Ahmed Warsama, John Whall, Lorraine Williams.

SPECIAL PHOTOGRAPHY
Geoff Dann 2, 3, 5, 6, 20, 35, 36, 37, 55, 58, 61, 73, 76, 96, 100, 105, 109, 120, 121, 124, 125, 136, 138, 145, 146, 153, 154, 155, 158, 159, 160, 162, 165.
Tim Ridley 2, 3, 5, 7, 18, 19, 27, 32, 33, 38, 39, 41, 57, 58, 75, 80, 86, 95, 101, 104, 112, 123, 138, 140, 141, 143, 167.
Dave Rudkin 1, 2, 3, 4, 5, 6, 7, 8, 9, 13, 15, 17, 21, 28, 29, 34, 37, 44, 45, 48, 49, 50, 51, 52, 53, 56, 60, 61, 64, 65, 66, 67, 72, 73, 74, 75, 76, 77, 80, 81, 82, 83, 84, 85, 87, 88, 89, 90, 91, 96, 100, 101, 105, 107, 108, 110, 111, 112, 113, 116, 117, 118, 121, 122, 127, 128, 129, 130, 131, 132, 133, 137, 142, 144, 147, 148, 149, 150, 151, 155, 156, 157, 161, 162, 163, 164, 166, 167, 171, 174, 175, 177, 178.
Spike Walker (Microworld Services) 13, 24, 29, 33, 34, 35, 36, 40, 48, 56, 57, 59, 81, 105, 107, 108, 110, 137, 170, 172.

Geoff Brightling 105. *Jane Burton* 111. *Andy Crawford* 116, 120, 137, 174. *Philip Dowell* 87. *Andreas von Einsiedel* 101. *Steve Gorton* 99, 144. *Frank Greenaway* 95. *Peter Hayman* 37. *Dave King* 12, 20, 24, 43, 44, 45, 69, 94, 127, 163. *Cyril Laubscher* 117. *Bill Ling* 170. *David Murray* 163. *Steven Oliver* 25. *Brian Pitkin* 71. *Tim Shepard at Oxford Scientific Films* 80. *Chris Stevens* 20. *Harry Taylor* 82. *Jeff Veitch* 44. *Jerry Young* 20, 33, 101, 127, 136.